Multiple Sclerosis
Therapeutics

Compliments
of

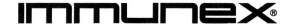

To our patients, colleagues, and supporters, who have worked together to make progress in the MS field possible.

The cover shows an immunofluorescent confocal micrograph taken from an active inflammatory lesion in the brain of a person with multiple sclerosis. On the left is an axon that has been partially demyelinated, as indicated by the loss of red fluorescence. The axon on the right is undergoing demyelination, but in addition the axon is transected, as indicated by the green swelling. The micrograph was generously provided by Dr Bruce D Trapp, Chairman of the Department of Neuroscience, Lerner Research Institute, Cleveland Clinic Foundation.

Multiple Sclerosis Therapeutics

Edited by

Richard A Rudick MD
Donald E Goodkin MD

MARTIN DUNITZ

© Martin Dunitz Ltd 1999

First published in the United Kingdom in 1999 by
Martin Dunitz Ltd
The Livery House
7–9 Pratt Street
London NW1 0AE

Tel: +44–(0)20–7482–2202
Fax: +44–(0)20–7267–0159
E-mail: info@mdunitz.globalnet.co.uk
Website: http://www.dunitz.co.uk

A CIP catalogue record for this book is available from the British Library

ISBN 1–85317–812–8

Composition by Wearset, Boldon, Tyne & Wear
Printed and bound in Great Britain by Biddles Ltd, Guildford and King's Lynn

Contents

Contributors

Douglas L Arnold MD, Department of Neurology and Neurosurgery Montreal Neurological Institute and Hospital 3801 University Street, Montréal PQ Canada H3A 2B4

Frederik Barkhof MD, MR Center for MS Research, Academisch Ziekenhuis Vrije Universiteit 1007 MB Amsterdam, The Netherlands

François Bethoux MD, Neuroimmunology Fellow, Cleveland Clinic Foundation, Mellen Center for Multiple Sclerosis Treatment and Research Cleveland OH 44195, USA

Anthony Bourdakis Director, Regulatory Affairs and Quality Assurance, Berlex Laboratories 15049 San Pablo Avenue, Richmond CA 94806 USA

William H Burns MD, Professor of Medicine and Microbiology, Director, Bone Marrow Transplant Program, Medical College of Wisconsin Milwaukee, WI 53226, USA

Richard K Burt MD, Assistant Professor of Medicine Director, Allogenic Bone Marrow Transplant Program Robert H Lurie Cancer Center, Northwestern University Medical School, Chicago IL 60611, USA

Giancarlo Comi MD, Professor and Head of Department of Clinical Neurophysiology San Raffaele Scientific Institute, Via Olgettina 60, 20132 Milano, Italy

Christian Confavreux MD, Professor of Neurology, Head of Department, Service de Neurologie EDMUS Co-ordinating Center, Hopital de l'Antiquaille 69321 Lyon Cedex 05, France

Patricia K Coyle MD, Department of Neurology and Director, Stony Brook Multiple Sclerosis Comprehensive Care Center, State University of New York at Stony Brook, Stony Brook NY 11794-8121, USA

Gary Cutter PhD, AMC Cancer Research Center 1600 Pierce Street, Denver CO 80214, USA

Franz Fazekas MD, Professor of Neurology Department of Neurology Karl-Franzens-Universität Graz, Auenbruggerplatz 22 A-8036 Graz, Austria

Massimo Filippi MD, Head, Neuroimaging Research Unit, Department of Neuroscience, San Raffaele Scientific Institute, Via Olgettina 60 20132 Milano, Italy

Jill S Fischer PhD, Director, Psychology Program Cleveland Clinic Foundation, Mellen Center for Multiple Sclerosis Treatment and Research Cleveland OH 44195, USA

Richard P Foa MD MA, Georgetown University Medical Center, 3800 Reservoir Road NW Washington DC 20007-2197, USA

Corey C Ford MD PhD, Medical Director, Clinical and Magnetic Resonance Research Center and Multiple Sclerosis Speciality Clinic, 1201 Yale NE Albuquerque NM 87131, USA

Gordon Francis MD, Medical Director MS/CNS
Serono Labs, 700 Longwater Drive
Norwell MA 02061, USA

Elliot M Frohman MD PhD, Assistant Professor of
Neurology and Ophthalmology, Director, Multiple
Sclerosis Program, University of Texas Southwestern
Medical Center, 5323 Harry Hines Boulevard
Dallas TX 75235, USA

Ralf Gold MD, Department of Neurology, Julius-
Maximilians-Universität, Josef-Schneider-Str. 11,
90780 Würzburg, Germany

Richard Gonsette MD, National MS Center
Melsbroek, Belgium

Donald E Goodkin MD, Associate Professor of
Neurology, Director, Mount Zion Multiple Sclerosis
Center, University of California at San Francisco
1701 Divisadero Street, Suite 480
San Francisco, CA 94115-1642, USA

Sylvie Grégoire DPharm, Vice President, Regulatory
Affairs, Biogen Inc, 14 Cambridge Center
Cambridge MA 02142, USA

Hans-Peter Hartung MD, Professor and Chairman
Department of Neurology, Karl-Franzens-Universität
Graz, Auenbruggerplatz 22
A-8036 Graz, Austria

Stephen L Hauser MD, Professor and Chairman,
Department of Neurology
University of California at San Francisco
San Francisco, CA 94143-0435, USA

Robert M Herndon MD, Neurology Service
GV Montgomery MA Medical Center
Jackson MI, USA

Ronald Kanner MD, Professor of Neurology
Chairman, Department of Neurology, Albert Einstein
College of Medicine, Long Island Jewish Medical
Center, New Hyde Park NY 11040, USA

R Philip Kinkel MD, Director, Medical Programs
Mellen Center for Multiple Sclerosis Treatment and
Research, Cleveland Clinic Foundation, Cleveland OH
44195, USA

Mariko Kita MD, Department of Neurology
Mount Zion Multiple Sclerosis Center, University of
California at San Francisco, 1701 Divisadero Street,
Suite 480, San Francisco, CA 94115-1642, USA

Hilmar Krapf MD, Department of Neuroradiology
Universitätsklinikum Tübingen, Tübingen, Germany

Lauren B Krupp MD, Department of Neurology
State University of New York at Stony Brook
Stony Brook NY 11794-8121, USA

Thomas A Lang MA, New England Medical Center
Division of Clinical Care Research, 750 Washington
Street, Boston MA 02111, USA

Siobhan M Leary MB BS MRCP, Institute of
Neurology
University of London, National Hospital for
Neurology and Neurosurgery, Queen Square
London WC1N 3BG, UK

Scott E Litwiller MD, Assistant Professor of Urology
and Neurology, Chief of Urology, North Texas VA
Medical Spinal Cord Injury Unit, University of Texas
Southwestern Medical Center, 5323 Harry Hines
Boulevard, Dallas TX 75235, USA

Fred D Lublin MD, Professor of Neurology, Director
Multiple Sclerosis Center, Department of Neurology
MCP Hahnemann School of Medicine
3300 Henry Avenue, Philadelphia PA 19129, USA

Henry McFarland MD, Chief, Neuroimmunology
Branch, National Institute of Neurological Disorders
and Stroke, (NINDS), Bethesda MD 20892-1400, USA

Joseph C McGowan PhD, Research Assistant
Professor of Radiology, University of Pennsylvania,
3400 Spruce Street, Philadelphia PA 19104, USA

Gianvito Martino MD, Head of Experimental Neuroimmunotherapy Unit DIBIT, San Raffaele Scientific Institute, Via Olgettina 60, 20132 Milano, Italy

Paul M Matthews MD, Centre for Functional Magnetic Research Imaging of the Brain, Department of Clinical Neurology, University of Oxford, Radcliffe Infirmary, Oxford, UK

David H Miller MD, The NMR Unit, Institute of Neurology, Queen Sqaure, London W5 5BG, UK

Deborah M Miller PhD LISW, Director Comprehensive Care, Mellen Center for Multiple Sclerosis Treatment and Research, Cleveland Clinic Foundation, Cleveland OH 44195, USA

Sarah L Minden MD, Assistant Professor of Psychiatry, Harvard Medical School, Brigham and Women's Hospital, 75 Francis Street, Boston MA 02115, USA

Sean Morrissey MD, Abteilung für Psychiatrie Universitätsklinikum Regensburg, Regensburg, Germany

Jorge R Oksenberg PhD, Assistant Professor Department of Neurology, University of California at San Francisco, San Francisco, CA 94143-0435, USA

Chris H Polman MD, Academisch Ziekenhuis Vrije Universiteit, 1007 MB Amsterdam The Netherlands.

Carlo Pozzilli MD, Clinica Neurologica, Università degli Studi 'La Sapienza', Roma, Italy

Stephen C Reingold PhD, Vice President, Research Programs, National Multiple Sclerosis Society 733 Third Avenue, New York NY 10017-3288, USA

George Rice MD, University of Western Ontario 339 Windermere Road, London ON Canada N6A 5A5

Richard A Rudick MD, Director, Mellen Center for Multiple Sclerosis Treatment and Research, Cleveland Clinic Foundation, Cleveland OH 44195, USA

Mona Salesse BSc, Manager, Regulatory Affairs Serono Canada, Oakville ON, Canada L6M 262

Lynn Sartori MA, Associate Director, Regulatory Affairs, Biogen France SA

Steven R Schwid MD, Assistant Professor of Neurology, Univeristy of Rochester School of Medicine Department of Neurology, 601 Elmwood Avenue Rochester NY 14642, USA

Valerie L Stevenson MB BS MRCP, Research Registrar, The NMR Unit, Institute of Neurology, Queen Sqaure, London W5 5BG, UK

Lael Stone, Staff Neurologist, Mellen Center for Multiple Sclerosis Treatment and Research, Cleveland Clinic Foundation, Cleveland OH 44195, USA

Siegrid Strasser-Fuchs MD, Department of Neurology, Karl-Franzens-Universität Graz Auenbruggerplatz 22, A-8036 Graz, Austria

William H Stuart MD, Medical Director, MS Center at Shepherd Center, 2020 Peachtree Road NW, Atlanta GA 30309, USA

Alan J Thompson MD FRCP FRCPI, Garfield Weston Professor of Clinical Neurology and Neurorehabilitation, Institute of Neurology, University College London, Queen Square, London WC1N 3BG, UK

Carla Tortorella MD, Neuroimaging Research Unit, Department of Neuroscience, San Raffaele Scientific Institute, Via Olgettina 60, 20132 Milano, Italy

Marianne AA van Walderveen MD, MR Center for MS Research, Academisch Ziekenhuis Vrije Universiteit, 1007 MB Amsterdam, The Netherlands

Emmanuelle L Waubant MD, University of California at San Francisco, Mount Zion MS Center 1701 Divisadero Street, Suite 480, San Francisco CA 94115-1642, USA

Brian G Weinshenker MD, Professor of Neurology, Mayo Clinic and Foundation, Rochester MN 55905, USA

Kate Whetten-Goldstein MPH PhD, Duke University Center for Health Policy, Law and Management Durham NC 27708, US

Preface

A little over 20 years ago it was thought by many that research into experimental therapies in multiple sclerosis (MS) was, at best, unlikely to provide valid or reproducible information relating to the treatment of the disease. This pessimistic opinion was reflected at the First International Conference on Therapeutics in Multiple Sclerosis, held in 1982. The concerns were based on many unsubstantiated claims for efficacy for treatments that could not be confirmed and on the failure to identify a significant treatment effect in the many trials that had been done prior to the meeting. While the failures were due in part to the highly variable and unpredictable clinical course, which is the clinical hallmark of the disease, there was also concern that a higher level of scientific quality was needed in experimental therapeutic research in MS. Today, research on new therapies in MS has become increasingly efficient and effective in identifying the effect of these therapies on the course of disease. In fact, research into the treatment of MS can be considered an example of excellence in experimental therapeutics in neurological disease. The change is evidenced by the approval in the USA of three therapies for the relapsing–remitting phase of the disease.

The change can be related to several factors. Certainly, demonstration that magnetic resonance imaging (MRI) can provide an objective means for monitoring MS, at least in some phases of the disease course, has provided a very powerful tool in experimental therapeutics in MS. Most important, however, has been the

growth of expertise in clinical research in MS. Impressive advances in the attention given to the design of clinical trials in MS ranging from early phase 1 or 2 studies to pivotal phase 3 studies are now evident. Examples of clinical trials with severe or fatal flaws in trial design, common in the past, are now unusual. These advances reflect the growing importance given to clinical research in MS.

Despite these advances, many unresolved questions relating to the study of new therapies in MS persist. Beginning with an important meeting focusing on clinical outcomes in MS research sponsored by the National Multiple Sclerosis Society and held in 1994, use of both clinical and MRI outcomes has been carefully studied. New approaches to the assessment of clinical disease progression have been described and are now beginning to be used in clinical trials. Further, use of MRI as an outcome measure has been and continues to be carefully evaluated. Thus, summary of the advances in MS experimental therapeutics, including detailed assessment of clinical and MRI outcomes, is especially timely.

Early in the use of MRI as an outcome measure, many investigators were convinced that measure of disease activity on MRI could replace clinical outcome measures completely. It was hoped that MRI was a direct measure of the disease activity occurring in MS and that monitoring changes in disease activity as seen on MRI during the use of a new treatment could establish the effectiveness of that treatment. It is now clear that, although MRI is a very powerful tool, the ability to translate changes in disease activity seen using conventional MR imaging directly to clinical outcomes is not perfect. It is becoming increasingly evident that the evolution of the MS lesion is complex and probably variable among patients. Further, the evolution of the pathological processes involved in the disease probably does not represent a continuum of a single process but, instead, various components each contributing in different ways to damage of the myelin sheath and the axon. Thus, it is likely that the correlation between various MRI modalities differs during various stages of the disease process. For example, the level of disease activity as measured on T2-weighted images or on post-contrast T1-weighted images early in the course of the disease may be helpful in predicting the severity of future disease. These same measures of disease activity, when examined later in the course of disease, may have little relationship to the level of disability existing at the time of study or to the future progression of the disease. It is likely that progression is closely related to irreversible damage to the myelin sheath and to axonal damage, neither of which are specifically reflected on T2-weighted images. Further, the level of new activity seen in contrast-enhanced T1-weighted images may have only a small impact on the overall level of disease once a large degree of diseased brain exists. Thus, it is hoped that imaging sequences, which have greater pathological specificity for the events contributing most directly to progression, will provide a more useful tool for monitoring new therapies in clinical trials.

The chapters incorporated in the first section of this book, written by individuals with particular expertise in their respective areas, will provide an up-to-date review of the assessment of clinical and MRI outcome measures that are and that will be used in clinical trials in MS. Overall, the reader will develop an understanding of the problems in experimental therapeutics that are unique to MS, knowledge about clinical outcomes that form the heart of clinical trials, and a solid foundation regarding the strengths and weaknesses of imaging as an outcome measure in clinical trials in MS. The interest in experimental therapeutics in MS is growing rapidly as advances in immunology and genetics point to therapies that may have potential for modifying the disease process. The issues discussed will provide the reader with the information necessary to assess and to participate in this exciting area of clinical research.

Following this basic foundation, subsequent chapters examine the results of the most important symptomatic and disease-modifying therapies in MS. As one reviews current understanding of many of these therapies, one can understand the importance of well-designed clinical studies. Unfortunately, in many cases, the effectiveness of these therapies is incompletely resolved. More important, the ability of many of the therapies to have a truly modifying effect on the course of disease is uncertain. As implied above, it is likely that the effect of some of these therapies will differ among patients and with respect to the stage of the disease process when they are administered. As the reader evaluates the results obtained with therapies that have been tested in MS, the need for continued improvement in trial design will become apparent. The decision as to whether and when to treat is dependent upon both the physician and the patient having a complete understanding of the effect of the therapy in relation to the stage of the disease and in relation to side effects. In many cases, considerable uncertainty still exists and assessment by both physician and patient of the risks in relation to the benefits is difficult.

It is hoped that careful attention to future trial design and the use of new imaging modalities to define better the effect of the therapies will lead not only to new, effective treatments but also to improved understanding of the disease process.

Henry F McFarland MD
Chief, Neuroimmunology Branch
National Institute of Neurological
Disorders and Stroke
National Institutes of Health
Bethesda MD
USA

Acknowledgements

Our thanks are due to all those who contributed towards this book. We appreciate expert secretarial and administrative assistance provided by Kim Law and Janet Perryman. The publishers have been a pleasure to work with; our thanks to Martin Dunitz for providing early advice, and to Alan Burgess and Tanya Wiedeking for all their efforts in co-ordinating the project and ensuring the expeditious publication of this book. Dr Bruce Trapp generously provided the beautiful micrograph on the cover.

PART I

Introduction

1
Aspects of multiple sclerosis that relate to clinical trial design and treatment

Richard A Rudick and Donald E Goodkin

INTRODUCTION

The purpose of this chapter is to discuss the most important aspects of multiple sclerosis (MS) that have an impact on clinical trial design, development of new therapies, and patient care. These aspects include the clinical course of disease, clinical heterogeneity, and the presence of subclinical disease activity during the early stage of disease. The presence of ongoing subclinical disease activity implies that sensitive, reliable, and valid surrogate markers will be required to develop more effective therapies.

The clinical course presents challenges, because MS is chronic and has strikingly heterogeneous clinical manifestations that evolve over decades. During the relapsing–remitting multiple sclerosis (RRMS) stage, periodic relapses occur at irregular and unpredictable intervals, averaging only about one per year. Relapses tend to become less conspicuous over the years, and the majority of patients evolve into a pattern of continuously progressive neurologic deterioration, known as secondary progressive multiple sclerosis (SPMS). During this stage, neurologic, cognitive, emotional, social, and economic decline is the rule, and the illness seems more refractory to treatment. This stage of the disease is also difficult to study, however, because deterioration occurs

over the course of years and because significant individual variability persists. In a minority of cases, categorized as primary progressive multiple sclerosis (PPMS), neurologic disability becomes progressively worse from the onset of the symptoms. A consensus has emerged that PPMS should be considered separately from the other groups for the purpose of controlled clinical trials, in part because of uncertainty about the etiologic relationship between PPMS and the other categories.

Clinical manifestations vary considerably between patients within a clinical disease category, and manifestations also vary over time in individual patients. Even within multiply affected families, there is striking clinical heterogeneity between affected family members. This presents significant challenges for the design of clinical trials. Multidimensional outcome measures can be used to capture the main ways that MS affects the patients (see Chapter 2), but separate trials and treatment arms within a given trial contain variable admixtures of clinical manifestations that are not necessarily evenly matched between study arms or across studies.

It has become increasingly clear that clinical manifestations of MS bear a loose relationship to the ongoing pathologic process, as measured with magnetic resonance imaging (MRI) scanning (see

Chapters 5–9). Particularly in RRMS patients, the disease is active by imaging criteria during the time between clinical relapses. Interestingly, some patients are entirely stable clinically but have active and progressive disease documented by serial MRI scans. Assuming that MRI disease activity and progression is meaningful, this suggests that a sensitive and meaningful surrogate marker for the disease process will be required, and most efforts to date have focused on the use of MRI for this purpose.

CLINICAL DISEASE CATEGORIES AND CLINICAL HETEROGENEITY

The disease classification mentioned above was developed by consensus (*Table 1.1*).[1] Eighty-five percent of patients have either RRMS or SPMS. In RRMS, episodic attacks of neurologic dysfunction are followed by recovery, and individual relapses are clearly separated by a stable clinical phase. Over 50% of RRMS patients eventually evolve into more or less continuous clinical deterioration in the SPMS disease stage. The transition from RRMS to SPMS does not occur at a precise point in time. Rather, the clinical relapses become less distinct episodes, recovery becomes

Table 1.1 Clinical Categories of MS[1]

Disease Category	Description
Relapsing–remitting MS (RRMS)	Episodic relapses with recovery and a stable phase between relapses. MS begins as RRMS in 80% of cases. Clinical relapses imply that the disease is active, but clinical remission does not mean the disease is quiescent. MRI studies have shown that the disease may be active when the disease is clinically inactive.
Secondary progressive MS (SPMS)	Gradual neurologic deterioration with or without superimposed acute relapses in a patient who previously had RRMS. Over 50% of patients with RRMS progress into this stage of the disease. A major goal of disease therapy in RRMS patients is to prevent SPMS.
Primary progressive MS (PPMS)	Gradual, nearly continuous neurologic deterioration from the onset of symptoms. Some patients with PPMS have onset in middle age and MRI and CSF findings identical to patients with SPMS. These patients probably have SPMS, but without evident clinical relapses during the early stage of disease. Other PPMS patients appear to have a degenerative process with minimal evidence of inflammation. These patients present as a gradually worsening gait disorder, and often have minimal cranial disease by MRI scans.
Progressive relapsing MS (PRMS)	Gradual neurologic deterioration from onset but with subsequent superimposed relapses. This is an unusual clinical pattern.

less robust, and the RRMS stage blends into the SPMS stage, commonly 10–20 years after the onset symptoms. The beginning of the SPMS stage can be dated only in retrospect, once it is clear that the patient has continuously worsened for months or years.

Approximately 10–15% of patients have PPMS, in which continuous clinical deterioration occurs from disease onset. Patients with PPMS have symptom onset at a later age, typically between ages 40 and 60 years, and the female preponderance seen with RRMS and SPMS is not evident. Some PPMS patients probably have the same disease as SPMS but without clinical symptoms during the early disease stage. Other PPMS patients present clinically with insidiously progressive spastic weakness, imbalance, and sphincter dysfunction, diffuse and less nodular lesions on T2-weighted MRI, no gadolinium-enhanced lesions, and little inflammatory change in the cerebrospinal fluid.[2] These cases may represent a type of MS that is less dependent on inflammation and that may be primarily degenerative. The explanation for the lack of female preponderance is unknown.

Common practice has been to define relatively homogeneous patient groups for inclusion in clinical trials, typically by defining disability limits using the Kurtzke Expanded Disability Status Scale (EDSS),[3] and by entering patients within specified disease categories. This strategy reduces between-patient variability, which increases the power to show therapeutic effects at any given sample size. There is also a theoretical concern that an intervention would be selectively applicable to a particular disease stage or type. This explains why separate trials have been conducted for patients with RRMS and SPMS. The distinction between these two categories is not precise, however, and the reliability of classifying patients

into these categories has never been tested. In all likelihood, there is an admixture of RRMS patients in SPMS trials, and vice versa. Because the exact patient composition of separate trials cannot be compared accurately, it is difficult to be certain that separate trials with the same entry criteria actually contain comparable patient populations. The problem of classifying patients is most difficult at the interface between RRMS and SPMS. As disease duration and EDSS increase, the patient is more likely to be categorized as SPMS, and the cut-point appears to be around an EDSS of 4.0. At this level and above, the large majority of patients are classified as SPMS.

Table 1.2 lists characteristics of patients entered into recent large clinical trials. Disease duration and disability level are clearly different in RRMS trials compared with SPMS trials. Because the utility of restricting entry by disease category is unclear, a study of sulfasalazine allowed entry of patients based only on disability criteria.[4] *Table 1.2* indicates that patients in the sulfasalazine trial were comparable to RRMS populations in terms of disability score and disease duration.

Studies in PPMS are problematic because these cases comprise only about 15% of the MS population and because the PPMS category contains a mixture of SPMS patients without a symptomatic RRMS stage as well as patients with non-inflammatory disease of the central nervous system with an uncertain etiological and pathogenic relationship to MS.

Clinical manifestations within disease categories are very heterogeneous. Individual patients may have predominantly cognitive impairments, cerebellar dysfunction, spastic paraparesis, sensory ataxia, visual impairment, or various combinations of these.[5] Treatment arms, therefore, can be expected to contain a mixture of

Table 1.2 Patient characteristics In selected controlled clinical trials

Clinical trial	Number of patients	Age (years)*	Disease duration (years)*	Mean EDSS
Trials with entry restricted to RRMS				
IFN-β-1b (Betaseron®)	123 (placebo)	36.0	3.9‡	2.8
	125 (1.6 × 10⁶IU)	35.3	4.7‡	2.9
	124 (8.0 × 10⁶IU)	35.2	4.7‡	3.0
IFN-β-1a (Avonex®)	143 (placebo)	36.9	6.4	2.3
	158 (treatment)	36.7	6.6	2.4
IFN-β-1a (Rebif®)	560 (total)	34.9†	5.3†	2.5
Glatiramer (Copaxone®)	126 (placebo)	34.3	6.6	2.4
	125 (treament)	34.6	7.3	2.8
Mean of RRMS trials		**35.5**	**6.4§**	**2.6**
Trials with entry restricted to SPMS				
IFN-β-1b (Betaseron®)	358 (placebo)	40.9	13.4	5.2
	360 (treatment)	41.1	12.8	5.1
IFN-β-1a (Avonex®)	416 (total)	47.6	16.4	5.2
Mean of SPMS trials		**43.2**	**14.8**	**5.2**
Trials without entry restricted by disease category				
Sulfasalazine	96 (placebo)	27	5.0	2.5
	103 (treatment)	28	6.0	2.5

*Mean, except where indicated.
†Median.
‡From diagnosis.
§Excluding Betaseron study because disease duration is unknown.

patients with various combinations of motor, sensory, visual, cognitive, affective, bowel, bladder, and sexual dysfunction. Outcome measures have been used that can be appropriately applied to a heterogeneous patient population, although traditional outcome measures have been heavily weighted in the direction of motor impairments (see Chapter 2).

VARIABLE DISEASE SEVERITY AND PROGNOSTIC MARKERS IN MS PATIENTS

Because of pronounced individual variability, there is a need for accurate prognostic markers that could be used for treatment decisions and to design clinical trials. Fifty percent of MS patients are unable to carry out household and employment responsibilities 10 years after disease onset, 50% are unable to walk unassisted after 15 years, and 50% are unable to walk after 25 years, even with assistance.[6] About 10% of patients have unusually bad disease and deteriorate to severe irreversible disability in only a few years. Another 10% have benign disease, with intermittent neurologic symptoms but little disease progression and minimal disability decades after the first symptoms.

During the time frame of a clinical trial (typically 2–3 years) most placebo patients do not show worsening on the EDSS scale. Moreover, most patients have either no relapses or only one relapse. In recent trials involving RRMS patients, one third or fewer of the placebo patients had EDSS worsening during 2 years.[7,8] Clinical stability in the majority of placebo treated patients results in large sample sizes. One approach to this problem has been to develop more sensitive clinical outcome measures and MRI-based surrogate measures (see below).

Another approach has been to enroll selectively patients at high risk of disease progression, excluding patients who are not likely to change during the trial. In groups of patients, benign disease has been associated with sensory symptoms or optic neuritis at onset, good recovery from relapses, and infrequent relapses during the first couple years.[9–12] Conversely, symptom onset at an older age, progressive disease from onset, or poor recovery from relapses mark a relatively worse prognosis. Clinical features are only weak predictors of subsequent disease severity, however, and their value for assigning prognosis for the purpose of informative enrollment in clinical trials has not been successful.[13] The presence of multicentric white matter lesions at the time of first MS symptoms has been associated with a higher risk of MRI and clinical disease progression in the subsequent 5 years.[14] Although it is not possible to predict the prognosis for individual patients accurately using MRI findings, the presence of multicentric white matter lesions is increasingly required as an entry criteria into clinical trials.

THE PRESENCE OF SUBCLINICAL DISEASE ACTIVITY DURING RRMS

The pathologic process in the brain is active in many RRMS patients during the periods of clinical remission between clinical relapses. Over 50% of RRMS patients have one or more gadolinium enhancing lesion on a single cranial MRI scan obtained when the disease is clinically inactive,[15,16] and over 70% of RRMS patients have at least one gadolinium-enhancing lesion evident on three successive monthly scans (see Chapter 5). Gadolinium enhancement represents an early event in development of a new T2-weighted MRI lesion[17] and marks sites of active brain inflammation.[18] However, the vast majority of new gadolinium-enhancing lesions are clinically silent.[19] Gadolinium enhancement resolves after 4–6 weeks and leaves behind T2 hyperintense lesions, leading to progressive increase in the volume of T2 lesions. Gadolinium-enhancing lesions are related to subsequent increase in T2 lesion volume,[20] are related to the frequency of clinical relapses,[20] and have been reported to increase the risk of enlargement of the third ventricle over the subsequent 2 years.[21] These findings suggest that MRI parameters can be used to quantify brain inflammation and predict subsequent MRI disease progression.

A number of investigators have found reduced

N-acetyl aspartate, a neuronal marker, in brain tissue from RRMS patients,[22–30] suggesting that recurrent brain inflammation occuring during the RRMS stage damages axons (see Chapter 9; Chapter 19). This has been directly confirmed through histologic analysis of MS lesions[18] demonstrating axonal transection at sites of active inflammation, regardless of the duration of MS in the individual case.

Taken together, the findings indicate that active inflammatory brain disease occurs during the RRMS stage and that this process is not reflected accurately by clinical relapses. One hypothesis[31] holds that irreversible brain tissue injury occurs repeatedly in the inflammatory lesions during the RRMS disease stage. This accumulates over the years, leading to progressive clinical deterioration in patients with SPMS. Progressive disability develops only after the amount of tissue loss has exceeded a threshold beyond which compensatory mechanisms are exhausted and functional decline ensues.

This view of MS has significant clinical implications for patients, particularly in view of approved disease therapies (see Chapter 30). First, there is an increasing consensus that disease modifying therapy should be used in RRMS patients to delay or prevent subsequent neurologic disability[32] rather than withheld until after disability has become advanced. Once a specific neurologic impairment has persisted for longer than 6 months, spontaneous recovery is uncommon and no therapies are known that promote recovery. Secondly, the poor relationship between clinical relapses and the severity of brain inflammation implies that more accurate and sensitive surrogate markers of the pathologic process in RRMS are needed.

TRADITIONAL CLINICAL OUTCOME MEASURES

Traditional clinical outcome measures include relapses and ratings of neurologic impairment or disability. Relapses are defined as neurologic symptoms lasting at least 48 hours accompanied by a change in the neurologic exam. This definition is inherently imprecise. Patients often report changes in their symptoms without clear changes on neurologic exam, or they have changes on the neurologic examination that are not associated with new symptoms. Different neurologists, using the broad definition above, almost certainly define relapses differently. Certain investigators have attempted to create operational definitions for relapses,[33] but this creates different types of problems and does not eliminate the element of patient self-report. Other investigators have graded clinical relapses as mild, moderate, or severe using the neurologic rating scale.[7,34] The definition of these categories is arbitrary, however, and has not been validated. The relapse rate remains useful as an outcome measure in controlled trials, but it is critical that the treatment be effectively masked from patients and evaluator because a relapse is in part patient-defined. It is also absolutely mandatory that disability data be collected so that the relapse data can be analysed in terms of disability data derived from the neurologic exam or quantitative tests of neurologic disability. This is particularly important because patients typically experience fewer relapses while converting to steadily progressive neurologic deterioration.

The EDSS has achieved widespread use as a primary clinical rating scale in recent years. The EDSS is an ordinal scale that comprises 19 steps between 0 and 10 (0.5 point increments), representing increasing disability as the EDSS score increases:

(a) between 0 and 3.5, the composite score represents the scores assigned to eight functional systems scales;

(b) between 4.0 and 5.5, the composite score represents the distance an individual patient can ambulate;

(c) 6.0 represents the use of unilateral assistance such as a cane to walk;

(d) 6.5 represents the need for bilateral assistance such as a walker to walk;

(e) and between 7.0 and 9.5 represent increasing degrees of immobility and dependence.

Groups of patients progress up the EDSS scale in a reasonably ordered and consistent way, and the EDSS has become well accepted as the standard method for categorizing patients for disease severity.

The EDSS has been extensively criticized because of several shortcomings related to its use as an outcome measure for controlled clinical trials. The main problems with the EDSS can be summarized as follows:

(a) In the lower range of EDSS, the definitions for the functional system scales gradations are vague and subjective, limiting the reproducibility of the functional system scales; additionally at the low end of the scale the definition of EDSS using the various functional system scores is somewhat arbitrary.

(b) In the mid-range of the scale, the EDSS is almost entirely an ambulation instrument, yet the information is truncated into a small number of discrete categories, discarding important information about change. For example, an individual patient may remain at the 6.5 level for several years, during which walking becomes increasingly limited. The patient changes, but the EDSS score does not reflect the change. For this reason, it has been argued that the EDSS is inadequately sensitive to change for the purposes of controlled clinical trials.

(c) In the upper range, EDSS steps are so vague and stable as to be almost useless as a rating scale for clinical trials.

(d) At any range of the scale, there are no cognitive assessments, even though cognitive impairments are common in MS patients (see Chapter 3).

(e) At the 4.0 to 6.5 range, the EDSS is insensitive to arm impairment.

In response to many of these concerns, a consensus workshop was held in Charleston, South Carolina in 1994. The consensus from the workshop[35] indicated that the majority of participants felt that an improved clinical outcome measure was required for future clinical trials. The new clinical outcome measure was to retain the best elements of the EDSS but should include measure(s) of cognitive impairment and should be quantitative, reproducible, and more useful in monitoring treatment effects in controlled clinical trials. To address this need, the National Multiple Sclerosis Society's Advisory Committee on Clinical Trials of New Agents in Multiple Sclerosis appointed a Task Force charged with making specific recommendations for improved clinical outcome measures. The Task Force articulated desirable attributes of a clinical outcome measure for MS trials:[36]

(a) the score should, as far as possible, be quantitative, and the distance between points on the scale should be known;

(b) the score should have a high intra-rater and inter-rater reliability, or for self-report measures should have high test–retest reproducibility;

(c) the measure should be sensitive to clinical change over a relatively short time interval, so that the outcome measure could be reasonably expected to show therapeutic effects;

(d) the clinical outcome measure should have demonstrated validity; and

(e) the measure should be easy and quick to administer, consistent with comfort, safety, and compliance, and should be cost- and time-efficient.

The need for increasingly sensitive clinical measures was considered to be extremely important by the Task Force in order to allow progress in the field. *Table 1.3* shows sample size calculations for two hypothetical clinical trials using the EDSS as the primary outcome. The first clinical trial is placebo-controlled. The sample size calculation assumes that 40% of placebo recipients will reach the clinical endpoint in 3 years, however that is defined. It is assumed that the active therapy will be 40% effective (i.e. only 24% of patients in the active treatment group will reach the clinical endpoint). Such a trial would require 132 subjects per arm, or a total of 264 subjects. Further assuming a 20% drop-out rate, the study would require 317 patients to achieve a power of 80% to show the therapeutic effect at the required significance level of $p < 0.05$. The second study in the table incorporates an active arm comparison, assuming the

availability of a partially effective therapy (e.g. assume that treatment 1 was effective and the second study is a follow-up to compare a newer promising therapy to the 'standard' treatment). For the active arm comparison study, 520 patients would be required to show a further 40% improvement in the number of patients on treatment 1 who reach the clinical endpoint, assuming that the outcome measure and all other assumptions remain unchanged. With a 20% drop-out rate, the active arm comparison study would require 624 patients. Thus, as partially effective therapies are developed, demonstrating effectiveness of better treatments would require longer trials, increased sample sizes, more sensitive clinical measures, or some combination of these approaches.

To arrive at recommendations, the Task Force analysed informative data sets from recent controlled clinical trials and from natural history studies to assess potential measurement techniques against the favorable attributes listed above (see Chapter 2).[37] From that analysis, the Task Force recommended a three-part composite, the Multiple Sclerosis Functional Composite

Table 1.3 Analysis of why more study subjects are required for active arm comparison trials when using the same clinical outcome measure[36]

	Placebo-controlled trial	*Active arm comparison trial*
Primary comparison	Treatment 1 versus Placebo	Treatment 2 versus Treatment 1
Rate of worsening for placebo	40%	NA
Rate of worsening for treatment 1	24%*	24%
Rate of worsening for treatment 2	NA	14.4%*
Sample size for 3-year study†	**317 subjects required**	**624 subjects required**

*Assumes a 40% treatment effect.
†Calculation uses a two-tailed test of significance with $\alpha = 0.05$ and $1\text{-}\beta = 0.80$, and a 20% drop out rate.
NA, not applicable.

(MSFC), for further testing and for use in controlled clinical trials.[38] The MSFC includes a timed 25-foot (8 m) walk,[39] the average time from two trials from either arm to complete the Nine-Hole Peg Test,[40] and the number of correct responses on the 3 second version of the Paced Auditory Serial Addition Test.[41] Results from each of the component measures is transformed to a Z-score, representing the number of standard deviation units away from the mean of a reference population, and the individual Z-scores are combined to create a single score. In the meta-analysis conducted by the Task Force,[37] there was a reasonably strong relationship between MSFC scores and the EDSS, and between change in the MSFC and change in the EDSS. Interestingly, the MSFC often changed before the EDSS did, suggesting the MSFC change could predict subsequent EDSS change. This might mean that the MSFC is more responsive than the EDSS, and it might therefore be more informative in demonstrating small amounts of change during the time frame of controlled clinical trials. Studies are ongoing to validate the MSFC further by comparing scores to MRI and quality of life outcomes, and to determine whether short term changes predict clinically significant changes in subsesquent years.

SURROGATE MARKERS OF THE DISEASE PROCESS

The poor relationship between clinical relapses and the severity of brain inflammation implies that more accurate and sensitive markers of the pathologic process in RRMS will be required for use as a surrogate marker(s). The United States Food and Drug Administration (FDA) defines a surrogate marker as any non-clinical measure that can reliably predict clinical changes 'within a reasonable amount of time'. Although certain biological markers (see Chapter 10) and conventional MRI parameters (see Chapters 6–9) correlate with disease activity, and MRI can be used to predict conversion from clinically isolated syndromes suggestive of MS to clinically definite MS,[14] no surrogate measure has acceptable validity for predicting eventual disability in patients who present with a diagnosis of MS.

It is generally agreed that MRI has the greatest potential to meet the FDA definition of a surrogate marker. Neurologists already obtain cranial MRI scans periodically to estimate MS disease activity and progression in some patients, to determine the need for disease modifying therapy in patients with clinically benign disease, and to follow the response to disease modifying therapy. The Advisory Committee on Clinical Trials of New Agents in Multiple Sclerosis of the United States National Multiple Sclerosis Society appointed a Task Force, which made recommendations about using MRI in clinical trials[42] (*Table 1.4*). The Task Force report was generally optimistic about the potential for using MRI parameters as surrogate markers. It made initial recommendations based primarily on analysing gadolinium-enhancing lesions and it indicated the rapid developments in the field that can be expected to result in future more specific recommendations in the future.

MRI lesion analysis faces a number of important challenges as a surrogate marker for controlled clinical trials:

(a) There are a number of candidate measures that are related, and it is not clear which should be used or how they should combine. The following are all of great potential importance:

T2 hyperintense lesions,

Table 1.4 Recommendations from the task force on use of MRI in MS clinical trials[42]

1. MRI is a highly sensitive marker of pathological activity in RRMS and SPMS.
2. There are significant correlations emerging between a number of MRI and clinical parameters, although in established MS the relationship between short-term MRI activity and long-term disability is uncertain.
3. High sensitivity makes MRI an excellent tool for rapid screening of therapies aimed at suppressing new pathological activity in RRMS and SPMS. Because the long-term relationship between MRI and disability is still uncertain, MRI data should not be the definitive determinant of therapeutic efficacy. A clinically significant endpoint must be shown. MRI should be used to select appropriate patients with clinically isolated syndrome for trials of therapy aimed at delaying the evolution to definite MS.
4. There are evolving major improvements in the resolution and sensitivity of MRI and in new techniques to monitor demyelination and neuronal damage and to quantify lesion load. Further studies are needed in ongoing treatment trials to determine whether these new techniques (fluid attenuated inversion recovery sequences, magnetization transfer imaging, proton-magnetic spectroscopic imaging, and diffusion-weighted imaging) will prove to be strongly predictive of clinical outcome.

T1 hypointense lesions, gadolinium-enhancing lesions, magnetization transfer ratios in lesions, in normal-appearing white matter, or in whole brain, and spectroscopic data applied to lesions, normal-appearing white matter, or regions of interest.

(b) A more global measure of the pathologic process, such as atrophy, is appealing, as this is likely to reflect the net effect of various pathologic processes, and the outcome is likely to be meaningful. However, atrophy measures are not expected to be sensitive to disease activity over short time intervals, and they will not provide insights into the mechanisms of tissue loss or the mechanisms of therapeutic responses.

(c) MRI lesions are characterized by a high degree of variability evident within individual patients in longitudinal studies. This leads to the problem of sampling error. If a patient is tested during a burst of disease activity, lesion analysis may suggest that the pathology is increasing when the overall pattern is decreasing. This results in large sample sizes or frequent MRI scans.

(d) The histologic substrate of most lesions remains uncertain, and there is likely to be histologic heterogeneity within lesions that all appear the same on the MRI scans.

(e) MRI lesion analysis has not yet been shown to predict subsequent clinical deterioration, although few studies have incorporated adequate methodology to establish predictive validity so far. Although MRI is promising as a surrogate, further studies are needed to define precisely how MRI is to be used as a surrogate marker in clinical trials, and to validate the precise methods using the FDA definition of surrogate marker.

FUTURE CONSIDERATIONS FOR THERAPEUTICS IN MS

Placebo control groups and active arm comparison studies

Placebo controlled trials in RRMS are now impractical, because effective therapies are available in most regions of the world. More importantly, placebo-controlled trials are ethically questionable, given convincing evidence for meaningful therapeutic benefits from the available treatments. The use of a placebo control group in patients with SPMS is increasingly problematic, with emerging reports of effective therapies. However, current therapies are only partly effective. Therefore, it will be necessary to define a methodology for active arm comparison studies and for studies of drugs given in combination. This will significantly increase the complexity and possibly the cost of controlled clinical trials unless more sensitive clinical measures or reliable surrogate markers can be identified.

The trend towards early treatment and cost benefit analyses

The trend in the direction of proactive preventive therapy designed to delay or stop SPMS will require novel outcome studies. The potential medical, economic, and society benefits of effective therapy in the early stages of MS may not be immediately evident. During the early disease stage, many patients feel reasonably well and are working. How will the need for and the benefits of aggressive early treatment used to prevent the devastating later effects of MS be demonstrated?

Rationally designed interventions

Most contemporary clinical trials are based on the concept that MS is caused by autoreactive T cells that injure the central nervous system (see Chapter 19). Interventions range from highly specific inhibition of the tri-molecular complex to more global forms of immune suppression. However, recent pathology studies[43] suggest that the pathology may vary significantly between individual patients. This raises the possibility that therapy could be individualized. Increasingly, axonal degeneration is considered a prominent feature of MS, providing a rationale for neuroprotective or neurotrophic factors in future clinical trials. Understanding of the mechanisms that lead to axonal degeneration and of strategies to monitor the process are lacking, however. Will adequate information related to pathogenic mechanisms to design rational therapeutic intervention eventually be developed? Or will development of MS therapeutics be entirely a trial-and-error process based on practical considerations about potential therapies?

Methodologies for individual patient treatment

Extrapolating from controlled clinical trials to clinical practice is an imprecise art (see Chapters 30–40). Increasingly, neurologists will be required to make decisions for the individual patient based on limited data from a clinical trial. By necessity, entry criteria for clinical trials are narrow in order to reduce heterogeneity and focus the question for the trial. However, in clinical practice only a tiny fraction of patients have the same characteristics as the clinical trial population. Additionally, methods for monitoring individual patients during open-label therapy are lacking. Can we develop methods to address a common clinical question: 'Is this drug working?' A valid definition of therapeutic response is needed for individual treatment decisions. Clinical studies at the interface between controlled clinical trials and clinical practice will be critical for optimizing therapy for individual MS patients.

REFERENCES

1 **Lublin FD, Reingold SC.** Defining the clinical course of multiple sclerosis: results of an international survey. *Neurology* 1996; **46**:907–911.

2 **Thompson AJ, Kermode AG, Wicks D et al.** Major differences in the dynamics of primary and secondary progressive multiple sclerosis. *Ann Neurol* 1991; **29**:53–62.

3 **Kurtzke JF.** Rating neurologic impairment in multiple sclerosis: an expanded disability status scale (EDSS). *Neurology* 1983; **33**:1444–1452.

4 **Noseworthy JH, O'Brien P, Erickson BJ et al.** The Mayo Clinic–Canadian Cooperative trial of sulfasalazine in active multiple sclerosis. *Neurology* 1998; **51**:1342–1352.

5 **Poser S, Wikstrom J, Bauer HJ.** Clinical data and the identification of special forms of multiple sclerosis in 1271 cases studied with a standardized documentation system. *J Neurol Sci* 1979; **40**:159–168.

6 **Weinshenker BG.** The natural history of multiple sclerosis (Review). *Neurol Clin* 1995; **13**:119–146.

7 **The IFNB Study Group.** Interferon beta-1b is effective in relapsing–remitting multiple sclerosis. I. Clinical results of a multicenter, randomized, double-blind, placebo-controlled trial. *Neurology* 1993; **43**:655–661.

8 **Jacobs LD, Cookfair DL, Rudick RA et al.** Intramuscular interferon beta-1a for disease progression in relapsing multiple sclerosis. The Multiple Sclerosis Collaborative Research Group (MSCRG). *Ann Neurol* 1996; **39**:285–294.

9 **Runmarker B, Andersen O, Anderson O.** Prognostic factors in a multiple sclerosis incidence cohort with twenty-five years of follow-up. *Brain* 1993; **116**:117–134.

10 **Runmarker B, Andersson C, Oden A, Andersen O.**
Prediction of outcome in multiple sclerosis based on multivariate models. *J Neurol* 1994; **241**:597–604.

11 **Weinshenker BG.** Natural history of multiple sclerosis. *Ann Neurol* 1994; **36 (suppl)**:S6–S11.

12 **Weinshenker BG, Rice GP, Noseworthy JH et al.** The natural history of multiple sclerosis: a geographically based study. 3. Multivariate analysis of predictive factors and models of outcome. *Brain* 1991; **114**:1045–1056.

13 **Weinshenker BG, Issa M, Baskerville J.** Meta-analysis of the placebo-treated groups in clinical trials of progressive MS. *Neurology* 1996; **46**:1613–1619.

14 **Filippi M, Horsfield MA, Morrissey SP et al.** Quantitative brain MRI lesion load predicts the course of clinically isolated syndromes suggestive of multiple sclerosis. *Neurology* 1994; **44**:635–641.

15 **Simon JH.** Contrast-enhanced MR imaging in the evaluation of treatment response and prediction of outcome in multiple sclerosis. *J Magn Reson Imaging* 1997; **7**:29–37.

16 **McFarland HF, Stone LA, Calabresi PA et al.** MRI studies of multiple sclerosis: implications for the natural history of the disease and for monitoring effectiveness of experimental therapies. *Multiple Sclerosis* 1996; **2**:198–205.

17 **Miller DH, Rudge P, Johnson G et al.** Serial gadolinium enhanced magnetic resonance imaging in multiple sclerosis. *Brain* 1988; **111**:927–939.

18 **Trapp BD, Peterson J, Ransohoff RM et al.** Axonal transection in the lesions of multiple sclerosis. *N Engl J Med* 1998; **338**:278–285.

19 **McFarland HF, Frank JA, Albert PS et al.** Using gadolinium-enhanced magnetic resonance imaging lesions to monitor disease activity in multiple sclerosis. *Ann Neurol* 1992; **32**:758–766.

20 **Simon JH, Jacobs LD, Campion M et al.** Magnetic resonance studies of intramuscular interferon beta-1a for relapsing multiple sclerosis. The Multiple Sclerosis Collaborative Research Group. *Ann Neurol* 1998; **43**:79–87.

21 **Simon JH, Jacobs LD, Campion M et al.** A longitudinal study of brain atrophy in relapsing MS. *Neurology* 1999; in press.

22 **Narayana PA, Doyle TJ, Lai D, Wolinsky JS.** Serial proton magnetic resonance spectroscopic imaging, contrast-enhanced magnetic resonance imaging, and quantitative lesion volumetry in multiple sclerosis. *Ann Neurol* 1998; **43**:56–71.

23 **Narayanan S, Fu L, Pioro E et al.** Imaging of axonal damage in multiple sclerosis: spatial distribution of

magnetic resonance imaging lesions. *Ann Neurol* 1997; **41**:385–391.

24 Matthews PM, Pioro E, Narayanan S et al. Assessment of lesion pathology in multiple sclerosis using quantitative MRI morphometry and magnetic resonance spectroscopy. *Brain* 1996; **119**:715–722.

25 Davies SE, Newcombe J, Williams SR et al. High resolution proton NMR spectroscopy of multiple sclerosis lesions. *J Neurochem* 1995; **64**:742–748.

26 Tourbah A, Stievenart JL, Iba-Zizen MT et al. In vivo localized NMR proton spectroscopy of normal appearing white matter in patients with multiple sclerosis. *J Neuroradiol* 1996; **2**:49–55.

27 Rooney WD, Goodkin DE, Schuff N et al. 1H MRSI of normal appearing white matter in multiple sclerosis. *Multiple Sclerosis* 1997; **3**:231–237.

28 De Stefano N, Matthews PM, Narayanan S et al. Axonal dysfunction and disability in a relapse of multiple sclerosis: longitudinal study of a patient. *Neurology* 1997; **49**:1138–1141.

29 Bruhn H, Frahm J, Merboldt KD et al. Multiple sclerosis in children: cerebral metabolic alterations monitored by localized proton magnetic resonance spectroscopy in vivo. *Ann Neurol* 1992; **32**:140–150.

30 Husted CA, Goodin DS, Hugg JW et al. Biochemical alterations in multiple sclerosis lesions and normal-appearing white matter detected by in vivo 31P and 1H spectroscopic imaging. *Ann Neurol* 1994; **36**:157–165.

31 Trapp BD, Ransohoff RM, Fisher E, Rudick RA. Neurodegeneration in multiple sclerosis: relationship to neurological disability. *The Neuroscientist* 1999; **5**:48–57.

32 Munschauer FE 3rd, Stuart WH. Rationale for early treatment with interferon beta-1a in relapsing–remitting multiple sclerosis. *Clin Ther* 1997; **19**:868–882.

33 Jacobs L, Cookfair DL, Rudick RA et al. A phase III trial of intramuscular recombinant beta interferon as treatment for exacerbating–remitting multiple sclerosis: design and conduct of study and baseline characteristics of patients. *Multiple Sclerosis* 1995; **1**:118–135.

34 Sipe JC, Knobler RL, Braheny SL et al. A neurologic rating scale (NRS) for use in multiple sclerosis. *Neurology* 1984; **34**:1368–1372.

35 Whitaker JN, McFarland HF, Rudge P, Reingold SC. Outcomes assessment in multiple sclerosis clinical trials: a critical analysis. *Multiple Sclerosis* 1995; **1**:37–47.

36 Rudick R, Antel J, Confavreux C et al. Clinical outcomes assessment in multiple sclerosis. *Ann Neurol* 1996; **40**:469–479.

37 Cutter GR, Baier ML, Rudick RA et al. Development of a multiple sclerosis functional composite as a clinical trial outcome measure. *Brain* 1999; **122**:874–882.

38 Rudick R, Antel J, Confavreux C et al. Recommendations from the National Multiple Sclerosis Society Clinical Outcomes Assessment Task Force. *Ann Neurol* 1997; **42**:379–382.

39 Hauser SL, Dawson DM, Lehrich JR et al. Intensive immunosuppression in progressive multiple sclerosis. A randomized, three-arm study of high-dose intravenous cyclophosphamide, plasma exchange, and ACTH. *N Engl J Med* 1983; **308**:173–180.

40 Goodkin DE, Hertsgaard D, Seminary J. Upper extremity function in multiple sclerosis: improving assessment sensitivity with box-and-block and nine-hole peg tests. *Arch Phys Med Rehabil* 1988; **69**:850–854.

41 Gronwall DMA. Paced auditory serial-addition task: a measure of recovery from concussion. *Percept Motor Skills* 1977; **44**:367–373.

42 Miller DH, Albert PS, Barkhof F et al. Guidelines for the use of magnetic resonance techniques in monitoring the treatment of multiple sclerosis. US National MS Society Task Force. *Ann Neurol* 1996; **39**:6–16.

43 Lucchinetti C, Bruck W, Rodriquez M, Lassmann H. Distinct pattern of multiple sclerosis pathology indicates heterogeneity in pathogenesis. *Brain Pathol* 1996; **6**:259.

PART II

Clinical trial methodology

2
Measures of impairment and disability

Gary R Cutter

INTRODUCTION

The goal of good patient care is to prevent problems, alleviate suffering, and effect a cure. For these purposes, clinical assessments are needed to identify problems, document the course of the disease, provide etiological clues, and evaluate therapeutic efficacy. Because of complexity of the disease process and the breadth of clinical consequences, clinical tools for multiple sclerosis (MS) can be effectively applied only by a skilled and experienced clinician. Good clinical care can be viewed as a series of informal clinical trials by an astute clinician using single patients as the study population. Individualized treatment is central to patient care, but it is generally not appropriate for experimental studies. Rather, clinical measurements derived from a population of patients are needed for controlled clinical trials. This chapter describes the measurement of impairment and disability for use in MS clinical trials from a population, rather than from a patient care perspective. Many of the concepts discussed here are relevant at the patient care level, but the reader should be cognizant that optimal measures for clinical trials may differ significantly from evaluative methods for individual patient care.

There are many approaches to measuring impairment and disability, resulting in confusion as to the concept being measured. The World Health Organization (WHO) developed the International Classification of Impairments, Disabilities, and Handicaps.[1] In this framework, a patient is classified in terms of disease, impairment, disability, and handicap. Disease represents the underlying diagnosis or pathologic process. Impairment is the loss of physical or psychosocial capacities. Disability refers to limitations in performing a usual activity of normal life. Handicap is a disadvantage resulting from impairment or disability that inhibits or prevents a role that is normal for that person. Nagi[2] developed a functional limitation model, which described pathology, impairment, functional limitation and disability. According to Nagi, pathology is the 'interruption or interference of normal bodily processes or structures.' Impairment is the 'loss or abnormality of mental, emotional, physiological, or anatomical structure or function.' A functional limitation is 'restriction or lack of ability to perform an action or activity in the manner or within the range considered normal.' Disability is the 'inability or limitation in performing socially defined activities and roles expected of individuals within a social or physical environment.' There are marked similarities between these two formulations of impairment and disability, although the WHO framework equates handicap to what Nagi calls disability.

These related classifications seem to encompass the spectrum of impairment and disability, but at the measurement level another dimension needs to considered. There is often great debate over the value of an outcome measure of disability in MS. For example, some experts believe that extensive cognitive testing is essential to characterize a patient's disability, whereas others are content with a more global assessment. Part of this debate stems from the perspective of observer. There are two general perspectives or models of disability that drive measurement approaches. The medical model of disability focuses on the individual and specifically on the individual's impairment. This is the most familiar and common approach. The goal of treatment is to alleviate consequences of the impairment and to return the individual to normal (or as close to normal as possible). This model requires accurate diagnosis of the impairment and its pathology. It relies on a detailed understanding of normal function in order to develop the goals of intervention. In this model, patients are commonly labeled in terms of disability (e.g. wheelchair-bound) rather than at the level of impairment. The second perspective is the health psychology perspective. This vantage point is heavily focused on coping behaviors and developing strategies to minimize the effects of impairment. The view is that a person is disabled not only by his or her impairment, but also by how he or she responds to it. From this perspective, an assessment of activities of daily living and how a patient plans to accomplish certain tasks would make up the tools for assessing a patient. Both approaches are valid for outcome measures in clinical trials. Interventions that seek to effect a cure are best measured from the medical model perspective. Interventions that are designed to ameliorate symptoms often can be approached using the health psychology perspective.

In this chapter the primary concern is with the measurement of impairment or disability from a medical model perspective. Although there is a wide range of measurement tools for application in MS, encompassing everything from fatigue to sleep to bowel and bladder functioning, this chapter focuses on global clinical trial outcome measures.

METHODOLOGICAL ISSUES IN MEASURING IMPAIRMENT AND DISABILITY

Measures can be grouped into four classes:[3]

(a) biologic assays, which use laboratory methods, such as the amount of neutralizing antibodies, to assess a particular function or parameter;

(b) performance measures, which are standardized procedures for testing human function, such as the nine-hole peg test;[4]

(c) rating scales, which are ordered (ordinal) scales requiring human assessment, the most common in MS being Kurtzke's Expanded Disability Status Scale (EDSS);[5] and

(d) self-report measures, which require the individual patient to provide information about his or her condition from his or her own perspective. The Incapacity Status Scale[6] is an example of a self-report measure in the MS field.

These four classes of measurement describe the types of measures and provide a framework for assessment. However, the purposes of the measurements are not restricted by the different classes. In other words, a particular research question could be addressed by a laboratory test, a measure of patient function, a clinical rating scale, or a self-report. In clinical medicine, more than one measure (and often many measures) are used to evaluate a patient's status, check progress, alter the course of therapy, or make other recommendations. In a clinical trial, however, a single measure must be identified as the primary outcome, and that measure is the focus of decision making. There is a natural conflict between a complete clinical assessment of a patient from a physician perspective and the summary or index measure used in a clinical trial. The conflict may not show in the choice of instruments, but it can and does influence the interpretation of the results.

Some instruments are used to measure disease specific functions or conditions. Examples are ambulation, bladder function, and angina. Other instruments aim at measuring disease dysfunction in a non-specific manner, thus enabling comparison across diagnostic conditions. The Adult Functional Independence Measure (FIM)[7] is a generic instrument used to measure impairment in a number of diseases or conditions. There are benefits and disadvantages to disease-specific instruments as well as to generic instruments, which must be related to the underlying research question. Clinicians generally prefer disease-specific instruments, except in areas of psychosocial evaluation, where disease specific approaches are often too narrow and broad-based assessments tend to be cumbersome or time consuming. In the context of a clinical trial, disease-specific approaches often have more merit with respect to the illness under investigation, while generic measures provide more generalizability and context for the results.

Another important measurement issue is whether to choose an instrument that measures a single dimension of impairment or one that addresses a broader spectrum of the patient's condition. For example, measures of ambulation focus on leg function in the MS patient, whereas the EDSS is a composite score capturing nine functional systems, at least at the lower end of the scale. For certain clinical trials, a more specific outcome measure is preferred, while in other trials, multiple responses may be important. In testing an anti-spasticity drug, for example, a measure of leg spasticity might be preferred over a multidimensional measure, because the outcome measure would be more responsive to the specific question being asked, in this case whether the drug reduces leg spasticity. Such a specific outcome measure may not address the overall patient response to the drug. In a trial of disease-modifying therapy (e.g. an interferon trial), a more global measure, such as EDSS, may be preferable because the principal question relates to the overall condition of the patient.

Thus, while no single measure will ever be completely adequate to characterize an MS patient, a given clinical trial must choose an endpoint that is felt to address the question being asked most appropriately. Because of the difficulty in characterizing impairments and disability associated with MS, and because the disease results in multiple clinical manifestations, optimal outcome measures in MS clinical trials are likely to be composite clinical measures or surrogate laboratory measures that have been shown to correlate with the clinical outcomes.

THE MULTIPLE SCLEROSIS FUNCTIONAL COMPOSITE

In February 1994, a meeting entitled 'Outcomes Assessment in Multiple Sclerosis Clinical Trials' was held in Charleston, South Carolina. A meeting summary was published by Whitaker et al.[8] The Charleston meeting recommended the development of an improved clinical outcome measure for MS clinical trials that met several criteria:

(a) the measure should be multidimensional to reflect the varied clinical expression of MS across patients and over time;

(b) the individual dimensions should change relatively independently over time; and

(c) measures of cognitive function should be included, in addition to those clinical dimensions already incorporated into the EDSS.[5,9]

The results and recommendations from this meeting led the National Multiple Sclerosis Society's Advisory Committee on Clinical Trials of New Agents in Multiple Sclerosis to appoint a Task Force on Clinical Outcome Assessment. This group convened its initial meeting in Chicago in October 1994 and published a detailed set of criteria for defining new clinical outcomes and a set of guidelines for developing the new measure.[10] Two key components of the guidelines were:

(a) the exploration of quantitative functional measures as components of a composite outcome measure; and

(b) the establishment of specifications for a meta-analysis of primary and secondary outcome assessments in existing MS clinical data sets to provide an objective basis for a multidimensional component outcome assessment.

Recommendations from the Task Force based on these guidelines have been presented elsewhere.[11]

The delineation of the Multiple Sclerosis Functional Composite resulted from a pooled data set of placebo control groups and natural history study databases. The use of multiple data sets ensured that decisions regarding the creation of a multiple sclerosis functional composite (MSFC) would not be dependent on any single data set with its potential biases. The Task Force developed six guiding principles for the composite development and analyses that are reported in this paper:

(a) to use measures that reflect the major clinical dimensions of MS;

(b) to avoid redundancy;

(c) to use simple rather than complex measures;

(d) to improve on the valuable characteristics of the EDSS;

(e) to emphasize measures sensitive to change; and

(f) to develop an outcome measure that will be useful in clinical trials (and may or may not be directly useful for clinical care).

These principles helped to structure the analysis plan. The process, drew by necessity, on the experiences of previous investigations. The Task Force, based on clinical expertise, identified the major clinical dimensions of MS and specified criteria by which to proceed.[11] The major clinical dimensions identified for evaluation were the arm, leg, cognitive, and visual dimensions.

The criteria established by the Task Force to select candidate component measures included:

(a) good correlation with the biologically relevant clinical dimensions;

(b) good reliability of the measurement (the ability to obtain the same result on repeat testing when no change occurred);

(c) the ability to show change over time; and

(d) availability of a minimum of two data points in time 1 year apart.

Construct validity (the extent to which the measure of interest correlates with other measures in predicted ways, but for which no true criterion exists) was used to reduce the number of candidate measures. This was based on the logic that individual measures within the same clinical dimension should correlate with each other (convergent validity) and not with measures of different clinical dimensions (discriminant validity).

Applying these criteria, a subset of candidate measures were selected. Reliability estimates observed from the literature, means and standard deviations of change and the relationship between changes in these candidate variables and changes in the EDSS were assessed. To ensure that the Task Force recommendations for a refined clinical outcome measure were satisfied, both concurrent and predictive validity of the composite measure were evaluated. Concurrent validity was defined as change in the composite measure compared with concurrent change in the EDSS over a 1-year period. Predictive validity was defined as change in the composite occurring over the first year of follow-up compared with subsequent change in EDSS among those patients with no sustained change in EDSS during the first year. Predictive validity was felt to best illustrate and validate the composite construction. Detailed discussion of this process has been reported elsewhere.[12]

The recommended MSFC is a unified score representing the combination of results from three performance tests, the Nine-Hole Peg Test (9HPT), the timed 25-foot (8 m) walk; and the 3-second Paced Auditory Serial Addition Test (PASAT3). These performance tests are combined to form a single score. To generate the MSFC scores, the following scores are generated:

(a) The scores from four trials on the 9HPT—two trials of the left hand and two trials of the right hand—are averaged separately. Then the reciprocals of the left and right hands' results are averaged.

(b) Scores from two trials of the timed 25-foot walk are averaged.

(c) The number of correct answers from the PASAT3 test is used.

The MSFC score thus incorporates three clinical dimensions representing arm, leg, and cognitive function to create a single score that can be used to detect change over time in a group of MS patients.

Because the underlying measurement variables differ between these tests (time for the 9HPT and timed 25-foot walk compared with the number of correct answers for the PASAT3), it was necessary to identify a sensible way of combining variables that measure a dimension differently. A Z-score was selected as a common measure for this purpose. The Z-score is a standardized number representing how close a test result is to the mean of a standard or reference population to which the result is compared. The Z-score is expressed in units of standard deviation and usually ranges from -3 to $+3$, although there are no restrictions on its values. The standard deviation of a measure is, on average, how far an observation is from the mean in the original units of measurement, whereas the Z-score is a relative measure (e.g. a Z-score of 2 always implies an observation is twice two standard deviatons from the mean, whereas the meaning of a standard deviation of 2 depends on what is being measured: seconds, minutes, number correct, etc. and would need to be known before the value could be considered as large or small). The Z-score is obtained by subtracting the mean of the reference population from the test result, and then dividing by the standard deviation of the reference population. Because the Z-score is a relative measure indicating how many standard deviation units the current observation is from the mean of the reference population, the units are the same irrespective of the underlying measurement scale. For example, the number of seconds required to perform a test can be represented on the same Z-score scale as the number of correct responses on the PASAT3. This allows the results from tests using different measures (e.g. seconds and number correct) to be combined.

The three components of the MSFC are combined by creating a Z-score for each component, then averaging the Z-scores to create the overall MSFC score. Implicit in this approach is the idea that patients who deteriorate or improve on all three component measures will have an overall larger change than patients who change on only one of the three measures. Furthermore, patients who deteriorate in one area but improve in another may show no change on the MSFC, because the MSFC represents the average change in the three tests.

Determining a Z-score for the timed walk

As an example, suppose we have five patients with 25-foot timed walk results of 20, 25, 30, 35 and 40 seconds. The mean time for the timed walk in this group of patients is 30 seconds, and the standard deviation is 7.906 seconds. To create a Z-score for the timed walk using these patients as the standard population, the mean is subtracted from each score and the result is divided by the standard deviation of the population (*Table 2.1*). Thus, in *Table 2.1*, patient 1 is 1.27 standard deviation units better than the mean, patient 2 is 0.63 standard deviation units better than the mean, patient 3 is 0 standard deviation units from the mean, patient 4 is 0.63 standard deviation units worse than the mean, and patient 5 is 1.27 standard deviation units worse than the mean.

The general formula for creating the composite is given in *Table 2.2*. Detailed formulae that allow creation of the composite Z-score are provided in *Tables 2.3* and *2.4*, and are further explained below.

Table 2.1 Creating Z-scores using the test patients to standardize scores

Patient	Formula for Z-score, 9HPT	Z-score$_{9HPT}$
1	$\dfrac{(20-30)}{7.906}$	-1.27
2	$\dfrac{(25-30)}{7.906}$	-0.63
3	$\dfrac{(30-30)}{7.906}$	0
4	$\dfrac{(35-30)}{7.906}$	0.63
5	$\dfrac{(40-30)}{7.906}$	1.27

Correcting Z-scores to indicate improvement by a positive number

In order to combine Z-scores from all three tests, it is necessary to insure that the Z-score sign (direction) representing worse or better performance is the same for all three tests. Increased raw scores represent worsening on the 9HPT and the timed 25-foot walk, whereas decreased raw scores represent worsening in the PASAT3. Therefore, the Z-scores for the timed 25-foot walk and the 9HPT are adjusted so that in both cases higher Z-scores correspond to an improved outcome, and lower Z-scores correspond to worsening, as is the case with the PASAT3. Changing the signs of the Z-scores for the timed

Table 2.2 Formula for creating the MSFC score

$$MSFC\ score = \frac{(Z_{arm,average} - Z_{leg,average} + Z_{cognitive})}{3.0}$$

Where Z_{xxx} = Z-score for xxx

Table 2.3 Formula for creating the MSFC score to compare groups within a study (the preferred method)

$$\text{MSFC score} = \frac{\text{Average (1/9HPT)} - \text{baseline mean (1/9HPT)}}{\text{baseline standard deviation (1/9HPT)}}$$

$$-\frac{\text{average (25-foot walk)} - \text{baseline mean (25-foot walk)}}{\text{baseline standard deviation (25-foot walk)}}$$

$$+\frac{\text{(PASAT3)} - \text{baseline mean (PASAT3)}}{\text{baseline standard deviation (PASAT3)}}$$

Average (1/9HPT) is the average of the inverse for the right and left hand trials from the test patient.

Baseline mean (1/9HPT) and standard deviation (1/9HPT) are the baseline values from all treatment groups combined at the baseline assessment.

Average (25-foot walk) is the score from the test patient; similarly, the baseline mean (25-foot walk) and the standard deviation (25-foot walk) are of all the baseline groups combined.

PASAT3 is the score from the test patient, and the baseline mean (PASAT3) and standard deviation (PASAT3) are from the baseline assessements of all patients.

25-foot walk to insure that a negative value implies worse function is called 'transforming' the data.

The Task Force has recommended two transformations based on the best performance for each. More information about these approaches are provided in the Scoring Manual,[13] but these account for the use of subtraction (the minus sign) for the timed walk and the inverse of the time for the 9HPT appearing in *Tables 2.3* and *2.4*.

Furthermore, Z-scores involve comparing each outcome to that found in a reference population, a process called standardizing the variable. This involves a decision about what population to use as the reference to derive the means and standard deviations to create the Z-scores. The preferred method for creating Z-scores provided in the

Table 2.4 Formula for creating the MSFC score using task force database to allow comparison between studies

$$\text{MSFC score} = \frac{\text{Average (1/9HPT)} - 0.0439}{0.0101}$$

$$-\frac{\text{Average (25-foot walk)} - 9.5353}{11.4058}$$

$$+\frac{\text{PASAT3} - 45.0311}{3.0}$$

Average (1/9HPT) is the average of the inverse for the right and left hand trials from the test patient, 0.0439 and 0.0101 are the mean and standard deviation of the inverse of the 9HPT for the reference population.

Average (25-foot walk) is the score from the test patient, 9.5353 and 11.4058 are the mean and standard deviation of the reference population.

PASAT3 is the score from the test patient, and 45.0311 and 12.0771 are the mean and standard deviation of the reference population.

Scoring Manual[13] is to use test results from the baseline assessments from all patients in a particular study cohort (see *Table 2.3*). An alternative method is to use the results from a representative database with a broad spectrum of MS patients. The equation for this method, using data from the National Multiple Sclerosis Society Task Force database, is shown in *Table 2.4*. This method allows a comparison of disease severity in patients participating in different studies because their scores are standardized against a common population. This method may not be the optimal method for demonstrating change in a particular population or for showing treatment effects.

The formula in *Table 2.4* uses values derived from all patients in the Task Force data set.[10–12] Composite scores created using this formula should be comparable across different trials. The results from the formulae presented in *Tables 2.3* and *2.4* will be similar but may not be identical. The recommended scoring rule for clinical trials is to use the study population baseline average for statistical comparisons of the two groups. When comparing among studies, using the Task Force database values for showing results relative to an external standard is appropriate. These recommendations result from the fact that many studies use a restricted range of subjects, which can yield different standard deviations. Different standard deviations cause the three components to be weighted slightly differently from study to study. A second advantage of using the average of all study participants' baseline measures in a clinical trial is that the means and standard deviations of the component Z-scores will be close to 0 for the mean and close to 1 for the standard deviation, making comparison of the treatments easier for assessing baseline comparability. Thus, in a clinical trial, it seems relevant to weight the Z-scores in the context of the study baseline data.

EXAMPLE OF THE MSFC IN A HYPOTHETICAL CLINICAL TRIAL

Suppose you are conducting a randomized clinical trial to compare drug B with a widely used therapy, Rx. A total of 699 patients complete the study out of 800 randomized patients (400 per group). The MSFC is computed using the combined baseline values for all 699 patients (*Table 2.5*).

Examination of the data on the patients completing the study shows that mean baseline EDSS averaged 2.7 and 2.8 (both groups showed a median EDSS of 2.5). Average EDSS did not change over 1 year for patients treated with drug B, but worsened by an average of 0.5 points for patients on Rx. Among patients treated with drug B, 16.2% experienced a 3-month sustained worsening from baseline EDSS (defined as two consecutive EDSS ratings at least 3 months apart that are 1 step worse than baseline for patients with a baseline EDSS of < 5.5, or 0.5 steps worse than baseline for patients with a baseline EDSS of ≥5.5). In comparison, 20.7% of the Rx group experienced sustained worsening of EDSS. The PASAT3 averaged about 45 and 47 at baseline and rose by nearly 2 and 3 correct responses, respectively. The timed 25-foot walk was completed in 7.8 and 7.1 seconds, respectively, at baseline. This slowed substantially at 12 months to 29.3 seconds and 13.7 seconds, respectively. The large standard deviations in the timed 25-foot walk are due to the increasing times to complete the measurement at follow-up with few people improving. The mean change in the 9HPT was about a 1.5-second increase for both groups as well as a larger standard deviation. The MSFC for the Rx group was slightly negative at baseline and declined almost 1 standard deviation unit after 12 months, compared to a decline of 0.2 standard

Table 2.5 Baseline and follow-up results for patients completing clinical trial of drug Rx versus drug B

Variable	Drug Rx N = 329		Drug B N = 370	
	Mean	Standard deviation	Mean	Standard deviation
EDSS baseline	2.7	1.7	2.8	1.5
EDSS at 12 months	3.2	1.8	2.8	1.5
Change in EDSS	0.5	1.2	0.0	0.9
% Sustained Change	20.7%		16.2%	
PASAT3 baseline	44.6	12.7	47.2	10.9
PASAT3 at 12 months	46.3	13.1	50.2	11.1
25-foot walk baseline	7.8	8.7	7.1	5.5
25-foot walk at 12 months	29.3	121.3	13.7	66.8
9HPT baseline	25.0	8.7	24.1	8.9
9HPT at 12 months	26.4	13.0	25.8	22.0
MSFC baseline	−0.073	0.767	0.084	0.630
MSFC at 12 months	−0.970	5.497	−0.115	3.070
Change in MSFC	−0.897	5.191	−0.199	2.827

deviation units for treatment B. The test of the hypothesis for a treatment effect is not statistically significant using the percentage with a sustained EDSS change ($p = 0.129$), but is significant for MSFC changes ($p = 0.030$). In this example, EDSS changes and MSFC changes move in a consistent direction over the first year of observation, but only the MSFC changes are statistically significant.

There are several additional points to note. The number of patients who completed the study differed in the two treatment arms (329 versus 370). Shown here are the baseline data for those completing the study. This differential dropout (17.8% versus 7.5%) should be examined. If the baseline data were presented on the entire randomized population, it is likely that the groups were balanced at the start of the trial. However,

comparing the data for each group shows potential selection biases. There were no differences on the EDSS at baseline. However, the baseline PASAT3 results showed a statistically significant higher score for drug B recipients ($p < 0.004$); there were no significant differences on the timed 25-foot walk or the 9HPT. The baseline MSFC in the drug B recipients was significantly better than the baseline MSFC in the Rx recipients ($p < 0.004$). Assuming that the groups were balanced at baseline when the entire randomized cohort was present, differences seen in subgroups completing the trial suggest that patients with higher MSFC scores in the Rx Group dropped out of the study. Such suggestions of potential differences should be investigated for a full assessment of trial results.

In the above example, the MSFC was more sensitive to change than was the EDSS. This may not always be the case, since the EDSS encompasses more clinical dimensions and could show changes in circumstances in which the MSFC does not. The MSFC is a continuous measure, however, which should increase its power for demonstrating differences in impairment and disability within the clinical dimensions included in it. The EDSS, an ordinal measure with differing duration of times between steps of the scale, often requires the use of a rule for sustained change that alters the size of the required step (i.e. 0.5 steps for those 5.5 and over). This is equivalent to a recognition of the unequal time intervals between later and earlier steps on the EDSS.

The MSFC score is a continuous variable that can be used like any numerical variable in analyses. The value is subject to tests appropriate for continuous variables, such as t-tests, analysis of variance and regression analyses. A composite based on such Z-scores can also measure change in performance over time. By computing the composite at one point in time and measuring the patient at a later point in time, the arithmetic difference between MSFC scores can be used to measure improvement or worsening.

SPECIAL CONSIDERATIONS REGARDING THE MSFC

Handling data where some data points are missing for reasons other than inability to perform the test

In the event that a particular patient does not complete some of the tests (e.g. the patient was running late so only one trial of the 9HPT per arm was completed), the available data can be used to calculate the MSFC. In this case, the MSFC is still the average of the three Z-scores as usual:

$$\text{MSFC score} = \frac{[Z_{arm,average} - Z_{leg,average} + Z_{cognitive}]}{3.0}$$

In the usual instance, the $Z_{arm,average}$ is computed as:

$$Z_{arm,average} = \{(1/\text{trial}_{arm,left} + 1/\text{trial}_{arm,right})/2.0 - \text{Baseline mean}(1/9HPT)\}/\text{Baseline Standard Deviation }(1/9HPT)$$

where $1/\text{trial}_{arm,left} = (1/(\text{average of the two times of the left arm trials})$ and similarly for $1/\text{trial}_{arm,right}$.

However, in the absence of two trials for each arm for the 9HPT, the $Z_{arm,average}$ would be computed based on the trials available, as follows:

$$Z_{arm,average} = \{(1/\text{trial}_{arm,trial \#1,left} + 1/\text{trial}_{arm,trial \#1,right})/2.0 - \text{Baseline mean }(1/9HPT)\}/ \text{Baseline Standard Deviation }(1/9HPT)$$

Handling data missing because the patient was unable to perform the test owing to disability

The author recommends using data from patients who were unable to perform the test because of disability. For example, suppose an individual completed the 9HPT in an average of 55 seconds at the beginning of the trial but was unable to complete the 9HPT at the end of the trial because of increasing disability. It is advantageous to capture the data in such a way that it indicates worsening, rather than leaving the data point missing, which would provide no information about change.

The 9HPT

In most datasets used in the meta-analysis,[3,4] the inability to perform the 9HPT was coded as 777. Keeping that convention, 1/777 was arbitrarily used to represent the inability to perform the test, providing a value close to 0, but one that is informative. Therefore, for the 9HPT, the following formula is recommended for a subject who could not complete either arm of the 9HPT because of disability:

$$Z_{arm,trial\ \#} = \{1/777 - mean\ (1/9HPT)\}/Baseline$$
$$Standard\ Deviation\ (1/9HPT)$$

Or in the case of standardizing to the Task Force Database the value would be:

$$Z_{arm,trial\ \#} = (1/777 - 0.0439)/0.0101 = -4.2191$$

If the patient could complete the right arm of the 9HPT in 20 seconds for the first trial of the 9HPT and 30 seconds on the second trial (a mean of 25 seconds for the right arm) and couldn't complete the left arm, the score would be computed using the average of the inverses of each arm minus the baseline mean for the study groups divided by the standard deviation of these values. Assuming that the overall baseline average was 0.0537 and the standard deviation 0.0191, the score to use would be:

$$Z_{arm,trial\ \#} = \{(1/777 + 1/25)/2 - 0.0537\}/0.0191;$$

which reduces to

$$Z_{arm,trial\ \#} = (\{0.00129 + 0.04\}/$$
$$2 - 0.0537)/0.0191;$$

and becomes

$$Z_{arm,trial\ \#} = (0.0206 - 0.0537)/0.0191;$$

which equates to

$$Z_{arm,trial\ \#} = -1.73$$

25-Foot walk

For the 25-foot walk, as noted above, the inverse transformation (1/time) yielded a very restricted range on the transformed Z-score (the smallest Z-score was −2) and thus it was decided to use the Z-score associated with the slowest time of any patient in the combined data set used by the Task Force in its meta-analysis. The largest Z-score in the Task Force dataset was 13.7. Although this is a very large Z-score, it represents an actual time that this patient took to complete the test. The range of values is sufficiently wide so that an extremely high value had to be chosen to enable a person with declining ambulation to deteriorate in terms of his or her Z-scores (i.e. there were patients whose baseline Z-score was over 5 and others who at 6 months had Z-scores of 8 or 9 completing the timed walk and yet by 18 months were unable to complete the test). Therefore, the following is recommended for a subject who could not complete the 25 foot walk:

$$Z_{leg,average} = -13.7$$

PASAT3

Data substitution is done only for 9HPT and the 25-foot walk; it is not recommended for the PASAT3. This is because nearly all patients can achieve some score on the PASAT3, even if it is close to 0 or even 0. In the event that an individual patient cannot complete the PASAT3 because of disability, a score of 0 is assigned.

SUMMARY

The measurement of impairment and disability requires the question being addressed to be sharply focused. Patient-specific clinical care questions may require measures of impairment and disability that are directed at guiding therapy. The approach is usually a measure of disease or specific physical ailment. When the question to be answered requires a controlled clinical trial, outcomes measures of group performance are generally preferred. Continuous measures of impairments and disability are preferred over ordinal scales, because they allow more precise measures and smaller sample sizes. However, these measures may result in therapeutic benefits without obvious clinical benefits, so related studies to explore the clinical meaning of the continuous impairment measures are important.

The MSFC is a new measure of impairment and disability. It is likely to undergo revision and improvement as information is collected about its use and as better measures are developed. However, the concept underlying the MSFC goes beyond the current component measures. If newer or more reliable measures of arm, leg, and cognitive function become available, they could be substituted for current MSFC components measures. If newer informative measures of dimensions not currently included in the MSFC are developed (e.g. vision) they could be added to the composite. Although the MSFC needs more complete testing in the realm of clinical trials, it represents a potential improvement over ordinal clinical rating scales. Of particular importance is the ability to show small changes in active arm comparison studies. Without increasingly sensitive measures, progress in MS will be constrained by cost and by the availability of patients for clinical trials.

REFERENCES

1 **World Health Organization.** *International Classification of Impairments, Disabilities, and Handicaps (ICIDH).* World Health Assembly Resolution 29.35, 1980.

2 **Nagi S.** Disability concepts revisited: implications for prevention. In: Sussman MG, ed. *Sociology and Rehabilitation.* Washington, DC: American Sociological Association, 1965, 100–113.

3 **La Rocca NG.** Statistical and methodological consideration in scale construction. In: Munsat TL, ed, *Quantification of Neurologic Deficit*, 49–67. Butterworth: Stoneham, Massachusetts, 1989.

4 **Mathiowetz V, Weber K, Kashman N, Volland G.** Adult norms for 9 Hole Peg Test of finger dexterity. *Occup Ther J Res* 1985; 5:24–38.

5 **Kurtzke JF.** Rating neurologic impairment in multiple sclerosis: an expanded disability status scale (EDSS). *Neurology* 1983; 33:1444–1452.

6 **International Federation of Multiple Sclerosis Societies.** MRD minimal record of disability for multiple sclerosis. New York: National Multiple Sclerosis Society, 1985.

7 **Granger CV, Hamilton BB, Keith RA et al.** Advances in functional assessemnent for medical rehabilitation. *Top Geriatr Rehabil* 1986; 1:59–74.

8 **Whitaker JN, McFarland HF, Rudge P, Reingold SC.** Outcomes assessment in multiple sclerosis clinical trials: a critical analysis. *Multiple Sclerosis* 1995; 1:37–47.

9 **Kurtzke JF.** A new scale for evaluating disability in multiple sclerosis. *Neurology* 1955; 5:580–583.

10 **Rudick R, Antel J, Confavreux C et al.** Clinical outcomes assessment in multiple sclerosis. *Ann Neurol* 1996; 40:469–479.

11 **Rudick RA, Antel J, Confavreux C et al.** Recommendations from the clinical outcome assessment task force of the National Multiple Sclerosis Society. *Ann Neurol* 1997; 42:379–382.

12 **Cutter GR, Baier ML, Rudick RA et al.** Development of the Multiple Sclerosis Functional Composite as a Clinical Trials Outcome Measure. *Brain* 1999; 122:101–112.

13 **Fischer J, Jak A, Kroker JE et al.** *Administration Scoring Manual for Multiple Sclerosis Functional Composite (MSFC).* New York: Demos Medical Publishing, Inc, 1999.

3
Assessment of neuropsychological function

Jill S Fischer

RATIONALE FOR ASSESSMENT OF NEUROPSYCHOLOGICAL OUTCOMES IN MULTIPLE SCLEROSIS TRIALS

Cognitive function is often impaired in multiple sclerosis (MS) patients. Prevalence estimates derived from two large-scale cross-sectional studies are similar: after adjusting for impairment rates in demographically matched healthy controls, 43% of a community-based MS sample[1] and 44% of a mixed clinic-based sample[2] were impaired on formal neuropsychological testing. Cognitive impairment is directly related to the presence and extent of cerebral MS lesions. Neuropsychological test performance correlates moderately with quantitated MS lesion burden on T2-weighted brain MRI,[3–5] as well as with newer MRI parameters that indicate parenchymal abnormalities (e.g. magnetization transfer ratios) and brain atrophy.[6,7] Furthermore, deterioration in neuropsychological test performance over a 1-year period has been associated with significant increases in cerebral lesion burden.[8] In contrast, correlations between neuropsychological test performance and conventional disease parameters such as MS duration, disease course, and EDSS are surprisingly weak.[1,9,10] Clinicians typically overestimate the magnitude of these relationships, however.[11]

The functional consequences of MS-related cognitive impairment can be striking. Compared to cognitively intact patients with comparable physical disability, cognitively impaired MS patients are significantly less likely to be employed and to engage in social activities, and they are significantly more likely to need assistance with daily activities such as personal care and household management.[3,12,13] Clinical experience suggests that cognitively impaired MS patients have difficulty performing complex multiple-step activities, including complex treatment regimens, and they are more prone to accidents at home and while driving. Thus, MS-related cognitive impairment is common, functionally disabling, and directly related to cerebral MS lesions. However, traditional MS clinical outcome measures are insensitive to MS-related cognitive deficits.[14]

The purpose of this chapter is to review natural history studies and clinical trials of disease-modifying and symptomatic medications in which neuropsychological outcomes have been explicitly assessed, and to make recommendations about the assessment of neuropsychological outcomes in future MS clinical trials. It extends concepts that have been previously advanced,[15] emphasizing work conducted in the last 3 years.

NATURE OF MS-RELATED COGNITIVE DYSFUNCTION

Not all cognitive functions are equally disrupted by MS. Learning and recall of new information are the most susceptible functions, with 22–31% of the patients in the sample of Rao et al.[1] exhibiting severe deficits (i.e. scoring below the 5th percentile for demographically matched healthy controls) in this domain. Deficits in information processing speed and flexibility are also common: severe deficits were observed in 22–25% of this sample. Although not as common as impaired information processing and recent memory, deficits in visuospatial abilities and in executive functions (i.e. reasoning, problem solving, and planning–sequencing) still occur with surprising frequency: 12–19% of this sample exhibited severe deficits. In contrast, auditory attention span and verbal abilities are typically spared.

Although general statements can be made about common cognitive deficits in MS patients as a group, individual patients vary considerably in their patterns of impairment. In early studies,[16,17] three different patterns of memory performance among MS patients were observed. Based on a cluster analysis of baseline performance on a comprehensive neuropsychological battery, the MS Collaborative Research Group (MSCRG) recently identified six cognitively distinct subgroups in our sample of relapsing MS patients entering the interferon-β 1a (Avonex) trial:[18]

(a) a cognitively intact group (34%);

(b) a group with circumscribed deficits in information processing and visuospatial abilities only (27%);

(c) a group with memory deficits in addition to deficits in information processing and visuospatial abilities (15%);

(d) a group with memory–word retrieval deficits alone (10%);

(e) a group with executive dysfunction only (12%); and

(f) a globally impaired group (2%).

Thus, MS-related cognitive impairment is heterogeneous.

NATURAL HISTORY STUDIES OF MS-RELATED COGNITIVE DYSFUNCTION

Relatively little is known about the evolution of MS-related cognitive impairment. To date, three controlled longitudinal studies comparing the performance of MS patients with that of healthy controls have been published (*Table 3.1*).[13,19,20] Each of these followed a relatively small sample of MS patients, although the studies differed substantially in terms of the disease characteristics of the patients, neuropsychological measures, and methods for statistical analysis. Nonetheless, several important observations can be derived from these natural history studies.

First, once MS-related cognitive impairment is present, it is unlikely to remit to any significant extent. At best, cognitive deficits remain stable over time; however, they may progress. Progression rates vary among patients and across functions, but rapid cognitive deterioration appears to be relatively rare. Finally, at least one longitudinal study[20] suggests that some patients remain cognitively intact despite substantial physical disability. Specific risk factors for the development of MS-related cognitive impairment and predictors of progression rates have not yet been identified.

In addition to these small longitudinal studies, the large cohort described by Rao and his col-

Table 3.1 Controlled natural history studies of MS-related cognitive dysfunction

Study	Sample	Design and analysis	Outcome
Jennekens-Schinkel et al, 1990[19]	33 patients (40% with relapsing–remitting MS) and 18 healthy controls Mean DSS = 4.0 (SD = 2.2) Mean age = 48 (SD = 13.5) Mean education = 12 (SD = 3.5)	4-year follow-up Cross-sectional between-group comparisons on individual tests Longitudinal within-group comparisons on individual tests	MS group was generally stable (except on choice RT, finger tapping, visual list learning, and reading speed); some patients (6–12%) deteriorated markedly, while one patient improved
Amato et al, 1995[13]	50 patients (88% with relapsing–remitting MS) and 70 healthy controls Mean EDSS = 2.6 (SD = 2.4) Mean age = 29.9 (SD = 8.5) Mean education = 11.4 (SD = 3.6)	4.5-year follow-up Cross-sectional between-group comparisons on individual tests	Group differences persisted over time on most measures; deficits in verbal fluency and auditory comprehension emerged at follow-up; for MS group only, performance variability increased over time
Kujala et al, 1997[20]	42 patients (86% with chronic–progressive MS) and 34 controls *'Intact' group (n = 20):* Mean EDSS = 5.7 (SD = 1.6) Mean age = 46.8 (SD = 8.7) Mean education = 11.9 (SD = 3.8) *'Impaired' group (n = 22):* Mean EDSS = 6.5 (SD = 1.1) Mean age = 45.9 (SD = 7.5) Mean education = 11.0 (SD = 3.0)	2.8-year follow-up Cross-sectional between-group comparisons on individual tests Longitudinal between-group comparisons of difference scores on individual tests	'Intact' group remained relatively stable but 'impaired' group continued to deteriorate on measures of attention span, processing speed, verbal fluency, verbal memory, visual memory, and susceptibility to interference; however, 7 out of 20 (35%) 'intact' patients deteriorated slightly, while 5 out of 22 (23%) 'impaired' patients remained stable or improved

The test battery in the study by Jennekens-Schinkel et al[19] consisted of: confrontation naming, word generation, reading (100 words), writing to dictation, figure copy, Knox Cubes, Wechsler Memory Scale (WMS), 10-item list learning task (auditory and visual), 7/24 Spatial Recall Test, Stroop test, Wisconsin Card Sort (Nelson version), Raven's Progressive Matrices, and finger tapping.

The test battery in the study by Amato et al[13] included: Blessed Information–Memory–Concentration Test, Token Test, figure copy, Digit Span (forward), Corsi Blocks, Randt Repeatable Memory Battery (5 words and paired words), Set Test, and Raven's Progressive Matrices.

Measures administered by Kujala et al[20] included: Mini-Mental State Examination, 20-item object naming, verbal fluency (letters), Benton Visual Retention Test (BVRT), Wechsler Adult Intelligence Scale-Revised (WAIS-R) Digit Span, WAIS-R Digit Symbol, WAIS-R Block Design, WAIS-R Similarities, Paced Auditory Serial Addition Test (PASAT), WMS Logical Memory, 20-item verbal paired associate recall, 7/24 Spatial Recall Test, 20-item object recall, and Stroop test.

SD, standard deviation.

DSS, Disability Status Scale; EDSS, Kurtzke Expanded Disability Status Scale leagues[1] was reassessed at 3-year and 8-year intervals, although these results have not been formally published. Early analyses indicated that, over the initial 3-year interval, the MS group deteriorated compared to controls on nearly all of the neuropsychological measures administered; statistically significant group differences were observed on seven measures, tapping a diverse array of cognitive functions.[21] However, only about 20% of the MS patient group met criteria for 'significant deterioration' over the initial 3-year interval (SM Rao, personal communication). Results of the 8-year follow-up have not been reported. Thus, data from this larger natural history study confirm the results of published studies based on smaller samples: MS-related cognitive impairment is often progressive, albeit at variable rates.

CLINICAL TRIALS OF DISEASE-MODIFYING MEDICATIONS

Assessment of neuropsychological outcomes is a relatively recent phenomenon in MS clinical trials. In fact, the first controlled clinical trial to incorporate neuropsychological measures was the double-blind, placebo-controlled phase 3 trial of cyclosporine.[22] Now that the prevalence and functional impact of MS-related cognitive impairment has become more widely recognized, it has become customary to include neuropsychological measures as secondary outcome measures in definitive trials of disease-modifying medications, particularly those initiated in North America since 1990.

Table 3.2 provides an overview of the five completed clinical trials in which neuropsychological outcomes have been assessed and formally reported.[22–30] In each of these trials, beneficial

treatment effects were demonstrated on at least one primary outcome measure. Consequently, it is reasonable to hypothesize that these medications would affect neuropsychological test performance as well. As with the natural history studies, there were important differences among these trials in terms of sample size, patients' disease course and level of disability at study entry, the breadth and timing of neuropsychological assessment, and the approach to statistical analysis. Furthermore, neuropsychological measures were not administered before initiation of treatment in one trial,[26] so neuropsychological results from this trial must be interpreted cautiously. Despite these caveats, these studies illustrate several important principles about neuropsychological outcome assessment in MS trials.

First, these studies confirm that the effects of disease-modifying therapies often extend to neuropsychological measures as well. In fact, data from the methotrexate trial suggest that neuropsychological measures may be able to detect treatment effects very early in a trial.[24] Secondly, currently available therapies often exert subtle or gradual effects. Consequently, the choice of neuropsychological measures and statistical methods is critical in determining whether a statistically significant treatment effect will be observed. For example, measures of learning–recent memory and information processing were administered in most trials, but not all were equally sensitive in detecting treatment effects. Furthermore, the three trials with statistically significant neuropsychological effects controlled for demographic variables that often affect neuropsychological test performance, either by converting raw scores to age-corrected and education-corrected scores based on published norms,[26] or by using demographic variables as covariates in the

Table 3.2 Completed clinical trials of disease-modifying medications with neuropsychological outcome assessment

Study	Overall sample	NP measures and design	Primary analysis	NP outcome
Cyclosporine (Multiple Sclerosis Study Group, 1990,[22] Syndulko, personal communication)	547 chronic progressive MS patients EDSS range = 3.0–7.0 Phase 3 trial	SDMT at baseline and every 3 months for 24 months (n = 317)	Two-way ANOVAs (Group × Test Time) of unadjusted Z-scores	No treatment effect (no significant Group × Test Time interaction)
Methotrexate (Goodkin et al, 1995;[23] Goodkin & Fischer, 1996[24])	60 chronic progressive MS patients EDSS range = 3.0–6.5 Phase 2 trial	Comprehensive NP battery at baseline, 12 months, 24 months (n = 40); focused NP battery every 6 weeks for 24 weeks (n = 35)	MANCOVA of 2-year change scores on BNT-15, WAIS-R Block Design, PASAT-2", CVLT LDFR, WCST Psv Rs (covariates were age, education)	Marginal overall treatment effect (p = 0.07), with most striking effects on PASAT-2" (p = 0.002); PASAT-2" effect significant at 12 weeks (p = 0.005)
Betaseron (interferon-β 1b) (IFNB Multiple Sclerosis Study Group, 1993;[25] Pliskin et al, 1996[26])	372 relapsing–remitting MS patients EDSS range = 0.0–5.5 Phase 3 trial	Focused NP battery (WMS Logical Memory, WMS Vis. Reproduction, Trails, Stroop) at 2 years and 4 years (n = 30)	Two-way ANOVAs (Group × Test Time) of demo-adjusted scores on individual variables	Significant treatment effect (Group × Test Time interaction) on Delayed Visual Reproduction (p < 0.03), favoring high-dose group (p < 0.003), with similar trend on Trails B (p < 0.14)
Avonex (interferon-β 1a) (Jacobs et al, 1996;[27] Fischer et al, 1998[28])	301 relapsing–remitting MS patients EDSS range = 0.0–3.5 Phase 3 trial	Comprehensive NP battery at baseline, 2 years (n = 166); focused NP battery every 6 months for 24 months	MANOVA of demo-adjusted 2-year change scores on three sets of variables identified through factor analyses	Significant treatment effects, most noticeably on memory and information processing variables (p = 0.036) and executive functions and visuospatial abilities (p = 0.043)*
Copaxone (glatiramer acetate) (Johnson et al, 1995;[29] Weinstein et al, 1999[30])	251 relapsing–remitting MS patients EDSS range = 0.0–5.0 Phase 3 trial	Focused NP battery (Buschke SRT, 10/36 SRT, PASAT, SDMT, and Word List Generation) at baseline, 12 months, and 24 months (n = 248)	Two-way ANCOVAs (Group × Site × Test Time) of individual variables (covariate = baseline score)	No significant treatment effects

A small (n = 20) 6-month phase 2 trial of interferon-α 2a also included measures of memory (Wechsler Memory Scale (WMS)) and visual construction (Bender–Gestalt Test). The investigators reported that these measures 'did not show any change from baseline', but no details regarding the statistical analyses were provided.[31]

*Memory and information processing measures included CVLT Total 1–5, RFFT Error Ratio, and CALCAP Sequential RT.
NP, neuropsychological; SDMT, Symbol-Digit Modalities Test; 10/36 SRT, 10/36 Spatial Recall Test; CVLT, California Verbal Learning Test; LDFR, Long Delay Free Recall (from the CVLT)

statistical analyses;[24,28] the other two trials[22,30] did not. Considerations in selecting neuropsychological measures and statistical techniques are discussed further below.

NEUROPSYCHOLOGICAL OUTCOME ASSESSMENT IN TRIALS OF SYMPTOMATIC TREATMENTS

Neuropsychological measures have also served as outcome measures in several small ($N < 50$) controlled trials of symptomatic treatments for MS. Criteria for patient selection varied greatly across studies. In some trials, cognitive deficits were the target of the intervention, so only patients with documented cognitive deficits were included (*Table 3.3*).[32–34] In other trials, neuropsychological effects of a given treatment had been anecdotally noted and objective neuropsychological measures were administered, but cognitive impairment was not a criterion for study participation (*Table 3.4*).[36–40] There were also important differences among these studies in terms of their design (cross-over versus parallel groups), choice of neuropsychological measures, and approaches to statistical analysis. Nonetheless, several important conclusions can be drawn.

First, statistically significant treatment effects were demonstrated in all three studies in which patients had documented cognitive deficits at study entry,[32–34] but in only three of the five trials in which cognitive impairment was not an explicit selection criterion.[38–40] This should not be surprising: patients whose neuropsychological test performance is intact at baseline are likely to have more limited room for improvement. Secondly, when statistically significant treatment effects were observed, these were present only on selected measures. Furthermore, no single measure consistently detected treatment effects across studies. Finally, these studies suggest that MS-related cognitive dysfunction may be amenable to symptomatic treatment. This observation is particularly encouraging, because as more effective disease-stabilizing therapies become available, interventions for MS-related cognitive function may be able to ameliorate a symptom that is a source of significant disruption in everyday function.

FACTORS COMPLICATING NEUROPSYCHOLOGICAL OUTCOME ASSESSMENT IN MS

Despite promising findings in both disease-modifying and symptomatic trials, several factors complicate neuropsychological outcome assessment in MS. Although these factors certainly pose methodological challenges, they are not insurmountable if they are taken into account in planning a clinical trial.

The first factor is the heterogeneity of MS-related cognitive dysfunction: only about half of all patients develop measurable cognitive impairment, and those who do vary considerably in terms of the specific cognitive functions that are impaired and the magnitude of impairment in any given cognitive domain. This has implications for both patient selection and choice of neuropsychological measures for an MS trial.

The second complicating factor is that MS patients' neuropsychological test performance fluctuates over time.[41] Some fluctuations in neuropsychological test performance are attributable to measurement error, which is inherent in any test instrument. Other fluctuations reflect transient changes in the patient's underlying disease.[42] In many respects, the variability in

Table 3.3 Controlled clinical trials of symptomatic treatments with neuropsychological outcome assessment: trials with documented cognitive deficits in patient selection criteria

Study	Sample	NP measures	Primary analysis	NP outcome
Intravenous physostigmine (Leo & Rao, 1988[31])*	4 patients with definite MS (EDSS = 3.0–6.0) and documented memory impairment 6-week placebo-controlled crossover (no washout)	Digit Span (forward) and Buschke SRT at baseline and weekly for 6 weeks	Paired t-tests (1-tailed) on individual measures	Significant treatment effects ($p < 0.05$) on selected Buschke SRT variables (LTS, LTR, STR) and consistent trends ($p < 0.10$) on others (Total Recall, CLTR, intrusions); no effect on Digit Span
Cognitive rehabilitation (Jonsson et al, 1993[32])	40 inpatients with definite MS (mean EDSS = 5.6, SD = 1.3) and documented cognitive impairment for the group as a whole 6-week parallel groups	Comprehensive NP battery administered at baseline, end of treatment, and 6 months later	T-tests of age-, sex-, and education-adjusted T-scores for different factors	Significant treatment effect on visual perception factor ($p < 0.04$) and trend on visuospatial memory ($p < 0.08$), but trend on visual information processing favoring non-specific treatment group ($p < 0.07$); gains were maintained at 6 months
Process-specific attentional retraining (Plohmann et al, 1998[33])	22 patients with definite MS (EDSS = 2.0–8.0) and documented attentional impairments 18-week parallel groups/cross-over	Battery of computerized attentional measures (TAP-1.02c) at baseline and every 3 weeks for 18 weeks	Wilcoxon-matched pairs tests comparing baseline and post-training; Mann–Whitney test comparing specific versus non-specific training conditions on individual measures (RTs, errors)	Significant process-specific and non-specific training effects ($p < 0.05$) for specific modules; gains maintained over a 9-week follow-up

*This group subsequently published an abstract on a small (n = 8) study of oral physostigmine.[35] They demonstrated a statistically significant benefit on one Buschke SRT variable (CLTR), no effects on other memory measures, and an adverse effect on information processing (PASAT3").

LTS, Long-Term Store; Buschke SRT, Buschke Selective Reminding Test; LTR, Long-Term Retrieval; STR, Short-Term Retrieval; CLTR, Consistent Long-Term Retrieval.

Table 3.4 Controlled clinical trials of symptomatic treatments with neuropsychological outcome assessment: trials without documented cognitive deficits in patient selection criteria

Study	Sample	NP measures	Primary analysis	NP outcome
4-aminopyridine (up to 10 mg qid) (Smits et al, 1994[34])	20 patients with definite MS (EDSS = 2.5–8.0) 4-week placebo-controlled cross-over (no washout)	Focused NP battery (16-item verbal learning, 10/36 SRT, PASAT, SDMT, Word List Generation) at baseline, 2 weeks, 4 weeks	T-tests comparing conditions on change scores for individual measures	No significant treatment effects, but trends on PASAT-2" ($p = 0.09$) and on 10/36 SRT Delayed Recall ($p = 0.06$), favoring 4-AP
3,4 diaminopyridine (DAP, up to 100 mg/day, divided) (Bever et al, 1996[35])	36 patients with definite MS (EDSS = 2.5–9.0) and leg weakness 90-day placebo-controlled crossover, including 30-day washout	Focused NP battery (Buschke Selective Reminding, 10/36 SRT, PASAT, SDMT, Word List Generation) at baseline and every 30 days	Paired Wilcoxon signed rank tests of post-test scores on individual measures	No significant treatment effects
Multimodal group therapy (Rodgers et al, 1996[36])	22 patients with definite MS (no EDSS given) 24-week parallel groups	Focused NP battery (10-item verbal list-learning, SDMT, Shipley) at baseline, 12 weeks, and 24 weeks	T-tests comparing groups on change scores for individual measures	Significant treatment effect on list-learning and abstraction measures ($p < 0.05$)
Amantidine (100 mg bid) versus pemoline (56.25 mg qd) (Geisler et al, 1996[37])	45 patients with definite MS (EDSS < 6.5) and documented fatigue 6-week placebo-controlled parallel groups	Focused NP battery (Digit Span, SDMT, Trails, Buschke SRT, BVRT) at baseline and 6 weeks	ANOVAs (Group × Test Time) of individual measures	Significant treatment effect on written SDMT ($p < 0.03$), favoring amantidine, and similar trend on oral SDMT ($p < 0.08$)
Intravenous methylprednisolone (2.5–10 g, divided doses) (Oliveri et al, 1998[38])	14 patients with definite relapsing–remitting MS, in acute relapse versus 12 healthy controls 1-week parallel groups	Focused NP battery (Rey AVLT, auditory span, visual span, Corsi blocks, verbal fluency, WCST) at baseline, 1 week, and 2 months	ANOVAs of within-group change over time on individual measures; ANCOVAs comparing groups at 1 week individual measures (Hamilton Depression and Corsi Blocks as covariates)	Significant adverse treatment effect on Rey AVLT at Week 1 ($p < 0.005$), which disappeared by 2 months

neuropsychological test performance is analogous to that observed on cerebral magnetic resonance imaging.[43] This variability in test performance over time must be anticipated in designing MS trials with neuropsychological outcome measures.

A third factor complicating the assessment of neuropsychogical outcomes in MS trials is the fact that many (if not most) neuropsychological measures are subject to practice effects, regardless of the length of the inter-test interval.[44–47] Practice effects may even differ across populations (e.g. patient groups versus healthy controls) and across patients within the same population.[45] Furthermore, practice effects are not entirely alleviated by using alternate forms.[41,48,49] Although the results of numerous trials suggest that neuropsychological measures that are susceptible to practice effects can detect differential change between groups over time,[24,26,28,32,34,38,40] practice effects must be taken into account in selecting a control group and establishing the timing of assessments.

A final complicating factor relates to the fact that measures with good discriminative properties (i.e. ones that can detect impairment in MS patients relative to healthy controls) do not necessarily have optimal evaluative properties (i.e. they may not be sensitive to change over time). Thus, although MS patients as a group are impaired on most measures of learning–recent memory and information processing, not all memory and information processing measures have been sensitive to treatment effects in clinical trials. Guyatt and colleagues[50] have developed a formula for determining the 'responsiveness' of a measure, or its sensitivity to change. This formula could be applied to neuropsychological data from recent MS clinical trials to identify measures with optimal psychometric properties for use in future trials.

DESIGN AND ANALYSIS OF NEUROPSYCHOLOGICAL OUTCOME ASSESSMENT IN MS TRIALS

The remainder of this chapter covers a number of issues concerning study design and statistical analysis in order to guide investigators who are interested in assessing neuropsychological outcomes in their clinical trials.

Is a single neuropsychological measure adequate?

This question applies principally to trials of disease-modifying medications, since trials of symptomatic interventions for MS-related cognitive dysfunction typically include multiple neuropsychological outcome measures. The National Multiple Sclerosis Society-sponsored Clinical Outcomes Assessment Task Force recently proposed a new multidimensional clinical outcome measure for disease-modifying clinical trials. The Multiple Sclerosis Functional Composite measure (MSFC) includes a measure of cognitive function, as well as quantitative measures of leg function and arm–hand function.[51–54] The primary measure of cognitive function in the MSFC is the Paced Auditory Serial Addition Test (PASAT),[55] a measure of information processing speed and flexibility as well as calculation ability.[56,57]

Although the MSFC represents an important advance in MS clinical outcome assessment, it was not designed to provide a comprehensive assessment of either cognitive function or physical function. Given the heterogeneity of MS-related cognitive impairment, no currently available neuropsychological measure is likely to detect all of the variants of MS-related cognitive impairment. Such a measure would either need to be multidimensional (i.e. covering the cognitive domains most often affected by MS) or, if it were domain-specific, it would need to be predictive of concurrent or future change in other cognitive domains. Until such a measure is identified, it is advisable to include more than one neuropsychological outcome measure in trials of disease-modifying medications.

Which neuropsychological measures should be used in future MS trials?

Neuropsychological batteries can be characterized as either broad spectrum (i.e. assessing multiple cognitive domains) or focused (i.e. assessing only one or two cognitive domains). The broad spectrum approach is desirable when little is known about either the potential effects of an experimental treatment or the psychometric properties of the measures. This approach was fruitfully applied in natural history studies of MS-related cognitive dysfunction,[13,19,20] trials of methotrexate[24] and interferon-β 1a,[28] and in a study of cognitive rehabilitation.[33] Although these studies have yielded invaluable psychometric data about diverse neuropsychological measures, the broad spectrum approach to neuropsychological outcome assessment is inherently time-consuming. Furthermore, the risk of type 2 statistical errors (i.e. failure to detect a true change in the underlying cognitive function) may be increased if unresponsive measures have been included or if adjustments to the alpha level have been made to compensate for multiple statistical tests.

For practical reasons, the focused approach has been used in most disease-modifying and symptomatic trials in MS to date. This approach is certainly optimal when specific hypotheses

about treatment effects can be formulated, as in studies of symptomatic interventions for MS-related memory or information processing deficits. However, the focused approach may be premature when relatively little is known about the psychometric properties of the measures themselves or about the range of potential treatment effects. To date, no single neuropsychological measure or set of measures has consistently detected treatment effects in every MS trial in which it has been administered.

However, evidence from recent trials of disease-modifying and symptomatic treatments suggests that the most promising measures are ones that tap the cognitive domains most susceptible to impairment in MS. These include measures of information processing speed and flexibility (as assessed by measures such as the PASAT, Trails A and B, Stroop, Symbol–Digit Modalities Test, and computerized complex reaction time tasks such as California Computerized Assessment Package (CALCAP) or the battery used in the study by Plohmann and colleagues[34]); visuospatial abilities (as assessed by visuospatial span tasks (e.g. Corsi Blocks or Wechsler Memory Scale-Revised (WMS-R) Visual Memory Span), Wechsler Adult Intelligence Scale-Revised (WAIS-R) Block Design, and Ruff Figural Fluency Test (RFFT)); verbal learning and memory (as assessed by 12- to 16-item list-learning tasks, such as the Buschke Selective Reminding Test, Rey Auditory Verbal Learning Test, and California Verbal Learning Test (CVLT)); and visual learning and memory (as assessed by WMS-R Visual Reproduction, 10/36 Spatial Learning Test, and the RFFT Error Ratio). Descriptions of these measures can be found in Lezak,[58] as well as in published articles on the trials in which they were used. Measures of executive functions such as planning and problem solving may also be useful, but these have not yet been implemented widely enough in MS trials to yield firm conclusions regarding their usefulness as outcome measures. Finally, measures of overall verbal abilities and attention span are of limited use in monitoring change over time in MS, at least over the brief periods involved in clinical trials. These measures may be useful in characterizing MS patients at study entry, however.

In the recent clinical trial of interferon-β 1a for relapsing MS,[28] three measures (PASAT, CVLT, and RFFT) proved to be an efficient means of capturing the major dimensions represented in the comprehensive neuropsychological battery. They also yielded a composite measure that was sensitive to relatively subtle treatment effects. While it would be premature to recommend a mandatory set of neuropsychological measures for future MS clinical trials, other investigators are encouraged to include these measures in their outcome assessment to determine if they are equally sensitive to the effects of other treatments and in MS patients with other disease courses.

Which patients should be assessed?

Ideally, all participants in a clinical trial of a disease-modifying medication would be administered a limited 'core' set of neuropsychological measures. Specific neuropsychological questions of interest could be investigated by administering additional measures to patients at selected sites with specialized neuropsychological expertise. If there are practical constraints on the number of clinical trial participants who can be monitored neuropsychologically, patients should be selected randomly or by site, not on the basis of their initial cognitive status.[15] Given the heterogeneity

of MS-related cognitive dysfunction and its weak relationship to physical disability, investigators should consider using initial cognitive status as a blocking factor to assign patients to treatment conditions. This is analogous to using the expanded disability status scale (EDSS) as a stratification variable, as has been done in previous trials. Finally, although random assignment of patients to treatment conditions may result in demographically comparable groups, particularly with large samples, there is no guarantee that this will occur. Consequently, methods for assigning patients to treatment conditions should ensure that groups are equated on demographic characteristics that can influence neuropsychological test performance (i.e. age, sex, and education).

When should neuropsychological measures be administered in MS trials?

The frequency of neuropsychological outcome assessment will depend in part on theoretical factors (such as the hypothesized action of an agent and the anticipated time course of treatment effects) and in part on practical considerations (such as the length of the neuropsychological battery and the number of other secondary outcome measures). As a minimum, neuropsychological outcome measures should be administered before initiating treatment to establish the neuropsychological equivalence of treatment groups at study entry, and at the end of the treatment phase to evaluate overall treatment effects. Under ideal circumstances, however, neuropsychological outcome measures would be administered several times before the initiation of treatment.[15,41] This 'run-in' period can not only stabilize neuropsychological test performance before the treatment phase but also allow estimation of the natural variability in neuropsychological test performance in clinically stable patients. Finally, neuropsychological change in MS is likely to be a continuous non-linear process rather than a one-time event. Consequently, neuropsychological measures should also be administered periodically during the treatment phase to determine the time course of treatment effects. In previous trials, the frequency of on-study neuropsychological assessments has ranged from every 6 weeks[24] to every 6 months.[28,30] Administering neuropsychological outcome measures at 3-month intervals seems to be a reasonable compromise.

What should be done to ensure the quality of neuropsychological data collected during clinical trials?

Several steps can be taken to increase the likelihood that neuropsychological data collection will be complete and accurate, thereby reducing error variance. First, the neuropsychologist responsible for this component of the clinical trial should ensure that examiners who will be administering and scoring the neuropsychological outcome measures are appropriately trained. Optimal reliability is achieved when training is centralized, and when a standardized manual and training procedures are used.[59] Secondly, examiners should practice administering and scoring the neuropsychological measures several times before administering them to study participants. Finally, all test protocols (including 'practice protocols') should be reviewed at a central neuropsychology co-ordinating center, which should provide timely feedback to examiners about the accuracy of test administration and scoring. The neuropsychology co-ordinating center should also be responsible for transcribing data on onto case report forms.

How should neuropsychological outcome measures be analyzed statistically?

In general, neuropsychological outcome assessment in MS clinical trials has consisted of analysis of the mean change in test performance from baseline to the end of the treatment phase, using analysis of variance-based (ANOVA) methods or analogous non-parametric procedures. In most trials, neuropsychological measures have been examined individually for evidence of treatment effects, and demographic factors that can influence neuropsychological test performance have not been controlled. However, the conventional approach to neuropsychological outcome assessment has not consistently yielded statistically significant results, even for treatments with demonstrable effects on other outcome measures. Several steps can be taken to improve the sensitivity of the statistical analyses used to assess neuropsychological outcomes.

First, it is essential to minimize irrelevant sources of variance ('noise') in order to be able to detect treatment effects ('signal'), which are often subtle. One method for minimizing error variance is to standardize test procedures and testing conditions, as recommended earlier. Irrelevant variance can be further reduced by statistically 'extracting' the effects of demographic factors that can affect neuropsychological test performance. Demographic adjustments to raw test scores are only appropriate when treatment groups are demographically comparable at baseline, however.

Secondly, unless a treatment is hypothesized to have differential effects across cognitive domains, it is generally advantageous to evaluate treatment effects on multiple neuropsychological outcome measures simultaneously. Analysis of individual variables may fail to detect subtle treatment effects that do not reach statistical significance on any single variable in isolation. Furthermore, it can increase the probability of making errors of statistical inference. Presuming that relatively independent outcome measures have been chosen, either a multivariate analysis of variance (MANOVA) can be performed, or a neuropsychological composite variable can be constructed: both yield identical results statistically if equal weightings are used in constructing the composite.

Thirdly, if neuropsychological outcome measures have been administered during the treatment phase, statistical techniques that make use of all available data should be employed. One such approach is random-effects regression modeling (also known as hierarchical linear modeling), in which slopes and intercepts are calculated for each individual patient in order to characterize different patterns of change over time.[61–64] Hierarchical linear modeling can not only accommodate variable follow-up intervals, but it also permits interpolation of missing data. Recent applications in neurologic disease have included analysis of neuropsychological progression in human immunodeficiency virus infection,[65,66] treatment outcome analysis in an amyotrophic lateral sclerosis clinical trial,[66] and in modified form, secondary analysis of neuropsychological outcome data from the interferon-β 1a trial.[28]

Another statistical approach that makes use of all available data is survival analysis, which calculates the length of time it takes for patients to reach a predetermined criterion for significant deterioration.[67,68] An extension of survival analysis that incorporates both deterioration and improvement, termed multistate analysis, has recently been proposed as well.[69] Survival analysis served as the primary outcome analysis in several recent MS clinical trials.[22,23,27] It was also used in secondary analyses of neuropsychological outcomes in two of these trials.[28,70] Although the criterion for significant neuropsychological deterioration in these trials was determined using conventional statistical cut-offs (change of at least 0.5 standard deviation relative to the baseline distribution), alternative approaches such as the reliable change index[71–73] could also be employed.

Finally, variations in treatment response among patients assigned to the same treatment condition can be obscured if analyses are confined to treatment groups as a whole. Consequently, subgroup analyses should also be performed. One simple method for subdividing patients neuropsychologically is to do a median split, based on patients' initial performance on one of the neuropsychological outcome measures. A more sophisticated method for grouping patients is to use cluster analysis to identify patients who differ in their baseline pattern of performance on several different neuropsychological measures (as done by Fischer et al.[18]). Neuropsychological subgroup membership can then serve as a between-subjects factor (or potentially a covariate) in analyses of treatment response.

CONCLUDING COMMENTS

The widespread prevalence of MS-related cognitive dysfunction, its direct relationship to cerebral MS lesions, and its devastating functional impact are now well recognized. There is convincing evidence from clinical trials of both disease-modifying therapies and symptomatic treatments that neuropsychological outcome measures can detect even subtle treatment effects, provided that sensitive measures are chosen and appropriate statistical techniques are applied. Assessment of neuropsychological outcomes has become an accepted, if not an expected, component of trials of disease-modifying therapies in MS. The next challenge will be to develop empirically supported criteria for clinically significant neuropsychological change and to identify risk factors for neuropsychological deterioration, which can be used to guide individual treatment planning and design of the next generation of MS clinical trials.

REFERENCES

1 Rao SM, Leo GJ, Bernardin L, Unverzagt F. Cognitive dysfunction in multiple sclerosis: I. Frequency, patterns, and prediction. *Neurology* 1991; 41:685–691.

2 Heaton RK, Nelson LM, Thompson DS et al. Neuropsychological findings in relapsing–remitting and chronic–progressive multiple sclerosis. *J Consult Clin Psychol* 1985; 53:103–110.

3 Rao SM, Leo GJ, Haughton VM et al. Correlation of magnetic resonance imaging with neuropsychological testing in multiple sclerosis. *Neurology* 1989; 39:161–166.

4 Huber SJ, Bornstein RA, Rammohan KW et al. Magnetic resonance imaging correlates of neuropsychological impairment in multiple sclerosis. *J Neuropsychiatry Clin Neurosci* 1992; 4:152–158.

5 Swirsky-Sacchetti T, Mitchell DR, Seward J et al. Neuropsychological and structural brain lesions in multiple sclerosis: a regional analysis. *Neurology* 1992; 42:1291–1295.

6 Rovaris M, Filippi M, Falautano M et al. Relation between MR abnormalities and patterns of cognitive impairment in multiple sclerosis. *Neurology* 1998; 50:1601–1608.

7 van Buchem MA, Grossman RI, Armstrong C et al. Correlation of volumetric magnetization transfer imaging with clinical data in MS. *Neurology* 1998; 50:1609–1617.

8 Hohol MJ, Guttmann CRG, Orav J et al. Serial neuropsychological assessment and magnetic resonance imaging analysis in multiple sclerosis. *Arch Neurol* 1997; 54:1018–1025.

9 van den Burg W, van Zomeren AH, Minderhoud JH et al. Cognitive impairment in patients with multiple sclerosis and mild physical disability. *Arch Neurol* 1987; 44:494–501.

10 Beatty W, Goodkin DE, Hertsgaard D, Monson N. Clinical and demographic predictors of cognitive performance in multiple sclerosis: do diagnostic type, disease duration, and disability matter? *Arch Neurol* 1990; 47:305–308.

11 Fischer JS, Foley FW, Aikens JE et al. What do we *really* know about cognitive dysfunction, affective disorders, and stress in multiple sclerosis? A practitioner's guide. *J Neuro Rehab* 1994; 8:151–164.

12 Rao SM, Leo GJ, Ellington L et al. Cognitive dysfunction in multiple sclerosis: II. Impact on employment and social functioning. *Neurology* 1991; 41:692–696.

13 Amato MP, Ponziani G, Pracucci G et al. Cognitive impairment in early-onset multiple sclerosis: pattern, predictors, and impact on everyday life in a 4-year follow-up. *Arch Neurol* 1995; 52:168–172.

14 Whitaker JN, McFarland, Rudge P, Reingold SC. Outcomes assessment in multiple sclerosis clinical trials: a critical analysis. *Multiple Sclerosis* 1995; 1:37–47.

15 Fischer JS. Use of neuropsychologic outcome measures in multiple sclerosis clinical trials: current status and strategies for improving multiple sclerosis trial desian. In: Goodkin DE, Rudick RA, eds. *Treatment of Multiple Sclerosis: Advances in Trial Design, Results, and Future Perspectives*. London: Springer, 1996, 123–144.

16 Rao SM, Hammeke TA, McQuillen MP et al. Memory disturbance in chronic progressive multiple sclerosis. *Arch Neurol* 1984; 41:625–631.

17 Fischer JS. Using the Wechsler Memory Scale-Revised to detect and characterize memory deficits in multiple sclerosis. *Clin Neuropsychol* 1988; 2:149–172.

18 Fischer JS, Jacobs LD, Cookfair DL et al. Heterogeneity of cognitive dysfunction in multiple sclerosis (abstract). *Clin Neuropsychol* 1998; 12: 286.

19 Jennekens-Schinkel A, Laboyrie PM, Lanser JBK, van der Velde EA. Cognition in patients with multiple sclerosis: after four years. *J Neurol Sci* 1990; 99:229–247.

20 Kujala P, Portin R, Ruutiainen J. The progress of cognitive decline in multiple sclerosis: a controlled 3-year follow-up. *Brain* 1997; **120**:289–297.

21 Bernardin L, Rao SM, Luchetta TL et al. A prospective, long-term, longitudinal study of cognitive dysfunction in multiple sclerosis (abstract). *J Clin Exp Neuropsychol* 1993; **15**:17.

22 Multiple Sclerosis Study Group. Efficacy and toxicity of cyclosporine in chronic progressive multiple sclerosis: a randomized, double-blinded, placebo-controlled clinical trial. *Ann Neurol* 1990; **27**:591–605.

23 Goodkin DE, Rudick RA, VanderBrug Medendorp S et al. Low-dose (7.5 mg) oral methotrexate reduces the rate of progression in chronic progressive multiple sclerosis. *Ann Neurol* 1995; **37**:30–40.

24 Goodkin DE, Fischer JS. Treatment of multiple sclerosis with methotrexate. In: Goodkin DE, Rudick RA, eds. *Treatment of Multiple Sclerosis: Advances in Trial Design, Results, and Future Perspectives.* London: Springer, 1996, 251–287.

25 IFNB Multiple Sclerosis Study Group. Interferon beta–1b is effective in relapsing–remitting multiple sclerosis: I. Clinical results of a multicenter, randomized, double-blind, placebo-controlled trial. *Neurology* 1993; **43**:655–661.

26 Pliskin NH, Hamer DP, Goldstein DS et al. Improved delayed visual reproduction test performance in multiple sclerosis patients receiving interferon β-1b, *Neurology* 1996; **47**:1463–1468.

27 Jacobs LD, Cookfair DL, Rudick RA et al. Intramuscular interferon beta–1a for disease progression in relapsing multiple sclerosis. *Ann Neurol* 1996; **39**:285–294.

28 Fischer JS, Priore RL, Jacobs LD et al. Neuropsychological effects of Avonex (IFN-β-1a) in relapsing multiple sclerosis (MS) (abstract). *Neurology* 1998; **50**:A33.

29 Johnson KP, Brooks BR, Cohen JA et al. Copolymer 1 reduces relapse rate and improves disability in relapsing-remitting multiple sclerosis: results of a phase III multicenter, double-blind, placebo-controlled trial. *Neurology* 1995; **45**:1268–1276.

30 Weinstein A, Schwid SR, Schiffer RB et al. Neuropsychological status in multiple sclerosis after treatment with glatiramer acetate (Copaxone). *Arch Neurol* 1999; **56**:319–324.

31 Durelli L, Bongianni MR, Cavallo R et al. Chronic systemic high-dose recombinant interferon alfa-2a reduces exacerbation rate, MRI signs of disease activity, and lymphocyte interferon gamma production in relapsing remitting multiple sclerosis. *Neurology* 1994; **44**:406–413.

32 Leo GJ, Rao SM. Effects of intravenous physostigmine and lecithin on memory loss in multiple sclerosis: report of a pilot study. *J Neurol Rehabil* 1988; **2**:123–129.

33 Jönsson A, Korfitzen EM, Heltberg A et al. Effects of neuropsychological treatment in patients with multiple sclerosis. *Acta Neurol Scand* 1993; **88**:394–400.

34 Plohmann AM, Kappos L, Ammann W et al. Computer assisted retraining of attentional impairments in patients with multiple sclerosis. *J Neurol Neurosurg Psychiatry* 1998; **64**:455–462.

35 Unverzagt FW, Rao SM, Antuono P. Oral physostigmine in the treatment of memory loss in multiple sclerosis (abstract). *J Clin Exp Neuropsychol* 1991; **13**:74.

36 Smits RCF, Emmen HH, Bertelsmann FW et al. The effects of 4-aminopyridine on cognitive function in patients with multiple sclerosis: a pilot study. *Neurology* 1994; **44**:1701–1705.

37 Bever CT, Anderson PA, Leslie J et al. Treatment with oral 3,4 diaminopyridine improves leg strength in multiple sclerosis patients: results of a randomized, double-blind, placebo-controlled, crossover trial. *Neurology* 1996; **47**:1457–1462.

38 Rodgers D, Khoo K, MacEachen M et al. Cognitive therapy for multiple sclerosis: a preliminary study. *Altern Ther Health Med* 1996; **2**:70–74.

39 Geisler MW, Sliwinski, Coyle PK et al. The effects of amantadine and pemoline on cognitive functioning in multiple sclerosis. *Arch Neurol* 1996; **53**:185–188.

40 Oliveri RL, Sibilia G, Valentino P et al. Pulsed methylprednisolone induces a reversible impairment of memory in patient with relapsing–remitting multiple sclerosis. *Acta Neurol Scand* 1998; **97**:366–369.

41 Bever CT Jr, Grattan L, Panitch HS, Johnson KP. The brief repeatable battery of neuropsychological tests for multiple sclerosis: a preliminary serial study. *Multiple Sclerosis* 1995; **1**:165–169.

42 Foong J, Rozewicz L, Quaghebeur G et al. Neuropsychological deficits in multiple sclerosis after acute relapse. *J Neurol Neurosurg Psychiatry* 1998; **64**:529–532.

43 Stone LA, Albert PS, Smith ME et al. Changes in the amount of diseased white matter over time in patients with relapsing–remitting multiple sclerosis. *Neurology* 1995; **45**:1805–1814.

44 Claus JJ, Mohr E, Chase TN. Clinical trials in

dementia: learning effects with repeated testing. *J Psychiatr Neurosci* 1991; 16:2–5.

45 McCaffrey RJ, Ortega A, Orsillo SM et al. Practice effects in repeated neuropsychological assessments. *Clin Neuropsychol* 1992; 6:32–42.

46 McCaffrey RJ, Ortega A, Haase RF. Effect of repeated neuropsychological assessments. *Arch Clin Neuropsychol* 1993; 8:519–524.

47 McCaffrey RJ, Cousins JP, Westervelt HJ et al. Practice effects with the NIMH AIDS abbreviated neuropsychological battery. *Arch Clin Neuropsychol* 1995; 10:241–250.

48 Hannay HJ, Levin HS. Selective Reminding Test: an examination of the equivalence of four forms. *J Clin Exp Neuropsychol* 1985; 7:251–263.

49 Benedict RHB, Zgaljardic DJ. Practice effects during repeated administrations of memory tests with and without alternate forms. *J Clin Exp Neuropsychol* 1998; 20:339–352.

50 Guyatt G, Walter S, Norman G. Measuring change over time: assessing the usefulness of evaluative instruments. *J Chron Dis* 1987; 40:171–178.

51 Rudick RA, Antel J, Confavreux C et al. Clinical outcomes assessment in multiple sclerosis. *Ann Neurol* 1996; 40:469–479.

52 Rudick RA, Antel J, Confavreux C et al. Recommendations from the National Multiple Sclerosis Society Clinical Outcomes Assessment Task Force. *Ann Neurol* 1997; 42:379–382.

53 Cutter GR, Baier MS, Rudick RA et al. Development of a Multiple Sclerosis Functional Composite as a clinical trial outcome measure. *Brain* 1999; 122:871–882.

54 Fischer JS, Rudick RA, Cutter GR, Reingold SC. The Multiple Sclerosis Functional Composite Measure (MSFC): an integrated approach to MS clinical outcome assessment. *Multiple Sclerosis*; in press.

55 Gronwall D. Paced auditory serial addition task: a measure of recovery from concussion. *Percept Motor Skills* 1977; 44:363–373.

56 Sherman EMS, Strauss E, Spellacy F. Validity of the Paced Auditory Serial Addition Test (PASAT) in adults referred for neuropsychological assessment after head injury. *Clin Neuropsychol* 1997; 11:34–45.

57 Hiscock M, Caroselli JS, Kimball LE. Paced serial addition: modality-specific and arithmetic-specific factors. *J Clin Exp Neuropsychol* 1998; 20: 463–472.

58 Lezak MD. *Neuropsychological Assessment* 3rd edn. New York: Oxford University Press, 1995.

59 Fischer JS, Cohen JA, Cutter GR et al. Intra- and inter-rater reliability of the Multiple Sclerosis Functional Composite (abstract). *Neurology* 1999; 52:A548.

60 Nich C, Carroll K. Now you see it, now you don't: a comparison of traditional versus random-effects regression models in the anlaysis of longitudinal follow-up data from a clinical trial. *J Consult Clin Psychol* 1997; 65:252–261.

61 Bryk AS, Raudenbush SW. Application of hierarchical linear models to assessing change. *Psychol Bull* 1987; 101:147–158.

62 Gibbons RD, Hedeker D, Elkin I et al. Some conceptual and statistical issues in analysis of longitudinal psychiatric data. *Arch Gen Psychiatry* 1993; 50:739–750.

63 Krause MS, Howard KI, Lutz W. Exploring individual change. *J Consult Clin Psychol* 1998; 66:838–845.

64 Selnes OA, Galai N, Bacellar H et al. Cognitive performance after progression to AIDS: a longitudinal study from the Multicenter AIDS Cohort Study. *Neurology* 1995; 45:267–275.

65 Stern Y, Liu X, Marder K et al. Neuropsychological changes in a prospectively followed cohort of homosexual and bisexual men with and without HIV infection. *Neurology* 1995; 45:467–472.

66 Lai EC, Felice KJ, Festoff BW et al. Effect of recombinant human insulin-like growth factor-I on progression of ALS: a placebo-controlled study. *Neurology* 1997; 49:1621–1630.

67 Greenhouse JB, Stangl D, Bromberg J. An introduction to survival analysis: statistical methods for anlaysis of clinical trials. *J Consult Clin Psychol* 1989; 57:536–544.

68 Luke DA, Homan SM. Time and change: using survival analysis in clinical assessment and treatment evaluation. *Psychol Assess* 1998; 10:360–378.

69 Hartmann A, Schulgen G, Olschewski M, Herzog T. Modeling psychotherapy outcome as event in time: an application of multistate analysis. *J Consult Clin Psychol* 1997; 65:262–268.

70 Fischer JS, Goodkin DE, Rudick RA et al. Neuropsychological outcomes in the clinical trial of methotrexate in chronic progressive multiple sclerosis: traditional pre-post analyses may fail to tell the tale (abstract). *J Int Neuropsychol Soc* 1997; 3:35.

71 Jacobson JS, Truax P. Clinical significance: a statistical approach to defining meaningful change in psychotherapy research. *J Consult Clin Psychol* 1991; 59:12–19.

72 **Speer DC, Greenbaum P.** A comparison of five methods for computing significant individual client chagne and measurement rates: an individual growth curve approach. *J Consult Clin Psychol* 1995; **63**:1044–1048.

73 **Chelune GJ, Naugle RI, Lüders H et al.** Individual change after epilepsy surgery: practice effects and base-rate information. *Neuropsychology* 1993; **7**:41–52.

4
Health-related quality-of-life assessment

Deborah M Miller

ROLE OF HEALTH-RELATED QUALITY-OF-LIFE ASSESSMENT IN THE CONDUCT OF EVIDENCE-BASED MEDICINE

Health-care providers are placing increasing emphasis on the practice of evidence-based medicine (EBM), which is 'a conscientious, explicit, and judicious use of current best evidence in making decisions about the care of individual patients.'[1] As with other chronic conditions of unknown cause or cure that demonstrate exacerbating and remitting courses, the practice of EBM for persons with multiple sclerosis (MS) is generally directed to one of three goals:

(a) preventing disease progression;
(b) reducing the duration and severity of exacerbations; and
(c) managing the symptoms.

The evidence that is or could be available to guide decisions about the use of these treatments is of three types:

(a) anatomical or biological (e.g. magnetic resonance imaging (MRI), cerebrospinal fluid measurement);
(b) clinical (e.g. the Expanded Disability Status Scale (EDDS), the Functional Composite Measure); and
(c)   patient derived.

This last category of evidence (patient derived) may be evaluated at several levels of complexity, including general quality of life (QoL), the more specific health-related quality of life (HRQoL), or in terms of discrete indicators of functional status (FS).

Patient-derived data are gaining increasing acceptance as an important assessment domain. For conditions that do not effect mortality but do produce morbidity, the goal of treatment is arguably to reduce disease impact on patients' lives and to ensure that interventions do not cause more overall harm than good. These goals can be achieved only with patient input.

It has been established emperically that measures of patient perception are not redundant to clinician-assessed disability data.[2–4] Moreover, it has been determined that patient functioning in the somewhat artificial setting of the treatment center is not always duplicated at home,[5] thus indicating that clinical assessment is not always generalizable to daily living.

Currently, most of the empirical evidence available to direct the practice of MS EBM is anatomical or biological in nature or derived from clinical data from clinical trials. The Multiple Sclerosis Council for Clinical Practice Guidelines notes that the relative lack of systematically acquired data regarding patient perceptions and preferences about treatment options has effectively left the recipients of care removed from the systematic clinical decision making that EBM represents.[6]

This chapter addresses these important patient perceptions in terms of HRQoL. The chapter defines HRQoL and provides overview of assessment techniques. Measures used in MS HRQoL are reviewed and MS HRQoL research findings are discussed. Finally, future directions for MS HRQoL assessment are recommended.

DEFINITION OF HRQoL

A universally accepted conceptual definition of HRQoL remains to be set—researchers are refining the construct and developing effective ways of measuring it. This is an evolutionary process, one that is as important to the study of MS and its treatments as the development of the MRI and immunologic markers of the disease. As with the immunology of MS, researchers and clinicians are in the process of understanding the meaning of HRQoL abnormalities in the MS population, and measurement of HRQoL remains an imprecise but important science. To extend this analogy: Traugott[7] notes that there are a number of quantitative and qualitative abnormalities of the immune system that have been associated with MS. The presence of these changes is considered important but neither the cause nor the meaning of the changes is completely understood. There are also questions about the ways in which these markers act in relation to each other and how important the change in a marker really is. Traugott also notes that changes in these markers and the relationships among them are not fully understood. So it is with HRQoL measurement.

Quality of life is considered to be but one domain of health as defined by the World Health Organization (WHO).[8] HRQoL is a discrete component of general quality of life. Guyatt[3] notes that, although general QoL can be affected by many factors beyond the scope of health care, including economic instability, civil unrest or poor environment, these have only an indirect relationship with HRQoL and are not included in its definition. Schipper and colleagues[9] agree that while such factors as equal opportunity and social security are important to community health, these factors extend beyond the more immediate goal of treating the sick. These authors offer the following HRQoL definition: '"Quality of life" in clinical medicine represents the functional effect of an illness and its consequent therapy upon a patient, as perceived by the patient.' They find that, although there is variation in terminology, this construct includes four broad domains: physical and occupational function, psychological function, social interaction and somatic sensation. They establish several operational characteristics of HRQoL assessment that help to further define the construct. First and foremost, HRQoL is subjective. As Schipper and colleagues[9] explain '... in clinical medicine the ultimate observer of the experiment is not a dispassionate third party but a most intimately involved patient.' They go on to note that, since the goal of treatment is to minimize the manifest consequences of disease, HRQoL represents 'the final common pathway of all the physiological, psychological and social inputs into the therapeutic process.' The second characteristic of HRQoL is multifactoriality. Having defined HRQoL operationally as the integration of four domains, it is important to ensure that patients' daily experiences in all these regards are explored in the questionnaire, albeit in a manner that is parsimonious and minimizes respondent burden. When using psychometric techniques, the items that assess these dimensions are then summarized into scale scores or into one global score. Econometric techniques (see below) present the data as a global score. The third characteristic is self-administration. Because HRQoL is subjective, there is concern that external administration would in some way influence patient reporting. The final characteristic is that HRQoL is time variable: it fluctuates. Consequently, assessment at specified intervals is necessary to establish patterns of change when response to treatment is the central question.

ATTRIBUTES OF HRQoL MEASURES

Reliability

It is generally agreed that HRQoL measures need to demonstrate certain attributes in order to be considered scientifically rigorous. The first of these is reliability. Hobart[10] describes reliability as the demonstration that the results produced by a measure are accurate, consistent, stable, and reproducible. He describes four types of reliability, including internal consistency, test–retest reliability, rater reliability (inter-rater and intrarater), and parallel forms. He notes that each of these assesses a different source of random error and all are important in establishing the value of a measure. Guyatt and colleagues[3] suggest that an additional form of reliability is relevant for measures used in evaluative studies. They refer to this as 'signal-to-noise ratio' and define it as the ability to detect actual changes in a measure over time (the signal) in relation to error that occurs in any measurement process (noise). For measures that evaluate

change, this signal-to-noise ratio is referred to as 'responsiveness.' It is the size of the difference in scores between subjects who have actually experienced change and those who have not. Concerns have been raised about this ratio in the case of ordinal measures because differences between discrete points along the scale may not represent equivalent amounts of change. This concern is similar to that which has been raised about the EDSS, namely that change scores at the low and high ends of the scale are not equivalent. To date, there is no effective means to establish the responsiveness of a measure.[10]

Another threat to reliability occurs when a measure is used for evaluative purposes and it demonstrates floor and ceiling effects. This may occur, for example, when a measure that is designed for use in a seriously ill population is implemented with a group of less ill people. In such a situation, respondents cluster at the top of the scale and share the maximum score—although they are in fact different in their states of well-being, the measure is not designed to demonstrate that range of difference.

Validity

Validity is the second necessary attribute in developing a HRQoL. It concerns the relationship between the concept that is being measured and the instrument that assesses it. There are three means of establishing evidence of validity: content-related validity, criterion-related validity, and construct-related validity.[10] Because there is no gold standard for HRQoL it is not possible to establish the criterion validity of these measures.[11] Consequently, the methods used to establish an instrument and to assess what it is intended to measure are drawn from clinical and experimental psychology. According to Guyatt and colleagues,[3] Feinstein integrates face validity and content validity into the construct 'sensibility,' which relates to the applicability of a measure, its clarity and simplicity, the likelihood of bias, its comprehensiveness, and the inclusion of redundant items.[12]

TYPES OF RESEARCH APPROPRIATE FOR HRQoL ASSESSMENT

HRQoL can be an appropriate target of investigation in many types of medical research. The three forms of investigation that are discussed in this section—epidemiological studies, health services research and clinical trials—are presented in a somewhat hierarchical order in terms of ability to establish causality from descriptive studies to predictive investigations and clinical trials.

Epidemiological studies

Much has been learned about the pathology of MS through the process of epidemiological studies. Using the same principles, important naturalistically obtained information can be gained about the evolution of HRQoL in the MS population. These data can be useful in their own right, as when they are used to describe the impact of the disease relative to other conditions. They can also be used for hypothesis generation, such as proposing interventions that are intended to improve patient well-being, as is the goal in MS comprehensive care centers. Cross-sectional data can be used to construct statistical norms that allow comparison of one disease group with other illness groups or the general population. Longitudinal assessments could help delineate the

temporal associations among biological, clinical and HRQoL measures in MS. For instance, it is possible that a longitudinal epidemiological study would reveal a delay between biological indications of disease activity and their manifestation in clinical and HRQoL outcomes. This sort of information would be important in designing clinical trials, providing indications for the timing of assessments in relation to interventions, the frequency at which assessments should be made, and the duration of studies necessary to demonstrate a hypothesized change.

Health services outcomes research

Health Services Research (HSR) 'is a field of inquiry that examines the organization, financing and management of health care and impact of these factors on access, delivery, cost, outcomes, and quality of such care.'[13] While much of HSR is conducted using the same methods employed in randomized clinical trials, a subset of this research—outcomes studies—is intended to investigate or improve the usual processes of care. These outcome studies take place in 'usual practice' settings, and they place as much emphasis on patient perceptions as on clinical assessment for end points.[14] Outcomes studies can test the potential uses of HRQoL measures to serve as screening instruments for patients reporting changes in symptom severity or functional ability that signal the need for rehabilitative interventions. These same HRQoL measures could be used in other outcomes studies to examine how quality of life data could be used to involve patients and families in clinical decision making.[15]

Hobart[10] outlines several reasons that outcome studies are particularly important in MS care at this time. He notes that the major impetus for these studies results from the recent approval and availability of several therapeutic pharmaceutical agents that are intended to alter the disease course and the consequent need to establish their relative effectiveness. Secondly, he indicates that because the relative benefits of these interventions are likely to be marginal, a detailed analysis of their relative benefits is needed. Thirdly, he notes that long-term assessments of these agents are necessary because the treatments are expensive and must themselves be used long term. Additionally, because there are finite resources for MS care, the importance of these pharmaceutical agents should be calculated in relation to other aspects of service provision, including rehabilitation and community support, and all of these interventions should be allocated appropriately and equitably.

Clinical trials

Clinical trials provide essential information about potential therapeutic interventions when optimal treatment for a condition is unknown.[16] In chronic conditions, such as MS, that have unknown cause or cure, the goals of treatment are to prevent disease worsening, reduce the severity and duration of exacerbations and provide symptom management. Clinical trials are intended to define emerging interventions that achieve these goals. They are conducted under rigorous conditions in order to eliminate external sources of bias and to ensure that the intervention alone causes change. The end-points used in these studies typically assess biological or anatomical features or objectively assessed functional status.

There are many reasons that HRQoL mea-

sures should be used in MS clinical trials.[17] The first of these is to determine if the intervention has an impact on subjective well-being, an important end-point in conditions that do not affect mortality. Given the progressive nature of MS, it is important that the direction and magnitude of this expected impact on HRQoL are clearly specified. In the case of interventions intended to provide symptom relief, the impact may be an immediate improvement in HRQoL. Alternatively, interventions intended to slow or halt the progression of disease are not as likely to improve the HRQoL for study subjects as they are to slow the decline or sustain the well-being of subjects over a number of years.

The second reason for including HRQoL assessment is to determine the potential negative effects of the treatment for subjects and to compare them to the benefits of treatment. As in the case of the available MS disease-modifying treatments, until the relative and ultimate benefits of the interventions are determined, the side effects of the medicines (e.g. the severity of flu-like symptoms) and of the method of administration (e.g. injection site reactions) are crucial aspects in comparing the treatments.

Because both the costs of life-long disability from MS and the disease-modifying treatments for MS can be very high, a third reason for including HRQoL assessments in clinical trials is to assess the cost–benefit and cost–utility of the treatments. Because patient well-being is as important as morbidity and mortality in chronic illnesses, a number of regulatory bodies responsible for the approval of new interventions rely on HRQoL data in their deliberations.[18–20] These data are considered so significant that the Oncologic Drugs Advisory Committee of the Food and Drug Administration (FDA) in the USA has recommended that QoL data, along with survival data, should be the major efficacy end-point in approving new anticancer agents.[18]

Thus, a fourth reason for using HRQoL data is that those organizations responsible for approving new interventions consider these data to be important in their deliberations. Finally, LaRocca and colleagues[17] note that because these HRQoL data can be important in helping patients who have been recommended to receive the treatments in the course of usual care to make decisions about accepting these interventions.

When planning to use HRQoL measures in clinical trials, the FDA[18] urges that both generic and disease-specific instruments with well-documented psychometric properties should be used. It notes that phase 3 randomized controlled trials are the 'obvious venue for QOL assessment, given that the findings of such trials will likely have an impact on future clinical practice ... Most importantly, these trials allow valid use of a highly subjective instrument.' It is important that the HRQoL measures used in clinical trials represent the multidimensional nature of the construct rather than a discrete aspect of well-being.

TYPOLOGIES OF HRQoL MEASURES

There are several topologies the can be used to categorize HRQoL measures. Two of the most commonly used are based on the type of research question that is being asked (the capacity of the measure to detect different types of relationships among study subjects) and the level of descriptive specificity that the measures can achieve. These two topologies are not mutually exclusive; rather, they describe two sets of criteria that should be considered in selecting an appropriate instrument for a particular study.

Relational typology

Guyatt[3] identifies three levels of measures within this typology, discriminative, predictive and evaluative. A discriminative index is used to differentiate among groups or individuals along a given dimension when there is not 'gold standard' to set a validation criteria as may be done in an epidemiological study. Assessing the HRQoL of persons with MS in comparison to persons with rheumatoid arthritis and inflammatory bowel disease requires a discriminative instrument. So does a study that compares MS patients who were divided into three levels of disability according to EDSS score.

A predictive index is used to classify patients into pre-established present or future categories. As was suggested in the preceding section, an appropriate use of a predictive index would be in an HSR study designed to predict the current need for rehabilitative services or a future job loss resulting from disability. In another sense, a measure may also be considered predictive when it is highly correlated with a longer or more cumbersome measure that is believed to assess the same construct.

Evaluative indexes are those that measure the amount of change in an individual or group over time as the result of disease progression or treatment intervention. Sugano and McElwee[21] note that these three types of instruments represent a developmental continuum from epidemiological measures that are a static means of classification (descriptive) through to risk factors (predictive) and outcome or response measurement.

Descriptive specificity

There are two broad categories within this typology:[2,3] generic and disease-specific. Generic measures are intended to be broad assessments that are relevant to persons in a wide variety of health states. They tap a wide range of health concepts and are useful in making broad comparisons across the general population or between persons with different conditions, or in comparing the relative benefit of different treatments.

There are two types of generic measures, health profiles and utility measures. Health profiles are based on psychometric techniques[22] and include several subscales that assess theoretically and empirically distinct domains of HRQoL. These subscales can be calculated into summary or global scores, or both. Three of the best-known health profiles are the Sickness Impact Profile (SIP),[23] the Medical Outcomes Study Short Form-36 (SF-36),[24,25] and the Medical Outcomes Study Short Form-12 (SF-12).[26]

The SIP is a behaviorally based, 138-item measure that includes 12 subscales, among which are: sleep and rest, emotional behavior, body care and movement, home management, mobility, social interaction, ambulation, alertness behavior, communication, work, recreation and pastimes, and eating. The physical dimension is composed of ambulation, mobility, and body care and movement. The psychosocial dimension incorporates communication, alertness behavior, emotional behavior, and social interaction. The remaining five categories are considered to be independent. Although they are not included in either of the summary scores, they are included in the total score. It is also appropriate to report individual subscale scores. Higher scores indicate poorer performance on all of the scales.

Two commonly used generic measures have emerged from the Medical Outcomes study. The SF-36 includes eight subscales:

(a) physical functioning (10 items), role-physical (four items), bodily pain (two items) and general health (five items) constitute the Physical Component Summary (PCS);

(b) vitality (four items), social functioning (two items) role-emotional (three items) and mental health (five items) are included in the Mental Component Summary (MCS).

The SF-12 is an empirically derived measure composed of the 12 most salient items of the SF-36; it is reported as the PCS and the MCS.

On a continuum of these generic measures, the SIP provides the greatest amount of detail and has the greatest demand on respondent burden (most appropriate when ability to detect change is a priority), while the SF-12 provides the least respondent burden and concurrently the least amount of detail concerning illness impact (best used for population monitoring). The SF-36 lies between the other two measures on both these counts. It is generally thought that these generic health profile measures are particularly useful in epidemiological studies that monitor the health of a diverse population or of individual patients with a medical condition that has a diverse set of signs and symptoms associated with it, such as MS. Because the SF-36 has had such extensive use and has accumulated longitudinal normative data in many different illness groups, the developers of this measure are able to set levels of change in the scores of its sub-scales that are considered clinically relevant in different sample sizes, including single samples.[25] Consequently, the SF-36 has been used both in studies of groups and to monitor the health of individuals. Both the SIP[27–29] and the SF-36[5,30] have been used in assessing the HRQoL impact in MS patients in clinical investigations. In one study of MS patients that compared the SIP and the SF-36, both measures were able to detect differences is levels of disability but the SF-36 demonstrated better scale reliability.[31] The results of these MS intervention studies are reviewed below.

Six other less commonly used generic health profiles have been used in descriptive studies of the MS population. Aronson and colleagues[32] used the Canadian General Social Survey. Lankhorst and colleagues[33] as well as Jonsson and colleagues[34] used the Disability and Impact Profile.[33] Gianino[29] used the Ferrans and Powers QLI. Rudick and colleagues[35] used the Farmer QoL Index. Murphy and colleagues[36] implemented the Functional Status Question-naire.[37] Gulick[38] used the Life Satisfaction Survey.[39]

Utility measures, the second type of generic measure, are derived from economic and decision theory. They reflect patient preferences for different health states and are summarized in a single summary score. These measures incorporate preference measurements and allow patients to assess their willingness to accept various health states in relation to death. Kaplan and Anderson[40] explain that they use the approach at the health policy level to explain the benefits of medical care, behavioral intervention, or prevention programs in terms of well-years in order to compare outcomes across very different interventions. At the individual level, this method is considered useful in helping patients with life-threatening conditions to make value judgements about their willingness to accept potentially life-saving treatments that have a high cost or profound negative effects on health status. LaRocca and colleagues[17] provide a detailed description of a commonly used method for calculating utilities.

There is some concern that the utility assessment approach may not be as useful as the health profile approach in MS assessments. First, the summary nature of the measure may blunt the impact of discrete symptoms. Secondly, this approach calls for subjects to select preferred health states. Given the variable nature of MS symptoms and the exacerbating and remitting nature of the disease, it may be difficult to develop representative health states to use in the modeling process. Finally, given the rather benign nature of MS treatments and the non-life-threatening nature of the disease, there are not the same relative risks in choosing between treatment and no treatment as is the case in assessing the impact of toxic doses of chemotherapy as are used in cancer interventions. Two of the best known utility measures are the Quality of Well Being Scale[40] and the Quality-Adjusted Time Without Symptoms and Toxicity (Q-Twist).[41] Of these, the Q-Twist has been used in an MS clinical trial.[41]

In contrast to generic instruments, disease-specific measures focus on aspects of health that are significant to the disease or intervention under consideration. The major reasons for adapting this approach is to ensure that the measure is sensitive to different health states within the condition.[3] This measurement approach is especially useful in clinical trials because it increases the ability to detect change produced by the intervention and, equally importantly, it allows intense assessment of both the positive and negative impacts of the intervention so that both the benefits and the costs can be evaluated. For this reason in particular, the use of disease-specific measures is especially important in conditions such as MS, which can manifest a broad range of symptoms that fluctuate over time. In order to allow both the detailed assessment inherent in disease-specific measures as well as a more general comparison of a study sample of MS patients with the general population or with other disease groups, it is commonly recommend that short generic measures are combined with disease-specific ones. Three instruments that integrate generic and disease-specific measures[2,42,43] have been developed for use in the MS population.

MS-SPECIFIC HRQoL MEASURES

Three different research teams independently began development HRQoL health profiles for use in the MS population in the mid-1990's. Although the Functional Assessment in MS (FAMS),[42] the QOL-54,[43] and the Multiple Sclerosis Quality of Life Inventory (MSQLI)[2] all integrate generic and disease-specific measures, they differ in development approach and intensity of assessment and may therefore may be most appropriate for different purposes.

FAMS

Cella and colleagues[42] used his Functional Assessment of Cancer Therapy (FACT) as the basis for the FAMS. The original version of the FAMS included 28 items from the general version of the FACT plus 60 MS-specific items generated by patients and providers and from a literature review. These additional 60 items assessed various physical, emotional, social, and functional consequences of MS. This 88-item measure was then administered by mail survey to 377 of 508 MS patients from two major midwestern USA hospitals (74% response rate) (survey subjects) and was completed during routine medical visits by 56 clinic attenders for whom partial clinical data were available. The final version of the FAMS includes 59 items, of which 44 are scored. These 44 items are contained in 6 subscales: mobility (seven items),

symptoms (seven items), emotional well-being (seven items) general contentment (seven items), thinking and fatigue (nine items), and family and social well-being (seven items). These six items demonstrated good internal consistency and test–retest reliability. The construct validity of the FAMS was supported by the predictable patterns of correlation among its subscales and other measures and self-assessed physical impairment.

MSQOL-54

Vickrey and colleagues[43] developed the MSQOL-54 using the SF-36[25] as the core generic measure. They supplemented the core measure with 18 items identified by MS experts as important in MS HRQoL assessment. These additional items included; overall quality of life (two items), health distress (four items), sexual function and satisfaction (five items), cognitive function (four items), energy (one item), pain (one item), and social function (one item). Validation of this measure was conducted on 179 of 231 consecutive clinic attenders who completed and returned the mail-out questionnaire along with sociodemographic, hospitalization and co-morbid conditions data as well as information used to estimate the EDSS score. In addition, 88 of 94 patients completed and returned a second administration of the measure a short time after the first mailing. Testing demonstrated adequate internal consistency reliability and test–retest reliability on all but the role-physical. Construct validity was established on the basis of moderate associations with self-reported symptom severity, ambulation status, employment-role status, and the presence of depressive symptoms.

MSQLI

The MSQLI was developed by a research group under the auspices of the Consortium of Multiple Sclerosis Centers.[2] Like the MSQoL-54, the MSQLI includes the SF-36 as its core measure. Unlike the QOL-54 or the FAMS, the MSQLI consists of the generic measure plus established scales (when available), rather than individual items to gain disease-specific sensitivity. This approach allows comparison with the general population and other illness groups using the generic instrument and comparison with other illnesses that share the same symptoms. The scales that comprise the MSQLI include: generic HRQoL (SF-36), general health (five-item SF-36 general health subscale), perceived physical functioning (SF-36 physical component summary and its 10-item physical functioning subscale), fatigue (21-item Modified Fatigue Impact Scale,[44] and four-item SF-36 vitality subscale), pain and disturbing sensations (six-item MOS Pain Effects Scale,[45] and two-item SF-36 bodily pain subscale), sexual functioning (four-item scale developed for the MSQLI), bladder function functioning (four-item scale developed for the MSQLI), perceived visual function (five-item scale adapted from the Michigan Commission for the Blind's Functional Capacity Assessment), perceived cognitive functioning (20-item Perceived Deficits Questionnaire),[46] emotional status (18-item Mental Health Inventory),[47] and social functioning (18-item MOS Social Support Survey).[48]

Details of the development process, which included two phases—instrument selection and content validation, and reliability assessment, construct validation and item reduction—are available in the MSQLI user manual[2] and a journal publication.[31] The instrument selection and content validation phase of this study began with a definition of the conceptual framework that is based on the World Health Organization's scheme of impairment, disability, and handicap, and then a review of the literature for established measures that assessed those domains. In cases when developed measures were not available, scales were developed. The adequacy of the model and the measures that made it operational were confirmed during a content validation process that included review by three expert panels comprising of neurologists specializing in MS care, allied health professionals specializing in MS care, and patients and their family caregivers. The reliability, construct validation, and item reduction phase included a pilot test of 15 subjects and a field test of 300 subjects from four MS clinics in the USA and Canada who were stratified by sex and disability. The instruments were administered in the clinic setting, and objective measures of physical and cognitive disability were completed on all subjects. Scale reliability was demonstrated for the SF-36 and all disease-specific scales. Content validity was established for the SF-36 when correlations among its subscale scores preformed in the predicted manner, as did the disease-specific scales for bladder, bowel, sexual, and visual function. Generally, construct validation was supported for the MSQLI.

Comparison of measures

These three MS HRQoL measures share several similarities but also have important differences.[31] All three include generic and disease-specific measures and demonstrate that their disease-specific components yield information that is not provided by the generic scores alone.

They use similar approaches in establishing internal consistency and construct validity. The MSQLI included a more detailed process in its development than the other two measures. Its sampling plan included a much broader range of disability and the validation process included comparison with self-reported measures as well as objective measures of physical and cognitive deficits for all subjects. The major difference between the measures themselves is that the FAMS and the MSQOL supplement their generic core with disease specific items whereas the MSQLI includes disease-specific measures. This allows the MSQLI when used in clinical trials to demonstrate more subtle changes over time and to assess in greater detail the unexpected negative consequences of an intervention. It also allows for possible comparisons across interventions that are targeted for specific MS symptoms. However, this flexibility and comprehensiveness has its price. The MSQLI is approximately twice as long as either the MSQOL-54 or the FAMS. It may be speculated that the MSQOL and the FAMS may be more appropriate for descriptive and epidemiological studies or for investigations designed to address health policy issues, while the MSQLI would probably be more appropriate for use in clinical trials because of its depth and breath. It is difficult to speculate which of these measures would be most effective as predictors of future or current needs. An actual comparison of these three measures for any of these purposes awaits their inclusion in clinical investigations. To date, there are no reports (other than those publications that describe their development) of their use in the literature.

REPORTS OF HRQoL ASSESSMENT IN MS-RELATED CLINICAL ASSESSMENT

The following is a review of interventional studies that have incorporated HRQoL assessments. The purpose of this review is to demonstrate the methods by which these instruments were used and to consider the impact of including the measures in the studies.

Health services research

Freeman and colleagues[5] assessed the long-term duration and carry-over of benefits gained after a short course of inpatient, multidisciplinary rehabilitation for patients with clinically definite, progressive MS using a single-group, prospective, longitudinal design. Routine demographic, diagnostic and disease severity data were collected for all patients. The two major end-points were disability as assessed using the Functional Independence Measure, and handicap, as assessed using the London Handicap Scale. HRQoL, as assessed using the SF-36, was included as a secondary end-point. Measures were taken at 3–month intervals for 1 year. The authors do not report any difficulties in obtaining data. Results indicate that HRQoL improvements were sustained for even longer than the disability and handicap measures, with improvements in emotional well-being sustained for 7 months and in the physical component for 10 months. These findings indicate that the HRQoL data make a unique contribution in this study. The authors do note that the HRQoL results are more complex and more difficult to interpret than the primary end-points and that they may be influenced by social and environmental factors that are not associated with the study intervention.

Clinical trials

Solari and colleagues[49] also conducted an assessment of the benefit of inpatient rehabilitation on impairment, disability, and QoL. In this assessment, subjects had been free of exacerbations for 3 months and the study used a randomized, single-blind, controlled design. Twenty-seven subjects were admitted to hospital for a 3-week course of intensive therapy while the remaining 23 subjects were given home exercise programs. Outcome assessments were made at baseline and at 3, 9, and 15 weeks. As in the previously reported study, the primary end-point was the Functional Independence Measure and the SF-36 was used to measure the secondary end-point. There were significant differences between the study and control groups on the Function Independence Measure at all assessment points. Overall, the SF-36 profile improved for patients who underwent the study treatment in all but the bodily pain scale. The difference between the study and control subjects was statistically significant for general health and mental health at all three assessment points, for vitality at 3 weeks and 15 weeks, and for role-emotional and social functioning at 9 weeks. The study group demonstrated clear but not statistically significant improvements in the PCS compared to the control group over the study period, while their improvement in the MCS was statistically significant in comparison to the study group. The authors note that the lack of significance in the PCS may be due to floor effects that it demonstrated at baseline. They note that the use of a disease-specific measure would most likely avoid this difficulty.

Petajan and colleagues[28] assessed the impact of outpatient aerobic training on fitness and HRQoL using the Sickness Impact Profile. Fifty-four subjects with an EDSS ≤ 6.0 were randomly assigned to treatment or control groups. The intervention consisted of three 40-minute sessions of aerobic exercise for 15 weeks. Control subjects agreed to not increase their activity level during the study period. Study assessments were taken at baseline and at 5, 10 and 15 weeks. A significant group-by-time interaction was found on the physical dimension of the Sickness Impact Profile for members of the study group, who reported significantly reduced disease impact at the end of the intervention. Study subjects improved on all three components of the physical dimension (ambulation, mobility, and body care and movement) at some point during the intervention. The control group demonstrated no change on the measure of the physical dimension during the study period. There were no changes in the psychosocial dimension for either the study group or the control group, although there was a general trend towards improvement in the study group. The total Sickness Impact Profile score was significantly improved at week 10 for the study group but did not change significantly for the control group.

In the one reported investigation of a disease-altering therapy (interferon-β 1b) that included HRQoL assessment, Schwartz and colleagues[50] collected clinical and QoL data in 79 subjects who participated in a random allocation lottery and were followed for 12 months. HRQoL data were analysed using the Extended Q-TWIST, the utility measure described above that evaluates treatment trade-offs by incorporating several QoL domains and patient preferences regarding these domains. They found that during the 12-month follow-up, the study patients reported 10.6 months of quality-adjusted time and the control subjects experienced 10.4 months of quality-adjusted time ($p = 0.50$). They concluded that during the first year the intervention did not improve or detract from HRQoL.

CONCLUSIONS

It has been established, that given the nature of MS and its treatments, HRQoL assessment is a unique and important component in assessing the best care for persons with this disease. Three assessment batteries that incorporate generic and disease specific elements have been developed for use in MS using well-established psychometric techniques. The validity of these measures will become better known when they are used in intervention studies. The relative value of these measures and the situations in which they are most appropriately will also be determined with experience.

There are a number of other issues that must be explored for HRQoL data to yield useful results and contribute the patient perspective to the practice of EBM. Among these are the development of methods of administering tests that accommodate the physical disability of the patients. There is much that MS researchers can learn from the assessment of HRQoL in patients with Alzheimer's disease so that QoL in MS patients who experience cognitive deficits can be measured. Although it is possible to determine the statistical significance of HRQoL scores, there is much we have to learn about the clinical significance of these scores. It is also essential that we become more precise in the hypotheses we construct about HRQoL change. It is anticipated that, in some instances, HRQoL will improve in study patients compared to controls. In other studies, it may be expected that HRQoL will initially stabilize and perhaps eventually improve compared to study patients, depending

on the amount of time it takes for the benefit of the intervention to be manifest. In summary, as more is learnt about HRQoL in MS patients better ways of monitoring will continue to be developed. While this developmental approach will lead to some temporary imprecision it is crucial that these measures of patients' reports of their well-being as it is effected by MS and treatment are systematically obtained.

REFERENCES

1 Sackett DL, Richardson WS, Rosenberg W, Haynes RB. *Evidence-based Medicine: How to Practice and Teach EMB*. Edinburgh: Churchill Livingstone, 1998, 2.
2 Ritvo PG, Fischer JS, Miller DM, et al. *Multiple Sclerosis Quality of Life Inventory: A User's Manual*. New York: National Multiple Sclerosis Society, 1997.
3 Guyatt GH, Jaeschke R, Feeny DH et al. Measurements in Clinial Trials: Choosing the Right Approach. In: Spilker B, ed. *Quality of Life and Pharmacoeconomics in Clinical Trials*, 2nd ed. Philadelphia: Lippencott–Raven, 1996, 41–48.
4 Rothwell PM, McDowell Z, Wong CK, Dorman PJ. Doctors and patients don't agree: cross sectional study of patients' and doctors' perceptions and assessments of disability in multiple sclerosis. *Br Med J* 1997; 314:1580–1583.
5 Freeman JA, Langdon DW, Hobart JC, Thompson AJ. Inpatient rehabilitation in multiple sclerosis. *Neurology* 1999; 52:50–56.
6 Kinkel RP, Conway K, Copperman L et al. *Fatigue and Multiple Sclerosis: Evidence-Based Management Strategies for Fatigue in Multiple Sclerosis*. Washington, DC: Paralyzed Veterans of America, 1998.
7 Traugott U. Evidence for immunopathogenesis. In: Cook S, ed. *Handbook of Multiple Sclerosis*. New York: Marcel Dekker, 1990, 101–127.
8 World Health Organization. *International Classification of Impairments, Disabilities and Handicaps (ICIDH): A Manual for Classification*. Geneva: World Health Organization, 1980.
9 Schipper H, Clinch JJ, Olweny CLM. Quality of life studies: definitions and conceptual issues. In: Spilker B,

ed. *Quality of Life and Pharmacoeconomics in Clinical Trials* 2nd edn. Philadelphia: Lippincott–Raven, 1996, 11–24.

10 Hobart JC. Measuring health outcomes in multiple sclerosis: why, which and how? In: Thompson AJ, Polman C, Hohlfeld R, eds. *Multiple Sclerosis: Clinical Challenges and Controversies.* St. Louis: Mosby, 1997, 211–226.

11 Spector WD. Functional Disability Scales. In: Spilker B, ed. *Quality of Life and Pharmacoeeconomics in Clinical Trials.* Philadelphia: Lippencott–Raven, 1996, 133–141.

12 Feinstein AR. *Clinimetrics.* New Haven: Yale University Press, 1987.

13 National Multiple Sclerosis Society. *Health Care Delivery and Policy Research (HCDPR) Program: Definition and Scope.* New York: National Multiple Sclerosis Society, 1995.

14 Spilker B. Introduction. In: Spilker B. *Quality of Life and Pharmacoeconomics in Clinical Trials* 2nd edn. Philadelphia: Lippencott–Raven, 1996, 1–10.

15 Rubenstein LV. Using quality of life tests for patient diagnosis or screening, or to evaluate treatment. In: Spilker B, ed. *Clinial Trials and Pharmacoeconomics in Clinical Trials* 2nd edn. Philadelphia: Lippencott–Raven, 1996, 363–374.

16 Hays RD, Sherbourne CD, Bozzette SA. Pharmacoeconomics and quality of life research beyond the randomized clinical trial. In: Spilker B, ed. *Quality of Life Research and Pharamcoeconomics in Clinical Trials* 2nd edn. Philadelphia: Lippencott–Raven, 1996, 155–160.

17 LaRocca NG, Ritvo PG, Miller DM et al. Quality of life assessment in multiple sclerosis clinicial trials: current status and strategies for improving multiple sclerosis clinical trial designs. In: Goodkin DE, Rudick RA, eds. *Multiple Sclerosis: Advances in Clinical Trial Design, Treatment and Future Perspectives.* London: Springer, 1996, 145–160.

18 Beitz J, Gnecco C, Justice R. Quality-of-life end points in cancer clinical trials: the U.S. Food and Drug Administration perspective. *J Natl Cancer Inst Monogr* 1996; 20:7–9.

19 Wiklund I. Quality of life and regulatory issues. *Scand J Gastroenterol Suppl* 1996; 221:37–38.

20 Turner S. Economic and quality of life outcomes in oncology: the regulatory perspective (review). *Oncology* 1995; 9(suppl 11):121–125.

21 Sugano DS, McElwee NE. An epidemiological perspective. In: Spilker B, ed. *Quality of Life and Pharmacoeconomics in Clinical Trials* 2nd edn. Philadelphia: Lippencott–Raven, 1996, 555–562.

22 Guyatt GH, Feeny DH, Patrick DL. Measuring health-related quality of life (review). *Ann Intern Med* 1993; 118:622–629.

23 Bergner M, Bobbitt RA, Carter WB, Gilson BS. The Sickness Impact Profile: development and final revision of a health status measure. *Med Care* 1981; 19:787–805.

24 Ware JEJ, Kosinski M, Bayliss MS et al. Comparison of methods for the scoring and statistical analysis of SF-36 health profile and summary measures: summary of results from the Medical Outcomes Study. *Med Care* 1995; 33 (suppl 4):AS264–AS279.

25 Ware JEJ; Snow KK; Kosinski M et al. *SF-36 Health Survey: Users Manual and Interpertation Guide.* Boston, Massachusetts: The Health Institute, New England Medical Center, 1993.

26 Ware JEJ, Kosinski M, Keller SD. A 12-Item Short-Form Health Survey: construction of scales and preliminary tests of reliability and validity. *Med Care* 1996; 34:220–233.

27 Cookfair DL, Fischer JS, Rudick RA et al. Quality of life in ambulatory MS patients from the phase III trial of avonex for relapsing MS. In press.

28 Petajan JH, Gappmaier E, White AT et al. Impact of aerobic training on fitness and quality of life in multiple sclerosis. *Ann Neurol* 1996; 39:432–441.

29 Gianino JM, York MM, Paice JA, Shott S. Quality of life: effect of reduced spasticity from intrathecal baclofen. *J Neurosci Nurs* 1998; 30:47–54.

30 Freeman JA, Langdon DW, Hobart JC, Thompson AJ. The impact of inpatient rehabilitation on progressive multiple sclerosis. *Ann Neurol* 1997; 42:236–244.

31 Fischer JS, LaRocca NG, Miller DM et al. Recent developments in the assessment of quality of life in multiple sclerosis (MS). *Multiple Sclerosis* 1999; in press.

32 Aronson KJ. Quality of life among persons with multiple sclerosis and their caregivers. *Neurology* 1997; 48:74–80.

33 Lankhorst GJ, Jelles F, Smits RC et al. Quality of life in multiple sclerosis: the disability and impact profile (DIP). *J Neurol* 1996; 243:469–474.

34 Jonsson A, Dock J, Ravnborg MH. Quality of life as a measure of rehabilitation outcome in patients with multiple sclerosis. *Acta Neurol Scand* 1996; 93:229–235.

35 Rudick RA, Miller D, Clough JD et al. Quality of life in multiple sclerosis. Comparison with inflammatory

bowel disease and rheumatoid arthritis. *Arch Neurol* 1992; **49**:1237–1242.

36 Murphy N, Confavreux C, Haas J et al. Quality of life in multiple sclerosis in France, Germany, and the United Kingdom. Cost of Multiple Sclerosis Study Group. *J Neurol Neurosurg Psychiatry* 1998; **65**:460–466.

37 Jette AM, Davies AR, Cleary PD et al. The Functional Status Questionnaire: reliability and validity when used in primary care (published erratum appears in *J Gen Intern Med* 1986; **1**:427). *J Gen Intern Med* 1986; **1**:143–149.

38 Gulick EE. Correlates of quality of life among persons with multiple sclerosis. *Nurs Res* 1997; **46**:305–311.

39 Chubon RA. *Manual for the Life Satisfaction Survey (1995 Revision)*. Columbia, South Carolina: University of South Carolina, School of Medicine, Department of Neuropsychiatry and Behavioral Science, Rehabilitation Counseling Program, 1995.

40 Kaplan RM, Anderson JP. The general health policy model: an integrated approach. In: Spilker B, ed. *Quality of Life and Pharmacoeconomics in Clinical Trials* 2nd edn. Philadelphia: Lippencott–Raven, 1996, 309–322.

41 Schwartz CE, Cole BF, Gelber RD. Measuring patient-centered outcomes in neurologic disease. Extending the Q-TWiST method (review). *Arch Neurol* 1995; **52**:754–762.

42 Cella DF, Dineen K, Arnason B et al. Validation of the functional assessment of multiple sclerosis quality of

life instrument. *Neurology* 1996; **47**:129–139.

43 Vickrey BG, Hays RD, Harooni R et al. A health-related quality of life measure for multiple sclerosis. *Qual Life Res* 1995; **4**:187–206.

44 Fisk JD, Ritvo PG, Ross L et al. Measuring the functional impact of fatigue: initial validation of the fatigue impact scale. *Clin Infect Dis* 1994; **18 (suppl 1)**:S79–S83.

45 Sherbourne CD. Pain measures. In: Stewart AL, Ware JEJ, eds. *Measuring Functioning and Well-Being: the Medical Outcomes Study Approach*. Durham, North Carolina: Duke University Press, 1992, 220–234.

46 Sullivan MJL, Edgley K, Dehoux E. A survey of multiple sclerosis. Part 1: Preceived cognitive problems and compensatory strategy use. *Can J Rehabil* 1990; **4**:99–105.

47 Veit CT, Ware JEJ. The structure of psychological distress and well-being in general populations. *J Consult Clin Psychol* 1983; **51**:730–742.

48 Sherbourne CD, Stewart AL. The MOS Social Support Survey. *Soc Sci Med* 1991; **32**:472–480.

49 Solari A, Filippini G, Gasco P et al. Physical rehabilitation has a positive effect on disability in multiple sclerosis patients. *Neurology* 1999; **52**:57–62.

50 Schwartz CE, Coulthard-Morris L, Cole B, Vollmer T. The quality-of-life effects of interferon beta-1b in multiple sclerosis. An extended Q-TWiST analysis. *Arch Neurol* 1997; **54**:1475–1480.

5
Measures of gadolinium enhancement

Massimo Filippi and Carla Tortorella

INTRODUCTION

Gadolinium (Gd) is a rare element of the lanthanide series, with strong paramagnetic properties. Its chelates are widely used as contrast agents in magnetic resonance imaging (MRI) of the brain and spinal cord. Gd administration markedly increases T1 relaxation time of adjacent mobile water protons, thus producing focal high signal intensity on T1-weighted images in areas where Gd is concentrated.[1] Data from animals studies[2] and from multiple sclerosis (MS) brain biopsy studies[3,4] have demonstrated that Gd enhancement is associated with histopathological evidence of blood–brain barrier (BBB) breakdown and inflammation. In animals, it has also been shown that Gd enhancement correlates with the number of inflammatory cells within the active lesions[5,6] and mainly represents macrophage activation.[7]

In MS patients, studies with serial enhanced MRI scans indicate that enhancement occurs in almost all the new lesions from patients with relapsing–remitting (RRMS) or secondary progressive MS (SPMS).[8–10] Focal enhancement can also be detected before the appearance of any abnormality on unenhanced T2-weighted scans.[11] Enhancement can also reappear in chronic lesions with or without a concomitant increase in size.[8] Enhancement duration, after a standard dose of Gd, usually lasts between 4 and 8 weeks.[8,12,13] However, lesions with shorter enhancing periods may be seen with weekly MRI.[9,10]

Although enhancing lesions also occur in clinically stable MS patients, the number and the extent of enhancing lesions are much higher in the presence of concomitant clinical activity.[8,14–17] Periods of increased lesion activity are associated, although weakly, with an increased risk of exacerbations, while no correlation is found with accumulation of disability.[18] However, activity on enhanced MRI is a relatively good predictor of further enhancement over at least the subsequent 2 years,[16,17,19] subsequent accumulation of T2 lesions[20] and development of brain atrophy as measured by ventricular diameter, brain width, or corpus callosum area.[19]

This chapter summarizes the major contributions of Gd-enhanced MRI to the planning and monitoring of treatment in MS. It also reviews the potential of new MRI strategies and techniques to increase the sensitivity for detecting MS active lesions and to improve our understanding of the evolution of the underlying pathological changes.

ENHANCED MRI AS A TOOL TO SELECT PATIENTS FOR TREATMENT TRIALS

MRI-based criteria for patient selection have acquired progressively increasing importance in MS treatment trials. They are particularly important for the selection of patients who present with clinically isolated syndromes (CIS)[21–23] that are suggestive of MS to be enrolled in trials assessing the efficacy of treatment in preventing the development of clinically definite MS (CDMS). Identifying patients at presentation with CIS with a high risk of developing CDMS has three major advantages. First, it allows patients with other neurological conditions to be excluded from trials. Secondly, by increasing the likelihood of CDMS in the patients who are enrolled, it allows reduced sample sizes and shorter trial durations to demonstrate a treatment effect. Thirdly, it protects patients with a low risk of developing CDMS from the potential side effects of the clinical trial interventions.

In patients at presentation with CIS, MRI is the best tool to identify those patients with a high risk of an unfavourable evolution. The presence of multiple abnormalities on T2-weighted scans (i.e. MRI demonstration of spatial dissemination of lesions) is a strong predictor of:

(a) the risk of developing CDMS;
(b) the time elapsing between the first and the second clinical manifestation of the disease;
(c) the accumulation of moderate to severe disability in the following 5–10 years; and
(d) the accumulation of other MRI abnormalities.[24–27]

The presence of enhancement on the MRI scans obtained from patients at presentation with CIS further improves the predictive value of MRI[21] by demonstrating lesions of different ages

(i.e. MRI demonstration of the temporal dissemination of the lesions). This can be useful in distinguishing MS from acute disseminated encephalomyelitis, a monophasic condition.

MRI-based criteria can also be used to select RRMS and SPMS patients for phase 2 clinical trials.[28] In this case, selecting patients with high baseline MRI activity can allow selective enrolment of patients who are likely to have persistent disease activity during the trial. This may reduce the number of uninformative scans, allowing smaller sample sizes and shorter follow-up durations to achieve adequate study power.[29] Such an approach is expensive, however, since a significant proportion of clinically eligible patients would have negative enhanced scans and therefore be excluded from the trial. Another caveat of such an approach is the increased risk of selecting patients during periods of relatively high disease activity, with subsequent regression to the mean, resulting in a decline in lesion activity during the trial in all subjects regardless of the treatment used. The magnitude of this effect would be proportional to the amount of activity required for trial entry, and is a particular problem if the study lacks a placebo arm.[29] In addition, the use of selection criteria makes the results of a trial less able to be generalized to all the potential subjects that might benefit from the treatment.[29,30]

ENHANCED MRI AS A TOOL TO MONITOR PHASE 2 CLINICAL TRIALS

Use of enhanced MRI to monitor treatment efficacy in MS is attractive for several reasons. First, serial monthly enhanced MRI scans are 5–10 times more sensitive in detecting MS activity than clinical relapses in RRMS and SPMS.[28,31,32] As a consequence, in these clinical subgroups, the number of patients required is much fewer and the study duration is shorter when using an MRI-derived end-point than when using a clinical outcome to monitor disease evolution.[29,30,33,34] Secondly, MRI provides objective measures on continuous scales, which are therefore amenable to robust statistical approaches. Thirdly, MRI changes may be more directly related to the pathology than clinical manifestations. Fourthly, counting the number of enhancing lesions is very reproducible in experienced hands.[35,36] Reproducibility in identifying enhancing lesions can be optimized by formal training and use of an ad hoc reading criteria.[35] Fifthly, it is important in clinical trials that the observers are unaware of the treatment regimen of individual patients in order to avoid bias caused by unblinding. This is easily achieved using MRI-derived end-points. Finally, MRI scans are retrievable, so the analyses can be easily audited and re-assessed as needed.

However, the use of MRI to monitor phase 2 clinical trials also has some problems and uncertainties.[37] The weak correlation between MRI-detected disease activity and long-term disease evolution[18] is the most important issue. Furthermore, lack of a treatment effect on a particular MRI parameter may not necessarily imply that the treatment has no beneficial effects on the clinical manifestations or evolution. Similarly, a treatment effect on MRI-monitored disease activity does not necessarily mean that clinical benefits will follow. For these reasons, outcomes derived from enhanced MRI are used as primary end-points only in monitoring phase 2 trials to obtain preliminary information about the effect of new treatments.[28,31] These studies are very important in providing a rationale for more definitive phase 3 clinical trials.[28,31]

Another caveat of this approach is that sample sizes and study durations should be determined not only by statistical considerations but also by characteristics of the experimental treatment used. Moreover, small studies may have enough statistical power but may not be fully representative of the general MS population. Short studies may miss a treatment effect that takes months to develop. Furthermore, small, short-term studies will be less likely to detect relevant side effects or early failure of treatment.[34]

ENHANCED MRI AS A TOOL TO MONITOR PHASE 3 CLINICAL TRIALS

The role of enhanced MRI in phase 3 clinical trials is much less relevant. Currently, clinical measures are used as the primary end-point in phase 3 clinical trials[28] and MRI end-points are considered secondary end-points. Secondary MRI end-points are usually derived from computer-assisted measures of disease burden on T2-weighted scans.[28,32] Nevertheless, enhanced MRI may be useful also in this context. Because of the high statistical power of Gd-enhanced MRI studies, enhanced MRI is commonly obtained in only a subgroup of patients (e.g. in patients enrolled in centres with adequate MRI facilities) to provide additional important confirmation of the clinical results. Serial monthly enhanced MRI may also be obtained for some time after the treatment to assess the duration of the treatment effects.[16,28]

NEW STRATEGIES TO INCREASE THE SENSITIVITY OF ENHANCED MRI

It has been demonstrated recently that there are at least seven possible strategies for further increasing the sensitivity of enhanced MRI for detecting active lesions in MS. In addition to benefits in the context of controlled clinical trials, increasing MRI sensitivity may help in the understanding disease pathogenesis.

Strategies to increase the sensitivity of Gd-enhanced MRI can be divided into three categories. The first strategy attempts to maximize the information that can be obtained by conventional scanning and includes more frequent MRI sampling (e.g. weekly instead of monthly),[9,10] evaluation of the brain and spinal cord instead of brain-only imaging[38] and an increased delay between Gd injection and scanning (e.g. 20–30 minutes instead of the conventional 5–7 minutes).[39,40] The second strategy aims at increasing the signal of enhancing lesions, and includes the use of higher doses of Gd (0.3 mmol/kg instead of 0.1 mmol/kg)[40–42] and acquisition of thin slices (e.g. 1 mm or 3 mm thick instead of the conventional 5 mm).[43] The third strategy is the use of techniques that increase the likelihood of detecting enhancing lesions by reducing the signal of the background tissue. This includes application of a magnetization transfer (MT) pulse to the Conventional Spin Echo (CSE) T1-weighted sequence[44–47] or the use of co-registration techniques.[48]

At present, there is a large body of evidence indicating that use of a triple dose of Gd (0.3 mmol/kg) is the strategy that allows the maximum improvement over conventional imaging.[40–42] Its use in combination with other strategies can lead to an increase in sensitivity of about 130% compared to the standard technique.[40] A recent longitudinal study[42] confirmed these findings and also showed that use of serial triple-dose MRI is safe and permitted the number of scans needed to show treatment effects to be reduced by 30% or more.[42]

Increasing the sensitivity of enhanced MRI to detect MS activity might improve our ability to monitor treatment, both for practical purposes (smaller sample sizes and shorter follow-up needed to show a treatment effect) as well as for a better understanding of the mechanisms of treatment. However, this must be weighed against other less favourable considerations, including difficulties in standardizing the newer techniques, increased costs, and the caveats mentioned above for conventional Gd-enhanced studies.

ASSESSMENT OF INDIVIDUAL LESION EVOLUTION

New MS lesions evolve in a variable manner, leading to different amounts of tissue damage. Therefore, monitoring the evolution of individual lesions may be relevant not only for the understanding of MS pathophysiology but also as a new approach for assessing treatment efficacy. In phase 2 trials, this approach might give information in a relatively short period of time about the efficacy of experimental treatment in preventing severe tissue destruction.

Although several other MRI techniques have been used to monitor individual lesion evolution,[49,50] the most valuable results have been obtained using magnetization transfer imaging (MTI). Several authors[50–58] have consistently showed that the opening of the BBB is associated with structural tissue changes, the magnitude of which is related to the severity[54] and duration[59] of BBB disruption. Such associated tissue changes may or may not show a partial or complete recovery 1–6 months after the cessation of the enhancement.[50–57] This suggests that the balance between damaging and repairing mechanisms may be highly variable during the early phases of MS lesion formation. Different proportions of lesions with different degrees of structural change may, therefore, contribute to evolution of the disease[58] and there may be weak correlations between enhancing lesions and the long-term disease evolution.[18]

CONCLUSIONS

Because of its unique sensitivity in detecting disease activity, enhanced MRI is extremely valuable for conducting phase 2 clinical trials in order to ascertain quickly and efficiently the effect of a therapy on pathological activity. Enhanced MRI also has a role in selecting patients for trials, particularly when assessing the efficacy of treatment in the early phases of the disease. Nevertheless, enhanced MRI provides restricted information about the BBB, and the relationship between Gd enhancement and the long-term evolution of the disease remains unclear. This means that the results of trials using enhanced MRI must be interpreted cautiously. It also indicates the need for multiple MRI approaches in clinical trials to obtain optimally informative MRI outcomes.

REFERENCES

1 Grossman RI, Gonzalez-Scarano F, Atlas SW et al. Multiple sclerosis: Gadolinium enhancement in MR imaging. *Radiology* 1986; **161**:721–725.

2 Hawkins CP, Munro PMG, Mackenzie F et al. Duration and selectivity of blood–brain barrier breakdown in chronic relapsing experimental allergic encephalomyelitis studied by gadolinium-DTPA and protein markers. *Brain* 1990; 113:365–378.

3 Bruck W, Bitsch A, Kolenda H et al. Inflammatory central nervous system demyelination: correlation of magnetic resonance imaging findings with lesion pathology. *Ann Neurol* 1997; 42:783–793.

4 Lucchinetti CF, Bruck W, Rodriguez M, Lassmann H. Distinct patterns of multiple sclerosis indicates heterogeneity of pathogenesis. *Brain Pathol* 1996; 6:259–261.

5 Seeldrayers PA, Syha J, Morrissey SP et al. Magnetic resonance imaging investigation of blood–brain barrier damage in adoptive transfer experimental autoimmune encephalomyelitis. *J Neuroimmunol* 1993; 46:199–206.

6 Namer IJ, Steibel J, Piddlesen SJ et al. Magnetic resonance imaging of antibody-mediated demyelinating experimental allergic encephalomyelitis. *J Neuroimmunol* 1994; 54:41–47.

7 Morrissey SP, Stodal H, Zettl U et al. In vivo MRI and its histological corelates in acute adoptive transfer experimental allergic encephalomyelitis. Quantification of inflammation and oedema. *Brain* 1996; **119**:239–248.

8 Miller DH, Rudge P, Johnson J et al. Serial gadolinium-enhanced magnetic resonance imaging in multiple sclerosis. *Brain* 1988; 111:927–939.

9 Lai M, Hodgson T, Gawne-Cain M et al. A preliminary study into the sensitivity of disease activity detection by serial weekly magnetic resonance imaging in multiple sclerosis. *J Neurol Neurosurg Psychiatry* 1996; 60:339–341.

10 Tortorella C, Rocca MA, Codella C et al. Disease activity in multiple sclerosis studied with weekly triple dose magnetic resonance imaging. *J Neurol* 1999; in press.

11 Kermode AG, Tofts P, Thompson AJ et al. Heterogeneity of blood–brain barrier changes in multiple sclerosis: an MRI study with gadolinium-DTPA enhancement. *Neurology* 1990; 40:229–235.

12 Thompson AJ , Kermode AG, MacManus DG et al. Patterns of disease activity in multiple sclerosis: clinical and magnetic resonance imaging study. *Br Med J* 1990; 300:631–634.

13 Harris JO, Frank JA, Patronas N et al. Serial gadolinium-enhanced magnetic resonance imaging scans in patients with early, relapsing–remitting

multiple sclerosis: implications for clinical trials and natural history. *Ann Neurol* 1991; **29**:548–555.

14 Smith ME, Stone LA, Albert PS et al. Clinical worsening in multiple sclerosis is associated with increased frequency and area of gadopentetate dimeglumine-enhancing magnetic resonance imaging lesions. *Ann Neurol* 1993; **33**:480–489.

15 Pozzilli C, Bastianello S, Koudriavtseva T et al. Magnetic resonance imaging changes with recombinant human interferon beta-1a: a short term study in relapsing–remitting multiple sclerosis. *J Neurol Neurosurg Psychiatry* 1996; **61**:251–258.

16 Molyneux PD, Filippi M, Barkhof F et al. Correlations between monthly enhanced MRI lesion rate and changes in T2 lesion volume in multiple sclerosis. *Ann Neurol* 1998; **43**:332–339.

17 Koudriavtseva T, Thompson AJ, Fiorelli M et al. Gadolinium enhanced MRI disease activity in relapsing–remitting multiple sclerosis. *J Neurol Neurosurg Psychiatry* 1997; **62**:285–287.

18 Kappos L, Moeri D, Radue EW et al. Predictive value of gadolinium-enhanced MRI for relapse rate and changes in disability/impairment in multiple sclerosis: a metaanalysis. *Lancet* 1999; **353**:964–969.

19 Simon JH. From enhancing lesions to brain atrophy in relapsing MS. *J Neuroimmunol* 1999; in press.

20 Simon JH, Jacobs LD, Campion M et al. Magnetic resonance studies of intramuscular interferon beta-1a for relapsing multiple sclerosis. *Ann Neurol* 1998; **43**:79–87.

21 Barkhof F, Filippi M, Miller DH et al. Comparison of MR imaging criteria at first presentation to predict conversion to clinically definite multiple sclerosis. *Brain* 1997; **120**:2059–2069.

22 Paty DW, Oger JJF, Kastrukoff LF et al. Magnetic resonance imaging in the diagnosis of multiple sclerosis: a prospective study of comparison with clinical evaluation, evoked potential, oligoclonal banding, and CT. *Neurology* 1988; **38**:180–185.

23 Fazekas F, Offenbacher H, Fuchs S et al. Criteria for an increased specificity of MRI interpretation in elderly subjects with suspected multiple sclerosis. *Neurology* 1988; **38**:1822–1825.

24 Morrissey SP, Miller DH, Kendall BE et al. The significance of brain magnetic resonance imaging abnormalities at presentation with clinically isolated syndromes suggestive of multiple sclerosis. A 5-year follow-up study. *Brain* 1993; **116**:135–146.

25 Filippi M, Horsfield MA, Morrissey SP et al. Quantitative brain MRI lesion load predicts the course of clinically isolated syndromes suggestive of multiple sclerosis. *Neurology* 1994; **44**:635–641.

26 O'Riordan JI, Thompson AJ, Kingsley DP et al. The prognostic value of brain MRI in clinically isolated syndromes of the CNS. A 10-year follow-up. *Brain* 1998; **121**:495–503.

27 Sailer M, O'Riordan JI, Thompson AJ et al. Quantitative MRI in patients with clinically isolated syndromes suggestive of demyelination. *Neurology* 1999; **52**:599–606.

28 Miller DH, Albert PS, Barkhof F et al. Guidelines for the use of magnetic resonance techniques in monitoring the treatment of multiple sclerosis. *Ann Neurol* 1996; **39**:6–16.

29 Nauta JJP, Thompson AJ, Barkhof F, Miller DH. Magnetic resonance imaging in monitoring the treatment of multiple sclerosis patients: statistical power of parallel-groups and crossover designs. *J Neurol Sci* 1994; **122**:6–14.

30 Truyen L, Barkhof F, Tas M et al. Specific power calculations for magnetic resonance imaging (MRI) in monitoring active relapsing–remitting multiple sclerosis (MS): implications for phase II therapeutic trials. *Multiple Sclerosis* 1997; **2**:283–290.

31 Barkhof F, Filippi M, Miller DH et al. Strategies for optimizing MRI techniques aimed at monitoring disease activity in multiple sclerosis. *J Neurol* 1997; **244**:76–84.

32 Filippi M, Horsfield MA, Adèr HJ et al. Guidelines for using quantitative measures of brain magnetic resonance imaging abnormalities in monitoring the treatment of multiple sclerosis. *Ann Neurol* 1998; **43**:499–506.

33 Trubidy N, Ader HJ, Barkhof F et al. Exploratory treatment trials in multiple sclerosis using MRI: sample size calculations for relapsing remitting and secondary progressive subgroups using placebo controlled parallel groups. *J Neurol Neurosurg Psychiatry* 1998; **64**:50–55.

34 Sormani MP, Molyneux, PD, Gasperini C et al. Statistical power of MRI monitored trials in multiple sclerosis: new data and comparison with previous results. *J Neurol Neurosurg Psychiatry* 1999; **66**:456–469.

35 Barkhof F, Filippi M, van Waesberghe JH et al. Improving intraobserver variation in reporting gadolinium-enhanced MRI lesions in multiple sclerosis. *Neurology* 1997; **49**:1682–1688.

36 Filippi M, Barkhof F, Bressi S et al. Inter-rater variability in reporting enhancing lesions on standard

and triple dose gadolinium scans in patients with multiple sclerosis. *Multiple Sclerosis* 1997; 3:226–230.

37 Miller DH, Grossman RI, Reingold SC et al. The role of magnetic resonance techniques in understanding and managing multiple sclerosis. *Brain* 1998; 121:3–24.

38 Thorpe JW, Kidd D, Moseley IF et al. Serial gadolinium-enhanced MRI of the brain and spinal cord in early relapsing–remitting multiple sclerosis. *Neurology* 1996; 46:373–378.

39 Filippi M, Yousry T, Rocca MA et al. Sensitivity of delayed gadolinium-enhanced MRI in multiple sclerosis. *Acta Neurol Scand* 1997; 95:331–334.

40 Silver NC, Good CD, Barker GJ et al. Sensitivity of contrast enhanced MRI in multiple sclerosis: effects of gadolinium dose, magnetization transfer contrast and delayed imaging. *Brain* 1997; 120:1149–1161.

41 Filippi M, Yousry T, Campi A et al. Comparison of triple dose versus standard dose gadolinium-DTPA for detection of MRI enhancing lesions in patients with MS. *Neurology* 1996; 46:379–384.

42 Filippi M, Rovaris M, Capra R et al. A multi-centre longitudinal study comparing the sensitivity of monthly MRI after standard and triple dose gadolinium-DTPA for monitoring disease activity in multiple sclerosis: implications for clinical trials. *Brain* 1998; 121:2011–2020.

43 Filippi M, Yousry T, Horsfield MA et al. A high-resolution three-dimensional gradient echo sequence improves the detection of disease activity in multiple sclerosis. *Ann Neurol* 1996; 40:901–907.

44 van Waesberghe JHTM, Castelijns JA, Roser W et al. Single dose gadolinium with magnetization transfer contrast versus triple dose gadolinium in detecting enhancing multiple sclerosis lesions. *AJNR* 1997; 18:1279–1285.

45 Petrella JR, Grossman RI, McGowan JC et al. Multiple sclerosis lesions: relationship between MR enhancement pattern and magnetization transfer effect. *AJNR* 1996; 17:1041–1049.

46 Hiehle JF, Grossman RI, Ramer NK et al. Magnetization transfer effect in MR-detected multiple sclerosis lesions: comparison with gadolinium-enhanced spin-echo images and non-enhanced T1-weighted images. *AJNR* 1995; 16:69–77.

47 Metha RC, Pike BG, Enzmann DR. Improved detection of enhancing and non-enhancing lesions of multiple sclerosis with magnetization transfer. *AJNR* 1995; 16:1771–1778.

48 Filippi M, Horsfield MA, Hajnal JV et al. Quantitative assessment of magnetic resonance imaging lesion load in multiple sclerosis. *J Neurol Neurosurg Psychiatry* 1998; 64 (suppl 1):88–93.

49 Davie CA, Hawkins CP, Barker GJ et al. Serial proton magnetic resonance spectroscopy in acute multiple sclerosis lesions. *Brain* 1994; 117:49–58.

50 van Waesberghe JH, van Walderveen MA, Castelijns JA et al. Patterns of lesion development in multiple sclerosis: longitudinal observations with T1-weighted spin-echo and magnetization transfer MR. *AJNR* 1998; 19:675–683.

51 Filippi M, Rocca MA, Martino G et al. Magnetization transfer changes in the normal appearing white matter precede the appearance of enhancing lesions in patients with multiple sclerosis. *Ann Neurol* 1998; 43:809–814.

52 Goodkin DE, Rooney WD, Sloan R et al. A serial study of new MS lesions and the white matter from which they arise. *Neurology* 1998; 51:1689–1697.

53 Silver NC, Lai M, Symms MR et al. Serial magnetization transfer imaging to characterize the early evolution of new MS lesions. *Neurology* 1998; 51:758–764.

54 Filippi M, Rocca MA, Rizzo G et al. Magnetization transfer ratios in MS lesions enhancing after different doses of gadolinium. *Neurology* 1998; 50:1289–1293.

55 Lai HM, Davie CA, Gass A et al. Serial magnetisation transfer ratios in gadolinium-enhancing lesions in multiple sclerosis. *J Neurol* 1997; 244:308–311.

56 Filippi M, Gomi G. Magnetization transfer ratio changes in a symptomatic lesion of a patient at presentation with possible multiple sclerosis. *J Neurol Sci* 1997; 151:79–81.

57 Dousset V, Gayou A, Brochet B, Caille JM. Early structural changes in acute MS lesions assessed by serial magnetization transfer studies. *Neurology* 1998; 51:1150–1155.

58 Rocca MA, Mastronardo G, Rodegher M et al. Long term changes of MT-derived measures from patients with relapsing–remitting and secondary–progressive multiple sclerosis. *AJNR* 1999; 20:821–827.

59 Filippi M, Rocca MA, Comi G. Magnetization transfer ratios of multiple sclerosis lesions with variable durations of enhancement. *J Neurol Sci* 1998; 159:162–165.

6

Measures of magnetization transfer

Joseph C McGowan

INTRODUCTION

The pathology of multiple sclerosis (MS) is characterized by myelin loss resulting from a recurrent or chronic angiocentric inflammatory process. Hallmarks of the disease include multifocal inflammatory lesions characterized by infiltration of lymphocytes and macrophages, demyelination, gliosis, and in some cases remyelination.[1] From an imaging perspective, multiple sclerosis is usually considered a disease of white matter, but that has recently been challenged by evidence suggesting that axonal transection may be widespread and to a degree responsible for neurologic impairment.[2] This observation is consistent with some earlier proposals that axonal damage is chiefly responsible for the permanent disability that characterizes later stages of MS.[3,4]

State-of-the-art magnetic resonance imaging is highly sensitive for detecting MS lesions and is certainly the standard methodology for confirming the diagnosis of MS. Macroscopic MS lesions are bright on images that are weighted to reflect the T2 relaxation time, and some lesions, but not all, enhance with gadolinium contrast agents when viewed with T1-weighted imaging. Magnetic resonance imaging (MRI) may be less than optimal in specificity, however, with regard to

MS. Neither MRI nor any competing modality can at present distinguish the various classifications of the disease (e.g. relapsing–remitting MS versus chronic progressive MS) or prognosticate outcomes. There also exists a paradox in that clinical and cognitive status may not be closely correlated with imaging results.

With regard to MRI in MS, there is a need for sophisticated measures that are surrogate markers for the disease in order to document progression and to assess the efficacy of treatment protocols. For these reasons there is current interest in quantitative imaging techniques. Quantitative analysis enables distinctions to be made within and among images when contrast differences are too subtle to be appreciated by conventional reading of the image. Longitudinal application of quantitative techniques allows 'tracking' of disease processes in a way that is not possible when image contrast is adjusted so as to optimize the viewing of the particular image under study. Appropriate techniques should be robust and reproducible, and ideally might reveal information about the underlying histopathology. Early experience with magnetization transfer (MT), as well as the theory that has been advanced to describe the technique, suggested that MT might be a non-invasive probe for pathological study in vivo. This would be desirable, since patients usually live for many years with the disease. Investigations employing MT techniques are being conducted in a variety of animal models of disease, and are expected to provide new insights that will allow investigators to differentiate the various pathological aspects of the disease. However, MT imaging as it is currently implemented is well suited to explore the natural history of MS, and analyses exploiting the MT effect may play a role in forthcoming treatment trials.

In this chapter the physical principles of MT are discussed, followed by an outline of MT techniques, a description of methods for analysing MT data, and examples in current use. An understanding of both the theory of the phenomenon and its application may serve to provide insight into the possibilities for use of the technique and for future research directions.

PHYSICAL BASIS OF MAGNETIZATION TRANSFER

Magnetic resonance techniques, including MRI, exploit the enhanced absorption of energy experienced by certain nuclei when they are exposed to radio energy at a particular frequency. These nuclei posses a small magnetic moment and can be described using a quantum-mechanical property known as spin; it is common to refer to the nuclei as 'spins'. The combined effect of the spins is referred to as 'spin magnetization' and is manipulated as an experimental parameter in all magnetic resonance (MR) studies. A clinical MR examination is nearly always designed to explore proton spins and can be used, for example, to investigate the spin density (proton density). Alternatively, MRI can be obtained with 'weight-ing' to reflect the relaxation parameters T1 or T2. These variables describe the rapidity with which the spin magnetization returns to a state of equilibrium after excitation. MRI with T1-weighting provides exquisite delineation of morphology, and T2-weighted images offer unmatched sensitivity to certain disease processes, including those of MS. In fact, MRI is arguably the most important test performed in the diagnostic workup of MS, with far greater impact than analysis of cerebrospinal fluid or testing of evoked potentials.[5]

Conventional MRI techniques with relaxation-time weighting incorporate the implicit assumption that a region of tissue may be fully described using the aforementioned parameters: T1, T2, and proton density. Thus, a region of hyperintensity on T2-weighted imaging is characterized by relatively longer T2. The determination of whether an area is hyperintense or isointense may be subjective and relies on the specific display parameters chosen as well as on the experience of the evaluator. Additionally, conventional MRI does not provide quantitative measurements on an absolute scale. Thus, a region may be described as hyperintense without any conclusions being drawn about the magnitude of change in T2 that was responsible for the observation.

By comparison, MT techniques in MRI begin with the assumption that more than one relaxation time may influence the MR observation in a region. Specifically, tissue is treated as a more complicated structure that includes not only protons in water molecules, but also non-water protons associated with proteins and other large molecules. The constraints of the MR experiment prevent non-water protons from being detected directly, but it has been postulated that the effects of non-water protons may be probed by way of their effects on the water protons. This assumption, confirmed in part by experimental work, forms the basis of current MT techniques.

MT theory holds that proton spins, which have well-known relaxation properties, can exchange spin magnetization with protons of much larger molecules. This theory was delineated using coupled Bloch[6] equations modified to incorporate chemical exchange of nuclear MR-visible spins[7] and was supported by pioneering experimentation in chemical exchange models probed via MR spectroscopy.[8–10] These experiments were based upon the idea that if nuclei were being exchanged in a chemical process, the spin magnetization associated with the nuclei would also be exchanged in the process.[11] The currently accepted view of MT relies on cross-relaxation of spins instead of actual physical exchange, but the mathematics needed to describe the effect are identical.[11] The consequence of these exchange processes in human MRI is that observed proton relaxation times may reflect not only the characteristics of water protons but also the characteristics of the macromolecular environment. The advantages of exploiting MT processes to influence MRI contrast are apparent. MT techniques can provide quantitative information but also, more importantly, MT analysis represents a window into the structure of tissue. Additionally, MT analysis may provide new MR-based tissue analysis complementary to T1, T2, and proton density. The availability of even a single new independent variable could be essential to improved sensitivity or specificity of the MR examination. In MS, where conventional MRI is highly sensitive, MT offers the potential of improved specificity, which could aid in diagnosis, in the evaluation of disease progression, or in the assessment of the therapeutic efficacy of novel treatments.

The two-site exchange model

In biological tissue, where proton spins are those typically of interest for MR study, there exist many 'relaxation environments' corresponding to a variety of proton-containing macromolecules as well as to water. Water protons are characterized by the relatively long values of T1 and T2 that are associated with liquids. The relaxation environment for protons attached to macromolecules is, by comparison, more solid-like, with correspondingly short transverse relaxation (T2) times. Direct observation of these spins is precluded by the shortness of T2 relaxation, which has the effect of making the signal decay too fast for observation. It is further complicated by the fact that the resonance frequency of the macromolecular protons is near or identical to that of water. A two-site model is useful in understanding the observed behavior and in formulating techniques for data acquisition and analysis. In the model (*Figure 6.1*), spins are determined to belong either to the 'water' compartment or the 'macromolecular' compartment. It is assumed that each compartment is associated with intrinsic relaxation times T1 and T2. These should be distinguished from observed relaxation times that are measured with standard techniques. Except in special cases, it should not be assumed that intrinsic and observed relaxation times are equal. With the addition of a rate constant, k, and a molecular ratio, f, the exchange characteristics of the two-site system can be completely described using six variables. More complex models are possible and may be desirable in some cases,[12] but applications to date have not required models incorporating more than two sites.

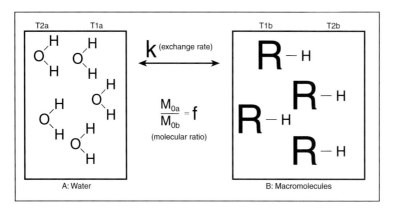

Fig. 6.1 A two-site model for MT, illustrating six parameters required for full characterization: intrinsic relaxation times T1 and T2 for 'a' and 'b' compartments, a pseudo first order exchange rate describing the transfer of magnetization between compartments, and a molecular ratio.

Selective saturation

As noted, MT methods seek to probe the macro-molecular protons in tissue by indirect means. A fundamental requirement for detecting the effects of one spin compartment as opposed to those of another is the ability to perform an MR study that is selective with respect to the spin compart-ment of interest. Saturation of spin magnetization is the historical method of choice for this purpose, as employed in the 'double resonance' experiments of Forsen and Hoffman,[8–10] who used a system of two chemically exchanging sub-stances for which the resonance frequencies dif-fered in the two spin systems. Briefly, saturating radio frequency excitation was applied at each spin resonance in turn while the magnetization of the opposite spin resonance was measured. The data obtained enabled the full characterization of the system. In contrast, the first 'MT' studies to be performed in vivo were based on selective inversion of the water spins, dubbed 'selective hydration inversion'.[13,14] Again, two experi-ments were performed in order to elucidate the behavior of the system with and without the inclusion of exchange effects.

With any of these methods, the analysis is similar. Comparison is sought between a baseline condition and a condition in which the spin system of interest has been perturbed in some way, and the extent of the effect is arrived at through measurement of the unperturbed system.

MAGNETIZATION TRANSFER IMAGING

MRI studies based on these ideas have been per-formed following the observation that radiofre-quency excitation, applied off-resonance, exhibits a preferential saturation effect on the short-T2 macromolecules. The first such study employed continuous radiofrequency excitation via a sepa-rate channel,[15] and subsequent experiments used off-resonance pulsed radiofrequency excitation, in which the MT saturation pulses were given in an interleaved fashion with the transmit and receive signals to and from the radiofrequency coil.[16] Another approach was introduced after the method of selective hydration inversion and was based on so-called on-resonance pulsed radiofrequency excitation,[17] in which a specific pulse combination given on-resonance produced the effect of a single off-resonance pulse. A theoretical treatment detailing off-resonance selective saturation has also been provided.[18]

The quantitative endpoint of any of the experimental MT techniques is a value representing the difference in spin magnetization of the observed nuclei between the baseline condition and the saturation condition. For example, one might add MT saturation pulses to a standard MRI sequence in order to study a sample exhibiting the MT effect and containing water and macromolecular spins. Assuming that the saturation is perfectly selective, meaning that the equilibrium magnetization of the macromolecular spins is reduced to zero while the water spin magnetization is not directly affected, the water spin magnetization will be maintained at a reduced value in the steady state. The decrease is attributable to the exchange of zero-magnetization spins for spins with finite magnetization. Moreover, the decrease will be larger in regions where the exchange of magnetization is more 'efficient', where efficiency is potentially a function of any of the six variables introduced above. In practice, despite the fact that selective saturation is never perfectly selective in vivo, contrast between areas exhibiting varying degrees of MT effect is developed and superimposed on the intrinsic contrast of the baseline image, be it proton-density weighting, T1 weighting, or some combination of these. In such an image, areas with highly efficient MT are dark, demonstrating that the saturation, or the reduced magnitude of longitudinal magnetization of the macromolecular spins, has been transferred to the water spins. MT contrast is used in a qualitative manner for applications including magnetic resonance angiography (MRA) and as a means of enhancing contrast visibility when exogenous contrast agents are given.

These techniques are successful because the MT effect is generally efficient in tissues and relatively ineffective in fluids. In MRA, this translates into reduced tissue intensity, while blood remains bright. In studies with injected gadolinium contrast agent, incorporation of MT pulses into the imaging sequence can provide additional tissue suppression to allow the contrast-affected tissues to appear brighter. Appropriate control studies should be used in this case to ensure that the two independent effects are not confused. These applications of MT are now well established and implemented on many commercial scanners, in conjunction with both gradient-echo and spin-echo pulse sequences.

Optimizing the magnetization transfer imaging examination

It should be noted that, although MT-prepared pulse sequences are now available to some degree on state-of-the-art clinical MR scanners, they may not be optimized for the acquisition of quantitative data and are almost certainly not optimized for all possible applications. Furthermore, there is great variability in the number of parameters that can be manipulated on any given scanner. MT saturation pulses can be added as a preparation to many pulse sequences used in clinical protocols. In order to make reasonable choices in acquisition parameters, it is useful to consider the pulsed off-resonance method of achieving MT saturation. It is well known that continuous application of radiofrequency energy at the resonance frequency will lead to saturation of the overall spin magnetization. That is, the spin magnetization will be near zero magnitude and thus examining the magnetization with an MRI sequence will yield zero signal. Similar results are obtained in the steady state under conditions of pulsed application of radiofrequency. As the radiofrequency excitation is moved off-resonance, the saturation effect diminishes and goes to zero for large offset frequencies. However, the saturation effect is dependent on the relaxation times of the affected spins, in such a way that solid-like macromolecular spins still experience some degree of saturation at relatively high offset frequencies.[18] This observation enables the selective saturation of the macromolecular spins, which makes the MT study possible. It is also observed that, for any given offset frequency, a larger magnitude of applied radiofrequency energy results in a greater degree of saturation for all spins.

The two essential parameters needed to describe the application of saturating radiofrequency energy are then 'effective offset frequency', and 'effective saturation amplitude'. The modifier 'effective' is added to generalize the argument and will be assumed in the discussion below. It is useful because in techniques other than pulsed off-resonance MT, including those where pulse trains are given on resonance to provide selective saturation, it is possible to establish the analogous equivalent frequencies and amplitudes to permit direct comparison with the continuous off-resonance radiofrequency case.[19] On MRI scanners where MT is implemented using off-resonance pulses, the offset frequency can usually be read directly and modified as a machine variable or a control variable. The amplitude, on the other hand, may be given in degrees as a flip angle, calculated by predicting the angle that spins would rotate if the pulse were given on-resonance. Although this flip angle does not have a physical basis, it can be used to calculate the strength of the MT saturation in more conventional units. Other possible variables

are saturation pulse shape and duration, which also must be included in the calculation of effective saturation amplitude. When these variables are taken into consideration, it is possible to generalize quantitative results from different groups that have been acquired with different scanning equipment.

An additional consideration is the possibility of approaching or exceeding limits on power deposition in the body, such as those established as guidelines by the US Food and Drug Administration. Under these circumstances it may be useful to decrease the effective saturation amplitude along with the offset frequency, recognizing that, in order to compare studies directly, both parameters must match.

Again, MT saturation can be implemented as a preparation to nearly any pulse sequence, but there is a reason to consider using a baseline scan that minimizes relaxation time weighting, in order to avoid competing or canceling effects. For rapid acquisition, some centers have opted for gradient–echo-based imaging with low flip angle to minimize T1 weighting, and the shortest possible echo time to minimize T2 weighting.

The saturation effects on both water and macromolecular spins continuously decrease as the offset frequency is increased and saturation amplitude is held constant. This response was dubbed the Z-spectrum and proposed as a means of characterizing tissue and of investigating the MT effect.[20,21] *Figure 6.2* provides examples of experimentally derived Z-spectra. There is no sharp boundary between regions where direct on-resonance saturation of the water spins is important, as opposed to regions where the transfer of saturated magnetization from macromolecular spins dominates the observation. Rather, both effects are likely to be present in any envisioned experiment. It follows that the observed MT effect is highly dependent on the experimental

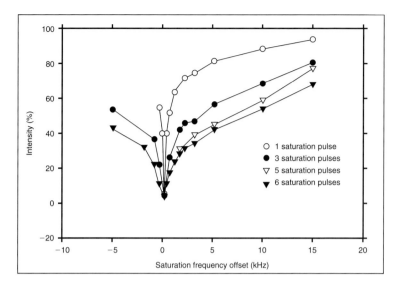

Fig. 6.2 *Intensity, expressed as a percentage of control intensity, varying with saturation offset frequency in an MT study of newborn piglet brain. Four 'Z-spectra' are shown, corresponding to 1, 3, 5 and 6 identical saturation pulses per repetition of the sequence. The saturation effect is non-linear in both effective saturation amplitude and offset frequency.[16] Reproduced with permission J Magn Reson 1994.*

parameters. On the other hand, theoretical prediction and experimental observation confirm that the technique is robust and reproducible when attention is paid to the acquisition parameters.

QUANTITATIVE ANALYSIS OF MT

Measurement of the MT ratio

The raw intensity of a region in an image obtained with MT contrast reflects the proton density in that region as well as relaxation-based weighting, which is always present to some degree, depending on the image acquisition parameters. For this reason it is desirable to normalize the MT data, and in so doing to calculate an index of MT effect, which may be independent of other tissue parameters. A typical practice is to calculate an MT ratio (MTR), given below in a form equivalent to that of the originators.[22]

$$\text{MTR} = \left(1 - \frac{M_s}{M_o}\right) \times 100\%$$

Here M_s refers to the intensity of a region of interest (ROI) or a pixel under conditions of MT saturation, and M_0 refers to the intensity of the same region or pixel as measured on the control study. In this equation, the ratio of intensities is subtracted from unity in order to establish MTR as a measure that increases with the MT effect. Since division is involved one must be careful to avoid small numbers in the denominator, so if the MT analysis is applied to an entire image, pixels with near-zero intensity values (including regions without tissue present) must be excluded. To the extent that the saturation is not perfectly selective, the MTR is not an absolute measure.

Rather, it is a function of the amplitude of the effective saturating radiofrequency as well as of its frequency offset.[18,21] The MTR can be explored with a variety of techniques, including ROI analysis,[22] contour mapping,[23,24] and histograms.[25,26]

Measurement of k and the effect of exchange on observed T1

The variation of observed T1 caused by the exchange of magnetization is understood and is fundamental to double resonance techniques. Specifically, in the presence of saturation pulses used to detect MT in vivo, the observed T1 relaxation time is shortened, consistent with theory and previous experimental results.[27] This observation suggests that the measurement of T1 in the presence of saturation (T1sat) can provide another MR parameter for study. Such data can be obtained through an inversion recovery experiment with and without incorporated saturation pulses. However, accurate measurement of T1 can be time consuming, and relatively few studies have probed the T1sat effect. An argument previously advanced for the measurement of T1sat suggested its use in obtaining an estimate of k, the pseudo first-order exchange rate. The attraction for doing so is clear, since k would represent an absolute number directly connected to the exchange process, as opposed to the MTR, which varies with the experimental conditions. The exchange rate k is unfortunately challenging to measure in vivo, owing to the difficulty of direct observation of the macromolecular spin system, which precludes a classic 'double resonance' approach. Although there are a number of published reports documenting calculation of k based on simplified coupled Bloch equations, the tech-

nique for doing so relies on the establishment of a perfect selective saturation condition, which is not possible in practice.[28] The result of this observation is that the parameters k and T1sat are, as is MTR, dependent upon acquisition conditions. Still to be answered are questions regarding their independence from one another and from other parameters measurable by MR.

Consideration should be given to the T1-shortening effects of MT saturation when experimental studies are designed. For example, if a scan protocol incorporates both T1 weighting and MT saturation, the eventual result may be difficult to interpret. A region with effective MT will tend to be darker on an MT-weighted image, owing to the transfer of saturated spins into the observed spin pool, but the same MT process will shorten T1, leading to a brighter appearance on the final image in accordance with the T1 weighting. In practice, the latter effect is relatively small, but different acquisition techniques may skew the importance of the competing effects. For this reason quantitative MT studies are often conducted in a way which minimizes T1 weighting of the acquired images.

ROI analysis

ROI analysis is typically the first method used to evaluate quantitative imaging results. To characterize the MT effect, it is desirable to obtain two images: an image acquired in the presence of selective saturation of the macromolecular spins and a control image identical in all respects except for omission of saturation. The images should be acquired at the same time with no motion of the subject between acquisitions. Alternatively, the images could be registered to one another via rotation and translation operations, although this is typically not essential.

If a particular structure is of interest, a simple ROI analysis of a defined area may be most useful. Homogeneity of the structure and clearly defined physical boundaries, which ideally will not overlap the boundaries of the ROI, will maximize the precision of the measurement. The selected pixel locations on both images should then be used to find corresponding intensities, which will be subjected to the equation above to find the MTR of the region.

If, on the other hand, the region is well defined or if the whole image must be examined, it is useful to compute a pixel-by-pixel MTR map. To do so one must exclude pixels of low (near-zero) intensity, which could cause the results of the equation to be very large. This can be done via segmentation of brain parenchyma for analysis. Alternatively, a simple threshold can be applied, perhaps to exclude any pixels that have intensities lower than 10% of the maximum intensity of the proton-density-weighted control image. Both techniques exclude pixels corresponding to noise, whether external to the body being studied or within voids such as sinuses. With either technique, an index of pixels subsequently analysed can be maintained so that the eventual results can be put back into image format and viewed as a map of MTR. An example of an image with MT weighting, together with its corresponding MT map, is given in *Fig. 6.3*. In this MS patient, one can see the high degree of variation present in the extent of abnormality of white matter, and also note that in fluids such as cerebrospinal fluid, the MT effect is small, as predicted by theory.

APPLICATIONS OF MT TO MS

The MTR in an ROI

ROI analysis of MT is commonly used in the study of MS and of animal models for the disease. Early experiments used MTR to characterize inflammatory lesions in a guinea pig model of experimental allergic encephalomyelitis (EAE) without demyelination.[22] Companion experiments in human volunteers and MS patients were carried out with identical techniques, allowing comparison of results. The initial observation was that MTR was reduced in all lesions detected via T2-weighted imaging. Further analysis suggested that MT might differentiate between inflammation and demyelination by virtue of smaller observed MT changes in the inflammatory lesions. Additionally, it was noted that some macroscopically normal tissue in MS patients appeared to be abnormal by MT findings. The observation of abnormal MTR in normal-appearing white matter (NAWM) was consistent with previous histopathological findings of microscopic damage caused by MS in macroscopically normal tissue.[29] The findings of reduced MT in MS as well as the presence of abnormal MT in NAWM were subsequently confirmed by other investigators, who noted areas of lowered MT in regions adjacent to lesions[30] and in frontal lobe NAWM.[31] More recently, it was suggested that changes in NAWM detectable by MTR analysis preceded the development of new MS lesion by several months.[32] These results were obtained in a study group of 10 patients who were imaged monthly employing MT imaging along with gadolinium-enhanced T1-weighted imaging, which is the 'gold standard' for detection of new MS lesion. In contrast other investigators found no significant MTR

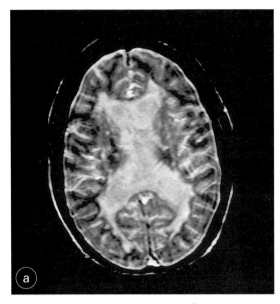 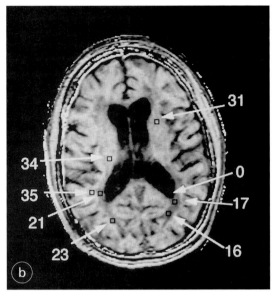

Fig. 6.3 *MT imaging in a patient with MS. (a) An image with MT contrast, where darker regions represent greater MT saturation effect. (b) The corresponding MT map, arrived at by normalizing the MT image using an image obtained without MT saturation (i.e. by obtaining the MT ratio). Higher intensity corresponds to greater MTR on the MT map. Regions of interest are shown with regional average MT values depicted, demonstrating the range and variance of abnormal tissue in MS.*

reduction before the appearance of lesions in three patients studied weekly.[33] Further study is warranted to resolve the discrepancy.

The natural history of MS lesions was probed by examining MTR in lesions differentiated by enhancement pattern, with the highest MTRs corresponding to homogeneously enhancing lesions, lower values in non-enhancing lesions, and the lowest values in the central portion of ring-enhancing lesions.[34] These results led to speculation on a pattern whereby homogeneously enhancing lesions, representing early inflammatory lesions, might evolve to ring-enhancing or non-enhancing lesions. The center portion of the ring-

enhancing lesion might subsequently deactivate, changing the lesion to non-enhancing status. Resumed activity in the lesion might return it to a ring-enhancing presentation, but as the tissue became demyelinated and devascularized there would eventually be no return to enhancement.[34]

ROI analysis was also used in a study that tested the sensitivity of MT to histopathological changes in a feline model of wallerian degeneration.[35] In this study, MT provided a reliable indication of structural changes at a time when such changes were not detected via conventional imaging or with light microscopy, but were able to be confirmed by electron microscopy. The biphasic response demonstrated by MT corresponded to known histologic phases of wallerian degeneration,[35] supporting the idea that quantitative MT imaging could provide a window on tissue structure. Finally, one study using ROI analysis of MT detected some correlation between MTR and clinical disability.[36]

Drawbacks of ROI analysis include potential difficulties in reproducibility resulting from the drawing technique and the operator dependence on placement of the ROI. Hand-drawn ROIs are particularly suspect, and ROIs of fixed shape may not be optimal for the structure being examined. If the ROI is near a boundary, partial volume effects may influence the results. Since MS is a disease that is characterized by focal lesions, small errors in placement of the ROI may result in relatively large errors. Finally, regions of different size may exhibit differences in variance, with contributions from both the heterogeneity of the tissue and the number of pixels included, which complicates statistical comparison.

Histogram analysis based on MTR

In MS, analysis of MT data by ROI yields information about disease progression and extent. However, ROI analysis is not well suited to global characterization of MS, in which both macroscopic and microscopic pathology are known to be present. Techniques that involve histogram analysis were developed as an alternative to using a series of ROIs. By constructing an MTR histogram, one gives up spatial information present in an image and instead looks at the distribution of MTR values. Histograms thus provide a means of estimating the relative volumes of tissues characterized by specific ranges of MTR and allow conclusions to be drawn regarding both focal and diffuse aspects of the disease.

A histogram is a graph showing the numbers of pixels on the vertical axis corresponding to specified ranges of values on the horizontal axis. The entire range of horizontal axis values is divided into 'bins', with 'bin size' used to describe the interval of values corresponding to a single bin. An MTR histogram can be drawn directly from an MTR map image obtained as described above. However, selection of an appropriate 'bin size' must be done consistently and will influence the appearance of the histogram as well as the numerical parameters used to describe it. Too many bins will produce a histogram with peak characteristics diminished and with excessive noise. Too few bins results in loss of the distribution information that the histogram is intended to provide. The optimal size may be the smallest number of bins that produces a smooth appearance of the histogram, and it is related to the noise present in the raw data. It is worthwhile to note that parameters which may be extracted from histograms for use as numerical indices, such as peak height and peak location, may be modulated by bin size.

MT histograms in the brains of MS patients reflect a weighted distribution of disease in tissue. They are typically characterized by a single relatively sharp peak, which is asymmetric, having a preponderance of pixels with lower MTR compared to the peak value. The location of the peak may be lower than in control subjects where it typically corresponds to normal MTR values in white matter. The histogram is weighted in that it reflects the presence of a small number of pixels with sharply lowered MTR, such as would be the case in an MS lesion, as well as the presence of many pixels with slightly lowered MTR, corresponding to MR occult disease in white matter.

In one study of 26 subjects,[25] MT histograms were constructed using MTR maps from the five consecutive MRI slices rostral from the anterior commissure. Thus, a slab with a total thickness of 2.5 cm was examined from a brain region where a relative minimum of extracerebral tissue was present. The chosen brain volume also contained the periventricular area, including the corona radiata and centrum semiovale, sites of prediliction for MS lesions. A bin size of 1% MTR was chosen and results were normalized to account for differences in brain volume and slice area. Results of this study indicated that, even with a relatively crude technique and no segmentation, the peak height of the histogram was a highly significant indicator of the presence of disease. Another observation was that, although the location of the peak was not different between groups, the distribution of pixels in the MS group was significantly shifted towards lower values. A longitudinal component of this study showed that peak height also decreased over time in a subgroup of seven patients, and that there did not appear to be a relationship between the peak height change and Kurtzke expanded disability status scale (EDSS) or ambulation index.[25]

Further study was conducted with a combination of highly observer-independent segmentation and MT histogram analysis, in order to develop histograms of the whole brain of patients with MS.[26] Results were similar, primarily limited to peak height changes with disease. Shape differences in the histograms were also quantified, using a new parameter MTR_x, defined as the xth percentile of the histogram (i.e. that MT value where the integral of the histogram was equal to x% of the total). In this study MTR_{25} and MTR_{50} were differed between patients and controls, whereas MTR_{75} did not differ. These results suggested a role for MTR histograms in monitoring disease progression, with potential application to therapeutic trials. On the other hand, there still existed the paradox that disease severity by MT was not strongly correlated to disease severity by clinical parameters.

A larger study in 44 patients indicated that certain MTR histogram parameters are correlated with clinical status and neuropsychological test results.[37] A new parameter was added: unnormalized histogram peak height (H_{ap}), which up to then had been normalized to exclude effects of atrophy, but was now left unnormalized in an effort to include those effects. The H_{ap} was found to exhibit significant correlation with disease duration. This result was in contrast with previous studies showing minimal correlations between duration of disease and MRI lesion load,[38,39] and it appeared to support the idea that the course of MS is characterized by long-term progression. Results also suggested that increasing physical disability was accompanied by an increasing shift of the MTR distribution in the direction of lower values, highlighted by changes in MTR_{50} and MTR_{25}. Correlations with clinical disability were weak, perhaps owing to the exclusion of spinal cord tissue from analysis and the relative high weighting of the EDSS and AI tests towards motor pathways. With regard to neuropsychological testing, the unnormalized histogram peak height was again the most sensitive indicator of clinical status, and it discriminated between patients classified as normal, moderately impaired, and severely impaired. This suggested that the clinical neuropsychological manifestations of MS were a function of both both atrophy and tissue disruption.

In a study designed to examine the effects of treatment with interferon-β 1b, the parameters most strongly correlated with disease duration were the location of the histogram peak and the global mean MTR[40]. In this population of nine patients with relapsing–remitting MS, who exhibited a high frequency of enhancing lesions, there was a reduction in both MTR parameters. During the first 6 months of treatment, there was no detectable change in the histogram parameters, although new enhancing lesions decreased in frequency. This study suggested that treatment with interferon-β 1b does not enhance improvement in the structure of the affected tissue.

Finally, in a rat model of spinal cord injury using a standard weight-drop paradigm, MTR histogram parameters were used to probe the extent of injury and correlation with histopathology. A new parameter was introduced, the area of the histogram corresponding to statistically 'normal' white matter as determined by control studies. It was found to be most highly correlated with weight drop in the model. All histogram parameters were found to be correlated with each other to some degree, and all were found to be highly correlated with histopathology, indicating the potential in this model for non-invasive measures of the extent of tissue injury. Finally, MTR-based parameters were noted to be slightly better than pathology at eliciting weight-drop height from the data. *Figure 6.4* is a composite MTR histogram from the study population, demonstrating the global shift that accompanied different drop-heights, and illustrating the 'normal range of white matter,' which was found to be a most successful analysis parameter.[41]

Contour plotting of MTR

A relatively novel method for viewing MTR data is to display the MTR values as an overlay on the MTR or another image, using contour mapping. The object of such a display is to enable the detection of gradients and boundaries of abnormal MTR that are too subtle to be detected by conventional 'reading' of the image. Contour plotting was applied in an animal study of diffuse axonal injury (DAI) designed to test the correlation between MTR histopathologic characteristics. Brain MRI of the injured animals was read as normal both immediately following the injury and 1 week later, making it unlikely that significant contributions from hemorrhage were present. MT ratio contours were used to identify areas of abnormal MTR that were statistically different from normal tissue (i.e. 2 standard deviations from normal). Selected regions were also constrained so as to be separate from boundaries where damage was expected to be worse but partial volume effects could contaminate the results. Results indicated that MTR analysis had a positive predictive value of 67% for pathology-positive lesions—89% if the MTR was abnormal on the acute MRI. Corresponding negative predictive values were 56% and 61%.[23] These results suggest that gains in sensitivity and specificity may be realized using contour plotting.

Contour plotting was employed to investigate the appearance of lesion boundaries in MS brain, and specifically to probe 'halo' lesions. Findings indicated that most or all MS lesions examined demonstrated a gradient of MTR at the boundaries, as opposed to a sharp delineation between diseased and normal tissue. This was also in contrast to observations in human DAI lesions, which were by comparison well-circumscribed.[42,43] *Figure 6.5* gives examples of two contour plots in MS.

A final observation that is consistent with the view of MTR as a window on tissue structure was found in a dog model of Krabbe disease. Here, known patterns of demyelination associated with the disease were clearly observed in an

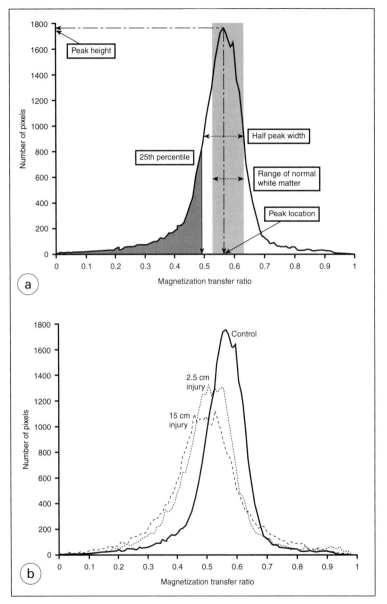

Fig. 6.4 *(a) An example MTR histogram labeled with analysis parameters employed for evaluation of injury and/or disease extent. (b) Histograms in a rat spinal cord injury model, including an average control histogram and average histograms corresponding to weight-drop injuries with 2.5 cm and 15 cm drop heights.*

affected animal and were found to be in sharp contrast to diffuse damage caused by radiation in a treated affected dog and a sham-irradiated animal.[44] Contour plotting revealed the charac-teristic inside-to-out demyelination in this model in a way that ROI analysis was unable to do, suggesting future applications of 'non-invasive histopathology'.

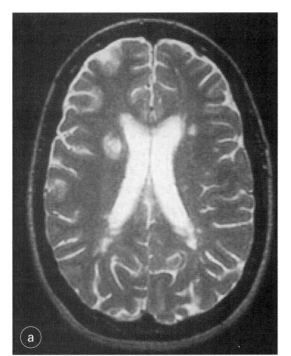

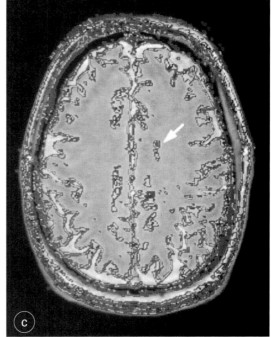

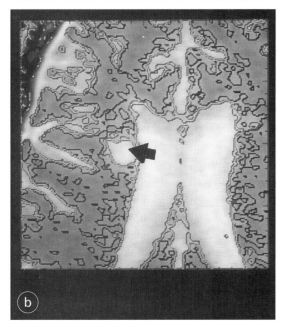

Fig. 6.5 *(a) An example of an MT image in MS with focal lesions in the periventricular white matter. (b) An MT contour plot demonstrating the gradation of MTR values from the low MTR center of the large focal lesion (thick arrow) to the NAWM. The contours are drawn at 2, 4, and 6 standard deviations below normal values as obtained from age-matched control subjects. A smaller lesion on the contralateral side is shown to be asymmetric with regard to MTR. (c) In another patient, a small focal MS lesion is demonstrated to be 6 standard deviations below normal (white arrow) but also to be extended into normal-appearing tissue by MT contours at 2 standard deviations below normal.*

SUMMARY

Analysis of MT effects provides a quantitative methodology for evaluation of disease progress in MS and potentially for monitoring therapeutic intervention. Advantages of the techniques discussed above include the inherent normalization of the MT ratio and the ability to use or discard the spatial information as appropriate to the application. Several studies have independently confirmed correlations between MTR and histopathology in brain tissue, offering the possibility of obtaining information about tissue structure in a non-invasive manner. Histogram techniques may be particularly appropriate for tracking global changes caused by novel treatments and therapeutic agents. Refinements in the techniques and equipment used for acquisition of MT images should result in more precise measures of the MT effect and eventually in more specific techniques for non-invasive MR based evaluation of MS patients.

ACKNOWLEDGEMENTS

Robert I Grossman, MD and Dennis L Kolson, MD PhD read the manuscript and provided valuable suggestions, and Mr Jeffrey Berman assisted in the preparation of the figures. Additionally, support of the National Institutes of Health (NS34353) is gratefully acknowledged.

REFERENCES

1 Prineas JW, McDonald WI, eds. Demyelinating Diseases. In: Graham DI, Lantos PL, eds, *Greenfield's Neuropathology*, 6th edn, London: Arnold, 1997, 813–896.

2 Trapp BD, Peterson J, Ransohoff RM et al. Axonal transection in the lesions of multiple sclerosis. *N Engl J Med* 1998; **338**:278–285.

3 Raine C. Axonal dystrophy as a consequence of long-term demyelination. *Lab Invest* 1989; **60**:714–725.

4 Ferguson B, Matyszak MK, Esiri MM, Perry VH. Axonal damage in acute multiple sclerosis lesions. *Brain* 1997; **120**:393–399.

5 Giang DW, Grow VM, Mooney C et al. Clinical diagnosis of multiple sclerosis. The impact of magnetic resonance imaging and ancillary testing. Rochester–Toronto Magnetic Resonance Study Group. *Arch Neurol* 1994; **51**:61–66.

6 Bloch F. Nuclear induction. *Phys Rev* 1946; **70**:460–474.

7 McConnell HM. Reaction rates by nuclear magnetic resonance. *J Chem Phys* 1958; **28**:430–431.

8 Forsen S, Hoffman R. A new method for the study of moderately rapid chemical exchange rates employing nuclear magnetic double resonance. *Acta Chem Scand* 1963; **17**:1787–1788.

9 Forsen S, Hoffman R. Exchange rates by nuclear magnetic multiple resonance. III. Exchange reactions in systems with several nonequivalent sites. *J Chem Phys* 1964; **40**:1189–1196.

10 Forsen S, Hoffman R. Study of moderately rapid chemical exchange reactions by means of nuclear magnetic double resonance. *J Chem Phys* 1963; **39**:2892–2901.

11 Hoffman RA, Forsen S. Transient and steady-state overhauser experiments in the investigation of relaxation processes. Analogies between chemical exchange and relaxation. *J Chem Phys* 1966; **45**:2049–2060.

12 McGowan JC, Schotland J, Leigh J. Oscillations, stability, and equilibrium in magnetic exchange networks. *J Magn Reson (A)* 1994; **108**:201–205.

13 Edzes HT, Samulski ET. Cross relaxation and spin diffusion in the proton NMR of hydrated collagen. *Nature* 1977; **265**:521–523.

14 Edzes HT, Samulski ET. The measurement of cross-relaxation effects in the proton NMR spin-lattice relaxation of water in biological systems: hydrated collagen and muscle. *J Magn Reson* 1978; **31**:207–229.

15 Wolff SD, Balaban RS. Magnetization transfer contrast (MTC) and tissue water proton relaxation in vivo. *Magn Reson Med* 1989; **10**:135–144.

16 McGowan JC, Schnall MD, Leigh JS. Magnetization

transfer imaging with pulsed off-resonance saturation: contrast variation with saturation duty cycle. *J Magn Reson* 1994; **4**:79–82.

17 Hu BS, Conolly SM, Wright GA et al. Pulsed saturation transfer contrast. *Magn Reson Med* 1992; **26**:231–240.

18 McGowan JC, Leigh J. Selective saturation in magnetization transfer experiments. *Magn Reson Med* 1994; **32**:517–522.

19 McGowan JC. *Characterization of Biological Tissue with Magnetization Transfer*. University of Pennsylvania, 1993.

20 Grad J, Mendelson D, Hyder F, Bryant RG. Direct measurements of longitudinal relaxation and magnetization transfer in heterogeneous systems. *J Magn Reson* 1990; **86**:416–419.

21 Grad J, Bryant RG. Nuclear magnetic cross-relaxation spectroscopy. *J Magn Reson* 1990; **90**:1–8.

22 Dousset V, Grossman RI, Ramer KN et al. Experimental allergic encephalomyelitis and multiple sclerosis: lesion characterization with magnetization transfer imaging (published erratum appears in *Radiology* 1992; **183**:878). *Radiology* 1992; **182**:483–491.

23 McGowan JC, McCormack TM, Grossman R et al. Diffuse axonal pathology detected with magnetization transfer imaging following brain injury in the pig. *Magn Reson Med* 1999; **41**:727–733.

24 Kasner SE, Galetta SL, McGowan JC, Grossman RI. Magnetization transfer imaging in progressive multifocal leukoencephalopathy. *Neurology* 1997; **48**:534–536.

25 van Buchem MA, McGowan JC, Kolson DL et al. Quantitative volumetric magnetization transfer analysis in multiple sclerosis: estimation of macroscopic and microscopic disease burden. *Magn Reson Med* 1996; **36**:632–636.

26 van Buchem MA, Udupa JK, McGowan JC et al. Global volumetric estimation of disease burden in multiple sclerosis based on magnetization transfer imaging. *AJNR* 1997; **18**:1287–1290.

27 Mann BE. The application of the Forsen–Hoffman spin-saturation method of measuring rates of exchange to the 13C NMR spectrum of N, N-dimethylformamide. *J Magn Reson* 1977; **25**:91–94.

28 Yeung H. On the treatment of the transient response of a heterogeneous spin system to selective RF saturation. *Magn Reson Med* 1993; **30**:146–147.

29 Allen I, McKeown S. A histological histochemical and biochemical study of the macroscopically normal white matter in multiple sclerosis. *J Neurol Sci* 1979; **41**:81–91.

30 Hiehle JFJ Jr, Grossman RI, Ramer KN et al. Magnetization transfer effects in MR-detected multiple sclerosis lesions: comparison with gadolinium-enchanced spin-echo images and nonenhanced T1-weighted images. *AJNR* 1995; **16** (**suppl 1**):69–77.

31 Filippi M, Campi A, Dousset V et al. A magnetization transfer imaging study of normal-appearing white matter in multiple sclerosis. *Neurology* 1995; **45**:478–482.

32 Filippi M, Rocca MA, Martino G et al. Magnetization transfer changes in the normal appearing white matter precede the appearance of enhancing lesions in patients with multiple sclerosis. *Ann Neurol* 1998; **43**:809–814.

33 Silver NC, Lai M, Symms MR et al. Serial magnetization transfer imaging to characterize the early evolution of new MS lesions. *Neurology* 1998; **51**:758–764.

34 Petrella JR, Grossman RI, McGowan JC et al. Multiple sclerosis lesions: relationship between MR enhancement pattern and magnetization transfer effect. *AJNR* 1996; **17**:1041–1049.

35 Lexa FJ, Grossman RI, Rosenquist AC. MR of wallerian degeneraion in the feline visual system: characterization by magnetization transfer rate with histopathologic correlation. *AJNR* 1994; **15**:201–212.

36 Gass A, Barker GJ, Kidd D et al. Correlation of magnetization transfer ratio with clinical disability in multiple sclerosis. *Ann Neurol* 1994; **36**:62–67.

37 van Buchem MA, Grossman RI, Armstrong C et al. Correlation of volumetric magnetization transfer imaging with clinical data in MS. *Neurology* 1998; **50**:1609–1617.

38 Edwards MK, Farlow MR, Stevens JC. Multiple sclerosis: MRI and clinical correlation. *AJNR* 1986; **7**:595–598.

39 Huber SJ, Paulson GW, Chakeres D et al. Magnetic resonance imaging and clinical correlations in multiple sclerosis. *J Neurol Sci* 1988; **86**:1–12.

40 Richert N, Ostuni J, Bash C et al. *Serial Monthly Magnetization Transfer (MT) Imaging in Relapsing Remitting Multiple Sclerosis Patients on Interferon Beta 1b: Analysis Using Whole Brain MT Histograms*. Vancouver: International Society of Magnetic Resonance in Medicine, 1997: 73.

41 Berman J, Hackney D, Ford J, McGowan J. *Magnetization Transfer Histograms to Determine the Severity of Spinal Cord Injury*. Chicago: Radiological Society of North America, 1998: 153.

42 **Bagley L, Grossman R, Lexa F et al.** *Magnetization Transfer Contour Plots: Measures of Multiple Sclerosis Lesion Extent.* Nice, France: Society of Magnetic Resonance, 1996: 282.

43 **Bagley LJ, Grossman RI, McGowan JC, Sinson G.** *Magnetization Transfer Imaging in the Detection of T2-Occult White Matter Lesions: a Predictor of Outcome in Traumatic Brain Injury?* Vancouver: International Society of Magnetic Resonance in Medicine, 1997: 76.

44 **McGowan J, Vite C, Wenger D et al.** Quantitative magnetization transfer imaging to monitor efficacy of bone marrow transplantation in globoid cell leukodystrophy. Chicago: Radiological Society of North America, 1998: 351.

7

Measures of T1 and T2 relaxation

Marianne AA van Walderveen and Frederik Barkhof

INTRODUCTION

In the last few years magnetic resonance (MR) technology has evolved rapidly, which has led to new insights in the pathology of multiple sclerosis (MS). MR imaging (MRI) shows abnormalities in more than 95% of patients with clinically definite MS.[1] In patients with suspected MS (who present with clinically isolated symptoms), an abnormal brain MRI scan has a positive predictive value of 65% for conversion to clinically definite MS after a follow-up of 5 years (and perhaps even higher with longer follow-up). On the other hand, a normal MRI scan of the brain *and* spinal cord can exclude the diagnosis of MS in nearly all cases.[2] Therefore, MRI is highly sensitive in the visualization of the pathology of MS and has a high negative predictive value in the diagnosis of MS.

Certain specific features on brain MRI make the diagnosis of MS more likely. MS lesions often have an irregular and confluent shape and are located in the periventricular region, especially around the frontal, occipital and temporal horn. A common feature is involvement of the corpus callosum, including the presence of subcallosal lesions and callosal atrophy. Furthermore, apart from scattering of lesions in the periventricular white matter, cortical and subcortical lesions can also be found. With improvements of MRI techniques, MRI of

the spinal cord has become common practice, and it shows focal and diffuse abnormalities.[3,4]

To improve the specificity of MRI in the diagnosis of MS, MR criteria have been defined. The diagnostic criteria of Paty et al,[1] consisting of the presence of four or more lesions on brain MRI scans or three lesions of which one is located in the periventricular region, has a sensitivity of 94% for MS but the specificity is rather low (57%). The specificity can be markedly improved if three or more lesions are visible on brain MRI with two of the three following features present:[5]

(a) size of a lesion ≥ 6 mm;

(b) lesion(s) abutting the ventricular bodies; or

(c) an infratentorial lesion.

More recently developed MR criteria showed that—in addition to infratentorial and periventricular lesions—the demonstration of gadolinium enhancement or the presence of a juxtacortical lesion are the most specific MRI characteristics for the diagnosis of MS in patients with clinically isolated syndromes.[6]

CONVENTIONAL PULSE SEQUENCES IN MS

The most commonly used MR pulse sequence in the diagnosis of MS is the spin echo (SE) pulse

91

sequence. In the SE sequence (*Fig. 7.1*), the magnetically aligned spins are brought to resonance with a 90° radiofrequency pulse. Dephasing of the spins, caused by magnetic field inhomogeneity and spin–spin interactions, lead to a gradual decay of the signal. This can partially be reversed by a rephasing 180° pulse, which produces a signal regain (or spin echo) after a time delay TE (the echo time). This pulse sequence (exciting 90° followed by a rephasing 180°) is repeated with a delay time TR (the repetition time) to collect sufficient information to create a high resolution MR image.

In SE imaging, image contrast is dependent on the TE and TR used, as well as on the inherent tissue parameters proton density (N(H)), T1 relaxation time and T2 relaxation time. The T1 relaxation time is the time constant that describes the transfer of energy from spins to their environment: the longitudinal or spin-lattice relaxation rate. The T2 relaxation time is the time constant that describes the transverse or spin–spin relaxation rate, a process that depends on spin–spin interactions and that induces dephasing of the MR signal. In biological tissues, typical T1 values range from about 50 msec to a few seconds. In general, the T2 relaxation time is shorter than the T1 relaxation time, and it ranges in biological tissues from a few microseconds in solids to a few seconds in liquids. The ability of MRI to create high contrast images of the brain depends on the differences in T1 and T2 relaxation times of the brain structures (see *Table 7.1*).

Apart from these inherent tissue parameters, MR contrast can be influenced by the user-selectable parameters TR and TE. Image contrast can be made T1-dominated ('T1-weighted') by using a short time interval between consecutive excitation pulses (short TR images). On the other hand, image contrast can be made T2-weighted (accentuating differences in T2 relaxation time) by allowing sufficient loss of phase coherence to occur before a refocusing pulse is applied to produce an echo (long TE images). To avoid T1 effects in the T2-weighted images the TR should be long, and therefore T2-weighted images have long TRs and long TEs. Proton density (PD) weighted images are obtained by choosing TR and TE so that T1 and T2 contrast effects are minimized; this is done by choosing long TRs and short TEs. In addition, one can add an extra inversion (180°) pulse to 'prepare' the magnetization before imaging. The time duration between

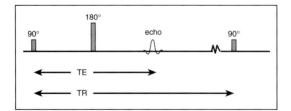

Fig. 7.1 Spin-echo pulse sequence. A 180° pulse is applied at time ½TE, causing the spins to get in phase at time TE (which leads to the formation of an echo). The repetition time (TR) is the time interval between two successive 90° pulses.

Table 7.1 Relaxation times for different brain tissues (determined at 1.5 Tesla).[7–11]

Tissue	T1 (ms)	T2 (ms)
White matter	521–718	63–67
Grey matter	858–1080	65–80
Putamen	826–1027	63–67
Thalamus	763–950	66–71
Internal capsule	555–700	61–77
CSF	2441–2610	345

this inversion pulse and the excitation pulse (the inversion time or TI) determines the image contrast (e.g. in short TI inversion recovery (STIR) imaging, the TI is very short, resulting in fat suppression).

MS lesions are detected as areas of increased T1 and T2 relaxation times relative to white matter of the brain. On PD-weighted images, the signal from cerebrospinal fluid (CSF) is suppressed, but T2 contrast is still preserved. Periventricular MS plaques can therefore easily be distinguished from adjacent CSF spaces because of greater signal intensity (*Fig. 7.2a*). On T2 weighted SE images, both CSF and MS lesions are displayed as very high-signal intensity (appearing bright), and there-

fore periventricular plaques can easily be obscured by partial volume effects (*Fig. 7.2b*).

Fluid-attenuated inversion recovery (FLAIR) sequences produce heavily T2-weighted images with suppression of the CSF signal by applying a long inversion time to produce nulling of CSF signal at the time of imaging. With the introduction of fast FLAIR, which is a more rapid imaging technique resulting in reduction of acquisition times, it is likely that this sequence may be increasingly used in the future for MS diagnosis and monitoring. Fast FLAIR is particularly sensitive in detecting juxtacortical lesions (*Fig. 7.3*), but lesions in the posterior fossa and spinal cord are more difficult to detect with fast

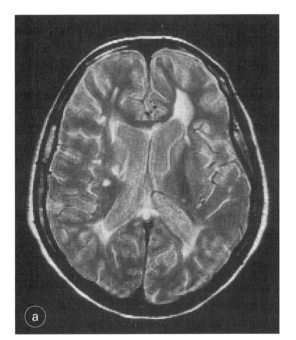 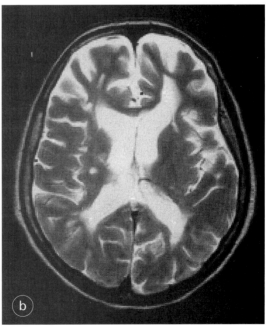

Fig. 7.2 *Proton density (PD) weighted (a) and T2-weighted (b) spin-echo MR images of an MS patient. On the PD-weighted MR image, the periventricular MS lesions (bright signal) are clearly distinguishable from the ventricles because of suppression of signal from cerebrospinal fluid (dark signal). On the corresponding T2-weighted MR image, cerebrospinal fluid has a high signal which hampers the distinction between the border of the ventricle and the border of the lesions.*

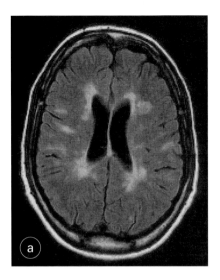
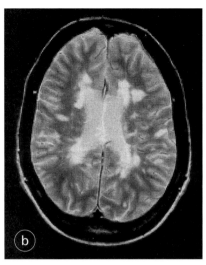

Fig. 7.3 Fluid attenuated inversion recovery (FLAIR) (a), and T2-weighted (b) images of an MS patient. Due to the reduced grey/white matter contrast on FLAIR images, and the low signal of CSF, cortical and subcortical lesions are more apparent than on the corresponding T2-weighted MR image.

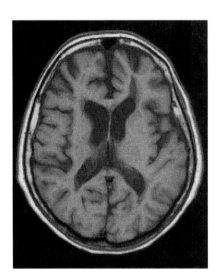

Fig. 7.4 Short TR/short TE (T1-weighted) MR image of an MS patient showing several severely hypointense lesions which are located around the ventricles. This T1-weighted image corresponds to the PD and T2-weighted images of Figure 7.2.

FLAIR than with conventional SE imaging.[12] This may be related to CSF pulsations (incomplete CSF signal suppression), the considerable inherent T1-weighting of this sequence (acting antagonistically to the T2 contrast), or to the difference in composition of lesions in the posterior fossa and spinal cord (resulting in a different imaging appearance).

On heavily T1-weighted images, obtained with an inversion recovery sequence, MS lesions are visualized as areas of reduced signal intensity (caused by the increased T1 relaxation time) compared to white matter of the brain. In general, inversion-recovery sequences take more time to acquire (for a given spatial resolution and signal-to-noise ratio), and lesions may be less conspicuous than on SE images, especially if they are located close to CSF spaces or grey matter. More commonly, moderately T1 weighted images (short TR and short TE) are used in MS patients in order to show contrast enhancement after the administration of gadolinium-DTPA in active lesions, indicating disruption of the blood–brain barrier in case of inflammation (see Chapter 5). In part of

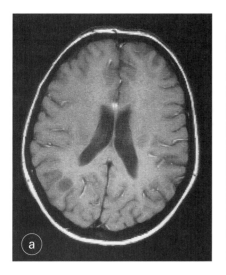 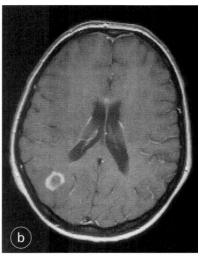

Fig. 7.5 Example of an acute (or 'wet') hypointense lesion. On the precontrast T1-weighted MR image (a) the lesion appears hypointense, whereas on the postcontrast T1-weighted MR image (b) ring-enhancement is visible after the administration of gadolinium DTPA.

the MS lesions, the T1 relaxation time is sufficiently prolonged to reduce signal intensity on T1-weighted MRI scans. These lesions are commonly known as hypointense T1 lesions or 'black holes' (*Fig. 7.4*), and their use to monitor disease progression in MS has recently been established.[13,14]

CONVENTIONAL SE MRI IN MS: WHERE DO WE STAND?

T2-weighted SE MRI

The most commonly used measure for disease burden in MS is the assessment of brain lesion load on unenhanced T2-weighted images. The quantitation of lesion volumes can be performed by manual tracing of lesion outlines or by semi-automated lesion detection, which provides an objective and reproducible measure of the amount of diseased brain tissue. Several studies have compared severity (extent) of disease on the MRI scan with the degree of clinical severity as measured with the expanded disability status

scale (EDSS) score. Overall, the link between T2-weighted lesion number or load and disability is weak (*Table 7.2*).[4,13–20]

Many factors may contribute to this clinico-radiological paradox. First, brain lesions that appear hyperintense on T2-weighted images may be histopathologically heterogeneous, consisting of oedema, inflammation, mild and severe demyelination, remyelination, gliosis and axonal loss. Although severe demyelination and axonal loss are probably the main factors that contribute to functional impairment, they have the same appearance as lesions consisting of oedema, mild demyelination and gliosis. Secondly, the EDSS is a subjective non-linear scale, which mainly represents spinal disease activity. Small lesions in the spinal cord may therefore be more important in determining disability than large lesions in the brain, whereas brain MRI lesions may correlate better with cognitive functioning. Thirdly, microscopic pathology in the normal-appearing white matter (NAWM) may contribute to disability, but this may be indiscernible on conventional T2-weighted scans or not included in the lesion load

Table 7.2 Correlation between T2 lesions and EDSS.

Study	Correlation	r-value
Mammi, 1996[15]	Change in T2 LL and change in EDSS	0.3
Gass, 1994[16]	T2 LL and EDSS	0.33
Filippi, 1995[17]	New T$_2$ lesions and change in EDSS	0.13
IFNB MS Study Group, 1995[18]	T2 LL and EDSS at entry	0.24
	T2 LL and EDSS at exit	0.27
van Walderveen, 1995[13]	Change in T2 LL and change in EDSS	0.19
Truyen, 1996[14]	Change in T2 LL and change in EDSS	0.11 (NS)
Lycklama à Nijeholt, 1998[4]	T2 LL and EDSS	0.21
Riahi, 1998[19]	T2 LL and EDSS	0.60
Gawne-Gain[20]	T2 LL and EDSS	0.49

LL, lesion load; EDSS, Expanded Disability Status Scale; NS, not significant.

measurement. In a recent study, the presence of diffuse abnormalities—defined as poorly demarcated high signal areas as seen on both PD and T2 images—in the brain was analysed.[4] This diffuse involvement of the NAWM seemed to be typical for primary progressive MS (PPMS) patients, indicating that in addition to the number and volume of T2 lesions, quantification of diffuse abnormalities may also be important in assessing the disease burden in MS patients more accurately.

At present, brain MRI lesion load is being used as a secondary outcome measure in definitive clinical trials, and clinical evaluations such as disability or relapse rate are still the accepted primary outcome measures.[21] New MR parameters have been analysed to improve the correlation with clinical disability or to improve the histopathological specificity. Apart from magnetization transfer imaging (see Chapter 6), MR spectroscopy (see Chapter 9) and brain and spinal cord atrophy (see Chapter 8), hypointense

T1 lesions have been shown to improve the association with clinical disability and to improve histopathologic specificity.

Hypointense lesions on short TR/short TE ('T1-weighted') MRI

Hypointense T1 lesions were first described by Uhlenbrock and colleagues,[22] who noted that hypointense lesions are common in MS but occur less frequently in subcortical arteriosclerotic encephalopathy. Uhlenbrock suggested that these lesions represent chronic MS plaques in which astrocyte growth and scarring is present. Autopsy[23,24] and biopsy[25] studies have confirmed this hypothesis: the degree of hypointensity on T1-weighted SE images correlates strongly with the degree of matrix destruction (widening of the extracellular space) and loss of axons. Compared to T2 lesion load, hypointense T1 lesion load correlates better with clinical disability in relapsing–remitting MS (RRMS) and secondary progressive MS (SPMS) in two follow-up studies.[13,14] In SPMS, the relative increase in hypointense T1 lesion load was highly related with disease progression (Spearman rank correlation coefficient $r = 0.81$). These studies indicate that hypointense T1 lesions are more specific than T2 lesions for identifying lesions that cause disability and may therefore be used as a surrogate marker for disease progression. Recent recommendations already include T1 lesions in addition to T2 lesions as a secondary outcome measure in clinical trials.[21]

However, some problems still need to be resolved. First, short TR and short TE images are usually referred to as T1 weighted, although the degree of T1 weighting is variable and highly sequence dependent. On T1-weighted SE images only part of the lesions appear hypointense, whereas all lesions appear dark on heavily T1-weighted images such as obtained with inversion recovery sequences. Apparently, T1 prolongation must be quite strong to result in the appearance of 'black holes' on short TR and short TE SE images. Therefore, the amount of hypointense T1 lesion load depends on the settings used to obtain the images which may make it difficult to standardize this sequence between sites. Secondly, the degree of hypointensity on T1-weighted MRI varies among lesions. Whereas some lesions have the same signal intensity as CSF (dark), others are closer to grey matter. These differences in appearance probably relate to a range of severity of tissue destruction. Furthermore, hypointense signal of CSF may obscure the identification of adjacent hypointense T1 lesions and, similarly, grey holes close to similar-appearing grey matter may go undetected. Therefore, standardization of acquisition parameters and the development of a clear definition of black holes (and grey holes) is mandatory.

One way of standardizing the measurement of lesion hypointensity in black holes is provided by precise relaxation time measurements. In order to be able to discuss this technically complex matter, the chapter first describes the methodology to measure T1 and T2 relaxation times.

MEASUREMENT OF T1 AND T2 RELAXATION TIMES

Methodological considerations in T1 and T2 measurements

The measurement of T1 relaxation times can be performed using several MR techniques. Difference in T1 dependence in successive images of the brain can be obtained by varying the TR (saturation recovery method), the TI (inversion recovery method) or the flip angle of the exciting radiofrequency pulse. In general, inversion recovery methods are preferred to saturation recovery techniques. A saturation recovery sequence requires a $TR \leq T1$, in which case the slice profile becomes very distorted and accurate measurements of T1 relaxation times are impossible. Inversion recovery methods can be run at long TRs, so that the slice relaxes completely between subsequent inversion pulses. Since T1 measurements obtained from images with different TI or TR values may be influenced by different transmitter and receiver gains of the scanner, these parameters should be kept constant during the whole measurement.

Until recently, T1 relaxation time measurements suffered from one major disadvantage: acquisition times tended to be very long, which limits the application in the clinical setting. Since more rapid acquisition techniques have become available, this problem may be circumvented.

Echoplanar imaging (EPI), for example, is the most rapid imaging technique available at present and provides complete spatial encoding of an MRI after a single 90° excitation pulse. The combination of rapidly switching magnetic field gradients and a high-speed data acquisition system allows a reduced examination time, typically to the order of a few minutes for the whole brain. Using EPI, T1 relaxation times can be measured by applying an 180° inversion pulse with varying inversion times to introduce a wide range of T1-dependent contrast in successive images.

T2 relaxation time measurements can be performed by using spin echoes at varying echo times. Most commonly, the Carr–Purcell–Meiboom–Gill (CPMG) sequence is used, in which any number of echoes can be collected by applying additional consecutive rephasing 180° pulses after an initial 90° pulse. The CPMG sequence is usually run in a single-slice mode since this allows the use of non-selective 180° pulses, which produce more accurate refocusing of the magnetization in the selected slice.

Interpretation of T1 and T2 measurements

In vivo measurement of T1 and T2 relaxation times of protons provides information about the tissue water environment. Research using gravimetric analysis of operative samples of patients with brain tumours has shown a linear correlation between total water content and T1 relaxation time.[26] Furthermore, relaxation time measurement gives information about the existence of two or more water compartments, in which case a bi- or multiexponential decay curve can be plotted. The possibility of multicomponent relaxation in the brain must always be considered when measuring T1 and T2 in the brain.

In normal brain tissue, the longitudinal relaxation decay curve follows a monoexponential function. Also, transverse relaxation of grey matter in normal brain is mono-exponential although bi-exponential decay curves can be found in cases of partial volume effects with CSF. In contrast, T2 of white matter is usually multicomponent in nature, and different T2 times correspond to three different water reservoirs:

(a) a minor fraction with a short T2 between 10 and 50 ms caused by water compartmentalized in myelin membranes (so called myelin water);

(b) a major fraction (approximately 80% of the water in normal brain) with T2 between 70 and 95 ms, caused by water in cytoplasmatic and extracellular spaces; and

(c) a small fraction with T2 values of 1 second or more, consistent with CSF (for example in perivascular spaces).[27–29]

Tissue characterization of T1 and T2 relaxation values: experimental results

In experimental studies correlations have been found between changes in T1 and T2 relaxation times (and their ratio) and histopathology. Triethyltin-induced cerebral oedema affects the brain white matter diffusely without enlargement of the extracellular space or astrocyte swelling.[30] T1 and T2 values lengthen with increasing water content of the oedematous white matter, and at all stages the percentage increase in T2 is almost twice that in T1. In vasogenic oedema the extracellular space enlarges and protein-rich fluid accumulates as a result of damage to blood vessels. This results in increased relaxation time values, but T2 increases in the same proportion as T1. Furthermore, the T2

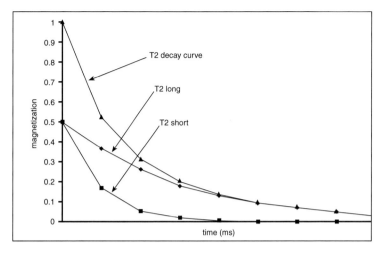

Fig. 7.6 *Example of a T2 decay curve that is fitted by a bi-exponential function (consisting of T2 long and T2 short component) according to the formula:*

$M_{xy}(t) = M_l \times e^{(-t/T2\ long)} + M_s \times e^{(-t/T2\ short)}$, *where M_l represents the magnetization of the T2 long component at time 0 and M_s represents the magnetization of the T2 short component at time 0.*

decay follows a bi-exponential function (*Fig. 7.6*) that consists of a short (intracellular water) and a long (oedematous fluid) T2 component.[31] The bi-exponential T2 decay in case of enlargement of the extracellular space is of interest, since this occurs—apart from in vasogenic oedema—in cases of axonal loss. This contrasts with findings in experimental gliosis in cats, where T1 relaxation time is increased without a corresponding increase in T2 relaxation time and the T2 magnetization decay remains mono-exponential.[32]

Several quantitative MR studies have been performed on animals with experimental allergic encephalomyelitis (EAE), an animal model for MS. The general conclusion that can be drawn from these studies is that, in the EAE lesion, prolongation of T1 and T2 relaxation times is particularly related to oedema. Furthermore, changes in relaxation time values can often be observed before onset of clinical symptoms or before onset of pathological changes.[33,34] In primate EAE, prolonged T1 and T2 values are associated with the presence of inflammation, demyelination and haemorrhagic necrosis.[34] In guinea pigs, prolongation of T1 has been observed during meningeal

and perivascular inflammation, whereas T2 increased with demyelination.[35] Stewart and colleagues[27] performed a multiexponential analysis of T2 data from EAE lesions in the spinal cord and brain of guinea pigs. They found a short T2 component, assigned to myelin water, which was smaller or absent in demyelinated lesions. Although these studies have provided some insights into the histopathological characteristics of changes in relaxation parameters, the results are often hampered by partial volume effects caused by the small size of the lesions and by difficulties relating the in vivo MR measurements and in vitro histological examination.

Relaxation time measurements in NAWM

Lacomis and colleagues[36] showed in 1986 that in patients with diagnosed MS, T1 relaxation time of NAWM is prolonged compared to control white matter and that this increase is most obvious in patients with longer disease duration. This finding was confirmed by

Haughton and colleagues,[37] who also observed that the T1 of NAWM increased progressively with increasing disability in MS patients, although this relation appeared only marginally significant. In other studies, consistent findings of increased T1 and T2 relaxation times in NAWM of MS patients have been found. In a more extensive study it was shown that, throughout the NAWM, discrete areas of abnormal T1 and T2 values are present, which often consist of only one or two pixels.[38] Barbosa and colleagues[38] hypothesized that these discrete areas may represent small areas of reactive astrocytes, oedema and perivascular cellular infiltration, which have also been described pathoanatomically. All these studies show that there are white matter abnormalities in MS that do not appear as discrete foci of abnormal signal intensity on conventional MRI. Since this 'invisible' lesion load may constitute a significant proportion of the total lesion load, an estimate of the disease burden might be more accurate if it were based on T1 and T2 calculations of white matter, in addition to the quantitation of number and volume of plaques.

Relaxation time measurements in focal MS lesions

Relaxation time measurements within MS lesions generally show increased T1 and T2 values. Larsson and colleagues[39] examined a group of patients with stable but severe disease. T1 relaxation was found to be mono-exponential in all MS lesions, but in seven of 33 lesions T2 relaxation curves were found to fit a bi-exponential function better than a mono-exponential function.

This study was extended to include patients suffering from an acute attack of MS.[40] A large overlap was shown between T1 and T2 values obtained in acute and chronic plaques. In acute plaques the T1 relaxation time was mono-exponential at all times, and T1 decreased with time. In contrast, a bi-expoential T2 relaxation process was observed after a time period of 23–187 days; this reversed to monoexponentiality in some cases. This study report suggested that, in the acute lesions, the increased number of inflammatory cells and the increased intercellular water probably accounts for the simultaneous increase in T1 and T2. The bi-exponential T2 decay curve would represent loss of myelin, which is replaced by water (accounting for the high mono-exponential T2 values) and gliosis (accounting for the T2 fast component). After resorption of oedema, only one component (gliosis) can be detected. Armsprach and colleagues[41] also showed that a bi-exponential T2 decay curve can usually be observed in lesions of MS patients, of which the short T2 component probably reflects remaining myelinated fibres. The long T2 values were spread out over a wide range, probably characterizing different pathological processes such as oedema, demyelination and gliosis. MacKay and colleagues[28] analysed T2 decay curves in MS lesions and focused on the short T2 component (between 10 and 55 ms), which is the myelin water component. In four MS cases, the average myelin water content in lesions was found to be significantly reduced compared to that of white matter in normal volunteers. MacKay and colleagues therefore noted that increased proton density, and elevated (overall) T2 relaxation time of a lesion do not necessarily relate to the state of myelination. The additional use of myelin maps, which is a representation of the very short T2 component, may therefore provide additional information on the myelinated state of lesions. Kidd and colleagues[42] postulated that T2 decay curve analysis may provide an insight into the pathological characteristics of lesions. A mono-exponential decay with a relatively short T2 would indicate lesions that consist predominantly of gliosis, whereas a bi-exponential decay or a mono-expontial decay with a long T2 may relate to an expanded extracellular space caused by loss of tissue structure (including axonal loss).

T1 relaxation measurements in chronic hypointense MS lesions

In an autopsy study,[23] hypointense lesions were shown to consist of axonal loss with matrix destruction as a prominent feature. In a more extensive histopathological sample,[24] 109 lesions were selected and examined using post mortem MR imaging and histopathology. Contrast ratio measurements on T1 weighted MRI scans were used as an in vivo MR index for tissue destruction, and magnetization transfer ratio (MTR) measurements were used as an in vivo MR index for demyelination. The histopathological outcome parameters were axonal density, degree of matrix destruction and degree of lesional activity (classification based on the presence of different myelin breakdown products, which reflect various stages of lesion development). In this large sample, a strong correlation was shown between MTR and T1 contrast ratio measurement and histopathological outcome parameters. In particular, the strong correlation with axonal loss indicates that quantitation of T1 and MTR may provide an in vivo tool for monitoring irreversible deficit in MS lesions and may be used as a surrogate outcome measure in clinical trials.

In vivo T1 relaxation time measurement in chronic hypointense T1 lesions has substantiated this hypothesis.[43] In a group of 14 MS patients, chronic hypointense lesions (more than 6 months old) were selected on previous T2-weighted images, and T1 relaxation time measurements were performed using an inversion recovery EPI sequence. MRS was performed to assess metabolite concentrations within the lesions. The highest values for T1 relaxation time were found for severely hypointense ('black') T1 lesions. Indeed, isointense and mildly hypointense ('grey') lesions have lower T1 relaxation times than severely hypointense lesions. Prolongation of T1 relaxation times in severely hypointense lesions was paralleled by a decrease in the concentration of *N*-acetyl aspartate (NAA), a brain metabolite that occurs exclusively in neurons and axons. This correlation was present for MS lesions, but remained significant after inclusion of NAWM into the analysis. These preliminary in vivo results indicate that measurement of T1 relaxation time provides an in vivo tool for monitoring disease progression (axonal loss) in lesions and NAWM of MS patients.

Can axonal loss in individual MS lesions be predicted?

Axonal loss is obviously the irreversible end-stage in the development of MS lesions and the main contributor to progressive neurological deterioration. Although axonal loss was thought to occur mainly in chronic MS, recent studies have shown that damage to axons also occurs in acute (inflammatory) lesions.[44,45] Trapp and colleagues[44] showed that axonal transection is an abundant feature in active and chronic active lesions from patients with duration of clinical disease ranging from 2 weeks to 27 years. Furthermore, the greatest degree of axonal transsection occurred in areas of active demyelination and inflammation. Bruck and colleagues[25] found various reductions in axonal density (ranging from 35% to 81% compared to periplaque white matter) in lesions showing massive gadolinium-DTPA enhancement. These enhancing lesions appear hypointense on unenhanced T1-weighted images, and the degree of hypointensity was shown to be affected mainly by two factors: the extent of axonal reduction and the amount of extracellular oedema.

Most (80%) enhancing lesions appear hypointense on unenhanced T1-weighted images[46] and are also known as acute (or 'wet') black holes. These acute hypointense lesions have the potential to reverse to isointensity at follow-up (55% do so), although some (45%) remain hypointense. Factors predicting the evolution of individual lesions are unknown at present. Hypointense appearance at 6 months' follow-up was in part determined by the MTR value at the time of initial enhancement and the duration of enhancement. Furthermore, ring-enhancing lesions were persistently hypointense in all cases, in contrast to nodular enhancing lesions.

The MTR value at the time of initial enhancement predicts the persistent hypointense appearance (indicating axonal loss) at follow-up, although in individual lesions this is difficult to predict since MTR values are generally decreased during the phase of enhancement;[47–49] in a large number of cases, they too tend to reverse to subnormal or normal values after enhancement ceases.[46,50] This shows great similarity to the observation of reversible decreases of NAA in acute lesions[51,52] and the decrease in T1 relaxation time at follow-up in acute lesions.[40]

At present, it is therefore not possible to indicate factors that predict the occurrence of axonal loss in MS lesions in a straightforward fashion.

Pattern and duration of enhancement, MTR, NAA concentration and T1 relaxation time measurement may all elucidate this issue to some extent. As far as individual patients are concerned, the percentage of enhancing lesions that evolve into black holes is only weakly related to the rate of enhancing lesions, and it is more strongly determined by whether or not black holes are present initially.[53] Therefore, apart from the amount of new inflammatory activity, other (possibly genetic) factors probably determine the development of axonal loss in MS lesions.

Measures of T1 and T2 relaxation: current perspectives

At present, conventional T2-weighted SE MRI is the most sensitive method for visualizing abnormalities in the brain of patients with suspected MS, since all pathological tissue alterations that occur in MS cause an increase in T2 relaxation. This histopathological heterogeneity probably accounts for the often only weak correlation that is found with clinical disability measures. Using T1-weighted SE MRI, a closer correlation with clinical disease progression can be obtained. Chronic hypointense T1 lesions ('black holes') correlate histopathologically with irreversible tissue destruction (i.e. matrix destruction and axonal loss). Experimental studies indicate that histopathological characterization of lesions may be improved using T1 and T2 relaxation time measurements. In MS lesions, a wide range of T1 and T2 times are observed, which probably reflect histopathological heterogeneity. Many plaques show bi-exponential or multiexponential T2 relaxation, which could be related to enlargement of the extracellular space. Although changes in T1 and T2 relaxation in MS lesions are not directly related to specific histological alterations (such as demyelination, expanded extracellular space, axonal loss, oedema and remyelination), these techniques may play a role in monitoring the degree of demyelination and axonal loss. The role of T1 relaxation time measurement as a marker of axonal loss seems to hold particular promise.

Table 7.3 MR parameters

T1 relaxation time	Time constant which describes the time required for longitudinal magnetization to return to 63% of its original value.
longtitudinal relaxation	Spin-lattice relaxation which refers to the return of the magnetization along the main axis of the field (due to the transfer of energy from spins to environment).
TR	Repetition time; the time between successive excitations (90° radiofrequency pulses).
T2 relaxation time	Time constant which describes the time required for transverse magnetization to fall by 63% of its original value.
transverse relaxation	Spin-spin relaxation which refers to the decay of magnetization in the transverse plane (due to interaction between adjacent nuclei which influence their precession frequency and phase coherence).
TE	Echo time; the time between the beginning of the 90° pulse and the maximum amplitude of the echo signal.
T1-weighted imaging	Contrast of the images is mainly based on differences in T1 relaxation times of tissues (commonly used sequence parameters are: TR 500–800 ms and TE 10–30 ms).
PD-weighted imaging	'Proton density'-weighted imaging; T1 and T2 contrast are minimized by choosing a long TR (2500–3000 ms) and a short TE (10–30 ms).
T2-weighted imaging	Contrast of the images is mainly based on differences in T2 relaxation times of tissues (commonly used sequence parameters are: TR of 2500–3000 ms and TE of 45–100 MS).
FLAIR	Fluid attenuated inversion recovery. Heavily T2-weighted images with suppression of signal from CSF by using a very long inversion time.
EPI	Echo planar imaging; very rapid scan technique which provides complete spatial encoding after a single excitation with use of rapidly switching read out gradients.
MTR	Magnetization transfer ratio; which can be calculated from the formula $(M_0-M_s)/M_0 \times 100$ to quantitate the amount of signal suppression which is caused by off-resonance irradiation (M_0 is signal intensity without off-resonance presaturation and M_s is the signal intensity with the presaturation pulse on).

REFERENCES

1 **Paty DW, Oger JJF, Kastrukoff LF et al.** Magnetic resonance imaging in the diagnosis of multiple sclerosis (MS): a prospective study of comparison with clinical evaluation, evoked potentials, oligoclonal banding, and CT. *Neurology* 1988; **38**:180–185.

2 **Morrissey SP, Miller DH, Kendall BE et al.** The significance of brain magnetic resonance imaging abnormalities at presentation with clinically isolated syndromes suggestive of multiple sclerosis. A 5-year follow-up study. *Brain* 1993; **116**:135–146.

3 **Lycklama à Nijeholt GJ, Barkhof F, Scheltens P et al.** MRI of the spinal cord in multiple sclerosis: relation to clinical subtype and disability. *AJNR* 1997; **18**:1041–1048.

4 **Lycklama à Nijeholt GJ, van Walderveen MAA, Castelijns JA et al.** Brain and spinal cord abnormalities in multiple sclerosis: correlation between MR parameters, clinical subtypes and symptomatology. *Brain* 1998; **121**:687–697.

5 **Fazekas F, Offenbacher H, Fuchs S et al.** Criteria for an increased specificity of MRI interpretation in elderly subjects with suspected multiple sclerosis. *Neurology* 1988; **38**:1822–1825.

6 **Barkhof F, Filippi M, Miller DH et al.** Comparison of MRI criteria at first presentation to predict conversion to clinically definite multiple sclerosis. *Brain* 1997; **120**:2059–2069.

7 **Grant Steen R, Gronemeyer SA, Taylor JS.** Age related changes in proton T_1 values of normal human brain. *J Magn Reson Imaging* 1995; **5**:43–48.

8 **Breger RK, Rimm AA, Fischer ME et al.** T_1 and T_2 measurements on a 1.5 T commercial MR imager. *Radiology* 1989; **171**:273–276.

9 **Kjaer L, Henriksen O.** Comparison of different pulse sequences for in vivo determination of T_1 relaxation times in the brain. *Acta Radiol* 1988; **29**:231–236.

10 **Darwin RH, Drayer BP, Riederer SJ et al.** T_2 estimates in healthy and diseased brain tissue: a comparison using various MR pulse sequences. *Radiology* 1986; **160**:375–381.

11 **Tong CY, Prato FS.** A novel fast T_1-mapping method. *J Magn Reson Imaging* 1994; **4**:701–708.

12 **Filippi M, Yousry T, Baratti C et al.** Quantitative assessment of MRI lesion load in multiple sclerosis: a comparison of conventional spin-echo fast-fluid-attenuated inversion recovery. *Brain* 1996; **119**:1349–1355.

13 **van Walderveen MAA, Barkhof F, Hommes OR et al.** Correlating MRI and clinical disease activity in multiple sclerosis: relevance of hypointense lesions on short-TR/short-TE ('T_1-weighted') spin-echo images. *Neurology* 1995; **45**: 1684–1690.

14 **Truyen L, van Waesberghe JHTM, van Walderveen MAA et al.** Accumulation of hypointense lesions ('black holes') on T1 SE MRI in multiple sclerosis correlates with disease progression. *Neurology* 1996; **47**:1469–1476.

15 **Mammi S, Filippi M, Martinelli V et al.** Correlation between brain MRI lesion volume and disability in patients with multiple sclerosis. *Acta Neurol Scand* 1996; **94**:93–96

16 **Gass A, Barker GJ, Kidd D et al.** Correlation of magnetic transfer ratio with clinical disability in multiple sclerosis. *Ann Neurol* 1994; **36**:62–67.

17 **Filippi M, Paty DW, Kappos L et al.** Correlations between changes in disability and T2-weighted brain MRI activity in multiple sclerosis: a follow-up study. *Neurology* 1995; **45**:255–260.

18 **The IFNB Multiple Sclerosis Study Group: University of British Columbia MS/MRI Analysis Group.** Interferon beta-1b in the treatment of multiple sclerosis: final outcome of the randomized, controlled trial. *Neurology* 1995; **45**:1277–1285.

19 **Riahi F, Zijdenbos A, Narayanan S et al.** Improved correlation between scores on the expanded disability status scale and cerebral lesion load in relapsing-remitting multiple sclerosis—results of the application of new imaging methods. *Brain* 1998; **121**:1305–1312.

20 **Gawne-Caine ML, O'Riordan JI, Coles A et al.** MRI lesion volume measurement in multiple sclerosis and its correlation with disability—a comparison of fast fluid attenuated inversion recovery (Fflair) and spin echo sequences. *J Neurol Neurosurg Psychiatry* 1998; **64**:197–203.

21 **Miller DH, Albert PS, Barkhof F et al.** Guidelines for the use of magnetic resonance techniques in monitoring the treatment of multiple sclerosis. *Ann Neurol* 1996; **39**:6–16.

22 **Uhlenbrock D, Sehlen S.** The value of T_1-weighted images in the differentiation between MS, white matter lesions, and subcortical arteriosclerotic encephalopathy (SAE). *Neuroradiology* 1989; **31**:203–212.

23 **van Walderveen MAA, Kamphorst W, Scheltens P et al.** Histopathologic correlate of hypointense lesions on T1-weighted spin-echo MRI in multiple sclerosis. *Neurology* 1998; **50**:1282–1288.

24 van Waesberghe JHTM, Kamphorst W, de Groot CA et al. Histopathologic correlate of MTR and hypointense signal intensity on T_1 SE in multiple sclerosis lesions. A direct postmortem study. Presented at the 14th Congress of the European Committee for Treatment and Research in Multiple Sclerosis (ECTRIMS). Stockholm, Sweden, 9–12 September 1998.

25 Bruck W, Bitsch A, Kolenda H et al. Inflammatory central nervous system demyelination: correlation of magnetic resonance imaging findings with lesion pathology. *Ann Neurol* 1997; **42**:783–793.

26 MacDonald HL, Bell BA, Smith MA et al. Correlation of human NMR T1 values measured in vivo and brain water content. *Br J Radiol* 1986; **59**:355–357.

27 Stewart WA, MacKay AL, Whittall KP et al. Spin-spin relaxation in experimental allergic encephalomyelitis: analysis of CPMG data using non-linear least-squares method and linear inverse theory. *Magn Reson Med* 1993; **29**:767–775.

28 MacKay AL, Whittall KP, Adler J et al. In vivo visualization of myelin water in brain by magnetic resonance. *Magn Reson Med* 1994; **31**:673–677.

29 Whittall KP, MacKay AL, Graeb DA et al. In vivo measurement of T2 distribution and water contents in normal human brain. *Magn Reson Med* 1997; **37**:34–43.

30 Barnes D, McDonald WI, Tofts PS et al. Magnetic resonance imaging of experimental cerebral oedema. *J Neurol Neurosurg Psychiatry* 1986; **49**:1341–1347.

31 Barnes D, McDonald WI, Johnson G et al. Quantitative nuclear magnetic resonance imaging: characterisation of experimental cerebral oedema. *J Neurol Neurosurg Psychiatry* 1987; **50**:125–133.

32 Barnes D, McDonald WI, Landon DN, Johnson G. The characterization of experimental gliosis by quantitative nuclear magnetic resonance imaging. *Brain* 1988; **111**:81–94.

33 O'Brien JT, Noseworthy JH, Gilbert JJ et al. NMR changes in experimental allergic encephalomyelitis: NMR changes precede clinical and pathological events. *Magn Reson Med* 1987; **5**:109–117.

34 Stewart WA, Alvord EC, Hruby S et al. Magnetic resonance imaging of experimental allergic encephalomyelitis in primates. *Brain* 1991; **114**:1069–1096.

35 Karlik SJ, Strejan G, Gilbert JJ et al. NMR studies in experimental allergic encephalomyelitis (EAE): normalization of T_1 and T_2 with parenchymal cellular infiltration. *Neurology* 1986; **37**:1112–1114.

36 Lacomis D, Osbakken M, Gross G. Spin-lattice relaxation (T_1) times of cerebral white matter in multiple sclerosis. *Magn Reson Med* 1986; **3**:194–202.

37 Haughton VM, Yetkin FZ et al. Quantitative MR in the diagnosis of multiple sclerosis. *Magn Reson Med* 1992; **26**:71–78.

38 Barbosa S, Blumhardt LD, Roberts N et al. Magnetic resonance relaxation time mapping in multiple sclerosis: normal appearing white matter and the 'invisible' lesion load. *Magn Reson Imaging* 1994; **12**:33–42.

39 Larsson HBW, Frederiksen J, Kjaer L et al. In vivo determination of T_1 and T_2 in the brain of patients with severe but stable multiple sclerosis. *Magn Reson Med* 1988; 7:43–55.

40 Larsson HBW, Frederiksen J, Petersen J et al. Assessment of demyelination, oedema, and gliosis by in vivo determination of T_1 and T_2 in the brain of patients with acute attack of multiple sclerosis. *Magn Reson Med* 1989; 11:337–348.

41 Armspach JP, Gounot D, Rumbach L, Chambron J. In vivo determination of multiexponential T_2 relaxation in the brain of patients with multiple sclerosis. *Magn Reson Imaging* 1991; 9:107–113.

42 Kidd D, Barker GJ, Tofts PS et al. The transverse magnetisation decay characteristics of longstanding lesions and normal-appearing white matter in multiple sclerosis. *J Neurol* 1997; **244**: 125–130.

43 van Walderveen MAA, Barkhof F, Pouwels PJW et al. Neuronal damage in T_1-hypointense multiple sclerosis lesions demonstrated in vivo using 1H MR spectroscopy. *Ann Neurol*; in press.

44 Trapp BD, Peterson J, Ransohoff RM et al. Axonal transection in the lesions of multiple sclerosis. *N Engl J Med* 1998; **338**:278–285.

45 Ferguson B, Matyszak MK, Esiri MM, Perry VH. Axonal damage in acute multiple sclerosis lesions. *Brain* 1997; **120**:393–399.

46 van Waesberghe JHTM, van Walderveen MAA, Castelijns JA et al. Patterns of lesion development in multiple sclerosis: longitudinal observations with T1-weighted spin-echo and magnetization transfer MR. *AJNR* 1998; **19**:675–683.

47 Lai HM, Davie CA, Gass A et al. Serial magnetisation transfer ratios in gadolinium-enhancing lesions in multiple sclerosis. *J Neurol* 1997; **244**:308–311.

48 Silver NC, Lai M, Symms MR et al. Serial magnetization transfer imaging to characterize the early evolution of new MS lesions. *Neurology* 1998; **51**:758–764.

49 Filippi M, Rocca MA, Comi G. Magnetization transfer ratios of multiple sclerosis lesions with variable durations of enhancement. *J Neurol Sci* 1998; **159**:162–165.

50 Dousset V, Gayou A, Brochet B, Caille JM. Early structural changes in acute MS lesions assessed by serial magnetization transfer studies. *Neurology* 1998; **51**:1150–1155.

51 Davie CA, Hawkins CP, Barker GJ et al. Serial proton magnetic resonance spectroscopy in acute multiple sclerosis lesions. *Brain* 1994; **117**:49–58.

52 Narayana PA, Doyle TJ, Lai D, Wolinskly JS. Serial proton magnetic resonance spectroscopic imaging, contrast-enhanced magnetic resonance imaging, and quantitative lesion volumetry in multiple sclerosis. *Ann Neurol* 1998; **43**:56–71.

53 van Walderveen MAA, Truyen L, van Oosten BW et al. Development of hypointense lesions on T1-weighted spin-echo magnetic resonance images in multiple sclerosis. Relation to inflammatory activity. *Arch Neurol* 1999; **56**:345–351.

8
Measures of brain and spinal cord atrophy

Valerie L Stevenson and David H Miller

BACKGROUND

Over recent years there have been major technological advances in magnetic resonance imaging (MRI), which have been applied to the field of multiple sclerosis (MS). MRI is now used routinely in the diagnosis of MS and it has become established as the main surrogate marker in the monitoring of efficacy in clinical trials in MS. Owing to the recent advent of several new therapeutic agents for MS, there has been considerable interest in correlating progressive disability with MRI findings.

Disability in MS results from two main causes —incomplete recovery from relapses and insidious disease progression. Although most patients follow an initial course of relapsing–remitting MS (RRMS), over half of these patients go on to the phase of secondary progressive MS (SPMS), in which disability accumulates steadily with or without superimposed relapses.[1] A smaller group of patients experience a progressive disease course from onset with the absence of any relapses or remissions; this is primary progressive MS (PPMS).

In the past, most therapeutic trials have focused on the rate of clinical relapses experienced by patients, and the monitoring of such trials has relied heavily on MRI measures of short-term disease activity. These measures include the rate of new lesion formation, which is known to be in the order of 10 times the frequency of clinical relapses[2–4] and (as a measure of inflammatory activity) the degree of gadolinium enhancement on MRI. Although these measures reflect acute inflammatory activity and blood–brain barrier breakdown, they are not wholly responsible for disease progression. This is illustrated well by the small group of patients with PPMS; these patients are known to have extremely low rates of new lesion formation and focal gadolinium enhancement, but they have considerable rates of accumulating disability.[5] In a small follow-up study[6] of patients with SPMS and PPMS, a correlation was demonstrated between gadolinium enhancement over a 6-month period and disability progression 5 years later in the SPMS patients but not in the PPMS group.[6]

The primary outcome measure in all definitive phase 3 therapeutic trials is clinical change.[7] The clinical outcome measures used include relapse rate and, more importantly, measures of disease progression, either sustained change in disability measures or the reaching of well-defined disability end-points. The clinical scales used to assess impairment and disability are not ideal with respect to reliability, validity and responsiveness, and consequently surrogate measures of disease progression that allow quantitative analysis are extremely valuable. All of the recent large therapeutic trials have relied upon serial MRI T2 lesion volume as a measure of the overall pathological extent of disease.[8–11] This is usually measured annually and has been shown to exhibit changes, in placebo arms of previous trials, in the order of a median increase of 5–10% per year in RRMS.[12]

The measurement of T2 lesion volume using semi-automated approaches[13] is reproducible (coefficients of variation less than 5%) and more sensitive than clinical scales; considerable changes in lesion loads are seen after only short time intervals when only minor alterations in the level of clinical impairment is measurable. However, as with any surrogate measure of disease progression, the measurement must reflect clinical change. Although the pathological correlations with individual lesions are good, demonstrating that plaques of demyelination correspond to areas of increased signal on T2-weighted scans,[14] the clinical correlations between disability scales and T2 lesion volumes in established MS are disappointingly low (r = 0.23 in the large IFNB MS study group in 1995).[8]

This discrepancy has been accounted for in several ways. First, the T2 lesion volume does not take into account the location of lesions within the brain, and it completely ignores the presence of disease in the spinal cord, which in itself may account for the majority of disability measured by scales that are typically weighted towards locomotor abnormalities. Secondly, increase in T2-weighted signal is non-specific pathologically. Areas of oedema, gliosis, demyelination or axonal loss cannot be distinguished from each other. This is demonstrated by the known vari-

ability of T2 lesion volumes, which fluctuate over short time periods, reflecting reversible changes. This variability limits their use for sporadic measures, particularly in the short term. Lastly, any pathological changes in the normal appearing white matter (NAWM) are ignored. Owing to these poor MRI–clinical correlations, more pathologically specific imaging techniques have been sought that reflect, in particular, global demyelination and axonal loss. One such technique is the measurement of atrophy of both the brain and spinal cord.

ATROPHY—A TOOL TO REFLECT DEMYELINATION AND AXONAL LOSS

When severe tissue destruction occurs, the central nervous system responds by shrinkage and reorganization—changes that are only visible at the edges of a structure—with widening of the sulci and ventricles in the brain and shrinkage of the circumference of the spinal cord. The measurement of the rate of shrinkage may therefore directly reflect the ongoing pathological process that results in disease progression. The nature of the process responsible for the atrophy is uncertain, but it is thought to be a combination of demyelination and, perhaps more importantly, axonal loss. Recent pathological studies have demonstrated axonal loss within both lesions and NAWM in MS,[15,16] observations that are supported by reductions of *N*-acetyl aspartate (NAA) in magnetic resonance spectroscopy studies.[17] Demyelination alone is known to result in a reduction of axonal diameter[18] and it could therefore contribute to atrophy by two mechanisms (loss of myelin per se and associated axonal shrinkage). Magnetization transfer (MT) studies of NAWM have demonstrated significantly lower MT ratios in patients with chronic progressive MS than in patients with RRMS, which probably reflects greater degrees of demyelination.[19,20] Measurement of central motor conduction times (CMCTs) has been shown to be related to spinal cord lesion load and hence reflects the degree of demyelination present. However, progressive motor deterioration has been documented despite the absence of new MRI lesions or further delay in the CMCT.[21] These findings further support the hypothesis that progressive axonal degeneration is an important contributor to increasing disability in MS. The suggestion that atrophy may have two mechanisms, one non-disabling (demyelination) and the other disabling (axonal loss), is supported by the considerable degree of atrophy that can occur in the minimally disabled patients with benign MS.[22]

The measurement of atrophy is not without its difficulties. The techniques used need to be sensitive and extremely reproducible over time to enable the measurement of very small volume changes. Techniques also should enable successful multiple-site implementation, a necessity in many clinical trials.

SPINAL CORD ATROPHY

Involvement of the spinal cord in MS has long been known to be extremely common and of particular importance in the development of disability.[23] Although MRI demonstrates lesions within the spinal cord in at least 75% of patients with MS, the number and extent of T2-weighted lesions has not been found to correlate with disability in cross-sectional or longitudinal studies.[24–26] However, atrophy, which may be focal at the site of lesions or may become generalized, has been noted.[27,28] The mechanisms of generalized atrophy include both the coalescence of focal destructive lesions and secondary wallerian degeneration within fibre tracts in which there has been axonal transection in distant lesions.

The first quantitative studies of spinal cord atrophy employed a T2-weighted gradient echo sequence and evaluated 5 mm axial slices taken at four vertebral levels (the fifth cervical, second thoracic, seventh thoracic and eleventh thoracic levels) in 80 patients. The cords were manually traced and atrophy was considered to be present when the measured area was two standard deviations below that of the mean for healthy controls. The mean cord areas of the patients were significantly smaller than that of the controls at each of the four levels. Those patients with atrophy were found to have significantly higher levels of disability as measured by Kurtzke's expanded disability status scale (EDSS) than those without atrophy.[24] In this study no difference in cord cross-sectional area was seen between the disabled SPMS and PPMS patients and the benign group who had relatively little disability. However, a further study using the same methodology concentrated on cord cross-sectional area at C5 and did demonstrate a significant difference between patients with benign MS and those with SPMS.[29]

In a follow-up study of PPMS and SPMS patients using the same technique, both groups showed a decrease in mean cord area over 1 year, which was greatest at C5, but there was no difference between the two groups and no significant correlation with clinical progression.[25] The intra-rater reliability of the measurement technique was 2%, but the scan–rescan variability was in the order of 6%. Changes detected were within the 95% confidence limits for measurement variation.

A further study[30] by the same investigators assessed RRMS patients over 1 year. No progressive atrophy was seen but the mean intra-rater variability was high, at 4.8% (intra-rater limits of agreement were −11.6 to 12.9%). A two year serial study of 60 patients using this technique failed to show any change in cord cross-sectional area, although this was not surprising considering the poor scan–rescan reproducibility (coefficient of variation of 6.0% in control subjects).[31]

All of the above studies depended on two-dimensional imaging with a T2-weighted gradient echo sequence and a manual outlining technique for cross-sectional area measurement. The poor reproducibility made impossible the detection of small change, which is an essential prerequisite for serial studies. Several factors contributed to this poor reproducibility. First, patient repositioning was partly responsible; although the intra-rater reproducibility for a single scan was good (2%), scan–rescan reproducibility was much worse at 6%. This is partly due to the anatomy of the spinal cord at the level of C5, which because of the cervical enlargement shows marked local variability in size at only slightly different levels. The cord is also at its most mobile here and is considerably affected by the degree of neck extension. Secondly, the cord boundary at C5 is often difficult to determine, the CSF space is small and the cord may be abutting the vertebrae. Cerebrospinal fluid (CSF) flow is often turbulent, which causes flow artefacts and can blur the cord–CSF boundary.

More recently, a technique has been developed to address these difficulties.[32] Spinal cord cross-sectional area is measured at the level of the intervertebral disc between the second and third vertebrae. This site was chosen because there is little variability in cross-sectional area over this segment and the cord is less mobile, reducing the effect of repositioning errors. The cord–CSF contrast is maximized because of the large CSF pool at this level, and due to the use of a volume-acquired inversion-prepared fast-spoiled gradient–echo T1-weighted sequence, which nulls the CSF (*Fig. 8.1*). This increased cord–CSF contrast allows the use of an automated measurement technique instead of manual outlining to define the edge of the cord.

Using this methodology, reproducibility was greatly improved, with a scan–rescan coefficient of variation of 0.79%. In a cross-sectional study, 30 controls and 60 patients were assessed (15 in each subgroup of early RRMS, PPMS, SPMS and benign MS patients). The cord cross-sectional areas of the benign MS, PPMS and SPMS patient

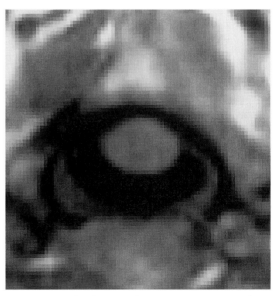

Fig. 8.1 Axial reformat of an inversion recovery fast-spoiled gradient–echo T1-weighted MRI sequence for assessment of spinal cord atrophy.

groups were significantly smaller than the controls, whereas the early RRMS group demonstrated no significant atrophy. Cord cross-sectional area correlated strongly with disability (r = −0.7, p < 0.001) and with disease duration ((r = −0.52, p < 0.001).[32] Despite the marked improvement in the measurement technique, further problems were encountered when this cohort was studied serially. During the study period a major hardware upgrade was undertaken, which resulted in minor changes in the pulse sequence and spatial signal intensity uniformity. As a consequence, all the control subjects in the study exhibited a small artefactual increase in their measured cord areas and no change was detectable in the patient group.[33] This experience emphasizes the need for quality assurance programmes to ensure that all parameters during data acquisition and analysis remain absolutely constant. This is particularly important since only extremely small changes in cord cross-sectional area are expected over a study period.[34]

A recent serial study[22] of 28 patients demonstrated that it is indeed possible to measure reproducibly and to detect change in cord cross-sectional area over a time period of 12 months using this technique in conjunction with a quality assurance programme. It also confirmed the previous findings of a strong cross-sectional correlation between a clinical measure of disability (the EDSS) and spinal cord atrophy. Cord atrophy was present at baseline in the benign MS and the PPMS groups, but it was most marked in the SPMS group. The early RRMS group had cords of normal size at baseline. Increasing atrophy over the 12-month period was detectable in the RRMS and the PPMS patient groups. No relationship was seen between the change in cord cross-sectional area and clinical progression; however, only eight of the 28 patients had a defi-

nite increase in their EDSS over the 12-month period. There were no significant differences, among these eight patients, in cord area at baseline (p = 0.69) or change in cord area over the 12 months (p = 0.51) compared to the 20 patients without a definite increase in EDSS.[22]

The findings in the PPMS group are of particular importance in relation to monitoring disease activity since this patient group show a much lower rate of new lesion development and enhancement than that seen in RRMS or SPMS. In a large multicentre study funded by the European Union involving 158 patients with PPMS, both brain and spinal cord atrophy correlated with the EDSS whereas T2 lesion volume or T1 hypointensity lesion volume did not.[35] Furthermore, over 1 year, progressive brain and cord atrophy was measurable in this cohort (VL Stevenson, 1999; personal communication). The fact that measurable rates of atrophy are present in this group despite the low rates of new lesion formation or gadolinium enhancement suggests that their slowly progressing disability is unlikely to be a direct consequence of focal inflammatory demyelinating lesions, but it may indicate a mechanism of more diffuse progressive axonal loss. This would be consistent with pathological[36] and MRI studies.[37,38]

BRAIN ATROPHY

The presence of brain atrophy in MS has been recognized for many years and has been associated with severe disability. In an early computed tomography (CT) study, brain atrophy was shown to develop early (within 1 year of diagnosis) in a subgroup of MS patients with a 'malignant' course.[39] With the advent of new MRI techniques more attention has been focused on increasing the understanding of the underlying pathological processes responsible for disability in MS. In an early spectroscopy study, NAA concentrations in cerebellar white matter were compared in controls, MS patients with cerebellar symptoms, MS patients without cerebellar involvement and patients with autosomal dominant cerebellar ataxia (ADCA), a condition in which there is loss of cerebellar neurones. Both the ADCA patients and the MS patients with cerebellar symptoms demonstrated significantly reduced NAA levels compared to controls, indicating axonal loss or dysfunction. There was no difference between the MS patients without cerebellar involvement and control subjects. On comparing their cerebellar volumes, calculated by using a semi-automated contour technique on 3 mm sagittal T1-weighted images, again only the ADCA patients and the MS patients with cerebellar symptoms demonstrated significant atrophy compared to the control subjects and MS patients without cerebellar involvement. Within the MS patient group there was a significant negative correlation between the degree of cerebellar atrophy and the NAA concentration (r = −0.44), thus demonstrating an important relationship between axonal loss and atrophy.[40]

Several other early studies looked at the relationship between cerebral atrophy and dementia, some finding a positive relationship[41,42] and others only a weak correlation or trend.[43,44] The major problem with cross-sectional studies of cerebral atrophy is the enormous natural variation in brain volume in normal subjects.[45] Serial assessments are essential to enable the measurement of progressive atrophy but since the changes expected to occur are extremely small the measurement technique needs to be both sensitive and highly reproducible. Other confounding factors that are known to influence cerebral volume must also be excluded: alcohol,[46] anorexia,[47] corticosteroids[48] and dehydration.[49]

The measurement of cerebral atrophy is more complicated than the measurement of cord atrophy since it involves both the extraction of the brain from the overlying tissues (scalp, skull and meninges) and the delineation of the lower border of the brain. The first study to measure changes in brain volume utilized two dimensional T1-weighted MRI and assessed serial change in four contiguous 5 mm slices with the most caudal at the level of the velum interpositum cerebri. This 20 mm thick slab was chosen because it covers a large proportion of the lateral ventricles and cortical sulci and because the velum interpositum cerebri is thought to be a stable landmark despite ongoing atrophy, thereby allowing accurate repositioning for serial assessment. The brain is extracted from the skull using a computer algorithm (e*XK*ull, © DS Yoo, Department of Medical Physics and Bio-engineering, University College, London, UK) and the area of each of the four slices was calculated. These were summed and multiplied by the slice thickness to give the volume of interest. Like the measurement of spinal cord atrophy, this was extremely reproducible—the scan–rescan coefficient of variation was 0.56%. A decrease in cerebral volume beyond the 95% confidence interval was seen in 16 of the 29 patients (who had RRMS or SPMS) in a time period of 18 months. The rate of atrophy was significantly higher in those with a definite change in disability, as measured by the EDSS, compared with those who did not.[50] Interestingly, there was no relationship between the rate of atrophy and the change in T2 lesion volume or volume of gadolinium enhancement, highlighting the disparity between markers of inflammatory disease activity (new lesions, gadolinium enhancement) and progressive tissue loss. In a small study of 12 patients using the same technique, cerebral atrophy was shown to correlate with the NAA concentration of NAWM.[51] This finding supports the theory that axonal loss is an important contributor to atrophy.

Other investigators have measured ventricular volume to reflect cerebral atrophy. In a study of 29 MS patients, ventricular volume was found to be significantly greater than in control subjects. No relationship was found between ventricular volume and the NAA:creatine ratio; however, this may be a consequence of the natural variation of brain parenchymal and ventricular volume in normal subjects.[52] Another cross-sectional study demonstrated higher ventricular volumes in SPMS than in RRMS or PPMS, but again no correlation was seen with the EDSS. The intra-rater reproducibility using a local thresholding technique on the same image was 6%, preventing its use in serial studies.[53] More recently, a serial study of patients with early RRMS (EDSS 1.0–3.5) demonstrated significant increases in third and lateral ventricle width at 1 or 2 years. These patients also showed significant decreases in brain width and sagittal corpus callosum area over the same period. Although only weak trends (not significant) were seen between the changes in these measures and the change in EDSS, the demonstration of atrophy developing in minimally disabled patients early in the disease process is very important.[54]

Whole brain volume can be calculated by reformatting a volume acquisition into 1 mm slices and performing simple manual segmentation of every slice.[55,56] This is obviously time consuming but allows the investigator to perform subanalyses on different brain structures. In one such study, 15 MS patients were compared to 15 controls (matched for age, sex, height and weight). Patients had significantly lower cerebral hemispheric, cerebellar and brainstem volumes than control subjects. By defining the presence of atrophy as a brain volume that is less than 2 standard deviations below that of the controls, cerebral atrophy was present in 47% of patients, while 40% had hemispheric atrophy, 20% had brainstem atrophy and 7% had cerebellar atrophy.[55] No correlations were demonstrated between the measures of brain volume and disability but again this was only a cross-sectional study. No reproducibility study was carried out to assess this technique, and therefore its usefulness for longitudinal assessment is unknown.

More automated methodology for cerebral volume quantification is obviously essential to improve reproducibility and to allow serial assessments. Many techniques are being developed, although most require some manual editing.[57,58] A recent study[59] combined a semi-automated atrophy quantification technique with measures of T2 lesion load and MT ratio histogram analysis. Brain parenchymal and CSF volumes were calculated from a T1-weighted volume acquisition. The first step of this process is the segmenting of extracranial contents, which requires the operator to 'train' the programme by identifying white matter, grey matter and CSF. Thresholding is then used to produce CSF-only mask images and hence enable CSF volume quantification. Brain parenchymal volume is calculated by subtracting the CSF volume from the total intracranial contents volume. To normalize for baseline differences in brain size, the percentage of brain parenchyma is calculated (the brain parenchymal volume divided by the intracranial contents volume, multiplied by 100). The MS patients had larger CSF volumes but smaller percentage brain parenchymal volumes than controls (but there was no difference in actual brain parenchymal volumes). There was also an interesting correlation between the peak height of the MT ratio histogram and the percentage brain parenchymal volume (r = 0.832, p = 0.0001); this was stronger than the relationship between the peak height of the MT ratio histogram and the T2 lesion volume (r = −0.728, p = 0.0001).[59] The increase in the strength of the relationship probably reflects the fact that a reduction of the MT ratio peak is in part due to lesions visible on T2-weighted imaging but it is also due to microscopic changes in the NAWM, which are incorporated in the atrophy measure.

The ideal methodology for cerebral atrophy assessment would be that of a fully automated technique that was capable of taking two or more serial image data sets from a patient and, by using subtraction techniques, could calculate the absolute change in volume of the brain or indeed any part of the intracranial contents. This is not without its problems: factors such as voxel size and shape may not remain constant over time and consequently if a simple subtraction is performed artefactual increases or decreases in brain volume may occur. As with spinal cord area measurements, a vigorous quality assurance protocol is essential to detect any 'machine drift'. It is, however, possible, using a technique currently in use in the field of Alzheimer's disease research, to overcome these problems by incorporating novel methodology to compensate for inconsistencies in voxel size.[60] Spatial scaling factors are applied by exactly matching the rigid outer surface of the cranium before precise registration takes place. Digital subtraction then occurs and a 'difference overlay image' is produced, in which pixels of significant change are coloured using alternate pixels to add colour without losing structural detail. An increase in pixel intensity ('gain' in tissue) is represented by green and a decrease ('loss' of tissue) in red. The reproducibility of this technique is excellent, with variability in the order of 1.7 ml (for a total average brain volume of 1150 ml) for controls scanned twice on the same day.[61] When this methodology was applied to Alzheimer's disease not only were patients clearly differentiated from controls but relatives of patients with Alzheimer's disease who were likely to develop the disease were also identifiable.[62]

This technique is currently being applied to MS (*Fig. 8.2*). In a small pilot study of 26 patients and 26 age- and sex-matched controls, patients demonstrated significantly smaller cerebral and ventricular volumes at baseline. The mean rate of brain atrophy (0.6%) per year in patients was twice the rate in the control group and ventricular growth was also significantly greater in the patient group (NC Fox, 1999; personal communication).

CONCLUSION

It is now possible to detect progressive atrophy of both the brain and spinal cord using increasingly automated, accurate and reproducible techniques. Through evidence from other MRI studies (spectroscopy and MT imaging) it appears that atrophy reflects a combination of both axonal loss and demyelination, both of which contribute to disease progression and accumulating disability in MS. The measures of spinal cord and cerebral atrophy are sensitive to change and show good correlations with disability; both should prove to be valuable tools in the monitoring of clinically relevant disease progression in MS.

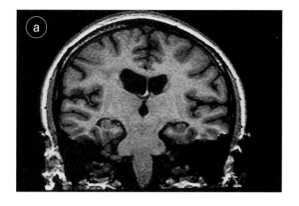

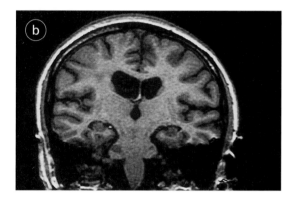

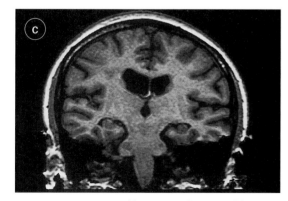

Fig. 8.2 Assessment of brain atrophy. (a and b) Equivalent coronal slices from two registered MRI scans of a patient with MS, one year apart. (c) Difference image.

REFERENCES

1 Runmarker B, Andersen O. Prognostic factors in a multiple sclerosis incidence cohort with twenty-five years of follow-up. *Brain* 1993; **116**:117–134.

2 Harris JO, Frank JA, Patronas N et al. Serial gadolinium-enhanced magnetic resonance imaging scans in patients with early, relapsing-remitting multiple sclerosis: implications for clinical trials and natural history. *Ann Neurol* 1991; **29**:548–555.

3 Thompson AJ, Miller D, Youl B et al. Serial gadolinium-enhanced MRI in relapsing/remitting multiple sclerosis of varying disease duration. *Neurology* 1992; **42**:60–63.

4 Barkhof F, Scheltens P, Frequin ST et al. Relapsing–remitting multiple sclerosis: sequential enhanced MR imaging vs clinical findings in determining disease activity. *Am J Roentgenol* 1992; **159**:1041–1047.

5 Thompson AJ, Polman CH, Miller DH et al. Primary progressive multiple sclerosis. *Brain* 1997; **120**:1085–1096.

6 Losseff NA, Kingsley DPE, McDonald WI et al. Clinical and magnetic resonance imaging predictors of disability in primary and secondary progressive multiple sclerosis. *Multiple Sclerosis* 1996; **1**:218–222.

7 Paty DW, McFarland H. Magnetic resonance techniques to monitor the long term evolution of multiple sclerosis pathology and to monitor clinical trials. *J Neurol Neurosurg Psychiatry* 1998; **64**:S47–S51.

8 IFNB Multiple Sclerosis Study Group, the University of British Columbia MS/MRI Analysis Group. Interferon β-1b in the treatment of multiple sclerosis: final outcome of the randomized controlled trial. *Neurology* 1995; **45**:1277–1285.

9 Jacobs LD, Cookfair DL, Rudick RA et al. Intramuscular interferon β-1a for disease progression in relapsing multiple sclerosis. The Multiple Sclerosis Collaborative Research Group (MSCRG). *Ann Neurol* 1996; **39**:285–294.

10 Simon JH, Jacobs LD, Campion M et al. Magnetic resonance studies of intramuscular interferon β-1a for relapsing multiple sclerosis. *Ann Neurol* 1998; **43**:79–87.

11 Miller DH, Molyneux PD, MacManus DG et al. A double-blind, placebo-controlled trial of Interferon β-1b in secondary progressive multiple sclerosis: magnetic resonance imaging results. *Ann Neurol* 1998; **44**:503–504.

12 Paty DW, Li DKB, Oger JJF et al. Magnetic resonance imaging in the evaluation of clinical trials in multiple sclerosis. *Ann Neurol* 1994; **36**:S95–S96.

13 Molyneux PD, Tofts PS, Fletcher A et al. Precision and reliability for measurement of change in MRI lesion volume in multiple sclerosis: a comparison of two computer assisted techniques. *J Neurol Neurosurg Psychiatry* 1998; **65**:42–47.

14 Stewart WA, Hall LD, Berry K et al. Magnetic resonance imaging (MRI) in multiple sclerosis (MS): pathological correlation studies in eight cases. *Neurology* 1986; **36**:320.

15 Ferguson B, Matyszak MK, Esiri MM, Perry VH. Axonal damage in acute multiple sclerosis lesions. *Brain* 1997; **120**:393–399.

16 Trapp BD, Peterson J, Ransohoff RM et al. Axonal transection in the lesions of multiple sclerosis. *N Engl J Med* 1998; **338**:278–285.

17 Fu L, Matthews PM, De Stefano N et al. Imaging axonal damage of normal-appearing white matter in multiple sclerosis. *Brain* 1998; **121**:103–113.

18 Prineas JW, Connell F. The fine structure of chronically active multiple sclerosis plaques. *Neurology* 1978; **28**:68–75.

19 Dousset V, Grossman RI, Ramer KN et al. Experimental allergic encephalomyelitis and multiple sclerosis: lesion characterization with magnetization transfer imaging. *Radiology* 1992; **182**:483–491.

20 Filippi M, Campi A, Martinelli V et al. A brain MRI study of different types of chronic–progressive multiple sclerosis. *Acta Neurol Scand* 1995; **91**:231–233.

21 Kidd D, Thompson PD, Day BL et al. Central motor conduction time in progressive multiple sclerosis. Correlations with MRI and disease activity. *Brain* 1998; **121**:1109–1116.

22 Stevenson VL, Leary SM, Losseff NA et al. Spinal cord atrophy and disability in MS: a longitudinal study. *Neurology* 1998; **51**:234–238.

23 Oppenheimer DR. The cervical cord in multiple sclerosis. *Neuropathol Appl Neurobiol* 1978; **4**:151–162.

24 Kidd D, Thorpe JW, Thompson AJ et al. Spinal cord MRI using multi-array coils and fast spin echo. II. Findings in multiple sclerosis. *Neurology* 1993; **43**:2632–2637.

25 Kidd D, Thorpe JW, Kendall BE et al. MRI dynamics of brain and spinal cord in progressive multiple sclerosis. *J Neurol Neurosurg Psychiatry* 1996; **60**:15–19.

26 Stevenson VL, Moseley IF, Phatouros CC et al. Improved imaging of the spinal cord in multiple sclerosis using three-dimensional fast spin echo. *Neuroradiology* 1998; **40**:416–419.

27 Tartaglino LM, Friedman DP, Flanders AE et al. Multiple sclerosis in the spinal cord: MR appearance and correlation with clinical parameters. *Radiology* 1995; **195**:725–732.

28 Thielen KR, Miller GM. Multiple sclerosis of the spinal cord: magnetic resonance appearance. *J Comput Assist Tomogr* 1996; **20**:434–438.

29 Filippi M, Campi A, Colombo B. A spinal cord MRI study of benign and secondary progressive multiple sclerosis. *J Neurol* 1996; **243**:502–505.

30 Thorpe JW, Kidd D, Moseley IF et al. Serial gadolinium-enhanced MRI of the brain and spinal cord in early relapsing–remitting multiple sclerosis. *Neurology* 1996; **46**:373–378.

31 Losseff NA, Lai M, Miller DH et al. The prognostic value of serial axial cord area measurement by magnetic resonance imaging in multiple sclerosis. *J Neurol* 1995; **242 (suppl 2)**:S110.

32 Losseff NA, Webb SL, O'Riordan JI et al. Spinal cord atrophy and disability in multiple sclerosis. A new reproducible and sensitive MRI method with potential to monitor disease progression. *Brain* 1996; **119**:701–708.

33 Losseff NA, Stevenson VL, Miller DH et al. Spinal cord atrophy and disability in multiple sclerosis: a serial MRI study. *Eur J Neurol* 1996; **3 (suppl 4)**:2.

34 Leary SM, Parker GJM, Stevenson VL et al. Quality assurance for serial studies of spinal cord atrophy. *Multiple Sclerosis* 1997; **3**:279.

35 Stevenson VL, Miller DH, Rovaris M et al. Primary progressive multiple sclerosis; a clinical and MRI cross sectional study. *Neurology* 1999; **52**:839–845.

36 Revesz T, Kidd D, Thompson AJ et al. A comparison of the pathology of primary and secondary progressive multiple sclerosis. *Brain* 1994; **117**:759–765.

37 Thompson AJ, Kermode AG, Wicks D et al. Major differences in the dynamics of primary and secondary progressive multiple sclerosis. *Ann Neurol* 1991; **29**:53–62.

38 Davie CA, Barker GJ, Thompson AJ et al. [1]H Magnetic resonance spectroscopy of chronic cerebral white matter lesions and normal appearing white matter in multiple sclerosis. *J Neurol Neurosurg Psychiatry* 1997; **63**:736–742.

39 Gross KR, Tomberg TA, Kokk AA et al. The prognosis of multiple sclerosis: computed tomographic

comparisons. *Zh Nevropatol Psikhiatr* 1993;
93:32–35.

40 Davie CA, Barker GJ, Webb S et al. Persistent
functional deficit in multiple sclerosis and autosomal
dominant cerebellar ataxia is associated with axon
loss. *Brain* 1995; **118**:1583–1592.

41 Rao SM, Glatt S, Hammeke TA et al. Chronic
progressive multiple sclerosis. Relationship between
cerebral ventricular size and neuropsychological
impairment. *Arch Neurol* 1985; **42**:678–682.

42 Comi G, Filippi M, Martinelli V et al. Brain magnetic
resonance imaging correlates of cognitive impairment
in multiple sclerosis. *J Neurol Sci* 1993; **115**:S66–S73.

43 Hageleit U, Will CH, Seidel D. Automated
measurements of cerebral atrophy in multiple sclerosis.
Neurosurg Rev 1987; **10**:32–35.

44 Huber SJ, Paulson GW, Shuttleworth EC et al.
Magnetic resonance imaging correlates of dementia in
multiple sclerosis. *Arch Neurol* 1987; **44**:732–736.

45 Blatter DD, Bigler ED, Gale SD et al. Quantitative
volumetric analysis of brain MR: normative database
spanning 5 decades of life. *AJNR* 1995; **16**:241–251.

46 Ron MA, Acker W, Shaw GK, Lishman WA.
Computerized tomography of the brain in chronic
alcoholism: a survey and follow-up study. *Brain* 1982;
105:497–514.

47 Kohlmeyer K, Lehmkuhl G, Poutska F. Computed
tomography of anorexia nervosa. *AJNR* 1983;
4:437–438.

48 Bentson J, Reza M, Winter J, Wilson G. Steroids and
apparent cerebral atrophy on computed tomography
scans. *J Comput Assist Tomogr* 1978; **2**:16–23.

49 Mellanby AR, Reveley MA. Effects of acute
dehydration on computerized tomographic assessment
of cerebral density and ventricular volume (letter).
Lancet 1982; **2**:874.

50 Losseff NA, Wang L, Lai HM et al. Progressive
cerebral atrophy in multiple sclerosis. A serial study.
Brain 1996; **119**:2009–2019.

51 Coles AJ, Wing MG, Paolillo A et al. Monoclonal
antibody treatment exposes three mechanisms
underlying the clinical course of multiple sclerosis.
Ann Neurol 1999; in press.

52 Matthews PM, Pioro E, Narayanan S et al. Assessment

of lesion pathology in multiple sclerosis using
quantitative MRI morphometry and magnetic
resonance spectroscopy. *Brain* 1996; **119**:715–722.

53 Lycklama à Nijeholt GJ, van Walderveen MAA et al.
Brain and spinal cord abnormalities in multiple
sclerosis. Correlation between MRI parameters,
clinical subtypes and symptoms. *Brain* 1998;
121:687–697.

54 Simon JH, Jacobs LD, Campion MK et al. A
longitudinal study of brain atrophy in relapsing
multiple sclerosis. *Neurology* 1999; in press.

55 Filippi M, Mastronardo G, Rocca MA et al.
Quantitative volumetric analysis of brain magnetic
resonance imaging from patients with multiple
sclerosis. *J Neurol Sci* 1998; **158**:148–153.

56 Hashimoto M, Kitagaki H, Imamura T et al. Medial
temporal and whole-brain atrophy in dementia with
Lewy bodies. A volumetric study. *Neurology* 1998;
51:357–362.

57 Stout JC, Jernigan TL, Archibald SL, Salmon DP.
Association of dementia severity with cortical grey
matter and abnormal white matter volumes in
dementia of the Alzheimer type. *Arch Neurol* 1996;
53:742–749.

58 Guttmann CRG, Jolesz FA, Kikinis R et al. White
matter changes with normal aging. *Neurology* 1998;
50:972–978.

59 Phillips MD, Grossman RI, Miki Y et al. Comparison
of T2 lesion volume and magnetization transfer ratio
histogram analysis and of atrophy and measures of
lesion burden in patients with multiple sclerosis. *AJNR*
1998; **19**:1055–1060.

60 Freeborough PA, Woods RP, Fox NC. Accurate
registration of serial 3D MR brain images and its
application to visualizing change in neurodegenerative
disorders. *J Comput Assist Tomogr* 1996;
20:1012–1022.

61 Fox NC, Freeborough PA. Brain atrophy progression
measured from registered serial MRI: validation and
application to Alzheimer's disease. *J Magn Reson
Imaging* 1997; **7**:1069–1075.

62 Fox NC, Freeborough PA, Rossor MN. Visualisation
and quantification of rates of atrophy in Alzheimer's
disease. *Lancet* 1996; **348**:94–97.

9

Measures for quantification of axonal damage in vivo based on magnetic resonance spectroscopic imaging

Douglas L Arnold and Paul M Matthews

INTRODUCTION

The clinical course of multiple sclerosis (MS) is highly variable, and pathological changes in the disease are heterogeneous between individuals. In recent years there has been increasing interest in developing approaches for characterizing the pathological substrates of disability in MS in the hope that quantitative indices of pathology in vivo would provide new, potentially more specific and sensitive end-points for treatment trials.

This chapter reviews magnetic resonance spectroscopy (MRS) studies of chemical pathology that is specific for axonal injury in vivo, and places these in context with respect to results from classical pathological investigations. It focuses on one of the most important of the hypotheses that have developed from magnetic resonance (MR) studies, namely that axonal damage may be the final common pathway causing disability in MS (*Fig. 9.1*).

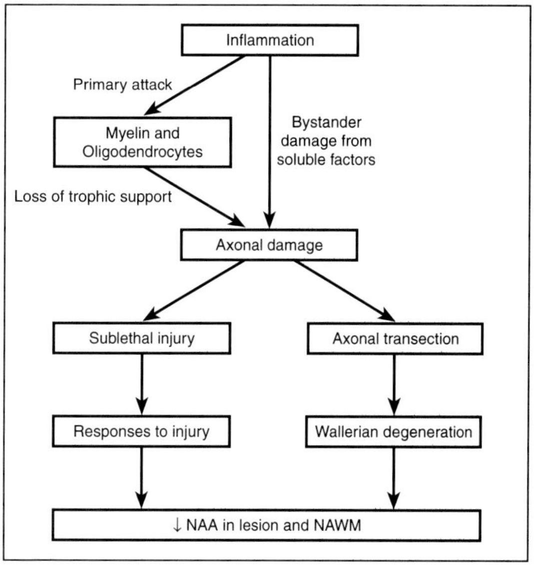

Fig. 9.1 The bases of axonal damage in lesions and NAWM of patients with MS.

THE CASE FOR AXONAL INJURY

Compared with the inflammatory lesions of encephalitis or ischemic infarction, microscopic examination of MS plaques shows demyelination with a relative preservation of axons. This observation, as well as experiments demonstrating that acute demyelination leads to conduction block, led to an earlier focus on demyelination as an explanation for functional impairments in MS.

119

Demyelination cannot account for chronic functional impairments in MS

However, demyelination alone does not adequately explain the functional impairments in MS. In patients with optic neuritis, although there may be early conduction block after acute inflammation, conduction recovers across chronically demyelinated regions of the optic nerve.[1] In the optic nerve of the myelin-deficient rat, action potential propagation is approximately five times slower than normal, but action potentials propagate securely and have frequency-following and refractory properties equivalent to myelinated axons in control rats.[2] Recently, Rodriguez and his colleagues have demonstrated that mice that are deficient in class I MHC (i.e. β-2-microglobulin deficient) and that are infected with Theiler's murine encephalomyelitis virus develop extensive demyelination without neurological deficits, whereas class II MHC-deficient mice develop demyelination and severe paralysis leading to early death.[3] A potentially important difference in the response of these two types of mice to inflammatory demyelination is that the class I MHC-deficient mice showed increased density of axon sodium channels after demyelination whereas class II MHC-deficit mice did not. Thus, demyelination alone is not sufficient for conduction block. Adaptations in the axon such as increased expression of sodium channels may contribute to maintenance of axonal function with chronic demyelination.

Mechanisms of acute conduction block are distinct from those for chronic functional impairment

It is important to distinguish acute from chronic impairment of axonal function. There are prob-ably multiple mechanisms of acute conduction block that are different from mechanisms causing chronic functional impairment. Acutely after demyelination, conduction block occurs because of the relatively sparse distribution of sodium channels in the normal internodal axon membrane. This effect appears not to be important with chronic demyelination, since sodium channels can be up-regulated along the demyelinated axon and conduction block recovers in more chronic models.[4] This phenomenon probably also operates in patients with MS, since demyelinated regions of white matter in MS patients have been shown to have an up to four-fold increase in sodium channels defined by autoradiographic binding of saxitoxin.[5]

The inflammatory response itself gives rise to additional potential mechanisms of acute conduction block in MS. Local inflammation can lead to injury or dysfunction of axons, even if axons are not the direct autoimmune target. Effects of the wide variety of locally released inflammatory mediators including, nitric oxide and reactive oxygen species, may cause metabolic dysfunction and conduction block[6,7] in axons projecting through areas of inflammation. Reversible dysfunction could also be mediated by local production of anti-neuronal antibodies. Central nervous system production of antibodies directed against a broad range of epitopes has been described in MS. Takigawa and colleagues have recently demonstrated that antibodies directed against GM1 gangliosides may suppress the axonal sodium current necessary for depolarization and cause conduction block.[8] Waxman has suggested that relative selectivity of antibodies for different sodium channel subtypes might account for the apparent variability of conduction block between different classes of axons.[9]

The axonal hypothesis

Defining the pathological changes that are ultimately responsible for functional impairments in MS is critical for the optimal targeting of new therapies. As demyelination is not a sufficient explanation, we have proposed the 'axonal hypothesis' for chronic disability in MS: 'Axonal damage or loss is **required** for **chronic** functional impairments and disability.'

One prediction of this hypothesis is that irreversible axonal loss must be associated with chronic, irreversible disability. A second prediction is that reversible axonal injury should be associated with functional recovery after relapse. Evidence supporting both predictions has come from MRS studies,[10,11] which provide quantitative tools for non-invasive detection of axonal injury and loss in patients with MS and allow dynamic correlations between pathology in vivo and disability (see *Fig. 9.1*).

Evidence of axonal injury from MRS and pathology

Introduction to MRS

A limitation of the use of conventional MRI to follow pathological changes is that image contrast is affected by too many factors to allow contrast changes to be interpreted in terms of specific pathological changes. In contrast, MRS studies can provide much more specific information about pathological changes in and around lesions, particularly regarding axonal loss or damage. Although the low concentrations of intracellular metabolites mean that the spatial resolution of the spectroscopic methods is much lower (currently in the order of 1 cm^3) than that of conventional MRI, statistical inferences from the two types of studies performed together can be pathologically specific and sufficiently well resolved.

Water-suppressed, localized proton MR spectra of the human brain (*Figs 9.2 and 9.3*) reveal major resonances from choline-containing phospholipids (Cho), creatine and phosphocreatine (Cr), N-acetyl groups, predominantly from N-acetylaspartate (NAA), and (under appropriate observational conditions) lactate and mobile lipids. Minor resonances from amino acids such as glutamate and γ-aminobutyric acid (GABA) and sugars such as glucose and inositol also can be identified. Two factors primarily determine which resonances can be usefully studied in the brain: mobility and concentrations. Only molecules that are freely mobile give rise to well-defined, discrete resonances, and only relatively abundant molecules with concentrations of the order of 1 mM lead to sufficient signal:noise ratio for adequate detection and quantification.

The N-acetyl group resonance has been particularly useful in studies of multiple sclerosis as a measure of NAA. NAA is found only in neurons and neuronal processes in the normal mature brain and therefore can be used as a specific axonal marker in white matter. Decreases in brain NAA in white matter reflect axonal pathology. Because MR spectra report on the density of NAA in a volume or 'voxel' of interest, decreases in the signal from NAA can occur as a result of either:

(a) decreased relative axonal density (volume per unit volume) in the voxel (caused by either axonal loss or axonal atrophy); or

(b) decreased concentration of NAA in axons (caused by axonal metabolic dysfunction).

Observed decreases in NAA may be either reversible or irreversible, depending on the nature of the responsible pathology (i.e. axonal loss secondary to axonal transection and wallerian

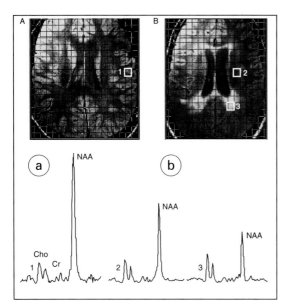

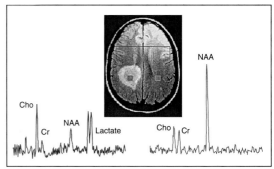

Fig. 9.3 *MR spectra from a large, isolated acute plaque. The conventional MRI shows the volume of excitation chosen for MRSI and indicates the locations from which sample spectra from the lesion (left) and contralateral normal-appearing brain (right) were chosen. Note the decrease in NAA in the lesion.*

Fig. 9.2 *(a) NAA in the NAWM of a normal subject. Conventional MRI shows the phase-encoding grid for the magnetic resonance spectroscopic image (MRSI). A sample spectrum from voxel 1 is shown below. (b) NAA in the NAWM of a patient with MS. Conventional MRI also shows the phase-encoding grid for the MRSI. A sample spectrum from a voxel with the appearance of lesion on MRI (2) and another from a voxel in NAWM (3) are shown below.*

degeneration, or reversible atrophy or metabolic dysfunction associated with sublethal injury).

MRS demonstrates substantial axonal injury in MS

The most striking observation made by the initial MRS studies of MS was that the brain NAA:Cr ratio was lower in patients with MS than in normal controls. As the Cr:Cho ratio is normal, it was concluded that brain NAA concentration must be reduced, implying that there was sub-stantial damage to axons throughout the white matter of patients with MS.[12–21] The decrease in NAA resonance intensity observed in normal-appearing white matter (NAWM) can approach 50% and the decrease of NAA in lesions can exceed 80%, presumably reflecting a proportional degree of axonal damage or loss (see *Fig. 9.2*). Direct measurements of the absolute concentrations of this metabolite has recently confirmed that NAA concentrations are reduced and that Cr concentrations are unchanged relative to normal controls.[22]

Histopathology also demonstrates substantial axonal damage in MS

This MRI evidence is consistent with a careful reading of post mortem pathological studies. Despite the emphasis in the past few decades on understanding myelin and oligodendroglial cell damage, even early neuropathological studies recognized axonal injury and loss in and around lesions in MS.[23] Charcot and many subsequent pathologists emphasized only that there was a relative preservation of axons (contrasting MS with highly destructive inflammatory diseases such as encephalitis). Axonal transection and damage in or around MS plaques have been assessed elegantly in recent studies that have demonstrated that axons are damaged in active lesions as well as in chronic lesions and that axonal damage (as assessed from expression of amyloid precursor protein) is far more extensive than is axonal transection.[24,25] Histopathology shows that loss of axons varies considerably between lesions[26] and extends substantially into the NAWM. For example, one study found that axonal density was decreased by a mean of 35% outside of lesions in the corpus callosum of eight patients with MS. In these cases there was a proportional loss of corpus callosum volumes, implying total axonal loss of as much as 50% in this NAWM (N Evangelou et al, unpublished).

The relationship between axonal damage, cerebral atrophy and disability

These observations emphasize that volume changes with loss of myelin and axons are not fully compensated by gliosis, so decreases in white matter volume should occur across the whole brain. In fact, a common observation from imaging of patients with MS is ventricular enlargement (and to a lesser extent, sulcal enlargement), as well as atrophy of the spinal cord.[27] Sensitive methods for detecting small volume changes from serially acquired structural brain (or spinal cord) images now are becoming more available.[28,29]

Total axonal loss can be assessed from the product of the axonal density and the brain volume loss (i.e. the relative decrease in NAA and the extent of atrophy). Since measures of spinal cord atrophy[30] and brain NAA[31] correlate strongly with disability, a combined index based on changes in spinal cord and cerebral volume and on decreases in the cerebral white matter NAA could prove to be a particularly sensitive index of change.

The relationship of axonal damage to disability

MRS measurements of NAA correlate with changes in disability

The axonal hypothesis (see above) posits that axonal damage is the major direct cause of chronic functional impairment in MS. If this is true, then there should be an inverse correlation between levels of brain NAA measured by MRS and disability both in cross-sectional studies and in longitudinal studies. One of the first MRS studies of MS suggested that this was indeed the case.[12] Davies and colleagues later showed that MS patients with high cerebellar dysfunction scores had lower cerebellar NAA than those with low cerebellar dysfunction scores and that normal controls had higher cerebellar NAA concentrations than either patient group.[32] More recent publications have shown strong negative correlations between cerebral white matter NAA concentrations and disability.[31]

Two studies have reported that the MRS measurement of white matter NAA concentrations is sensitive to the increasing axonal loss and damage expected from increasing disease burden with time. An informative early serial study of patients with MS in which single volume spectra were taken from a volume centered on the corpus callosum demonstrated a progressive decrease in the relative NAA resonance intensity over 18 months.[15] This was confirmed in a follow-up study with a larger group of patients, although the mean rate of decrease of NAA in the larger study was slower.[31] These and other studies[33] have emphasized that quantitative MRS studies are reproducible and that small changes can be detected reliably.

The importance of axonal damage in the NAWM

The earliest MRS studies in MS showed substantial decreases in brain NAA, even though lesions occupied only a small fraction of the magnetic resonance spectroscopic image (MRSI) volume. This suggested that axonal loss in MS was widespread. With the exception of the unpublished work on the corpus callosum cited above, we are aware of no direct pathological studies that have assessed the extent of axonal damage in NAWM. Because the NAWM constitutes the greatest bulk of white matter, even though axonal loss and damage are less severe overall than in individual lesions, it may be proportionally more significant in determining disability. The potential importance of these changes was suggested by a comparison of imaging changes in a group of patients with relapsing–remitting MS and a rather more disabled group with secondary progressive MS. The two groups did not have a significant difference in total T2-weighted lesion volume. However, the average extent of axonal injury assessed by brain NAA per unit lesion volume was significantly greater in those secondary progressive MS patients who had the longer disease duration and higher disability.[34] Follow-up

work showed definitely that this difference was due to relatively greater changes in the NAWM in the secondary progressive patients, rather than differences in the chemical pathology of the lesions themselves (see *Fig. 9.2*).[35] The strong correlation of decreases of NAA in NAWM with disability have been confirmed more recently and extended with measurements of absolute concentrations of NAA.[22]

In order to determine the relationship between progression of chronic disability and brain NAA, information from MRSI and conventional imaging studies have been combined using statistical models that allow precise correlations over time to be determined between the spatial distribution of chemical changes and changes on conventional MRI.[35,36] In this way, the time course of NAA changes can be followed with respect to the spatial distribution of NAA across the brain and the presence or absence of T2-weighted lesions in the same areas. This approach confirms our earlier reports of progressive decreases in NAA with time[15] and the correlation between generalized axonal damage in white matter and progression of disability in patients with MS.[35]

Reversible axonal dysfunction and clinical remission in MS

A striking and unexpected observation (which has since been confirmed by several research groups) has been that acute MS lesions (see *Fig. 9.3*) can be associated with reversible decreases in white matter NAA.[37,38] These reversible decreases in NAA are strongly correlated with reversible functional impairments in MS.[31] In small series of cases, serial studies of individual MRSI voxels have shown NAA decreases of between 30% and 80% in the center of lesions, with variable recovery of NAA towards normal concentrations after the acute phase of the relapse. NAA recovery was most rapid during the first few months. In these studies there was a striking direct correlation between the relative level of NAA in lesions and disability.

Only a small proportion of the apparent recovery of NAA in these large lesions can be related to resolution of local oedema, since the volume changes even in large lesions are relatively modest. Most of the change therefore must result from axonal volume loss or decreases in axonal NAA concentration. Axons can shrink in diameter with demyelination, because demyelination is associated with dephosphorylation of neurofilaments that help to maintain axonal diameter.[39] Increases in the diameter of reversibly atrophied axons should occur with remyelination. Alternatively, NAA recovery could reflect reversible metabolic dysfunction in axons, possibly associated with reversible mitochondrial damage. Mitochondrial toxins have been shown to cause decreases in NAA,[40] and in vitro studies of a neuronal cell line have demonstrated that decreases in NAA after serum deprivation can be fully reversed by further incubation in serum containing medium.[41] Several other acute, resolving pathologies have also been defined in which there are reversible changes in brain NAA.[38]

Integration of multiple measures of pathology and functional impairment

Recent pathological studies have emphasized heterogeneity in the pathology of MS. Defining this heterogeneity is important since it may be expected to contribute to the considerable clinical heterogeneity of MS. Lucchinetti and col-

leagues,[42] for example, have proposed that there are five distinct patterns of lesion pathology that can be discriminated in post mortem materials based on the nature of myelin, oligodendroglial cell and axonal changes. Just as the classical pathologist employs a range of cell and tissue markers together in order to develop a composite picture of pathological changes in lesions, so those studying MS pathology by MR must simultaneously apply and integrate multiple techniques. Combined use of MRSI and novel water-based imaging sequences that are more sensitive to different aspects of pathological changes than current, conventional MRI sequences are, should better define the pathological heterogeneity in lesions. Calculation of the extent of brain atrophy in conjunction with MRSI measures of axonal density should provide a better index of axonal damage.

Implications of MRS studies for understanding the natural history and treatment of MS

Evidence (as reviewed briefly above) is accumulating that chronic, progressive changes in disability may reflect directly the chronic progressive damage to axons that now is appreciated as such a key feature of multiple sclerosis. A principal conclusion of recent MRS studies has been that this damage is manifest *throughout* the white matter of the brain, not just in the focal lesions where the most prominent inflammatory changes occur.[22,25] Axonal metabolic dysfunction also seems likely to play a role in the acute, reversible functional impairments associated with relapses. These effects can be both local to new inflammatory lesions and much more widespread.[43]

These observations have important implications for the treatment of MS. First, they suggest that a given treatment strategy may not be equally efficacious for all patients even with the same clinical syndrome (e.g. relapsing–remitting MS). If there is significant heterogeneity of pathological mechanisms between individuals, it may be rational to tailor treatments for particular pathological subgroups. MR methods could provide a clinically practical way of stratifying patients for different treatments. There is clearly an urgent need to co-ordinate classical pathological and MR studies in an effort to address this question.

Secondly, new drugs or combinations of drugs that are targeted against multiple mechanisms responsible for the progression of the pathology need to be developed. Current approaches are directed primarily towards limiting the acute inflammatory responses. Modulation of mechanisms underlying acute and chronic axonal injury or enhancing functional reorganization of the brain may clearly also be important. The lack of enthusiasm for axonal potassium channel blockade by aminopyridines may be tempered by recognition that effects may only be expected for a limited period in lesion evolution (e.g. during the period of acute conduction block). Further development of strategies based on use of neurotrophins and other neuronal survival factors may be important for enhancing axonal survival and recovery potential in the longer term. Efforts to control specific mechanisms of axonal injury, such as those that might be mediated by anti-sodium channel antibodies, also need to be explored.

A third major conclusion from the work reviewed above arises from the observation that axonal injury occurs even in acute lesions. With this in mind, the rationale for reducing relapse rate and treating acute relapses changes from that of short-term enhancement of the quality of life to preventing the accumulation of later, more severe axonal loss and associated disability. The sensitivity of clinical measures in short trials designed to detect such changes is understandably limited, suggesting that the use of a surrogate marker such as brain NAA may be the only practical approach to defining effects of new drugs on the progression of axonal damage. Appreciation of the role of axonal injury in chronic disability progression should enhance enthusiasm for early treatment of patients to reduce inflammation.

Ultimately, the development of multiple, complementary methods for defining the pathological changes in MS may contribute to rational approaches towards the preparation of in vivo strategies for simultaneous targeting of multiple pathological stages with combined therapy. Such approaches also should allow improved trial designs, not only by increasing the precision with which trial end-points based on such surrogate markers can be reached, but also by providing pathological specificity to allow trials of new agents even in populations being treated with agents targeting other stages in the pathological progression of the disease.

SUMMARY

Recent MRS techniques have focused the attention of the MS research community on the importance of axonal injury in this primarily demyelinating disease. Axonal injury most likely results mainly from 'innocent bystander' damage to axons associated with the inflammatory response directed against myelin. However, because axons depend on glia for trophic and other support, glial damage alone may also lead to axonal atrophy or dysfunction. MRS studies have emphasized that axonal damage in MS can be substantial and that it occurs early on in the development of the disease. The dynamic observations of axonal pathology that are possible with MRS have demonstrated direct correlations between measures of axonal damage and disability. These observations suggest that new treatments for MS may be able to be directed towards limitation of damage to axons or the salvage of injured axons.

ACKNOWLEDGEMENTS

DLA is grateful for support from the Medical Research Council of Canada and the Multiple Sclerosis Society of Canada. PMM acknowledges support from the Medical Research Council of Great Britain.

REFERENCES

1 Youl BD, Turano G, Miller DH et al. The pathophysiology of acute optic neuritis. An association of gadolinium leakage with clinical and electrophysiological deficits. *Brain* 1991; 114:2437–2450.

2 Utzschneider DA, Thio C, Sontheimer H et al. Action potential conduction and sodium channel content in the optic nerve of the myelin-deficient rat. *Proc R Soc London [Biol]* 1993; 254:245–250.

3 Rivera-Quinones CMD, Schmelzer JD, Hunter SF et al. Absence of neurological deficits following extensive demyelination in a class I-deficient murine model of multiple sclerosis. *Nature Med* 1998; 4:187–193.

4 England JD, Gamboni F, Levinson SR, Finger TE. Changed distribution of sodium channels along demyelinated axons. *Proc Natl Acad Sci U S A* 1990; 87:6777–6780.

5 Moll C, Mourre C, Lazdunski M, Ulrich J. Increase of sodium channels in demyelinated lesions of multiple sclerosis. *Brain Res* 1991; 556:311–316.

6 Redford EJ, Kapoor R, Smith KJ. Nitric oxide donors reversibly block axonal conduction: demyelinated

axons are especially susceptible. *Brain* 1997; 120:2149–2157.

7 Brosnan CF, Litwak MS, Schroeder CE et al. Preliminary studies of cytokine-induced functional effects on the visual pathways in the rabbit. *J Neuroimmunol.* 1989; 25:227–239.

8 Takigawa T, Yasuda H, Kikkawa R et al. Antibodies against GM1 ganglioside affect K⁺ and Na⁺ currents in isolated rat myelinated nerve fibers (see comments). (Comment in: *Ann Neurol* 1995; 37:421–423). *Ann Neurol* 1995; 37:436–442.

9 Waxman SG. Sodium channel blockade by antibodies: a new mechanism of neurological disease? *Ann Neurol* 1995; 37:421–423.

10 Miller DH, Kesselring J, McDonald WI, eds. *Magnetic Resonance in Multiple Sclerosis.* Cambridge: Cambridge University Press, 1997.

11 Arnold DL, Matthews PM, De Stefano N. MRI and proton MRS in the evaluation of multiple sclerosis. In: Bachelard HS, ed. *Magnetic Resonance Spectroscopy and Imaging in Neurochemistry*, New York: Plenum Publishing, 1997: 267–288.

12 Arnold DL, Matthews PM, Francis G, Antel J. Proton magnetic resonance spectroscopy of human brain in vivo in the evaluation of multiple sclerosis: assessment of the load of disease. *Magn Reson Med* 1990; 14:154–159.

13 Matthews PM, Francis G, Antel J, Arnold DL. Proton magnetic resonance spectroscopy for metabolic characterization of plaques in multiple sclerosis (published erratum appears in *Neurology* 1991; 41:1828). *Neurology* 1991; 41:1251–1256.

14 Arnold DL, Matthews PM, Francis GS et al. Proton magnetic resonance spectroscopic imaging for metabolic characterization of demyelinating plaques. *Ann Neurol* 1992; 31:235–241.

15 Arnold DL, Riess GT, Matthews PM et al. Use of proton magnetic resonance spectroscopy for monitoring disease progression in multiple sclerosis. *Ann Neurol* 1994; 36:76–82.

16 Miller DH, Austin SJ, Connelly A et al. Proton magnetic resonance spectroscopy of an acute and chronic lesion in multiple sclerosis (letter). *Lancet* 1991; 337:58–59.

17 Van Hecke P, Marchal G, Johannik K et al. Human brain proton localized NMR spectroscopy in multiple sclerosis. *Magn Reson Med* 1991; 18:199–206.

18 Bruhn H, Frahm J, Merboldt KD et al. Multiple sclerosis in children: cerebral metabolic alterations monitored by localized proton magnetic resonance spectroscopy *in vivo. Ann Neurol* 1992; 32:140–150.

19 Grossman RI, Lenkinski RE, Ramer KN et al. MR proton spectroscopy in multiple sclerosis. *AJNR* 1992; **13**:1535–1543.

20 Davie CA, Hawkins CP, Barker GJ et al. Serial proton magnetic resonance spectroscopy in acute multiple sclerosis lesions. *Brain* 1994; **117**:49–58.

21 Husted CA, Goodin DS, Hugg JW et al. Biochemical alterations in multiple sclerosis lesions and normal-appearing white matter detected by in vivo 31P and 1H spectroscopic imaging. *Ann Neurol* 1994; **36**:157–165.

22 Sarchielli P, Presciutti O, Pelliccioli GP et al. Absolute quantification of brain metabolites by proton magnetic resonance spectroscopy in normal-appearing white matter of multiple sclerosis patients. *Brain* 1999; **122**:513–521.

23 Charcot JM. Histologie de le sclerose en plaques. *Gazette des Hopitaux* 1868; 554–558.

24 Ferguson B, Matyszak MK, Esiri MM, Perry VH. Axonal damage in acute multiple sclerosis lesions. *Brain* 1997; **120**:393–399.

25 Trapp BD, Peterson J, Ransohoff RM et al. Axonal transection in the lesions of multiple sclerosis. *N Engl J Med* 1998; **338**:278–285.

26 Barnes D, Munro PMG, Youl BD et al. The longstanding MS lesion; a quantitative MRI and electron microscopic study. *Brain* 1991; **114**:1271–1280.

27 Losseff NA, Miller DH. Measures of brain and spinal cord atrophy in multiple sclerosis. *J Neurol Neurosurg Psychiatry* 1998; **64**(suppl 1):S102–105.

28 Freeborough PA, Fox NC. The boundary shift integral: an accurate and robust measure of cerebral volume changes from registered repeat MRI. *IEEE Trans Med Imaging* 1997; **16**:623–629.

29 Liu CK, Edwards S, Gong Q et al. Three dimensional MRI estimates of brain and spinal cord atrophy in multiple sclerosis. *J Neurol Neurosurg Psychiatry* 1999; **66**:323–330.

30 Losseff NA, Webb SL, O'Riordan JI et al. Spinal cord atrophy and disability in multiple sclerosis. A new reproducible and sensitive MRI method with potential to monitor disease progression. *Brain* 1996; **119**:701–708.

31 De Stefano N, Matthews PM, Fu L et al. Axonal damage correlates with disability in patients with relapsing remitting multiple sclerosis: results of a jongitudinal MR spectroscopy study. *Brain* 1998; **121**:1469–1477.

32 Davie CA, Barker GJ, Webb S et al. Persistent functional deficit in multiple sclerosis and autosomal dominant cerebellar ataxia is associated with axon loss. *Brain* 1995; **118**:1583–1592.

33 Kalra S, Cashman NR, Genge A, Arnold DL. Recovery of N-acetylaspartate in corticomotor neurons of patients with ALS after Riluzole therapy. *NeuroReport* 1998; **9**:1757–1761.

34 Matthews PM, Pioro E, Narayanan S et al. Assessment of lesion pathology in multiple sclerosis using quantitative MRI morphometry and magnetic resonance spectroscopy. *Brain* 1996; **119**:715–722.

35 Fu L, Matthews PM, De Stefano N et al. Imaging axonal damage of normal appearing white matter in multiple sclerosis. *Brain* 1998; **121**:103–113.

36 Fu L, Wolfson C, Worsley KJ, De Stefano N et al. Statistics for investigation of multimodal MR imaging data and an application to multiple sclerosis patients. *NMR Biomed* 1996; **9**:339–346.

37 Arnold DL. Reversible reduction of N-acetylaspartate after acute central nervous system in damage (abstract). *Proc Soc Magn Reson Med* 1992; **1**:643.

38 De Stefano N, Matthews PM, Arnold DL. Reversible decreases in N-acetylaspartate after acute brain injury. *Magn Reson Med* 1995; **34**:721–727.

39 Prineas JW, Connell F. The fine structure of chronically active multiple sclerosis plaques. *Neurology* 1978; **28** (suppl 2):68–75.

40 Bates TE, Strangward M, Keelan J et al. Inhibition of N-acetylaspartate production: implications for 1H MRS studies in vivo. *NeuroReport* 1996; **7**:1397–1400.

41 Matthews PM, Cianfaglia L, McLaurin J et al. Demonstration of reversible decreases in N-acetylaspartate (NAA) in a neuronal cell line: NAA decreases as a marker of sublethal neuronal dysfunction (abstract). *Proc Soc Magn Reson Med* 1995; **1**:147.

42 Lucchinetti CF, Bruck W, Rodriguez M, Lassmann H. Distinct patterns of multiple sclerosis pathology indicates heterogeneity on pathogenesis (review). *Brain Pathol* 1996; **6**:259–274.

43 De Stefano N, Matthews PM, Narayanan S et al. Axonal dysfunction and disability in a relapse of multiple sclerosis: longitudinal study of a patient. *Neurology* 1997; **49**:1138–1141.

10
Body fluid markers for disease course and activity

Patricia K Coyle

INTRODUCTION

Most of the disease activity in multiple sclerosis (MS) is subclinical. Frequent brain magnetic resonance imaging (MRI) studies performed in relapsing and secondary progressive MS patients document that the rate of new lesion formation is five to 10 times greater than the clinical attack rate.[1] This silent and ongoing disease activity contributes to the total brain burden of disease, which increases by approximately 10% annually.[1]

The obvious conclusion from neuroimaging data is that dependence on clinical parameters alone to evaluate disease activity in MS will be misleading. Although MRI is considered the best current biologic marker of MS disease activity, it is not used in routine care to follow patients. Frequent scans are costly and impractical.

Body fluid markers for MS disease activity would be a major advance. Assays to detect such markers would need to be sensitive, specific, reproducible, economical, and repeatable at multiple timepoints.[2] Markers would not just allow accurate assessment of MS activity; they would also help to select the appropriate treatment on the basis of disease course and severity, and they would provide a measure of response to therapy. At the current time there are no standardized

criteria to determine treatment failure. Validated disease activity markers could be used in therapeutic trials, in place of multiple MRI scans, at significant cost savings. Markers for different MS disease courses, such as the transition stage from relapsing to secondary progressive MS, would also be invaluable. Although relapsing and progressive MS subtypes have been defined, it is not known whether they have true biologic differences. Identification of distinguishing markers for relapsing and progressive disease, as well as for the transition phase between the two, could offer important pathogenic clues to MS.

There is no accepted body fluid assay for MS disease activity or course. Many factors make development of such a marker difficult.[2] MS involves multiple pathologic processes (edema, inflammation, blood–brain barrier damage, demyelination, remyelination, gliosis, and axonal damage). Each of these processes may have different markers. MS also involves simultaneous destructive and repair mechanisms, so that the state being measured is rarely solely a damaging one. MS is highly variable and dynamic, which mandates frequent sampling. One would really want to validate markers in early patients who have minimal confounding factors created by a chronic disease state. MS takes a finite time to diagnose, however, so that very early (asymptomatic) patients are never studied. Finally, many of the proposed markers are immunologic ones. They have multiple different actions and are influenced by diverse extrinsic and intrinsic host factors. The immunology of MS is complex and is not likely to be measured by any single test.

BODY FLUIDS

A number of different body fluids have been examined in MS to look for immune, inflammatory, or other markers (*Table 10.1*). Both blood and urine have the advantage of being very easy to sample on multiple occasions, with little discomfort or risk. However, both body fluids are remote from the central nervous system (CNS), the site of the MS disease process. An additional disadvantage is that many different processes produce changes in blood and urine. They are

Table 10.1 Body fluids examined in MS

Blood
    Cells
    Non-cell components (serum, plasma)

Cerebrospinal fluid
    Cells
    Non-cell components

Urine

Mucosal fluids
    Tears (cells, non-cell components)
    Saliva (cells, non-cell components)

complex fluids that contain a number of components at significant levels. These components can contribute to the background noise and interfere with detection systems. Fluid components are also subject to diurnal variations.

Urine

Urine is an ideal fluid to study when a marker is excreted, since it will be enriched.[3] Urine is best suited to examining substances that are excreted with minimal tubular reabsorption. Examples of such substances are neopterin, nitrites, and nitrates. Urine is theoretically less suitable for the measurement of peptides and proteins. There are many factors to consider if urine is used as a sample source. The actual concentration of a marker in urine depends on urine output, which is highly variable over a 24-hour period. Therefore, creatinine, which has no appreciable tubular reabsorption, is generally used as an internal reference to correct for concentration. Urine values are expressed as the ratio of the measured factor to creatinine. Men have creatinine concentrations that are 1.2–1.4 times higher than those of women, so that a correction factor of 1.2 has been used to normalize for sex.[3] In the case of peptides and proteins, albumin serves as a better internal reference standard than creatinine. A number of factors can influence urine protein excretion and thus final results, including exercise, posture, and renal disease. The timing of sampling is another variable, and it has been suggested that the first morning urine may be the best source to use in neurologic disease.[3] The frequency of sampling is another consideration. To evaluate inflammatory factors, daily or weekly urine samples are probably better than twice-weekly or monthly urine samples. A final variable to consider, particularly in MS, is that bladder infection can influence urine components and should be excluded.

Cerebrospinal fluid

Cerebrospinal fluid (CSF) offers the advantage of direct access to the intrathecal compartment, since it consists of extracellular fluid from the brain and spinal cord as well as being the product of intraventricular choroid plexus. Unlike blood and urine it is 99% water, and it contains fewer components that are at much lower concentrations than seen in these other fluids. The major disadvantage of CSF is that collection requires lumbar puncture. Although minimally invasive, repeat lumbar punctures are problematic and never likely to be widely accepted.

Mucosal fluids

Mucosal fluids allow study of the mucosal immune system. This major systemic immune system is not well characterized in MS. External fluids such as tears and saliva are readily accessible, but with limitations. It is difficult to obtain large volumes of tears to study, there are dilutional factors to consider, and inadvertent ocular trauma during collection can confound results. Saliva also involves dilutional factors, and it must be collected by cannulation of the parotid gland duct if one wishes to avoid contamination by mouth debris. Other mucosal fluids, such as breast milk, bronchial secretions, and gastrointestinal fluids, are not easily available. There are no major studies of these body fluids in MS.

Measurement standardization

There is one final practical consideration. For any proposed disease marker it will be important to standardize measurement to account for daily fluctuations, and to quantify the ranges of values found in matched controls. This will help to define both variability and the degree of overlap with the normal population.

BLOOD

Although pathologic changes in MS are confined to the CNS, MS patients show many systemic immune disturbances. Immune components have been studied in blood to attempt to define a disease marker (*Table 10.2*). The difficulty has been that supportive studies are limited, there are often conflicting results, there have been limited longitudinal studies, and the markers are not specific to MS but can be elevated by a number of immune or inflammatory processes.

One potential blood marker involves an enzyme. Matrix metalloproteinases (MMPs) are a

Table 10.2 Blood disease markers studied in MS

Matrix metalloproteinases and tissue inhibitors

Circulating adhesion molecules

Cytokines and cytokine receptors

Cell subpopulations

Antibodies

S-100

Neopterin

family of enzymes that degrade basement membrane and extracellular matrix. They can also degrade myelin basic protein to release immunogenic fragments.[4] These enzymes are produced by leukocytes, astrocytes, and microglia, among other cells. Production is induced by cytokines that are released during an inflammatory reaction. MMPs appear to play an important role in allowing immune cells to penetrate the blood–brain barrier in MS. They are inactivated by tissue inhibitors (TIMPs). A recent study of 24 relapsing MS patients reported that increased serum levels of MMP-9 (gelatinase B), accompanied by low levels of TIMP-1, predicted occurrence over the following month of gadolinium-enhancing lesions on brain MRI.[5] Another study of 21 relapsing MS patients found elevated levels of MMP-9 compared to controls. Elevated levels were associated with both clinical and MRI disease activity, and the MS patients showed a distinctive TIMP response pattern compared to control subjects with inflammatory neurological disease.[6]

Another potential marker involves adhesion molecules. The data is strongest that soluble forms of intercellular adhesion molecule type I (sICAM-1) and vascular cell adhesion molecule type I (sVCAM-1) may correlate with disease activity.[2] In contrast, adhesion molecule expression on mononuclear cells does not correlate with activity. ICAM-1 belongs to the immunoglobulin superfamily. It is expressed on activated endothelial cells, lymphocytes, and monocytes. Elevations in sICAM-1 are found in clinically active MS patients, while clinically stable patients have much lower levels that are similar to those in healthy controls.[7] Two longitudinal studies of sICAM-1 have been performed. One study reported a significant association between relapses and elevated levels.[8] In the other study, sICAM–1 levels were variable, and there was no

consistent association with relapses.[9] Soluble ICAM-1 levels are also elevated in patients with contrast-enhancing lesions on brain MRI.[7] A recent cross-sectional study documented a correlation between sVCAM-1, and to a lesser extent sICAM-1, and the number and volume of enhancing lesions on MRI.[10]

VCAM-1 is another member of the immunoglobulin superfamily that is shed by activated macrophages and endothelial cells. Correlations with MS disease activity are not as strong as for sICAM-1.[7] Some studies have found elevated levels associated with active disease, but other studies have failed to confirm this association.[7,8,11,12]

There is also some data on selectins. E-selectin is shed from activated endothelial cells. Levels are reported to be higher in progressive MS patients than in relapsing MS patients, and appear to correlate with clinical disease progression.[11,13,14] L-Selectin is shed from activated leukocytes. Two groups have reported significant correlations between serum levels and contrast enhancing lesions on brain MRI.[12,15] Unfortunately, current assays do not differentiate L-selectin shed from lymphocytes from that shed from neutrophils. Lymphocyte L-selectin is likely to be much more pertinent to the MS disease process.

Other potential blood markers are cytokines and their receptors. Cytokines are soluble immunomodulators that play an important role in MS. There are many different cytokines, but they can be broadly divided into pro-inflammatory cytokines, anti-inflammatory and regulatory cytokines, and chemokines. There are several different ways of measuring cytokine levels. One way is to quantitate levels in serum or plasma at a single point in time. This can be misleading, since the half-life is short and levels can vary widely over time. Another way is to examine individual cell production of cytokines through intracellular staining, immunologic assays such as Enzyme Linked ImmunoSPOT (ELISPOT), or detection of cytokine gene message. Reverse transcriptive polymerase chain reaction or in situ hybridization can be used to measure cytokine messenger RNA (mRNA). A third way is to look at in vitro production of cytokines by isolated cells, by measuring their release into culture medium. Levels of pro-inflammatory cytokines such as tumor necrosis factor (TNF)-α, interleukin (IL)-1, IL-2 and interferon (IFN)-γ have been reported to be elevated in the serum of MS patients.[12,16,18] In contrast, cells expressing transforming growth factor (TGF)-β, an anti-inflammatory and regulatory cytokine, are higher in mild disease than in severe disease.[19] The data linking a blood cytokine to disease activity is strongest for TNF-α.[16,17,20–22] Another pro-inflammatory cytokine, IFN-γ, has been shown to increase in serum before clinical attacks in a northern European MS population.[16] A pro-inflammatory cytokine receptor, soluble IL-2 receptor, is also reported to be increased in active MS.[23,24] The difficulty with using cytokines or their receptors to assay disease activity in MS involves, in part, choosing the best way to measure them. However, cytokines belong to a network that involves multiple interactions. Every cytokine has multiple actions, which can be both good and bad for the MS disease process. They are also affected by many host factors. This explains, at least in part, why results of the various studies have been inconsistent.

Blood cells have also been proposed as potential markers. Lymphocyte subsets do not give consistent results when correlated with disease activity, although activated T cells as measured by specific surface markers are increased.[25] Functional suppressor (CD8+ T cell) activity is decreased, particularly in secondary progressive MS.[26,27] Immune cells produce cytokines. Using intracellular staining, there are increased subsets of CD4+ and CD8+ T cells producing IFN-γ in secondary progressive MS patients compared to relapsing patients.[28] T cell lines from MS patients with active disease produce less TGF-β than cells from patients with stable disease.[19] There is also a higher expression of TGF-β mRNA and IL-10 mRNA in mononuclear cells of stable MS patients than in relapsing MS patients.[18] Patients with progressive MS are said to show significantly increased IFN-γ production compared to relapsing MS patients when T cells are stimulated with anti-CD3 antibody (a T-cell receptor mediated process). This increased production is IL-12 dependent, and progressive MS patients show increased T-cell-receptor mediated IL-12 production compared to relapsing MS patients.[29]

Natural killer (NK) cells are large, granular lymphocytes that do not have a surface antigen receptor. They mediate antibody-dependent cell-mediated cytotoxicity, and they lyse virus infected and tumor cells. They can also release a variety of cytokines, activate phagocytic cells, and promote antigen specific T-helper 1 (TH$_1$) cells.[30] Both NK cell numbers and functional activity (typically based on in vitro assays of cell killing, with measurement of chromium 51 release) have been measured in MS. The results are conflicting and indicates fluctuations in both cell numbers and activity. A recent study did report a correlation between reduction in functional NK activity and appearance of active MRI lesions.[30] The authors of this study suggested that low functional NK activity provided a risk factor for clinical attacks and MRI lesions. However, the number of NK cells did not correlate with this decrease in functional activity. Measurement of NK cell numbers and functional activity is not sufficiently established and standardized to be useful as a biologic marker.

Antibodies have also been proposed as disease markers. Elevated levels of antibodies to cardiolipin have been associated with a slower progressive course, and atypical clinical features for MS (persistent headache and absent CSF oligoclonal bands).[31] Elevated levels of anti-GM3 ganglioside antibodies have been reported in progressive MS compared to relapsing MS.[32]

A number of miscellaneous markers have also been looked at. S-100 is an astrocyte protein. A recent study reported that plasma S-100 levels were increased in MS relapses.[33] Neopterin is also reported as increased in MS blood.

At the current time, enzymes and adhesion molecules appear to be the most promising blood markers of disease activity, but much more evidence needs to be presented.

CEREBROSPINAL FLUID

CSF is the body fluid that is most pertinent to the MS disease process. Unfortunately, it is not practical to do repeated CSF samples unless they provide invaluable information on the MS disease process. No CSF assay offers such information, with the exception of the diagnostic implications of CSF oligoclonal bands and intrathecal IgG production (*Table 10.3*). CSF examination is recognized as important in the diagnosis of MS. A high proportion (90–95%) of patients ultimately develop CSF oligoclonal bands, and 70–90% develop intrathecal IgG production. These tests are most likely to be negative early in the disease course, but once positive they remain positive. Therefore, they do not correlate with disease activity, although limited data suggests that persistent oligoclonal band negativity is more likely with a mild MS disease course. Early studies suggested that the number of T cells in the CSF might correlate with disease activity, but in subsequent studies CSF cell count has not correlated with activity. With regard to cell count, only a minority of MS patients have a pleocytosis. However, activated CD4+ T cells increase during clinical disease activity.[34]

Myelin basic protein (MBP) and its peptides can be detected in CSF. This assay correlates with acute myelin damage within the CNS, and has been extensively studied in MS.[35,36] CSF MBP is not disease-specific, and larger forms appear in CSF after stroke and head injury, to name two examples. In MS patients, MBP is most likely to be elevated in clinical relapses, and it can remain elevated for up to 6 weeks.[36] It is likely that the location as well as size of the lesion is a factor. MBP is more likely to be positive in polyregional attacks, and it is often negative in optic neuritis attacks. In clinically stable MS patients, CSF MBP is usually undetectable, while progressive MS patients can have negative or low positive values. In one study, the concentration of CSF MBP correlated with attack severity.[37] A recent study also found that MBP levels correlated with clinical disease activity measures.[38] In clinically definite MS patients, the CSF MBP concentration correlated with the patient's Kurtzke Expanded Disability Status Scale. In optic neuritis, CSF MBP levels correlated with visual acuity. MBP positivity may predict response to glucocorticoids.[39] In another study MBP positivity correlated with MRI disease activity.[40] The real problem is that the assay is not truly standardized. It remains a radioimmunoassay using polyclonal reagents, and it has not been converted to an enzyme-linked immunosorbent assay or a monoclonal based assay.

There is no clear-cut correlation between

Table 10.3 CSF disease markers studied in MS

CNS tissue markers

    Myelin basic protein

    S-100

    Neuron specific enolase

    Glial fibrillary acidic protein

    Neurofilaments

    Neural cell adhesion molecule

    Ciliary neurotropic factor

Immune markers

    Free light chains

    Cytokines and cytokine receptors

    Oligoclonal bands

    Intrathecal immunoglobulin production (IgD, IgM)

    T cells

    Adhesion and other surface molecules (HLA class I, CD27)

    Co-stimulatory molecules (B7-1)

Inflammatory and other markers

    Gliotoxin

    Neopterin

    Matrix metalloproteinases (MMP9/gelatinase B)

intrathecal IgG production and disease activity.[35] It is not uncommon to see CSF immunoglubulin levels increase with disability and disease duration, as a measure of blood–CSF barrier impairment. The immunoglobulin measures that have been suggested to correlate with disease activity are free immunoglobulin light chains, intrathecal IgD production, and intrathecal IgM production.[41–43] These assays are not routinely available. Free light chains in CSF appear to be useful in the diagnosis of MS.[44,45] Free κ chains tend to be more prominent than free λ chains and have greater specificity for

MS.[46] Some studies suggest that intrathecal synthesis of free light chains correlate with disease activity.[47–49] In the recent phase 3 trial of IFN-β 1a (Avonex®), baseline CSF free κ chains, IgG index, and oligoclonal bands showed a weak correlation with MRI parameters of contrast-enhancing lesion volume and T2-weighted burden of disease.[50] These CSF parameters were not affected by treatment.

Gliotoxin is a glycoprotein that is cytotoxic to primary cortical brain culture and glial cell lines. It causes disruption of the cytoskeletal structure, with cell death of glia through apoptosis (programmed cell death).[51] This protein appears to be specific to MS CSF.[52] It increases permeability of the blood–CSF barrier, leading to increased immunoglobulin levels. It has also been reported in MS urine. Neopterin is an IFN-γ-induced product of activated macrophages; it is a marker for inflammation. Neopterin is also reported to be increased in MS CSF.[53]

Pro-inflammatory cytokines have been reported to be increased in the CSF of MS patients. TNF levels have been associated with contrast-enhancing lesions on brain MRI[54] and with disease activity.[22] IL-15 mRNA-expressing cells were found to be up-regulated in the CSF of MS patients compared to aseptic meningitis patients.[55] There is increase in mRNA expressing cells for TNF-α and IFN-γ.[56,57]

Soluble adhesion molecules are also increased in MS CSF. CSF sICAM-1 levels, and the serum-to-CSF ratios, were associated with blood-brain barrier damage and disease activity as measured by MRI.[58] The data on whether sVCAM-1 is elevated in active MS are conflicting.[7]

S-100 is an astrocyte protein. In a preliminary report, CSF levels of S-100 were elevated following clinical relapse. Elevated levels persisted for at least 5 weeks.[59] In another preliminary report, neurofilaments were elevated in CSF of relapsing patients; levels correlated with disability and attack rate.[60] Glial fibrillary acidic protein is found in astrocytes. It is reported to be increased in the CSF of 9–39% of MS patients.[61] A recent study reported that CSF levels correlated with clinical deficit.[62] CSF levels of neural cell adhesion molecule and ciliary neurotrophic factor are also reported to be elevated after MS relapse.[63]

Overall, CSF markers have been disappointing to date with regard to offering a way to monitor MS disease activity. It does not seem likely that any assay will be developed to justify routine serial CSF sampling in MS.

URINE

Urine is an accessible fluid that can be collected on multiple occasions, although time of day, the volume collected, and the presence of infection may influence results. Several urinary markers have been looked at (*Table 10.4*).

The best established of these is an MBP-like material, which is detected using a highly selected antiserum.[64] It is immunochemically different from CSF MBP. The material detected in urine is smaller than that found in CSF, and it contains a cryptic epitope that is not exposed in the native

Table 10.4 Urine disease markers studied in MS

Myelin basic protein-like material

Free light chains

Neopterin

Gliotoxin

Neuron-specific enolase

molecule. The urine molecule is not attached to any other, and may actually represent a small peptide. MBP-like material is found as a normal urine constituent, and values fluctuate independent of acute relapses.

Diet, renal status, and MS disease activity do not seem to influence urine levels. However, recent studies suggest that MBP-like material in urine markedly increases in patients with the secondary progressive form of MS.[65] In the phase 3 trial of IFN-β 1b (Betaseron®), levels were elevated in relapsing MS patients who went on to develop secondary progressive MS.[66] In this group of patients, increased MBP-like material in urine did correlate with the number and volume of T2-weighted MRI brain lesions.[35] In a prospective study of 131 relapsing and 35 secondary progressive MS patients treated with IFN-β 1b, urine MBP-like material was higher in the progressive group, and in the 13 relapsing patients who converted to secondary progressive disease during the evaluation period.[67] These findings raise the possibility that this urine assay could be a marker for transition from relapsing to progressive disease. Unfortunately the assay is currently performed at only one research centre. Urine MBP-like material may reflect ongoing synthesized material that is not incorporated into the myelin sheath.

Neopterin is another potential urine disease marker. Urinary neopterin levels were studied in 31 relapsing, primary progressive, and secondary progressive MS patients, and compared to 14 healthy controls.[68] Urine samples were collected daily for up to 12 weeks. Urine neoplasm and creatinine levels were measured by high-pressure liquid chromatography. The urine neopterin-to-creatinine ratio was elevated in all the MS groups compared to the controls. All clinically apparent disease relapses were associated with elevated urine neopterin excretion. Neopterin excretion increased with infection, and this lasted longer in MS patients than in controls. The results of the study were interpreted as suggesting that urinary neopterin might be a marker for the inflammatory component of MS disease activity. The relapsing and secondary progressive MS patients tended to have high but fluctuating levels, while the primary progressive patient tended to have low levels. Although systemic infections resulted in increased neopterin excretion in MS patients as well as in healthy controls, the MS patients had increased excretion independent of infections.

Gliotoxin is also increased in MS urine as measured by an assay to detect in vitro gliotoxic activity.[69] Urine was studied from 35 MS patients, 35 healthy controls, and 34 patients with other neurologic diseases. Among the urine samples from the MS patients, 91% induced glial cell apoptosis. None of the urine samples from the healthy control and only 3% of the urine samples from the patients with other neurologic diseases had similar gliotoxic activity. These studies of gliotoxin are cross-sectional. At the current time there is very little data from longitudinal studies of gliotoxin.

Free light chains have also been studied in MS urine.[70–72] Both κ and λ chains are increased in MS urine; in preliminary studies, urinary κ chains increased with clinical disease activity.

Finally, neuron-specific enolase, a protein found in neurons, neuroendocrine cells, and platelets, is reported to be elevated in a subset of MS patients.[61]

Urine is an interesting and accessible body fluid. Several promising markers for MS activity and disease course have been proposed, but at the current time no definitive urine assay is established to evaluate MS.

OTHER FLUIDS

Other fluids have been studied in MS in a limited fashion. Tears are an interesting mucosal excretion of the lacrimal gland and conjunctiva. One group found increased immunoglobulin levels, cell counts, and oligoclonal IgG in MS tears.[73–76] Other groups were either unable to confirm these results or found much lower rates of these abnormalities.[77–79] The data on saliva is even more limited.[75,76,80]

RESPONSE TO THERAPY

It would be very helpful to have body fluid assays that measured response to disease modifying therapy. There are a number of biologic response modifiers that are induced by IFN-β in a dose dependent manner (*Table 10.5*). They consist of serum proteins, cell enzymes and markers, and metabolites. In theory, measuring these markers should allow evaluation of dosing response, provided that there is an accurate baseline level and knowledge about individual variability. These modifiers are being proposed as blood tests to determine IFN-β efficacy. There is also data that sVCAM-1 levels increase in IFN-β responders.[10] No equivalent studies have been reported for glatiramer acetate.

Table 10.5 Proposed biologic response modifiers to evaluate IFN-β therapy

β2-microglobulin
Neopterin
IL-10
MxA protein
Human leukocyte antigen (on monocytes)
2',5' oligoadenylate (2-5a) synthetase

SUMMARY

At the current time there is no reliable body fluid marker for disease activity or course in MS, but there are several promising ones. A marker unique to MS would be the most helpful, but to date no such marker has been discovered. Blood and urine are the easiest fluids to sample, but they offer potential problems with regard to reflecting effects of systemic inflammatory and immune conditions that may have nothing to do with MS.

A recent review on the status of body fluid markers in MS made several useful recommendations.[2] These included international standardization of reagents and assays, evaluation of candidate assays at multiple centers, and validation through longitudinal and cross-sectional comparisons with both clinical and MRI parameters. It is hoped that the increasingly sophisticated approach to analysis of inflammatory, immune, and CNS components in MS will lead to development of a number of useful body fluid assays to measure specific pathologies, disease stages, and disease activity.

REFERENCES

1 Miller DH, Albert PS, Barkhof F et al. Guidelines for the use of magnetic resonance imaging techniques in monitoring of the treatment of multiple sclerosis. *Ann Neurol* 1996; 39:6–16.

2 Laman JD, Thompson EJ, Kappos L. Body fluid markers to monitor multiple sclerosis: the assay and the challenges. *Multiple Sclerosis* 1998; 4:266–269.

3 Giovannoni G, Thompson EJ. Urinary markers of disease activity in multiple sclerosis. *Multiple Sclerosis* 1998; 4:247–253.

4 Chandler S, Coates R, Gearing A et al. Matrix metalloproteinases degrade myelin basic protein. *Neurosci Lett* 1995; 201:223–226.

5 Waubant E, Sloan R, Gee L et al. Serum level of matrix metalloprotease-9 (MMP-9) and natural tissue inhibitor of MMP type 1 (TIMP-1) in patients with relapsing–remitting multiple sclerosis (RRMS): Relationship to MRI activity. *Multiple Sclerosis* 1998; 4:507.

6 Lee MA, Palace J, Stabler G et al. Serum gelatinase B, TIMP-1 and TIMP-2 levels in multiple sclerosis. *Brain* 1999; 122:191–197.

7 Archelos JJ, Hartung HP. Adhesion molecules in multiple sclerosis: a review. In: Siva A, Kesselring J, Thompson AJ, eds. *Frontiers in Multiple Sclerosis*, vol 2. London: Martin Dunitz, 1999, 85–116.

8 Riekmann P, Martin S, Weichselbraun I et al. Serial analysis of circulating adhesion molecules and TNF receptor in serum from patients with multiple sclerosis: cICAM-1 receptor in serum from patients with multiple sclerosis: cICAM-1 is an indicator of relapse. *Neurology* 1994; 44:2367–2372.

9 Giovannoni G, Lai M, Thorpe J et al. Longitudinal study of soluble adhesion molecules in multiple sclerosis. Correlation with gadolinium enhanced magnetic resonance imaging. *Neurology* 1997; 48:1557–1565.

10 Rieckmann P, Altenhofen B, Riegel A et al. Correlation of soluble adhesion molecules in blood and cerebrospinal fluid with magnetic resonance imaging activity in patients with multiple sclerosis. *Multiple Sclerosis* 1998; 4:178–182.

11 Dore-Duffy P, Newman W, Balabanov R et al. Circulating, soluble adhesion proteins in cerebrospinal fluid and serum of patient with multiple sclerosis: correlation with clinical activity. *Ann Neurol* 1995; 37:55–62.

12 Hartung HP, Reiners RH, Archelos JJ et al. Circulating adhesion molecules and TNF receptor (60 kDa) in multiple sclerosis: correlation with MRI and comparison with viral encephalitis. *Ann Neurol* 1995; 38:186–193.

13 Tsukuda N, Miyagi K, Matsuda M et al. Soluble E-selectin in the serum and cerebrospinal fluid of patients with multiple sclerosis and human T-lymphotropic virus type-1 associated myelopathy. *Neurology* 1995; 45:1914–1918.

14 Giovannoni G, Thorpe JW, Kidd D et al. Soluble E-selectin in multiple sclerosis: raised concentrations in patients with primary progressive disease. *J Neurol Neurosurg Psychiatry* 1996; 60:20–26.

15 Mossner R, Fassbender K, Kuhnen J et al. Circulatory L-selectin in multiple sclerosis patients with active, gadolinium-enhancing brain plaque. *J Neuroimmunol* 1996; 65:61–65.

16 Beck J, Rondot P, Catinot L et al. Increased production of interferon gamma and tumor necrosis factor precedes clinical manifestations in multiple sclerosis: do cytokines trigger off exacerbations? *Acta Neurol Scand* 1988; **78**:318–323.

17 Trotter JL, Collins KG, Van der Veen RC. Serum cytokine levels in chronic progressive multiple sclerosis: interleukin-2 levels parallel tumor necrosis factor-alpha levels. *J Neuroimmunol* 1991; **33**:29–36.

18 Link J, Soderstrom M, Olsson T et al. Increased TGFβ, IL-4 and IFNγ in multiple sclerosis. *Ann Neurol* 1994; **36**:379–386.

19 Mokhtarian F, Shi Y, Shirazian D et al. Defective production of antiinflammatory cytokine, TGFβ by T cell lives of patients with active multiple sclerosis. *J Immunol* 1994; **152**:6003–6010.

20 Monteyne P, Sindic DJM. Data on cytokine mRNA expression in CSF and peripheral blood mononuclear cells from MS patients as detected by PCR. *Multiple Sclerosis* 1998; **4**:143–146.

21 Riekmann P, Albrecht M, Kitzke B et al. Tumor necrosis factor-α messenger RNA expression in patients with relapsing remitting multiple sclerosis is associated with disease activity. *Ann Neurol* 1995; **37**:82–88.

22 Sharief MK, Hentges R. Association between tumor necrosis factor-α and disease progression in patients with multiple sclerosis. *N Engl J Med* 1991; **325**:467–472.

23 Adachi K, Kumamoto T, Araki S. Elevated soluble interleukin-2 receptor levels in patients with active multiple sclerosis. *Ann Neurol* 1990; **28**:687–691.

24 Hartung HP, Hughes RA, Taylor WA et al. T cell activation in Guillain–Barré syndrome and in MS: elevated serum levels of soluble IL-2 receptors. *Neurology* 1990; **40**:215–218.

25 Hafler DA, Fox DA, Manning ME et al. In vivo activated T lymphocytes in the peripheral blood and cerebrospinal fluid of patients with multiple sclerosis. *N Engl J Med* 1988; **312**:1405–1411.

26 Antel JP, Bania MB, Reder A, Cashman N. Activated suppressor cell function in progressive multiple sclerosis. *J Immunol* 1986; **137**:137–141.

27 Balashov KE, Khoury SJ, Hafler DA, Weiner HL. Inhibition of T cell responses by activated human CD8⁺ T cells is mediated by interferon-gamma and is defective in chronic progressive multiple sclerosis. *J Clin Invest* 1995; **95**:2711–2719.

28 Becher B, Giacomini PS, Pelletier D et al. Interferon gamma secretion by peripheral blood T-cell subsets in multiple sclerosis: correlation with disease phase and interferon beta therapy. *Ann Neurol* 1999; **45**:247–250.

29 Balashov KE, Smith DR, Shoury SJ et al. Increased interleukin 12 production in progressive multiple sclerosis: induction by activated CD⁺ T cell via CD 40 ligand. *Proc Natl Acad Sci U S A* 1997; **94**:599–603.

30 Kastrukoff LF, Morgan NG, Zecchini D et al. A role for natural killer cells in the immunopathogenesis of multiple sclerosis. *J Neuroimmunol* 1998; **86**:123–133.

31 Karussis D, Leker RR, Ashkenazi A, Abramsky O. A subgroup of multiple sclerosis patients with anticardiolipin antibodies and unusual clinical manifestations: do they represent a new nosological identity? *Ann Neurol* 1998; **44**:629–634.

32 Sadatipour BT, Greer JM, Pender MP. Increased circulating antiganglioside antibodies in primary and secondary progressive multiple sclerosis. *Ann Neurol* 1998; **44**:980–983.

33 Missler U, Wandinger RP, Niesmann M et al. Acute exacerbation of multiple sclerosis increases plasma levels of S-100 protein. *Acta Neurol Scand* 1997; **96**:142–144.

34 Noronha A, Richman DP, Arnason BW. Detection of in vivo stimulated cerebrospinal fluid lymphocytes by flow cytometry in patients with multiple sclerosis. *N Engl J Med* 1980; **303**:713–717.

35 Whitaker JN, McFarland HF, Rudge P, Reingold SC. Outcomes assessment in multiple sclerosis clinical trials: a critical analysis. *Multiple Sclerosis* 1995; **1**:34–47.

36 Lamers KJB, de Reus HPM, Jongen PJH. Myelin basic protein in CSF as indicator of disease activity in multiple sclerosis. *Multiple Sclerosis* 1998; **4**:124–126.

37 Thomson AJ, Brazil J, Feighery C et al. CSF myelin basic protein in multiple sclerosis. *Acta Neurol Scand* 1985; **72**:577–583.

38 Sellebjerg F, Christiansen M, Garred P. MBP, anti-MBP and anti-PLP antibodies, and intrathecal complement activation in multiple sclerosis. *Multiple Sclerosis* 1998; **4**:127–131.

39 Whitaker JN, Layton BA, Herman PK et al. Correlation of myelin basic protein-like material in cerebrospinal fluid of multiple sclerosis patients with their response to glucocorticoid treatment. *Ann Neurol* 1993; **33**:10–17.

40 Barkhof F, Frequin STFM, Hommes OR et al. A correlative trial of gadolinium–DTPA MRI, EDSS, and CSF MBP in relapsing multiple sclerosis patients

treated with high dose intravenous methylprednisolone. *Neurology* 1992; **42**:63–67.

41 Vakaet A, Thompson ET. Free light chairs in the cerebrospinal fluid: an indicator of recent immunological stimulation. *J Neurol Neurosurg Psychiatry* 1985; **48**:995–998.

42 Sharief MK, Hentges R. Importance of intrathecal synthesis of IgD in multiple sclerosis. A combined clinical, immunologic, and magnetic resonance imaging study. *Arch Neurol* 1991; **48**:1076–1079.

43 Sharief MK, Thompson EJ. Intrathecal immunoglobulin M synthesis in multiple sclerosis. Relationship with clinical and cerebrospinal fluid parameters. *Brain* 1991; **114**:181–195.

44 Rudick RA, Peter DR, Bidlack JM, Knutson DW. Multiple sclerosis: free light chains in cerebrospinal fluid. *Neurology* 1985; **35**:1443–1449.

45 Rudick RA, French CA, Breton D, Williams GW. Relative diagnostic value of cerebrospinal fluid κ chains in MS: comparison with other immunoglobulin tests. *Neurology* 1989; **39**:964–968.

46 Krakauer M, Nielsen HS, Jensen J, Sellebjerg F. Intrathecal synthesis of free immunoglobulin light chains in multiple sclerosis. *Acta Neurol Scand* 1998; **98**:161–165.

47 Vakaet A, Thompson EJ. Free light chains in the cerebrospinal fluid: an indicator of recent immunological stimulate. *J Neurol Neurosurg Psychiatry* 1985; **48**:995–998.

48 Fagnart OC, Sindic CJM, Laterre C. Free κ and λ light chain levels in the cerebrospinal fluid of patients with multiple sclerosis and other neurological diseases. *J Neuroimmunol* 1991; **33**:63–72.

49 Sharief MK, Thompson ET. Immunoglobulin in the cerebrospinal fluid: an indicator of recent immunological stimulation. *J Neurol Neurosurg Psychiatry* 1989; **52**:949–953.

50 Rudick RA, Cookfair DL, Simonian NA et al. Cerebrospinal fluid abnormalities in a phase III trial of Avonex (IFNβ1a) for relapsing multiple sclerosis. *J Neuroimmunol* 1999; **93**:8–14.

51 Menard A, Amouri R, Dobransky T et al. A gliotoxic factor and multiple sclerosis. *J Neurol Sci* 1998; **154**:209–211.

52 Rieger F, Amouri R, Bentellounn N et al. Gliotoxicity in multiple sclerosis. *C R Acad Sci [III]* 1996; **319**:343–350.

53 Fredrikson S, Link H, Eneroth P. CSF neopterin as a marker of disease activity in multiple sclerosis. *Acta Neurol Scand* 1987; **75**:352–355.

54 Spuler S, Yousry T, Scheller A et al. Multiple sclerosis: prospective analysis of TNF-alpha and 55 kDa TNF receptor in CSF and serum in correlation with clinical and MRI activity. *J Neuroimmunol* 1996; **66**:57–64.

55 Kivisakk P, Matusevicius D, He B et al. IL-15 mRNA expression is upregulated in blood and cerebrospinal fluid mononuclear cells in multiple sclerosis (MS). *Clin Exp Immunol* 1998; **111**:193–197.

56 Riekmann P, Albrecht M, Kitze B et al. Cytokine mRNA levels in mononuclear blood cells from patients with multiple sclerosis. *Neurology* 1994; **44**:1523–1526.

57 Navikas V, He B, Link J et al. Augmented expression of tumor necrosis factor-α and lymphotoxin mRNA in mononuclear cells in multiple sclerosis and optic neuritis. *Brain* 1996; **119**:213–223.

58 Riekmann P, Nunke K, Burchhardt M et al. Soluble intercellular adhesion molecule-1 in cerebrospinal fluid: an indicator for the inflammatory impairment of the blood–cerebrospinal fluid barrier. *J Neuroimmunol* 1993; **47**:133–140.

59 Massaro AR, Carnevale P, Tonali P, Bock E. Glia cell pathobiology in multiple sclerosis detected by CSF markers. *J Neurochem* 1996; **66**(suppl 2):S28.

60 Lycke JN, Karlsson JE, Andersen O, Rosengren LE. Neurofilament protein in cerebrospinal fluid: A potential marker of activity in multiple sclerosis. *J Neurol Neurosurg Psychiatry* 1998; **64** (suppl 3): 402–404

61 Giovannoni G, Green AJE, Thompson EJ. Are there any body fluid markers of brain atrophy in multiple sclerosis? *Multiple Sclerosis* 1998; **4**:138–142.

62 Rosengren LE, Lycke J, Andersen O. Glial fibrillary acidic protein in CSF of multiple sclerosis patients: relation to neurological deficit. *J Neurol Sci* 1995; **133**:61–65.

63 Massaro AR. Are there indicators of remyelination in blood or CSF of multiple sclerosis patients? *Multiple Sclerosis* 1998; **4**:228–231.

64 Whitaker JN. Myelin basic protein-like material in the urine of multiple sclerosis patients: relationships to clinical and neuroimaging changes. *Multiple Sclerosis* 1998; **4**:243–246.

65 Whitaker JN, Williams PH, Layton BA et al. Correlation of clinical features and findings on cranial magnetic resonance imaging with urinary myelin basic protein-like material in patients with multiple sclerosis. *Ann Neurol* 1994; **35**:577–585.

66 Whitaker JN, Kachelhofer RD, Bradley EL et al. Urinary myelin basic protein-like material as a

correlate of the progression of multiple sclerosis. *Ann Neurol* 1995; **38**:625–632.

67 Whitaker JN, Layton BA, Bartolucci AA et al. Urinary myelin basic protein-like material in patients with multiple sclerosis during interferon-β 1b treatment. *Arch Neurol* 1999; **56**:687–691.

68 Giovannoni G, Lai M, Kidd D et al. Daily urinary neopterin excretion as an immunological marker of disease activity in multiple sclerosis. *Brain* 1997; **120**:1–13.

69 Malcus-Vocanson C, Giraud P, Broussolle E et al. A urinary marker for multiple sclerosis. *Lancet* 1998; **351**:1330.

70 Mehta PD, Cook SD, Troiano RA, Coyle PK. Increased free light chains in the urine of patients with multiple sclerosis. *Neurology* 1991; **41**:540–544.

71 Constantinescu CS, Mehta PD, Rostami AM. Urinary free κ light chain levels in chronic progressive multiple sclerosis. *Pathobiology* 1994; **62**:29–33.

72 Mehta PD, Cook SD, Coyle PK et al. Free light chains in multiple sclerosis urine. *Multiple Sclerosis* 1998; **4**:254–256.

73 Coyle PK, Sibony P. Tear analysis in multiple sclerosis. *Neurology* 1986; **36**:547–550.

74 Coyle PK, Sibony P, Johnson C. Oligoclonal IgG in tears. *Neurology* 1987; **37**:853–856.

75 Coyle PK. Molecular analysis of IgA in multiple sclerosis. *J Neuroimmunol* 1989; **22**:83–92.

76 Coyle PK, Bulbank M. Immune-reactive cells in multiple sclerosis mucosal secretions. *Neurology* 1989; **39**:378–380.

77 Mavra M, Thomson EJ, Nikolic J et al. The occurrence of oligoclonal IgG in tears from patients with MS and systemic immune disorders. *Neurology* 1990; **40**:1259–1262.

78 Liedtke W, Weller M, Wietholte H, Dichgans J. Immunological abnormalities in the tears of multiple sclerosis patients. *Acta Neurol Scand* 1992; **85**:228–230.

79 Martino G, Servalli C, Filippi M et al. Absence of oligoclonally restricted immunoglobulins in tears from multiple sclerosis patients. *J Neuroimmunol* 1993; **44**:149–156.

80 Pietz K, Haas J, Wurster U. Protein composition, IgG, and IgA analysis in the saliva of patients with multiple sclerosis. *Ann N Y Acad Sci* 1993; **694**:305–307.

11

The use of cost analyses to improve our understanding of the therapeutic trade-offs for multiple sclerosis

Kathryn Whetten-Goldstein

Examining the costs, the benefits, and the effectiveness of therapeutic technologies is essential to the decision making process about which therapies to use in which types of patients. The clearest example occurs when two therapies or technologies are equivalent in terms of effectiveness but differ in terms of cost. The decision as to which therapy to use can then be based primarily on the cost. However, in reality, decisions are not so clear-cut. Therapies are rarely equivalent in terms of effectiveness. Costs analyses differ by the type of costs that are included (e.g. direct medical costs, direct non-medical costs, indirect costs, intangible costs), the perspective of the payer, and whether the researchers use cost identification, cost-effectiveness, cost-utility, or cost-benefit analyses. This chapter helps clinical researchers to understand better the differences in cost analyses and identifies specific analyses that have been conducted for multiple sclerosis (MS).

TYPES OF COSTS

Cost analyses may include different types of costs, which are assigned weights depending on the perspective of the payer. In general, there are

four types of costs that might be included in a cost analysis: direct medical costs, direct non-medical costs, indirect costs, and intangible costs.

Direct medical costs

The first is direct medical costs. Such costs include the actual charges for resources associated with the therapy being examined and should be compared with the best therapeutic alternative. Such costs might include all clinical time, laboratory time, research and development, the need for ambulance services, visits to emergency rooms, hospital stays, radiological procedures, medications, or durable medical equipment. Researchers can include downstream costs such as nursing home admissions, hospital readmissions, or other more expensive treatment. Direct costs reflect the value of the resources used to prevent, diagnose, treat, and rehabilitate patients.

Direct non-medical costs

Direct non-medical costs are costs that are direct in nature but are not medical. Some examples of direct non-medical costs are the costs to the criminal justice system, the cost of paying disability income, transportation, lodging, child care, family counseling, home aids, alterations to homes or vehicles, and clothing. An examination of the impact of treatment of substance-abusing mentally ill patients might include an examination of the impact on costs to the criminal justice system and the welfare system (K Whetten-Goldstein, T Nguyen, A Heald. Are rural providers prepared to care for the chronically ill?; unpublished work).

A comprehensive examination of the costs of MS and the effect of particular therapies might examine if there are increases or decreases in the direct non-medical cost associated with the need for child care, transportation, home aids, or alterations to the family home or vehicle. A benefit of a therapy might be that it increases the ability of patients to return to work and that the patients therefore no longer need disability income or help with domestic chores. Researchers should be careful not to underestimate the value that such cost impacts can have for different payers. Direct non-medical costs are more difficult for clinical researchers to obtain than direct medical costs because they often require in-depth surveys and the use of secondary data sources to estimate the costs.

Indirect costs

Indirect costs are those that are not actually paid and do not reflect the use of resources. Included in this category are losses that result from job absenteeism, decreased earning ability of the person who is disabled and possibly the person who is the primary caregiver, changes in occupation resulting from illness or injury, the time costs of patient travel to appointments and waiting time in clinics, and informal caregiving. Indirect mortality costs due to premature deaths can be included in this category.

Intangible costs

Intangible costs represent the value that either those experiencing the illness, or society, place on the pain and suffering associated with a particular condition. Such losses are experienced as a result of a loss in the ability to perform activities of daily living and decreased social functioning.

THE PERSPECTIVE OF THE DECISION MAKER

The perspective of the decision maker is essential in determining which types of costs are most important. A health-care provider is often primarily concerned with direct medical costs that specifically affect the budget of the provider's organization. Providers will not ordinarily be concerned with direct non-medical, indirect, or intangible costs. However, social-service providers would be interested in direct non-medical and possibly indirect costs as a way of better understanding how to assist patients and how to justify the work that they perform.

The third-party payer is interested in the costs that pertain to reimbursement. Such a payer is very interested in medical expenses incurred or avoided as a result of a therapy. Some public third-party payer, such as Medicaid in the USA, may be interested in direct non-medical cost offsets, because such payers may in fact pay for some social services such as transportation or case management.

The patient and the patient's family are primarily interested in the amount of payments that are required of the patient or the family for medical care, alterations to the home and vehicle, lost work, informal caregiving, and intangible losses. Such decision makers are not so interested in direct medical costs.

Finally, the society perspective should be the most comprehensive and complex perspective. Society at large should be interested in valuing each of the cost components for all diseases and disabilities.

TYPE OF COST ANALYSIS

Simple cost identification can be used when the effects of the therapeutic interventions being compared are observed to be minimal. In such a case, costs can be added without a direct relationship to the effectiveness or benefits of the therapeutic interventions.

In cost–effectiveness analyses, alternative interventions are compared in terms of cost per unit change in health outcome. All relevant costs and benefits are measured and the ratio between the two is calculated. All other things being equal, an alternative with a lower cost:benefit ratio is preferable to an alternative with a higher cost:benefit ratio. When interventions are very different the issue may simply be whether the additional improvement in benefits is worth the cost. Examples of a unit of health outcome are the number of years of life saved, the decrease in the number of injuries, the increase in CD4+ lymphocyte or the counts decrease in viral load count. The direct comparison of the cost to the increase or decrease in unit of effectiveness creates a cost:effectiveness ratio (CER). Such ratios are relevant only when compared to at

least one other alternative therapeutic intervention. The great difficulty in comparing CERs is that, as seen by the preceding discussion, there is a vast array of costs that may or may not be included in any particular analysis. One must be very careful that the same costs have been included in the comparator CERs and that those costs were measured in the same way.

The six basic steps in cost–effectiveness analysis are as follows:[1]

1 Define the intervention. This includes specifying the nature of the intervention (e.g. provision of personalized cancer risk information), the types of people who will receive the intervention (e.g. patients, healthy adult volunteers, adolescents), and what alternative the intervention is replacing (e.g. usual care, less intensive administration of personalized risk information, current interventions used to achieve the same goal as the alternative intervention). In some cases, an intervention is compared to the natural history of a disease without any treatment, but more commonly an intervention is compared to an alternative intervention that could be used.

2 Identify relevant costs. These usually include direct costs, such as paper for copying brochures and the purchase of computers, but they may also include indirect costs, such as patient time spent in counseling, lost earnings, or other social costs associated with the intervention.

3 Identify relevant benefits. These include the net health benefits to the person receiving the intervention (after deducting any adverse side effects), but they may also include indirect benefits such as greater productivity.

4 Measure costs. This requires attaching a monetary value to all components of costs, which entails placing a value on medical inputs and

an individual's time. In the case of costs that occur in the future, a discount rate is typically used to convert all costs into present-value terms.

5 Measure benefits. Convert all benefits into a single benefit. In the case of benefits that occur in the future, a discount rate is sometimes used to convert all benefits into present-value terms.

6 Account for uncertainties. This entails using sensitivity analysis, Monte Carlo simulations, or other methods to test the robustness of conclusions to uncertainties in the measurement of costs and benefits.

Cost–utility is a form of cost–effectiveness analysis where the measure of effectiveness is life years gained adjusted by a series of 'utilities' or quality-of-life weights to reflect the relative values or worth that individuals place on different states of health. The outcome measure commonly used in cost–utility analyses is quality-adjusted life-years (QALYs). The cost:utility ratio is then expressed as the cost per QALY gained.

Cost–benefit analyses attempt to place monetary values on the set of outcomes resulting from each alternative. The outcomes are translated into units of currency through approaches such as 'willingness to pay.'

COST ANALYSES IN MS RESEARCH

Several studies have examined the cost of MS and as such provide a base for cost–effectiveness analyses for new therapeutic interventions. A comprehensive study in Canada was conducted to determine the cost of MS to the Ministry of Health, private third-party payers, patients, and society.[2] Patients were recruited from 14 clinics across Canada. Patients were classified according

to the Expanded Disability Status Scale (EDSS) as: mild (EDSS ≤ 2.5), moderate (EDSS = 3.0–6.0), or severe (EDSS ≥ 6.5). This retrospective study found that costs increased with severity and that the annualized society costs per patient were \$CDN14 523 for mild MS, \$CDN21 698 for moderate MS, and \$CDN37 024 for severe MS. The study found that most of the (74% to 88%) financial burden was borne by patients and that indirect costs from lost daily activity and leisure time and lost productivity were the major society cost drivers.

A second study assessed the utilization of medical services and community assistance for people with MS.[3] This study classified 184 patients into four grades of disability according to a simplified EDSS and examined direct health-care costs to society. The retrospective study surveyed patients on their sociodemographic status, their use of inpatient and outpatient medical services and pharmaceutical products during the previous year, their use of social assistance, their purchase of prostheses, and charges for house adaptations during the previous 5 years. Data were also collected prospectively by means of a diary over 1 month. The annual costs for the 5500 patients with MS in Flanders was estimated to be European Currency Unit (€) 13 106 000 for ambulatory care and €3 234 000 for pharmaceutical products. Added to these costs are €3 491 000 for social assistance and €4 938 000 for prosthetics and adaptations.

A study of the cost of MS in the USA (adjusted to the value of the dollar in 1994) found the average annual cost per person to be approximately \$US34 000.[4] This figure translates into a conservative estimate of national annual cost of \$US6.8 billion, and a total lifetime cost per case of \$US2.2 million. Major components of cost were lost wages (\$US17 900 per person per year) and informal care. Total health care costs averaged $US15 122 per person. Health-care costs included $US6452 worth of caregiving provided by family members, $US1247 for home care and personal assistance provided by paid caregivers, $US2485 in hospital costs, $US1746 in physician costs, $US847 for medications, $US845 for nursing home care, $US944 for retraining, and $US556 for other costs. Health insurance covered 51% of costs for services, excluding informal care. Although most people had health insurance, close to 25% had been denied private health insurance. On average, compensation for earnings loss was 27%.

In addition to lost wages and health care, $US1081 per person was spent on home and automobile alterations and special equipment. This study was completed before the widespread use of new disease-modifying agents, which can add $US10 000 or more to the cost of medications for those using one of these drugs. Those with the progressive form of MS had much higher costs, averaging $US49 084.

In a separate analysis, the same researchers examined the intangible cost of MS.[5] Much of the burden of MS, such as fatigue, numbness, mood changes, paralysis, and the anxiety of not knowing what tomorrow will be like, does not result in capital expenditures or outlays. However, in a court of law in the USA, intangible loss is recognized when a settlement or a piece of a settlement is awarded for pain and suffering. The researchers used risk–dollar and risk–risk to recover the intangible loss associated with MS. Results indicated that persons with MS were willing to give up more real income to reduce the risk of acquiring MS than were persons in the general population. However, persons with MS were less willing to undergo a hypothetical operation that entailed a mortality risk than the general population. The value of intangible loss of a case of MS derived from response from the general population was $US350 000–$US500 000, whereas persons with MS were willing to pay somewhat more than this amount.

Only a handful of studies have published cost–effectiveness, cost–utility, or cost–benefit analyses as part of their evaluation of a new therapy or technology in relation to MS. One such study[6] sought to determine the incremental cost–effectiveness of magnetic resonance imaging (MRI) and computed tomography (CT) in young adults presenting with equivocal neurological signs and symptoms. The researchers followed a decision analysis of long-term survival[7] using accuracy data from a diagnostic technology assessment of MRI and CT in patients with suspected MS. It was found that in the baseline analysis, at 30% likelihood of an underlying neurological disease, MRI use had an incremental, or additional, cost of $US101 670 for each additional quality-adjusted life-year saved, compared with $US20 290 for CT use. As the probability of neurological disease increased, researchers found that MRI use was a cost–effective alternative, with the cost dropping to $US30 000 for each quality-adjusted life-year saved. The researchers considered that if a negative MRI result provides reassurance, then the incremental costs of immediate MRI use decreased and fell below $US25 000 for each quality-adjusted life-year saved no matter what the likelihood of disease was. This study provides a very effective example of how such analyses can be used by providers and payers in the decisions over the type of care to provide patients.

In a study in 1981,[8] the researchers examined the costs and the effectiveness of providing multidisciplinary inpatient rehabilitation to 20 patients with MS. The researchers measured total direct medical costs of the intervention and a variety of functional status effectiveness measures: behavioral, cognitive, visual and perceptual, communication, sensation, muscle strength, spasticity, inco-ordination and involuntary movements, balance, arm and leg functional status, self-care activities, bowel and bladder incontinence, bed mobility, wheelchair transfers and management, ambulation status, homemaking, and performance in real-life activities. Researchers found that of the 20 areas rated, intensive multidisciplinary therapy produced statistically significant improvements in balance, self-care activities, bladder control, bed mobility, wheelchair transfers, ambulatory transfers, homemaking, and the ability to perform real-life activities. The average cost for rehabilitation was $US14 175. Home aid services diminished from $US25 909 to $US8680 following the intervention. It was concluded that such intensive therapy was cost–effective.

CONCLUSION

Cost analyses strengthen the ability of decision makers at different levels (e.g. providers, payers, family members) to determine which of a host of therapeutic interventions to engage. To date, such studies for MS have been sparse. Future comprehensive studies of the cost and burden of MS on society, providers, and families should give researchers a basis for the use of cost–effectiveness or cost–benefit analyses in their examination of new therapies. Researchers should ask not only, 'Does this new drug reduce some of the symptoms of MS?' but also 'Will this therapy reduce the need for informal care from loved ones?' 'Will this therapy allow patients to return to the work force?' or 'Will this therapy reduce the pain and suffering that patients endure (and how will these losses or gains be measured)?'

REFERENCES

1 **Sloan FA.** Introduction. In: Sloan FA. *Valuing Health Care: Costs, Benefits, and Effectiveness of Pharmaceuticals and Other Medical Technologies.* Cambridge: Cambridge University Press, 1995, 1–14.

2 **The Canadian Burden of Illness Study Group.** Burden of illness of multiple sclerosis. Part I: cost of illness. *Can J Neurol Sci* 1998; **25**:23–30.

3 **Carton H, Loos R, Pacolet J et al.** Utilisation and cost of professional care and assistance according to disability of patients with multiple sclerosis in Flanders (Belgium). *J Neurol Neurosurg Psychiatry* 1998; **64**:444–450.

4 **Whetten-Goldstein K, Sloan FA, Goldstein LB, Kulas ED.** A comprehensive assessment of the cost of multiple sclerosis in the United States. *Multiple Sclerosis: Clin Lab Res* 1998; **4**:419–425.

5 **Sloan FA, Viscusi KW, Chesson HW et al.** Alternative approaches to valuing intangible health losses: The evidence for multiple sclerosis. *J Health Econ* 1998; **17**:475–497.

6 **Mushlin AI, Mooney C, Holloway RG et al.** The cost–effectiveness of magnetic resonance imaging for patients with equivocal neurological symptoms. *Int J Technol Assess Health Care* 1997; **13**:21–34.

7 **Mooney C, Mushlin AI, Phelps CE.** Targeting assessments of magnetic resonance imaging in suspected multiple sclerosis. *Med Decis Making* 1990; **10**:77–94.

8 **Feigenson JS, Scheinberg L, Catalano M et al.** The cost–effectiveness of multiple sclerosis rehabilitation: a model. *Neurology* 1981; **31**:1316–1322.

12

The application of ethical principles to clinical trials in multiple sclerosis

Richard P Foa

INTRODUCTION

Large scale multicenter controlled clinical trials have now virtually transformed medical research and clinical medicine. In neurology they have had indelible effects in epilepsy, stroke, and multiple sclerosis (MS). They seem to be the accepted path to future progress in these areas as well as with even more intractable illnesses such as amyotrophic lateral sclerosis. So profound and pervasive is the influence of these trials that they now routinely extend themselves into the offices of small group and solo practices, where many clinicians have redefined their endeavors as private research institutes. In the field of MS, increasing numbers of phase 3 and phase 4 treatment trials are expected to look not just at relapsing–remitting MS and secondary progressive MS, but also at disease prevention. Trials of new treatments for suppression of acute exacerbations, specific symptom management, and functional recovery can also be safely predicted.

As the relative support for such trials from federal and not-for-profit coffers shrinks, a new entrepreneurial spirit has been kindled in researchers and we have entered an era of renewed trust and co-operation with for-profit pharmaceutical industry sponsors. But with the growth in the cost and complexity of clinical trials, there is increasing awareness of the need for restraints both for the protection of scientific integrity and for what sometimes seem to be only intuited 'ethical considerations.' There is now sufficient experience with large multicentered trials in MS that methodologies have been refined and guidelines have been created for the design and conduct of future trials.[1]

The ethical problems of large trials, whether for MS or any other disease, are principally about the protection of the persons who are simultaneously the participants in, the subjects of, and the ultimate beneficiaries of the trials. Research participants are by necessity the afflicted and therefore those to whom society and the medical community have special obligations to protect and heal. The ethical conflicts that may arise involving the interests of investigators and sponsors are relatively less important.

Contemporary sensitivity to the need for ethical guidelines in the conduct of clinical research arises from growing awareness of historical abuses such as Nazi experimentation during the Second World War, from the promulgation of several international and national codes of ethics pertaining to the conduct of research on human subjects, and from an intense effort over the past few decades to apply the discipline of ethical analysis to biomedical research and clinical medicine. The Nuremburg Code, emphasizing the basic requirement of the voluntary informed consent of research participants, was formulated in response to the revelation of Nazi medical atrocities before and during the War.[2] This was followed in 1964 by the World Medical Association's Declaration of Helsinki, since revised in 1975 (Tokyo), 1983 (Venice), and 1989 (Hong Kong).[3] Guidelines promulgated in 1993 by the Council for International Organizations of Medical Sciences together with the World Health Association[4] also emphasize the protection of vulnerable groups, appropriate inducements to participate in research, safeguards to confidentiality, the conduct of research in developing countries, and the importance of outside ethical review.[5] In the USA, the 1979 Belmont Report of the National Commission for the Protection of Human Subjects of Biomedical and Behavioral Research grounds clinical trials on the principles of respect for persons, beneficence, and justice.[6]

Yet, for all the authority of such declarations and guidelines, they still seem to be little known among the growing legions of physicians for whom participation in clinical trials has started to blend with daily clinical practice—perhaps a motivation for review and reiteration of clinical research guidelines in 1998 by the Ethics and Humanities Subcommittee of the American Academy of Neurology.[7]

The US medical community was startled by revelations of the unethical research conducted in the early 1960s at several pre-eminent medical centers.[8] Public awareness of research misconduct awaited disclosure in the 1970s of the now infamous Tuskegee syphilis study.[9–11] Since then there have been occasional revelations of research misconduct. Notable among them are federally sponsored or military studies in the early cold-war era that involved the biological effects of radiation exposure performed on unwitting or misinformed participants. Although such studies may reasonably be regarded as aberrant by contemporary standards, they are an historical basis for mistrust of research by patients, and they are reminders to us all that well-intentioned studies are not automatically ethical in either their design or execution.

Patients are commonly ambivalent about participation in clinical research. They all want what they believe will result in the best outcome. This, for many, means what is newest. However, patients are understandably reluctant to place their health at even greater risk to receive what is unproven. The old and yet still often heard expression, 'I don't want to be a guinea pig,' reflects not only the reluctance to take a leap into the unknown but also some mistrust of the researcher and the research. The explicit comparison is to the laboratory animal with no control over its fate – caged by circumstance, uninformed of choices, and unable to say 'no.' Those who gather themselves to make that leap into a clinical research protocol may be held back by the threat of being randomized to suboptimal treatment or, worse, to no treatment. From their misunderstanding of the requirements of research or from their need to equate 'new' with 'better', randomization to the control group may feel like a betrayal of their willingness to risk their fragile well-being for the goal of medical advancement.

We are approaching an era when it is conceivable that virtually every patient known to have MS will be a potential candidate for a research protocol. This will be an era when the competition to enroll patients from a finite pool will be enormous, particularly for studies directed at specific patient subpopulations defined by clinical pattern, disability score, characteristics on magnetic resonance imaging (MRI), or laboratory markers. It will be an era when increasing numbers of practicing neurologists will have to be drawn into increasingly extended multicenter trials. And so it must be an era in which trials, to achieve a near universal level of trust, are meticulously attentive to both scientific validity and to the respect for participants that is the ethical foundation of any trial.

ETHICAL FOUNDATIONS

To arrive at an understanding of the ethical foundations of clinical trials, it is helpful to review quickly the different approaches to ethical analysis. An individual confronting an ethical dilemma will naturally ask, 'How do I properly act?' or 'What is the correct moral response?' To answer these questions, one may turn to a variety of sources that reflect different teachings, traditions, or experience. For example, one may turn to a moral tradition grounded in a particular religion or philosophy, or one might rely on a conception of moral character exemplified by the behavior of an historical, contemporary or even mythical leader—if he were in my shoes, what would Jesus, or Ghandi, or Martin Luther King do? This is the realm of situation ethics. It places the individual in a position of having to respond to a situation probably not of his or her own creation. Guidance about how properly to respond then comes from comparisons with how others have responded in similar circumstances (an approach called 'casuistry') or by reference to how a particular moral character trait would be manifested in that situation (an approach called 'virtue ethics'). Still another approach is to look beyond the immediate circumstances in order to look at distant outcomes and to act in a way that is most likely to bring about the most desirable general outcome (an approach called 'teleological ethics' or 'utilitarianism'). Take, for example, the familiar dilemma of deciding whether it is better to control the pain or prolong the life of a patient with terminal cancer. One could follow the example of a trusted teacher, acting as this person did under similar circumstances. One might, like a warrior, fight to prolong life or, like a priest, elect to comfort and ease passage. One might also look beyond the immediate patient to consider what is best for all dying patients, thereby seeking a general rule.

Although utilitarian thinking (seeking what yields the greatest good for the greatest number in the end) may certainly be used to justify a commitment to research in general, none of these types of ethical reasoning is ideally suited to help with the problems of clinical research. In the design and conduct of clinical trials, most ethical conflicts are of our own creation since they are inherent in the structure of the trial itself. They are foreseeable and should therefore be avoidable. When ethical conflicts within a trial are unavoidable, the trial should be designed so that choices are clear and so that researchers or participants are not penalized for the choice that they make. The type of ethical reasoning that is best suited to the design and conduct of clinical trials is therefore grounded in principles or rules of conduct (an approach called 'deontological ethics' or 'principle-based ethics').

It is widely accepted the three ethical principles pertinent to research on human subjects are respect for autonomy, beneficence, and justice. Each of these warrants a brief explanation.

Respect for autonomy

Respect for autonomy means recognition of an individual's ability to deliberate about personal goals and to act to protect self-interest on the basis of that deliberation. In order to act autonomously, an individual must have adequate information about a proposed action and freedom to act voluntarily and without restraint.[12,13] The principle of autonomy is often expressed as respect for persons in order to cover the obligation to protect those in a condition of diminished autonomy, such as children, the mentally incompetent, or those who through illness have diminished decision-making capabilities. One must distinguish between autonomous persons and autonomous actions, since the actions of autonomous persons are not always autonomous.[12]

Actions may be autonomous by degrees depending on the availability of information and the voluntariness of the decision process. At a fundamental level, autonomy is considered a 'negative right.' To be fundamentally autonomous means having the basic and inviolable ability to say 'no' to any other person who would impose his or her will. The principle of autonomy is most frequently recognized in research as the basis for the obligation to obtain informed consent.

Beneficence

The principle of beneficence expresses the obligation to do what is right and best for a patient from a medical perspective. Beneficence carries the obligation to maximize benefits and the complementary obligation to minimize harms. Beneficence is also subject to degrees. At one end of a moral continuum is the principle of non-maleficence, the obligation to avoid harm. This is expressed in the often-stated dictum *Primum non nocere* ('First do no harm'). In this form it is a call to inaction. Further along the continuum is the obligation to act for the benefit of the patient with little or no risk or expense to the physician or researcher. Further still along this continuum is a call to act at some personal risk, and at the moral extreme is the call to act in order to benefit the patient at great personal cost or self-sacrifice.[14] As the potential risk to the provider rises, the obligation to act beneficently weakens. However, at the level of non-maleficence it remains absolute. The principle of beneficence is relevant to clinical research in the obligations to maximize patient benefit through protocol design, to risks properly balanced against intended treatment benefits, and to protect participant safety throughout the data monitoring process.

Justice

The third principle is justice. Unlike autonomy, the principle of justice is termed a 'positive right' because it expresses a claim by an individual to a share of what others may have. The type of justice to which we refer in the biomedical context is distributive justice. It pertains to how we decide each person's share of the total goods and services available to society as a whole. It is to be distinguished from the rules that we make to govern social behavior (civil justice) or that we make to punish violators of those rules (retributive or criminal justice). Justice in the biomedical setting is a difficult principle to apply because there is no universally accepted notion of what an individual is entitled to claim from society.

Confronted with limited resources, we may all agree that 'goods' should be distributed 'fairly.' But there are widely divergent views about what methods of distribution are fair. Differing notions include first-come, first-served, reward most who work the hardest, give to those who are best able to help others, redistribute wealth to the least well-off, give equal shares to all, etc. All these notions have vocal proponents and find support in different religious or political philosophies.

Issues of justice are readily discernible in the problems of access to scarce medical resources, maldistribution of services, and lack of universal health insurance. In the realm of clinical trials, issues of justice arise in considering access to a study (study size, enrollment criteria, distribution of participating centers), the selection of investigators, and internal issues such as data sharing or publication rights.

A CODE OF ETHICS

The author has previously proposed a code of ethics for the conduct of clinical trials in MS.[4] This shares with other modern codes a concern for the rights and welfare of participants, an emphasis on the examination of an important question answerable only by the study, and a search for results that can be generalized to patients outside the study. The essential elements with reference to the ethical principles that support them are now discussed.

Substantial new information must be sought and the trial must be capable of yielding that information

This requirement is grounded mainly in the principle of justice because of the enormous financial and human resources committed to the completion of a large scale clinical trial, especially to the extent that the trial receives public funding. Talent and resources committed to a trial that is poorly conceived and executed are wasted. Issues of justice are at stake even with commercially sponsored trials to the extent that the efforts and resources of investigators and patients are drawn away from other productive activity. The duty to maximize benefits and minimize risks under the principle of beneficence is also relevant, since one cannot justify taking any risk, however small, for futile research.

The research must address a question that can be answered only through the use of human subjects

This requirement is grounded in the principle of beneficence. Although it may be assumed that a clinical trial alone can reveal information about the efficacy and effectiveness of new therapies, there may be premature pressure at the phase 1 and phase 2 levels to undertake a large-scale clinical trial before basic questions about safety, therapeutic potential, or dosing are adequately addressed. Here again, the ethical issues revolve around the balance of risk and benefits. If research questions are answerable through animal experimentation, mathematical modeling, or computer simulation then no risks to human subjects are justifiable.

Benefits from the trial must outweigh harms

This requirement encompasses not only benefits and harms to an individual patient or, in the broader context, all patients with MS, but also benefits and harms to society. This is a matter of justice. It requires a balancing of the interests of a patient group or a research group against the wider interests of society in order to be sure that trials benefiting small numbers of people warrant their costs and to insure that a broad claim of social benefit is not used to impose enormous risks on a small number of study participants. This element of the code should force trial planners to consider whether the methodologies to be used or the data acquired could, in another context, become harmful. An example might be breaches of confidentiality that could occur with data sharing or the development of large patient registries.

It is not unimaginable that a well- but narrowly conceived MS clinical trial could have unintended harmful consequences unrelated to the primary outcome measure. Think, for example, about the interest we have in studies of strategies to prevent MS through early use of drugs now approved for treatment of established disease. Such a study must rely on recruitment of participants who do not have MS according to traditional criteria—perhaps a single episode of optic neuritis or a suggestive lesion on MRI alone. A trial protocol might expose the study subject to a potentially harmful treatment. Furthermore, trial enrollment may be misconstrued as indicative of the diagnosis of MS. Data sharing through a combined patient registry might then make that individual identifiable to people with no connection to the research for which they volunteered. Imagine also a future trial of this nature on people found to have a genetic marker

for MS (if one is discovered). It becomes easy to imagine pressure placed upon those perceived to be genetically 'at risk' to be swept into the whole process. And could preventive treatment trials in MS become models for similar trials with Parkinson's disease or Alzheimer's disease? This might be an exciting new frontier. But the question for ethics is, 'Might this be bad?'

There must be equity in the selection of research subjects

This requirement is obviously grounded in the principle of justice, and it depends on our understanding of what it means to be equitable. It was previously suggested that an ethical trial should offer 'an equal opportunity to participate ... according to gender, race, and ethnic background.'[15] But such democratic inclusion criteria may have no inherent scientific validity and therefore may ultimately be just as counter-productive as criteria that might exclude important groups for purposes of simplicity. Another aspect of equity in the selection process is protection of people who are unable to avoid conscription into a trial because they are desperately ill, poor, uninsured, or otherwise unable to say 'no.' This is a requirement grounded in both respect for persons and beneficence.

Clinical research must be conducted with the informed consent of participants

Properly obtained, voluntary informed consent is the sine qua non of respect for autonomy. Ideally, the provision of informed consent is a wholly autonomous act by an autonomous person. Even though this ideal is rarely achievable, it does not follow that 'consent' consisting of a signature on a lengthy and ill-understood legalistic contract is an acceptable alternative. Morally valid informed consent is essentially a process of communication that conveys a sufficient understanding of the research to enable a potential participant to enter a trial willingly and free of external, controlling influences.[12,13,16]

SPECIFIC ISSUES ARISING IN CONTEMPORARY CLINICAL TRIALS

Committees

There has been uncertainty and debate about the relative roles and composition of committees that oversee the development, conduct, and completion of multicenter MS clinical trials;[17,18] this has perhaps been quietened for the moment by the National MS Society Advisory Committee guidelines (see Chapter 16).[1] A few cautionary comments about ethical issues related to the function of these committees is warranted.

Ethically sound clinical trials require attention to ethical issues from the start. Well-conceived and well-designed trials should then encounter few problems when they are conducted. Responsibilities assigned to the advisory or steering committee include such ethically relevant tasks as ensuring the use of placebo controls wherever possible, the determination of entrance and exclusion criteria, attention to the protection of research subjects, and informed consent. This committee is, in effect, the guarantor of trial ethics. The data and safety monitoring committee is given overlapping responsibility for protecting study participants from harm through the power

to recommend early termination of a study 'for ethical considerations' as well as on the basis of safety and efficacy.[1] However, a study should never have to be stopped because of ethical considerations alone. Deciding to stop, an inherently ethical decision, should depend on safety and efficacy data. Predetermined statistical safeguards should be built into the study design and there should be no imaginable unethical trends leading to study termination.

Much is implicitly left to the local Committee of Human Research (CHR) or Institutional Review Board (IRB), to which individual investigators must submit a protocol in order to participate. IRBs at established universities or the National Institutes of Health stand as another layer of protection for research subjects. They offer an important review backed by the established character of the institution and its known values. The appearance of new, private IRBs apparently created solely to review commercially sponsored multicenter phase 4 studies warrants careful scrutiny. These studies may be conducted by office-based physician–researchers. A brief survey of studies conducted in this fashion in Maryland and Virginia identified three different private IRBs approving three trials sponsored by pharmaceutical companies.[19] None of these committees had recognizable affiliation to a larger research institution or established independence from the trial sponsor. This allows room for concern about the credentials of the committee members and the rigor of their review process. There must be reassurance that a private committee on human research will protect the rights and safety of study subjects. This may include the ability to require modification of study procedures or modification of a consent document drafted by a commercial sponsor for widespread use.

Issues intrinsic to trial design

Placebos

Opportunities for placebo controls in clinical trials for MS should sharply decline. All clinical trials should begin from a position of equipoise in which there is a genuine uncertainty about the relative benefits of the treatment arms.[20] But it is not enough for clinician–researchers alone to be in a position of equipoise. Patients must also have no reason to prefer one treatment over another. If an experimental treatment and its control have different impacts on patient lives (e.g., oral therapy versus parenteral therapy, inhalant versus injection, daily versus weekly) then patient preferences must also be considered in trial design. If there is likely to be a substantially different effect on the perceived quality of life for different treatment arms, then prior randomization or non-randomized controls may be considered.[21]

It is unethical to randomize patients to a placebo group if this means even temporarily depriving them of access to effective treatment.[22,23] Much depends on the trial design and the targeted study population. In the past, with no treatments of established efficacy, the study of a new therapy required comparison with a placebo. Now that partial efficacy is established for the β-interferons and for glatiramer acetate, trials of new agents for relapsing–remitting MS should be conducted using one of these agents as a control unless the clinical circumstance under study is one where the efficacy of these agents is unknown.

With little yet known about treatment for primary progressive and secondary progressive MS, placebo-controlled trials are probably essential. Use of placebos in trials of early, relapsing and remitting disease that look at different primary outcome measures from those used to date is a trickier undertaking. Imagine, for argument's sake, that someone wants to do such a trial looking at a primary outcome other than exacerbation rate, progression to disability or MRI changes. This trial would, instead, look at an end-point for which treatment effects are unknown. The researcher would be in a position of equipoise with respect to the chosen outcome measure, and a placebo control might be scientifically important. However, use of a placebo group in such a trial would probably be unethical because the participants might lose the benefits of a treatment with established effectiveness on other dimensions of the disease.

Blinding and randomization

Noseworthy and colleagues[22] have previously emphasized the importance of blinding both the investigators and the research subjects so that enthusiasm for the possibility of benefit does not lead to biased assessment of those in an experimental group. However, blinding highlights the inherent conflict between the investigator's role as a treating physician and his or her role as a research scientist. As a treating physician, there is an ethical obligation under the principle of beneficence to not give treatments with unknown benefits and risks. Protocols that designate different participating investigators as 'treating' and 'examining' physicians, the first with a primary obligation to the patient and the other with a primary obligation to the protocol, do not free either of them from these obligations. Furthermore, as previously argued, the system of divided responsibilities may impose extra burdens on participants, who, in the event of a clinical change or adverse reaction, may have to undergo duplicate clinical examinations. Wherever possible, provisions should be made for the provision of treating physicians who are uninvolved with the study.[15]

Participants can be guaranteed access to a new treatment only in studies with a cross-over design. Randomization, therefore, may divide a study population into the winners and losers of a small lottery. Patients who may be willing to undertake risks with the hope of something new may be unwilling to participate if given only a 50:50 or less chance of receiving the experimental treatment. Out of respect for participant autonomy, recruiters for a study must make the procedures for randomization and the differences between treatment arms apparent to all potential participants at the outset. Furthermore, if a study is designed to compare a new treatment with one of established efficacy, the requirement of equipoise dictates that there must be reasonable evidence to support the hope that new treatment will be as good as or better than the established treatment. Investigators have an additional obligation to inform participants of what they might lose if they are randomized into an experimental group.

Stopping and dropping out

As is appropriate in the longitudinal study of chronic illness, the recent controlled trials of interferon-β 1b and 1a and glatiramer acetate have been multiyear projects. Predictably, the same will be true for the studies currently in progress and for those on the drawing board. A lot can and will change for participants as these studies continue. New therapies will appear and old therapies will be abandoned. Patients involved in a long clinical trial must, out of respect for autonomy, be informed of any new treatment that might benefit them even if this jeopardizes their continued participation. If there

is an opportunity for a new treatment and this does not affect the ability of a trial to reach its primary outcome, the new treatment should be permitted even if modifications must be made in the protocol. If a new treatment is incompatible with the trial, participants must be given the option to withdraw from the trial. Either decision will require a modification of the consent document so that both the patients who decide to stay in a trial and those who decide to leave can be assured that they are given equal and balanced information on which to base their choice.

If investigators decide to continue a trial beyond the primary end-point in a way that restricts choices for treatment by participants, there must also be the option to withdraw. If an initial commitment has been made by a sponsor to make the study drug available to participants after a trial reaches its planned end, this commitment should be honored for those who elect to stop rather than stay in an extension of the trial. As with other significant protocol changes, informed consent with a new or addended consent document must be obtained from those participants who elect to participate in an extended study. The decision about whether to continue a treatment after the trial has ended is of course a clinical decision. It depends not merely on the availability of the drug if not yet approved for use, but also on an assessment of the benefits and harms to the patient based on that individual's experience. A patient who has received a placebo with promise of receiving the experimental treatment at the end or in the 'open label' phase of a study should be given access to the new drug even if he or she elects not to participate in an extension of the trial. This, of course, presumes that efficacy and safety data from the first part of the trial indicate the superiority of the trial drug to the placebo.

Issues extrinsic to trial design

Recruitment of study participants

As larger and more numerous phase 3 and phase 4 clinical trials compete for a finite patient population, and as individual centers are increasingly involved in more than one trial enrolling patients from the same pool, questions about appropriate inducements to participate naturally arise. The power of an inducement may range over a spectrum from persuasion to manipulation to coercion. Frankly coercive measures, such as a threat to discontinue care, are clearly unethical because participation is no longer voluntary. But the boundary between ethical persuasion and ethically questionable manipulation is unclear.[13] To persuade means to influence someone else's choice by means of reasoned argument and is respectful of autonomy. Manipulation may occur by limiting the available choices, by altering understanding through the deceptive limitation of information, or by application of psychological pressure. Deciding for a patient what ought to be done by invoking therapeutic privilege is an example of manipulation that is traditionally defended as beneficent. An implicit promise of early access to a new treatment or to care not covered by insurance is an inducement that may be manipulative but is not necessarily unethical. It may offer what a patient would choose freely under different circumstances.

Payment to patients for enrollment in a trial is not unethical so long as the amount paid is not large enough to lure a patient to enroll against his or her better interests or with loss of voluntariness.[4] In other words, monetary compensation should not be irresistible and therefore not likely to influence an individual to take risks they would not otherwise take.[13] However, the boundary between appropriate payment and excessive payment is also vague and irresistibility, of course, depends on an individual's needs and values. It is generally acceptable to reimburse patients small sums for time and expenses but payment of larger amounts to ill patients for participation in therapeutic trials should be viewed critically. Payment offered in proportion to risk is inappropriate exactly because it will encourage excessive risk taking for money alone.

Direct payment to an investigator or research center for enrollment of patients and indirect payment in the form of increased general financial support by study sponsors are other important financial inducements. Direct payment to investigators for enrollment and patient follow-up are, in fact, standard. This has become a common method for supplementing practice income and is changing the complexion of clinical practice as payment for clinical care diminishes. Although not inherently wrong, such payments may influence the care that is made available to a patient, especially if the physician is better paid to enroll the patient in a study than to provide standard treatment. Financial incentives such as these should be disclosed to study candidates as part of the consent process.

Researchers at universities or other large centers trying to conduct two competing trials should disclose to potential participants the nature of the financial incentives they receive from study sponsors. This will help minimize the influence of payment on a center's or researcher's preference for one trial over the other. Similarly, researchers or institutions that have a financial stake in a product that is being studied should disclose that interest, not only to patients who might participate but to the scientific community whenever trial outcomes are presented.[25]

Confidentiality

The guarantee of confidentiality is essential in the conduct of a clinical trial under the principle of respect for persons. Traditionally, confidentiality has been protected by the removal of all patient identifiers from data reports. Of course, in the clinical setting patients are not anonymous and there is little concern by most participants in a study that their name is known to the investigator if the study is viewed as an extension of clinical care. However, the development of extensive patient registries raises concern about the development of proprietary lists of names that might later be used to directly recruit patients for future studies and for marketing purposes. This concern has been sustained by attempts by commercial sponsors to identify MS patients at educational and support group meetings. It is to be hoped that open concern about the existence of such registries and resistance to their development by clinical investigators, practicing neurologists, and MS societies will remain a powerful deterrent to their use.

For the same reasons, there must be concern about possible breaches of confidentiality with the development of international computer databases on MS. Such data pools offer previously unimagined opportunities for sharing and exchanging information. These will enable pooling of data from small studies to enhance statistical power and create the opportunity to explore data sets for answers to questions not directly addressed in previous studies. Truly international trials will become easier. Developers have emphasized the importance of protecting a user's independence,[25] but such large data pools may make all MS patients unwitting participants in research. Although few patients may object, there must still be as much emphasis on the protection of patient confidentiality as on the protection of user access and independence. If such databases are shared on the Internet rather than on closed computer networks, there must be controlled access and the removal of any information that might permit the identification of individuals. Who will have access and what is considered appropriate use of the information will then be matters of debate.

Access to research data

In commercially sponsored trials, there must be full access to study data by participating investigators even when data is collected and initially analysed entirely by the sponsor.[17] This does not mean release of data into the public domain nor does it entail violations of confidentiality. It recognizes that all trials are collaborations between participants, investigators and sponsors. No single party should have proprietary control over the information generated. Investigators must be able to reanalyse data and perform subanalyses. This will ensure maximum scientific benefit and assure participants and the public that future trials are solidly grounded in past experience.

Trials on patients with cognitive impairment

There are now reliable measures of cognitive performance in MS that will enable trials that look at neuropsychological outcomes.[27] Prospective treatment trials for patients with secondary progressive MS will also inevitably involve patients with cognitive deficits. Protocols involving such vulnerable patients will require specific appropriate safeguards for the protection of participants. Existing regulations do not spell these out.[7] Under the principle of beneficence, clinical trials that examine cognitive performance or that include patients with dementia require a more careful balancing of the roles of treating physician and investigator.

The requirement for voluntary informed consent has often been seen as a serious impediment to enrolling cognitively impaired patients in a trial. Although inclusion of such patients depends on their ability to understand the proposed research and to distinguish between participating in a study and receiving routine care, valid informed consent does not require a comprehensive understanding of the research protocol and attendant risks. This ideal is, in fact, rarely reached in the consent process even with the most intelligent patients. The critical element is the voluntary nature of consent. The requirement should be that a patient is capable of understanding the trial well enough to participate voluntarily.

Will it then be impossible to conduct future trials with patients who are too impaired to understand the research process? Or will participation in future trials of advanced MS be possible with consent from a surrogate decision maker? For treatment, spouses, parents, and other close family members are given authority to make critical decisions in situations of temporary incapacity. More enduring decision-making authority is generally assumed by families for patients that are demented without turning to a court for a legally designated guardianship. People are also made surrogates through a durable power of attorney for health care that is written before incapacity occurs. A surrogate must act on behalf of the patient according to the patient's previously expressed wishes if these are known. This is the standard of substituted judgement. A surrogate must otherwise act under the principle of beneficence by a best interests standard. An obligation to minimize risks may make it difficult for a surrogate to enroll a demented patient in a clinical trial. However, if the physical risks are small and the requirements of participa-tion not burdensome, ethically valid consent by a surrogate seems reasonable. Enrollment is easier if a patient has previously expressed a willingness to participate in research; therefore, thought might be given to including an explicit statement concerning research in a document granting durable power of attorney for health care. If a patient is known to have been a risk taker, a surrogate applying substituted judgement may more easily provide valid consent.

CONCLUSION

Beecher concluded in 1966 that the greatest safe-guard to ethical research is 'the presence of a truly responsible investigator ... intelligent, informed, conscientious, compassionate.'[8] In his article, Beecher is careful not to identify the investigators and institutions of his examples of unethical research. But clearly he wrote of small trials conducted almost entirely within single institutions by a few researchers.[28] Typical numbers of patients involved were 20 or 30, and many studies involved fewer. There was one study that involved 500 but with a control group of 15, and the unethical practice cited involved that control group. Beecher expressed skepticism of the very possibility of truly informed consent. There continues to be frequent criticism of the way that consent is obtained for participation in clinical trials, and this fosters periodic calls to return to the virtue ethic that Beecher advocated.

However, the modern multicenter clinical trial has grown to a size far beyond the possibility of control by a single virtuous investigator. And the ethical character of a trial rests on far more than the steps taken to insure that consent is adequately informed and voluntary. To be sure, a virtuous investigator remains an immeasurably valuable asset and no trial can be ethical without due attention to obtaining the valid consent of participants. But the ethical requirements of contemporary and future clinical trials in MS, as in all other fields of medicine, are more complex and varied. They require an understanding of the principles of autonomy, beneficence, and justice as well as diligent attention to the application of those principles throughout all phases of the trial, from conception through funding, enrollment, treatment, data collection, analysis, and publication. Only in this way can we be sure that clinical trials will continue to enjoy the public support that they have acquired; and only then can we be confident that they will fulfil their promise as the best means to conquer MS and other intractable diseases.

REFERENCES

1 **Lublin FD, Reingold SC, and the National Multiple Sclerosis Society Advisory Committee on Clinical Trials of New Agents in Multiple Sclerosis.** Guidelines for Clinical Trials of New Therapeutic Agents in Multiple Sclerosis: Relations between Study Investigators, Advisors and Sponsors. *Neurology* 1997; **48**:572–574.

2 **Grodin MA.** Historical origins of the Nuremburg Code. In: Annas G, Grodin M. *The Nazi Doctors and the Nuremburg Code.* New York: Oxford University Press, 1992, 121–144.

3 **World Health Organization.** *Declaration of Helsinki.* Recommendations Guiding Doctors in Clinical Research. In: Annas G, Grodin M. *The Nazi Doctors and the Nuremburg Code.* New York: Oxford University Press, 1992, 331–342.

4 **Council for International Organizations of Medical Sciences (CIOMS) in collaboration with the World Health Organization.** *International Ethical Guidelines for Biomedical Research Involving Human Subjects.* Geneva: CIOM, 1993.

5 **Perley S, Fluss S, Bankowski Z, Simon F.** The Nuremburg Code: an historical overview. In: Annas G, Grodin M. *The Nazi Doctors and the Nuremburg*

Code. New York: Oxford University Press, 1992, 149–173.

6 **National Commission for the Protection of Human Subjects of Biomedical and Behavioral Research.** *The Belmont Report: Ethical Principles for the Protection of Human Subjects of Research.* Washington, DC: US Department of Health and Human Services, Government Printing Office publication GPO 1979, 807–809.

7 **Ethics and Humanities Subcommittee of the American Academy of Neurology.** Ethical issues in clinical research in neurology, advancing knowledge and protecting human research subjects. *Neurology* 1998; **50**:592–596.

8 **Beecher HK.** Ethics and clinical research. *N Engl J Med* 1966; **274**:1354–1360.

9 **Kampmeier R.** The Tuskegee study of untreated syphilis. *South Med J* 1972; **65**:1247–1251.

10 **Kampmeier R.** Final report the 'Tuskegee Syphilis Study'. *South Med J* 1974; **67**:1349–1353.

11 **Curran W.** The Tuskeegee syphilis study. *N Engl J Med* 1973; **289**:730–731.

12 **Faden R, Beauchamp T.** *A History and Theory of Informed Consent.* New York: Oxford University Press, 1986, 235–269.

13 **Beauchamp T, Childress J.** *Principles of Biomedical Ethics.* New York: Oxford University Press, 1989, 122–125, 194–203, 366–372.

14 **Foa R.** Ethical considerations raised by clinical trials. In: Goodkin DE, Rudick RA. *Multiple Sclerosis. Advances in Clinical Trial Design, Treatment and Future Perspectives.* London: Springer, 1996, 335–349.

15 **Katz J.** 'Ethics and clinical research' revisited: a tribute to Henry K Beecher. *Hastings Cent Rep* 1993; **23**:31–39.

16 **Whitaker J, McFarland H, Rudge P, Reingold S.** Outcomes assessment in multiple sclerosis clinical trials: a critical analysis. *Multiple Sclerosis* 1995; **1**:37–47.

17 **Spilker B.** *Guide to Ethical Clinical Trials.* New York: Raven, 1991, 124–128.

18 **Freedman B.** Equipoise and the ethics of clinical research. *N Engl J Med* 1987; **317**:141–145.

19 **Angell M.** Patients preferences in randomized clinical trials. *N Engl J Med* 1984; **310**:1385–1387.

20 **Rothman K, Michels K.** The continuing unethical use of placebo controls. *N Engl J Med* 1994; **31**:394–398.

21 **Goodkin D, Kanoti G.** Ethical considerations raised by

the approval of interferon beta-1b for the treatment of multiple sclerosis. *Neurology* 1994; **44**:166–170.

22 **Noseworthy J, Ebers G, Vandervoort M et al.** The impact of blinding on the results of a randomized, placebo-controlled multiple sclerosis clinical trial. *Neurology* 1994; **44**:16–20.

23 **Emanuel E, Steiner D.** Institutional conflicts of interest. *N Engl J Med* 1995; **332**:262–267.

24 **Confavreaux C, Paty D.** Current status of computerization of multiple sclerosis data for research in Europe and North America: the EDMUS/MS-COSTAR connection. *Neurology* 1995; **45**:573–576.

25 **Fischer JS.** Use of neuropsychologic outcome measures in multiple sclerosis clinical trials: current status and strategies for improving multiple sclerosis clinical trial design. In: Goodkin DE, Rudick RA. *Multiple Sclerosis. Advances in Clinical Trial Design, Treatment, and Future Perspectives*. London: Springer, 1996, 123–144.

26 **Rothman D.** Ethics and human experimentation. *N Engl J Med* 1987; **317**:1195–1199.

13

The process of drug approval and labeling in the USA

Anthony Bourdakis

COMPARISON OF THE REGULATION OF NEW DRUGS AND BIOLOGICS BY THE FOOD AND DRUG ADMINISTRATION

Conventional new drugs are usually synthetic, organic compounds having defined structures and physical and chemical characteristics. Typically, they are produced through chemical synthesis and are usually micromolecules with molecular weights of less than 500 kDa. In contrast, biologics are usually protein- or carbohydrate-based products, viral or bacterial entities for use as a vaccine, an isolated therapeutic protein, or a blood component. They are macromolecules by nature, and usually have much greater molecular weights than drugs.[1]

Conventional new drugs may be evaluated in standard pharmacological screens, and generally their activities may be based on the similarity of overall chemical structures to those of other compounds. They are relatively very stable and can be studied in short-term and long-term toxicology studies to assess safety. Conversely, since biologics are generally very large molecules, there is increased complexity associated with determining their characteristics. As a result, they tend to be less well defined.

The regulation of new drugs and biologics evolved from different regulatory agencies. In the USA, the foundation of the approval process for new drugs comes from the provisions of the Federal Food, Drug and Cosmetic Act,[2] which is regulated by the Food and Drug Administration (FDA). Until 1972, biologic products were regulated by the Public Health Service (PHS), based on the Public Health Services Act.[3] In 1972, the FDA assumed the added responsibility for regulating biologics. As a result, biologic products are governed under both laws and sets of regulations.

Currently, a new drug approved for the treatment of multiple sclerosis (MS), such as Copaxone® (glatiramer acetate), is regulated by the FDA's Center for Drugs Evaluation and Research (CDER), whereas biologics such as Betaseron® (interferon-β 1b) and Avonex® (interferon-β 1a) are regulated by FDA's Center for Biologics Evaluation and Research (CBER). Although significant differences do exist between new drugs and biologics, as discussed above, the FDA's evaluation and approval processes for both are similar.

PRE-CLINICAL SAFETY EVALUATION OF NEW DRUGS AND BIOLOGICS

A sponsoring company's primary goal in conducting pre-clinical studies is to obtain the necessary data to allow for the initiation of clinical trials. These data provide useful information for developing clinical monitoring parameters, the rationale for selection of an initial safe starting dose, dose escalation, duration of use, route of administration, and potential target organs for toxicity.

Components of pre-clinical development programs usually include studies to assess pharmacologic activity, pharmacokinetic parameters (including absorption, distribution, metabolism, and excretion (ADME)), and toxicity.

The investigational new drug or biologics application

During the early pre-clinical development of a new drug or biologic, the sponsoring company's primary goal is to determine if the product is reasonably safe and exhibits activity that justifies commercial development.[4] Should the product prove to be a viable candidate for further development, the sponsor then focuses on collecting the data and information necessary for establishing that the product will not expose human subjects to unreasonable risks when used in limited, early-stage clinical studies.[4] Generally, such data are grouped into three broad areas:

(a) Animal pharmacology and toxicology studies —pre-clinical data to permit an assessment as to whether the product is reasonably safe for initial testing in humans.

(b) Chemistry, manufacturing and controls information—descriptions of the product's composition and source, and methods used for its manufacture and control to allow an assessment as to whether the sponsoring company can adequately produce and supply consistent batches of the product.

(c) Clinical information and plans—detailed protocols for proposed clinical studies to permit an assessment as to whether the initial clinical trials will expose subjects to unnecessary risk.

Before initiating any clinical trials with a new drug or biologic, the sponsoring company must first compile and submit such information to FDA in the form of an Investigational New Drug application (IND).[5] The IND is a proposal through which the company obtains the FDA's permission to begin clinical testing. It is not an application for marketing approval but, rather, a request for an exemption from the federal statute prohibiting an unapproved drug or biologic from being shipped in interstate commerce.

THE FDA'S REGULATION OF PRE-CLINICAL TESTING: GOOD LABORATORY PRACTICES

When the sponsoring company begins to compile safety data for submission of an IND to the FDA, a set of FDA standards called Good Laboratory Practices (GLP) applies.[6] To ensure the quality and integrity of data derived from non-clinical testing, the FDA requires that all non-clinical laboratory studies designed to provide safety (i.e. toxicity) data for an IND must comply with such GLP. This includes studies performed in a sponsoring company's laboratories, private toxicology laboratories, academic and government laboratories, and all other facilities that conduct animal testing. Examples of safety studies that are subject to the requirements of GLP include acute, subacute, chronic, reproductive, and carcinogenicity studies.

THE FDA AND THE IND REVIEW PROCESS

When a sponsoring company submits an IND, it must agree not to begin clinical investigations until 30 days after the FDA's receipt of the IND, unless the sponsor receives earlier notification by FDA that the studies may begin.

THE PHASES OF CLINICAL INVESTIGATION

Once the FDA has approved the IND, clinical development for a new drug or biologic may commence generally proceeding in three phases.

Pilot and phase 1 clinical studies

Clinical development often begins with pilot studies, which are designed to explore the clinical safety and activity of the product before more formal phase 1 or combination phase 1 and 2 studies begin. Generally, such studies are performed in a small number of patients and may accelerate the process of identifying products for further testing.

In the absence of pilot studies, phase 1 investigations represent the first human exposure to a new drug or biologic. These studies are used to determine, for example, the product's metabolism and pharmacologic actions, as well as side effects. Typically, phase 1 tests are closely monitored studies that involve healthy male volunteers, usually with a small number of patients (between 10 and 20).

Phase 2 clinical trials

Phase 2 clinical trials generally represent the first controlled clinical trials designed to measure a product's effectiveness in its intended use or uses. They also present an opportunity to evaluate appropriate study end-points for pivotal trials. As researchers gain experience with the product, however, placebo controls are usually integrated into subsequent studies. Often divided into phase 2a (early) and phase 2b (later) trials, phase 2 studies are usually conducted in a limited number of patients (between 100 and 300), and they are generally used to establish an effective dose and regimen for further study in larger clinical trials.

Phase 3 clinical trials

Phase 3 clinical trials are usually performed to establish the safety and effectiveness of a new therapeutic product in the intended patient population. These studies often involve large number of patients (1000 or more) and are conducted under conditions more closely resembling those under which the drug is to be eventually marketed. They not only provide key evidence of the product's safety and effectiveness, but also provide important insights for the proposed product insert labeling.

Given their importance to the FDA's product approval decision, these 'pivotal' studies must meet particularly high standards. They are usually randomized, controlled, double-blind, multicenter trials designed to provide statistical proof of effectiveness and they normally constitute the so called 'adequate and well-controlled' clinical investigations that FDA requires to support eventual approval.

THE FDA'S REGULATION OF PRE-CLINICAL TESTING: GCP

Because the FDA's approval of any new therapeutic agent is based largely on clinical data provided by the sponsoring company, there are also regulations and guidelines governing the conditions under which these data are obtained. Through regulations and guidelines, known as GCP, the FDA sets minimum standards for clinical trials relating to responsibilities of Institutional Review Boards, informed consent of clinical subjects, and Sponsor–Monitor responsibilities.

Institutional Review Boards

The function of the Institutional Review Board is to ensure that risks to human subjects are minimized and that subjects are adequately informed about the clinical trial and its implications for their treatment.[7] Accordingly, any research program approved by an Institutional Review Board must meet the following criteria, which are specified in FDA regulations:

(a) risks to subjects must be minimized;

(b) risks to subjects must be reasonable in relation to the anticipated benefits and the importance of the knowledge that may be expected to be gained;

(c) subject selection must be equitable;

(d) informed consent must be sought from each prospective subject or the subject's legally authorized representative;

(e) informed consent must be appropriately documented;

(f) when appropriate, the research plan must make adequate provisions for monitoring the data collected to ensure the safety of subjects; and

(g) when appropriate, there must be adequate provisions to protect the privacy of subjects and to preserve the confidentiality of data.

Protection of human subjects

Informed consent is designed to ensure that patients do not enter a clinical trial either against their will or without an adequate understanding of their medical situation and the implications of the clinical study itself.[8] In this regard, FDA regulations require that, except under special circumstances, no investigator may involve a human being as a subject in research unless the investigator has obtained the legally effective informed consent of the subject or the subject's legally authorized representative. The following information must be provided to clinical subjects before they are involved in a trial:

(a) a description of any reasonably foreseeable risks or discomforts to the subject;

(b) a description of any benefits that the subject or others may reasonably expect from the research;

(c) a disclosure of appropriate alternative procedures or courses of treatment, if any, that might be advantageous to the subject;

(d) a statement that describes the extent, if any, to which confidentiality of records identifying the subject will be maintained and that notes the possibility that the FDA may inspect the records;

(e) an explanation as to whether any compensation or medical treatments are available if injury occurs during research involving more than minimal risk, and, if so, what the treatments and/or compensation consist of, or where further information may be obtained;

(f) the identity of the person to contact for

answers to pertinent questions about the research and research subject's rights, and the person to contact if the subject suffers a research-related injury; and

(g) a statement that participation is voluntary, that refusal to participate will involve no penalty or loss of benefits to which the subject is otherwise entitled, and that the subject may discontinue to participate at any time without penalty or loss of benefits to which the subject is otherwise entitled.

The NDA or Biologics License Applications

Before a company can legally market a new therapeutic agent in the USA, it must hold an approved NDA[9] or Biologics License Applications (BLA).[10] To obtain such an approval, the sponsor files an application, which usually consists of several hundred volumes of non-clinical and clinical data, chemical and biological information, and product manufacturing and control information. The application is intended to allow FDA reviewers to determine:

(a) Whether the drug or biologic is safe and effective for its indicated use, and whether the benefits of using the product outweigh the risks;

(b) whether the proposed labeling of the drug or biologic is appropriate; and

(c) whether the methods used in manufacturing and quality control are adequate to preserve the new drug or biologic's identity, strength, quality, potency, and purity.

During the FDA's review, great emphasis is placed on the extent to which the proposed insert labeling reflects the results of the submitted data. In this connection, FDA regulations require that the insert labeling shall constitute a summary of

the essential scientific information needed for the safe and effective use of the new drug or biologic. It must be informative, accurate, and neither promotional in tone nor 'false or misleading.' It is to be based on data derived from human experience with 'no implied claims or suggestions of drug use based on a lack of substantial evidence of effectiveness.'

Over the years, the FDA has set down very specific requirements for the content and format of labeling.[11] This is because, in addition to providing physicians with needed information for prescribing the new drug or biologic, labeling also serves other purposes. For example, although its role in patient reimbursement is well known, labeling also sets out the boundaries or limits as to how far the sponsoring company may go in advertising its product, and often the approved insert labeling may play a critical role in various legal proceedings such as in product liability or malpractice suits. For the sponsoring company and the FDA, labeling represents the culmination of endless hours of data review and deliberations in an effort to produce a document that fairly serves many important purposes.

ORPHAN DRUG ACT OF 1983

In 1983, the Orphan Drug Act[12] established for the federal government to provide assistance to sponsors in the development of new treatments for rare diseases. To qualify for such assistance, an 'orphan drug' ('orphan or biologic') has to be one that is intended to treat a condition that affects fewer than 200 000 persons in the USA or one that will not be profitable within 7 years of marketing approval by the FDA. A few examples of rare conditions that met the first criterion are multiple sclerosis (MS), cystic fibrosis, anemia of end-stage renal disease, amyotrophic lateral sclerosis, and phenylketonuria.

The Orphan Drug Act also allowed a single drug or biologic to receive multiple orphan drug designations. In making such a drug eligible for multiple orphan drug designations, the FDA took the position that not allowing for multiple designations would be a disservice to people suffering from such conditions, since it would create a disincentive for drug development.

For a new drug or biologic, the process of securing orphan status is fairly straightforward. The sponsor submits a request for designation to the FDA's Office of Orphan Products Development, citing the treatment it seeks to develop, the population to be treated, how the population was ascertained, and how the drug or biologic will treat the disease. When the submission is approved, orphan status is granted.

Orphan drugs must meet the same FDA standards as non-orphan drugs in that they must undergo controlled trials to prove safety and efficacy. However, the FDA is somewhat more flexible in the amount of data it will request because of, for example, the difficulties inherent in performing adequate and well-controlled trials with small populations. Currently, there are at least eight drugs that have been granted orphan drug designations in MS.

Once a drug that has an orphan drug designation receives marketing approval the developer is entitled to a number of significant benefits, including:

(a) shelter from competition for a period of seven years,
(b) tax credits for clinical research expenses; and
(c) a waiver of the filing fee resulting from Prescription Drug User Fee Act, which now exceeds $250 000.

In the 10 years before the Orphan Drug Act of 1983 was passed, only 10 products were approved for rare disorders. Since then, over 173 orphan products have been approved, of which 53 are new uses approved for previously marketed products, and 65 are new molecular entities.[13] With the success of the Orphan Drug program in the USA, a number of similar international initiatives have taken place in countries such as Australia, Japan, and Singapore. In addition, in 1998 the European Union passed its own guidelines for regulating orphan drug products in a manner similar to that in the USA.

RECENT INITIATIVES TO IMPROVE THE REVIEW PROCESSES OF THE FDA

The Food and Drug Administration Modernization Act of 1997

The Food and Drug Administration Modernization Act (FDAMA) of 1997,[14] which was passed on 9 November 1997, represents a comprehensive legislative reform effort designed to streamline regulatory procedures within the FDA and to improve the regulation of drugs, biologics, medical devices, and food.

The legislation was principally designed to ensure the timely availability of safe and effective drugs, biologics, and medical devices by expediting the pre-market review process for these products, while maintaining FDA's 'gold standard' for product approval.

The legislation improves FDA's public accountability and establishes, for the first time, an FDA mission statement that helps define the scope of the agency's regulatory responsibilities. It amends the Federal Food, Drug and Cosmetic Act by requiring FDA to prepare a plan for implementing their statutory compliance in consultation with appropriate scientific and academic experts, health-care professionals, representatives of patient and consumer advocacy groups, and the regulated industry. The FDA's compliance plan must be published in the Federal Register and reviewed twice a year. It is intended to eliminate backlogs in the drug and biologics approval process and to ensure the timely review of applications. As part of the FDA's new mission statement, the FDA must also review clinical research promptly and efficiently and take appropriate action on the marketing of regulated products so that innovation and product availability are not impeded or discouraged.

A key provision of FDAMA is the re-authorization of the Prescription Drug User Fee Act of 1992, which permits the continued collection of user fees from prescription drug and biologics manufacturers to augment the resources of the FDA that are earmarked for the review of such applications. Other important provisions of the legislation include the creation of a statutory 'fast-track' approval process for products for serious or life-threatening diseases and conditions, the authorization of the use of expert scientific panels in the review of clinical investigations, and the expansion of the rights of manufacturers to disseminate treatment information.

The legislation reflects congressional concern that the FDA's past regulatory practices hindered the innovative growth of the USA's pharmaceutical, biotech, and medical device industries, and that the FDA has been out of step with recent scientific and technological advances in the development and testing of new products.

During the past few years, these concerns became more pressing for both the US Congress and the President, particularly in the light of efforts in the USA to harmonize regulatory requirements with other national regulatory authorities, and the European Union move to adopt a uniform approval system for such products. By streamlining functions at the FDA and eliminating out-dated regulatory requirements, the legislation addressed what was regarded by many as an overly complex, burdensome, and expensive regulatory system.

Computer-assisted INDs, NDAs, and BLAs

In recent years, the FDA has faced increasing pressures on resources owing to the increasing number, size, and complexity of INDs, NDAs, and BLAs. This made the need for computer-based solutions more urgent, and the FDA has moved to ensure that computer-assisted applications would become a reality. Since then, the FDA has adopted a systems-based approach to allow sponsoring companies to submit computer-assisted submissions, which has greatly reduced voluminous paper submissions and average review times.

FDA's 'managed review' process for Marketing Applications

The FDA has implemented new 'managed review' processes for Marketing Applications. These processes include advance planning for and scheduling of reviews, tighter application tracking, and much closer communication both within the FDA and with the sponsoring company. These tighter controls are essential if the FDA is to meet the ambitious review time frames set by the Prescription Drug User Fee Act and the FDAMA of 1997.

REFERENCES

1 Mathieu M, ed. *Biologics Development: a Regulatory Overview*. (Parexel, Waltham, Massachusetts, 1993).

2 Federal Food, Drug and Cosmetic Act, as amended. 21 US Code (USC) (321).

3 Public Health Service Act, Biological Products. 42 USC (262).

4 Mathieu M, Evans A.G. (Eds) *New Drug Development: a Regulatory Overview*. (Parexel, Waltham, Massachusetts. 1994).

5 21 Code of Federal Regulations (CFR), Part 312.

6 21 CFR, Part 58.

7 21 CFR, Part 56.

8 21 CFR, Part 50.

9 21 CFR, Part 314.

10 21 CFR, Part 600.

11 21 CFR, Part 201.57.

12 Orphan Drug Act, Public Law 97–414.

13 Haffner M. The Impact of the Orphan Drug Act. *Mod Drug Discovery* 1998; 1:45–52.

14 The Food and Drug Administration Modernization Act of 1997.

14

The process of drug approval and labeling in Canada: the case of Rebif® (inteferon-β-1A)

Mona Salesse and Gordon Francis

INTRODUCTION

Phase 3 clinical testing of Rebif® began in Canada during the spring of 1994, leading ultimately to approval of Rebif® at two doses for patients with relapsing–remitting multiple sclerosis (RRMS). The drug was approved for use in 1998 and covered both relapse and disability indications in the target population. The approval process as outlined below was relatively rapid, requiring only 24 months, for a standard application. Other products approved for multiple sclerosis (MS) in Canada include Betaseron®, approved via a fast-track application, Copaxone®, and Avonex®. Canada is the first country in which approval was granted for all four disease-modifying therapies in MS. The details of approval for Rebif® are summarized to describe the drug approval process in Canada.

OVERVIEW OF THERAPEUTIC PRODUCTS PROGRAM REGULATION OF DRUGS AND BIOLOGICS IN MS

Health Canada is the federal department responsible for helping the people of Canada improve and maintain their health. Within Health Canada, the Therapeutic Products Program (TPP) is the national authority that regulates drugs, medical devices, and other therapeutic products used in Canada. The Director of each Bureau within the TPP reports to the Director General of the TPP, who in turn reports to the Deputy Minister and ultimately to the Minister of Health. The TPP is supported through the contributions of more than 700 scientists, doctors, technicians, administrators, inspectors, and managers. In addition to these government employees, expertise from outside is occasionally required for the review of some documents.

Overview of the structure of the Canadian TPP

The TPP comprises seven bureaus: Biologics and Radiopharmaceuticals; Compliance and Enforcement; Drug Surveillance; Pharmaceutical Assessment; Policy and Coordination; Medical Devices; and Drug Analysis Services. The Bureau of Pharmaceutical Assessment and the Bureau of Biologics and Radiopharmaceuticals are involved in review and approval of drug submissions. The Bureau of Pharmaceutical Assessment is responsible for the pharmaceutical drugs, and has units dedicated to the central nervous system, cardiovascular diseases, infection and immunology, acquired immunodeficiency syndrome and viral diseases, endocrinology, metabolism and allergy, gastroenterology, and hematology and Oncology, among others.

The Bureau of Biologics and Radiopharmaceuticals is divided into three divisions responsible for the review of submissions, namely Biotherapeutics, Vaccines, and Blood and Tissues. Drug submissions are routed to either Biologics and Radiopharmaceuticals or Pharmaceutical Assessment on the basis of the nature of the medication. Submissions are further routed to a specific division in the Bureau of Biologics and Radiopharmaceuticals or one of the three units in the Bureau of Pharmaceutical Assessment on the basis of the recommended indication (for pharmaceutical drugs) or the nature of the medication (for biologics).

Preclinical development and safety assessments

The molecule interferon-β 1a, is a unique compound with significant anti-viral, anti-proliferative and anti-inflammatory properties. Rebif® is a recombinant form of interferon-β 1a with an amino acid structure identical to that of natural β-interferon; like the natural product, it is gycosylated. The molecule is produced in mammalian cells. Preclinical development took place in Europe and consisted of six pharmacological studies, including pharmacodynamic and pharmacokinetic studies, as well as pharmacological studies of absorption, distribution, metabolism and elimination (ADME) of the drug. Additionally, 12 studies focused on the acute and long-term toxicity of the drug, and its mutagenicity, reproduction, and teratogenicity effects. These studies were completed in 1996 and provided evidence that the drug was safe and well tolerated, and showed benefit in animal models of disease.

Preclinical work in Canada must be done according to the International Conference on Harmonization (ICH) guidelines. None of the preclinical development for Rebif® took place in Canada. The TPP has no stipulation about mandatory testing of products in Canada at any stage of development and accepts data obtained world-wide related to products under review.

Special Access Program (Emergency Drug Release Program)

Rebif® was first made available to Canadians with MS in 1993 via the Special Access Program (SAP), formerly known as the Emergency Drug Release Program. This program allows the use of drugs not approved in Canada for patients with a serious or life-threatening illness when conventional therapies have failed or are unsuitable. In 1993 there were no approved therapies for MS. In such situations, the SAP unit of the TPP is responsible for authorizing the sale of pharmaceutical, biologic, and radiopharmaceutical products that are not approved in Canada.

A manufacturer has the final word on whether or not a drug will be supplied. Once the request has been approved and the manufacturer has supplied the drug, it is the physician's responsibility to report to the manufacturer and the TPP the results of the use of the drug, including information about adverse events.

The Investigational New Drug Submission

As defined by the TPP, a clinical investigation occurs when a drug or placebo is administered to healthy human subjects or patients for any purpose other than solely to prevent, diagnose, or treat disease in each recipient.[1] To evaluate the rationale for use of a product in a clinical investigation, an Investigational New Drug Submission (IND) is required.

The IND is a document that describes the drug to be used in the proposed clinical trial, previous preclinical and clinical studies (including information on adverse reactions and observed toxicological manifestations), and the protocol for the proposed clinical trial. A pre-IND meeting to discuss the upcoming submission can be scheduled at the sponsor's request. Before a clinical investigation is initiated, an IND must be approved by Health Canada. The only time an IND submission is not required is when a practitioner or research institution initiates a clinical trial for a drug marketed in Canada, independently of the manufacturer of the drug. This may be within or outside the parameters of the Notice of Compliance (NOC), a document issued by TPP to confirm approval of a New Drug Submission (NDS) or Supplementary New Drug Submission (S/NDS) for the drug.[2] Examples for a study outside the parameters of the NOC would include investigating an unapproved indication or an unapproved route of administration. Additionally, a sponsor undertaking post-marketing clinical trials within the parameters of the NOC for a drug may perform clinical investigations without an IND.

In early 1994, two INDs for Rebif® were filed with Health Canada to enable Canadian participation in multinational phase 3, placebo-controlled, clinical trials sponsored by Ares-Serono. The two clinical trials, one investigating Rebif® in RRMS (the PRISMS study[3]) and the other investigating Rebif® in secondary progressive multiple sclerosis (SPMS) were initiated in Canada in the spring of 1994. The IND files were submitted in parallel with similar filings in Europe. Approval was granted in Canada and Europe at approximately the same time. A third IND was filed in January 1995 to allow Canadian participation in a study of Rebif® investigating a once-weekly dosing regimen (the OWIMS study[4]).

Review of an IND submission consists of several stages. When the submission is received, the information undergoes screening for acceptability within 7 calendar days from receipt of the file in the Bureau. Once the file has passed the initial screening, it is accepted for review and placed in the queue, awaiting review by the Bureau. During review of the submission, the Bureau may require additional information. A 'clarifax' (clarification request) is issued when there is a need to expand, add precision, or reanalyse existing information or data in the submission. A response is required within 10 calendar days. A Not Satisfactory Notice (NSN) is issued if deficiencies are found during the review of the file. Response to a NSN must be submitted as a new IND. Review of an IND submission is subject to a 60-day review period. Following this, the study may begin if Health Canada does not raise objections or put forth questions.

Clinical drug testing

Pharmacological studies are designed to evaluate the pharmacological properties of a drug in healthy subjects or patients. Pharmacological studies also obtain information regarding tolerance and potential adverse effects. Therapeutic studies (clinical trials) are designed primarily to determine the appropriate manner for administering a drug to produce a prophylactic action, a diagnostic property, or a significant beneficial effect against a disease process. Coincident to demonstration of effectiveness is collection of all information possible to promote the safe use of the drug and to detect adverse effects that may be encountered.

To conduct clinical trials in Canada, submission of an IND is required. Once an IND has been approved by the TPP and the trial has been approved by the Ethics Committees from the clinical site(s), a trial can be initiated. IND Reports describing the status of the clinical trials in Canada and including all adverse events must be submitted to the TPP annually. Should the trial be ended prematurely, the TPP must be informed.

In the Rebif® NDS, there were a total of three clinical pharmacology studies and 26 clinical trials for MS or other, unrelated indications. In all, nine clinical trial sites, all university affiliated, participated in at least one of the MS studies with Rebif® in Canada. These sites were Vancouver, British Columbia; Calgary, Alberta; London, Ontario; Toronto, Ontario; Ottawa, Ontario; Montreal Neurological Institute, Montreal, Quebec; Hôpital Notre Dame, Montreal, Quebec; Quebec City, Quebec; and Halifax, Nova Scotia. This represents nine of 15 MS centers of excellence in the country. Of these centers, three participated in the RRMS PRISMS study; five were in the SPMS study, and seven were in the OWIMS study.

All clinical trials in Canada must be conducted under Good Clinical Practices (GCP). The guideline in use in Canada is the international 'Good Clinical Practice: Consolidated Guideline,' which was developed from the ICH tripartite guideline.

New drug submission

Before a drug can be sold in Canada, a New Drug Submission (NDS) must be submitted to, reviewed by, and approved by the TPP. Upon approval, a Notice Of Compliance (NOC) is issued. A NDS includes chemistry and manufacturing information (i.e., a description of the drug, a list of ingredients, method of manufacture, test methods), clinical and preclinical information (i.e. animal pharmacology and toxicology, human pharmacology and therapeutic studies). In addition, the master volume of the submission contains information such as the proposed labels and the proposed product monograph and package insert.

Upon receipt of a NDS submission, the information undergoes screening for acceptability, with a 45 calendar day target for completion of the screening by the Bureau. Once the file has passed the initial screening, it is accepted for review and placed in the queue, awaiting review by the Bureau. The target for initiation of review of a NDS, which contains clinical, chemistry, and manufacturing information, is 300 days after the file has passed the initial screening. Should the review not start during that time period, the reviewing Bureau issues an update notice for the manufacturer, thus providing the manufacturer with the possibility of updating the file. The manufacturer has 30 days to confirm its intentions in writing, and another 60 days from receipt of the response to the notice by the Bureau to file the update.

During review of the submission, the Bureau may require additional information. The request for additional information might be issued either as a clarifax, a Notice of Deficiency or a Notice of Non-Compliance, depending on the nature of the information that is required. A clarifax is issued when there is a need to expand, add precision to, or reanalyse existing information or data in the submission. A response is required within 15 calendar days. Should deficiencies that prevent the continuation of the review of the file be found, a Notice of Deficiency (NOD) is issued, with the response due in 90 calendar days. If the file is found to be deficient or incomplete after the review of the file is finished, a Notice of Non-Compliance (NON) is issued. As for a NOD, the response is due in 90 calendar days.

Responses to NODs and NONs are screened for acceptability, and review by the Bureau follows. Once the information is considered acceptable, the drug is approved and a NOC is issued.

Interaction with the Canadian Health Authorities during the preparation of the Rebif® NDS

While the submission was under preparation, a pre-NDS meeting was scheduled with the TPP. The purpose of the meeting, which took place in Ottawa in October 1995, was to introduce the file to the TPP. This early familiarization with the file can streamline the initial screening process and address some of the broader questions that arise in early technical review. Representatives from Ares-Serono, representing technical, medical, regulatory and marketing departments, representatives from the Bureau of Biologics and Radiopharmaceuticals, representing the Submission Management Division, the Vaccines Division and the Biotherapeutics Division, and one leading Canadian neurologist involved in the Rebif® clinical program were in attendance.

The meeting included presentation of the drug development program, overview of clinical trials, and an epidemiological study (presented by the physician). General information about the indications sought and the presentations to be submitted were also disclosed.

Based on positive results from an open crossover study of Rebif® in RRMS,[5]. Ares-Serono prepared a new drug submission for Canada, and Europe. Preparation of the submission was a collaborative process between Europe and Canada. Since Canada was the first country to submit, the submission could not be prepared on the basis of an existing file. Information was received from the corporate office, located in Switzerland, and the submission was assembled in Canada. The clinical section was prepared in Canada based on European Expert Reports and dozens of study reports, protocols and summaries. The clinical database was surveyed to make a list of all studies involving Rebif®. Information from these studies was combined with additional information from study reports, protocols, and study summaries. All information was reviewed and summarized according to the Canadian guidelines.

The Chemistry and Manufacturing section was prepared on the basis of information obtained from the manufacturing site. Since the study that formed the basis for the NDS[5] examined a different dosage than was included in the subsequent studies it was decided to submit with a broad dosage recommendation, which could be refined as more clinical information became available. The original study[5] used doses of either 11 μg or 33 μg three times weekly. The subsequent studies were conducted with the

22 µg or 44 µg format three times weekly (PRISMS)[3] or once weekly (OWIMS).[4] The NDS for Rebif® was submitted to the TPP on 30 January 1996. According to the regulations in place at that time, priority review ('fast-tracking') of the file could not be granted because one interferon-β (interferon-β 1b; Betaseron®) was already on the market in Canada. Initial screening of the file was completed by the TPP and acknowledged on 24 April 1996. The Vaccines Division, the division that has traditionally managed interferons, undertook review of the file. After the in-depth review of the submission, the first set of questions was issued by the Division on 29 May 1997, over 1 year from the application date. The questions and comments were addressed and a response was issued on 9 June 1997.

A reorganization of the Bureau took place during the summer of 1997, at which time review of interferons was transferred from the Vaccines Division to the Biotherapeutics Division. This reorganization meant a delay in the review of the file because the Biotherapeutics Division had to familiarize themselves with the submission.

During the review of the submission, a number of changes took place in chemistry and manufacturing as well as in clinical research. Although the dossier was submitted later in Europe than Canada, the review was initiated there earlier. Following comments from the European authorities, a change in the presentation using prefilled syringes and a change in the concentration of the product was introduced. This presented a predicament for the Canadian file, since the presentations for approval in Canada were no longer the ones that would be manufactured. The issue was discussed with Health Canada and Ares-Serono was allowed to submit the information

for the new presentations as part of a response to a clarifax from the Bureau.

Once this issue was resolved, registration samples from three consecutive batches were submitted to the Bureau for testing in October and November 1997. These registration samples were tested for batch to batch consistency. Inspection of the manufacturing plants by the Bureau took place during that time.

During the review of the file, the results of the second study of RRMS (PRISMS)[3] became available in the summer of 1997. PRISMS was a double-blind placebo-controlled study that tested two doses of interferon-β 1a in RRMS patients (22 µg three times weekly or Rebif® 44 µg three times weekly for 2 years). PRISMS demonstrated efficacy on relapse rate, accumulating disability, MRI activity measures and accumulation of disease burden (see Chapter 20). These results were shared with the TPP and, although PRISMS supported and expanded on the success of the first study,[5] the dosage and duration of treatment were different. The improved trial design and outcomes led to the PRISMS results subsequently forming the basis of the product monograph and labeling requests.

Before final approval, Health Canada performs review of labels and Prescribing Information, which in Canada is called the Product Monograph. The Drug Identification Numbers (DIN) were issued on 2 February 1998, and the Notice of Compliance followed on 5 February 1998, 22 months after acceptance of the NDS and almost 4 years after the initiation of the PRISMS study.

Throughout the review of the file, a number of commitments were requested of Ares-Serono, such as submission of validation reports and any additional information as it became available.

COST RECOVERY

Cost recovery was introduced in 1995 to cover some of the costs of Health Canada's activities. With implementation of cost recovery, the Canadian Health Authorities have begun invoicing sponsors of drug submissions for the evaluation process. The fees are dependent on the nature of the file (i.e. NDS, S/NDS, and Abbreviated NDS) and take into account the number of indications, dosage forms, and other features of the application. The NDS for Rebif® was the first large file that Ares-Serono Canada had submitted under these new rules, and the total cost of submission was about $CDN225 000 (payable in installments; 25% when submitted, and 75% when review is complete). If a submission is deemed incomplete or rejected, the manufacturer can only redeem a portion of their payment.

SUMMARY

The approval process for Rebif® illustrates the nature of the process in Canada and serves to highlight the fact that either party involved in the submission process, although it is structured, can alter certain aspects of it. The time frame for approval for Rebif® was similar to that for Copaxone®, slower than that for Betaseron®, which had fast-track status, and faster than that for Avonex®. The NDS was initiated in the case of Rebif® with results from one study but eventual approval and labeling indications were based on results of a larger, more comprehensive study that was ongoing at the time of the NDS. Ultimately, this permitted the availability of the dosing regimen that was in the best interest of MS patients based on available data.

REFERENCES

1   **Health Protection Branch, Health Canada.** *Preparation of Investigational New Drug Submission.* Ottawa: Canada Communication Group Publishing, 1991.

2   **Health Protection Branch, Health Canada.** Clinical trial review and approval. Ottawa: Canada Communication Group Publishing, 1997.

3   **PRISMS Study Group.** Randomised double-blind, placebo-controlled study of interferon β-1a in relapsing/remitting multiple sclerosis. *Lancet* 1998; 352:1498–1504.

4   **Freedman MS, for the OWIMS Study Group.** Dose dependent clinical and magnetic resonance efficacy of IFN β-1a (Rebif®) in multiple sclerosis (abstract). *Ann Neurol* 1998; **44**:992.

5   **Pozzilli C, Bastianello S, Koudriavtseva T et al.** Magnetic resonance imaging changes with recombinant human interferon-β-1a: a short term study in relapsing–remitting multiple sclerosis. *J Neurol Neurosurg Psychiatry* 1996; **61**:251–258.

15

The process of drug approval in the European Union

Sylvie Grégoire and Lynn Sartori

INTRODUCTION

The European Community was established by the Treaty of Rome in 1957. The European Community changed its name to the European Union (EU) in 1992. Currently, there are 15 member states: Austria, Belgium, Denmark, Ireland, Finland, France, Germany, Greece, Italy, Luxembourg, The Netherlands, Portugal, Spain, Sweden and the UK, sharing 11 official languages. Additional countries seeking to join the EU include Estonia, Hungary, Poland, Slovenia and the Czech Republic. The influences of the Treaty of Rome still guide much of the current legislation in the EU regarding the free movement of goods, persons, services and capital, the maintenance of fair competition and the co-ordination of national economic policies. In 1995, two approval procedures for medicinal products were established in the spirit of this Treaty: the Mutual Recognition and the Centralized Procedures. Developed because of the desire for rapid and consistent recognition of approvals within the EU and in order to ensure that innovative drugs of high interest become available to the whole EU simultaneously, these initiatives represent a significant step towards uniform national approval timelines, which could previously vary from 1 year to over 4 years.

In the EU, several multiple sclerosis (MS) treatments have recently been made available. Betaferon® (Schering AG), Avonex® (Biogen) and Rebif® (Serono) are recombinant interferon-β treatments that have been approved via the European Centralized Procedure during the last 4 years. Glatiramer acetate has been filed through the Mutual Recognition Procedure and the outcome of this is pending. This chapter provides an overview of the development and registration of such medicinal products in the EU.

OVERVIEW OF EU LEGAL FRAMEWORK REGARDING MEDICINAL PRODUCTS

The legal framework on medicinal products in the EU is divided into three main categories: Council regulations, Council and committee directives and decisions, and Committee of Proprietary Medicinal Products (CPMP) guidelines.

Council regulations

Adopted by the Council of the European Communities, Council regulations take immediate

179

effect throughout the EU and over-rule national laws of individual member states.

Council and Commission directives and decisions

Issued by the European Commission, decisions are binding on those to whom they are addressed. Directives must be incorporated into national laws within a specified time period; a certain degree of flexibility is possible in their implementation and national laws so arising may therefore vary in their detail.

CPMP guidelines

Issued by the European Medicines Evaluation Agency (EMEA), CPMP guidelines (or notes for guidance) are not legally binding, but provide useful regulatory guidance for EU filings; the CPMP also adopt the International Conference on Harmonization (ICH) Guidelines.

Legislation governing medicinal products also varies depending on the stage of product development. Although a harmonization effort is under way, requirements for clinical trial applications are under national authority control and each individual country maintains local procedures. Requirements and procedures for medicinal product development, dossiers and registration are governed at the EU level. Provisions for post-approval activities, such as pricing and reimbursement, are managed by national legislation or industry self-policing. In contrast to countries such as the USA, where the Food and Drug Administration (FDA) provides not only guid-

ance but also enforcement, the EU relies on a tradition of voluntary efforts and self-policing. Despite recent reforms, the European regulatory authorities are still largely funded by the EU. With fewer permanent staff than their USA equivalent, they rely on external assessors to provide scientific advice and assess Marketing Authorization Applications (MAA).

The ICH, initiated in 1990, has been a significant development in harmonizing requirements for product registration within the three major trading blocks of the USA, Japan and the EU. The primary goal was to agree to a single set of scientific data needed to demonstrate the safety, quality and efficacy of a new product that meets the regulatory requirements in these three regions. Areas where requirements are similar or differ have therefore been identified and addressed in tripartite, harmonized guidelines; the aim being to reduce or eliminate the need to duplicate studies. The guidelines are an intricate part of all development stages of the product, beginning with the preclinical stage. Current ICH guidelines can be found on the ICH website.[1]

PRECLINICAL DEVELOPMENT AND SAFETY ASSESSMENTS

In order to initiate clinical trials, animal data must provide the scientific rationale to support the use of the investigational product in the proposed human studies. Such rationale include the appropriate starting dose and dose escalation, the appropriate duration of drug use, the route of administration and the necessary safety parameters to be monitored, including the identification of potential target organs for toxicity.

As in the USA, the standards controlling these practices in the EU are known as Good Laboratory Practices (GLP), which seek to ensure the quality and integrity of data by establishing the basic standards of conduct and reporting of non-clinical testing. The principles of GLP in Europe date back to 1987 (Council Directive 87/18/EEC), are a well established part of the ICH process and are detailed in various European guidelines. The policing of these standards occurs at the national authority level. A current list of guidance documents can be found on the EMEA website.[2]

A preclinical safety guideline entitled *Safety Studies for Biotechnical Products* (S6, 3/98) was established to address the specific issues that exist for biotechnological products, their inherent nature preventing their regulation as conventional medicines. Of particular importance is the relevance and justification of animal species and models, antigenicity, specialized immunohisto-chemical procedures and safety pharmacology tests designs. Standard absorption, distribution, metabolism and excretion studies are generally not appropriate. For reproductive performance/developmental toxicity, carcinogenicity, or geno-toxicity studies, standard study designs may not be applicable for biological and biotechnology products, and the development of alternative models that can assess potential toxicity better is encouraged.[3]

CLINICAL TRIAL APPLICATIONS

Clinical trial application procedures in the EU are complex owing to the abundance and variability of national regulations. As mentioned earlier, legislation is at the national level, so timelines and documentation requirements vary by country. However, once study sponsors understand these national requirements, the EU can be an effective

choice for clinical trials for global registration and commercialization.

Before clinical trial initiation, the study sponsor must obtain ethical approval via local hospital Ethics Committees, as well as meet national administrative requirements, which can include importation authorization procedures. Additional requirements are often necessary for biotechnology and biological products in certain countries (e.g. viral safety committee submissions in France).

National requirements for regulatory authorities can generally be divided into notifications or authorizations. Notifications may occur in parallel to Ethics Committee submissions (e.g. in Belgium, Denmark and The Netherlands) or after them (e.g. in Finland, France and Germany). Similarly, authorizations can be obtained in parallel with Ethics Committee approvals (e.g. in Norway, Spain, Sweden and the UK) or afterwards (e.g. in Greece).[4]

A sponsor wishing to submit a clinical trial application in various EU countries assembles a core set of information, all or part of which satisfies regulatory requirements in all countries. Approval times for most EU countries are between 4 and 12 weeks, but some countries can take up to 1 year (e.g. Italy). Timelines can also vary by the study and medicinal product type. The UK is exceptional in differentiating between studies on healthy volunteer and studies on patients; an authorization for healthy volunteer (Phase 1) studies is not required in the UK, although the Ethics Committee approval is still required. Phase 2, 3 and 4 (post-marketing) studies in Denmark, Finland, France, Germany, Ireland, Spain and the UK all follow the same procedures.[5]

Good Clinical Practice (GCP) rules, which set the standards for the conduct and performance of clinical studies, are applicable in the EU as they are in the other ICH regions.[6] In order to be considered as part of the registration dossier at any authority, studies must have been performed in accordance with GCPs.

An initiative to harmonize clinical trial procedures is currently under way in the form of a directive on clinical trials and good clinical practices. The goal is to harmonize regulatory systems by rationalizing documentary and administrative procedures in European multicenter studies. There is no formal date for the adoption of this directive and many details of its content are yet to be defined.

TESTING FOR QUALITY OF THE MEDICINAL PRODUCT

Since 1991, European Directives require companies producing proprietary medicinal products to operate their facilities under current Good Manufacturing Practices (GMPs), which set basic standards for manufacturing facilities and their production controls and operations, to ensure that the products meet the standards of identity, strength, quality and purity.

The EU follows the rules outlined in a basic GMP Directive 91/356/EEC and its appendixes. The manufacturer of finished products is required to have a manufacturing authorization in Europe, as outlined in Directive 75/319/EEC as amended, and manufacturing plants are subject to regular national inspections.

The requirement of a 'qualified person', as defined by Directive 75/319/EEC, is central to the provision of a Marketing Authorization Application (MAA) in the EU. This person is responsible for each batch release, ensuring that each batch is manufactured and controlled in accordance with the laws of the member state in which the manufacturing takes place and in accordance with the requirements of the MAA.

As with the US Pharmacopeia, the European Pharmacopoeia (EP) is an influential regulatory body responsible for developing monographs and reference standards for substances, containers, excipients and chemical and biological products, among others. Applications for both development products and marketing authorizations, particularly for biologics, must meet EP requirements; if a product is not referenced in an EP monograph, a Master Drug File must be submitted for its authorization.

The requirements for the chemical, pharmaceutical, and biological documentation (Part II) of the marketing authorization application have been central to the ICH discussions, and many harmonized guidelines have been issued over the past 6 years. In addition, many European guidelines, which predate the ICH effort, are available, and a current list can be found on the EMEA website.[2]

The quality evaluation of biotech products is covered by a series of quality guidelines that are part of the ICH process. Owing to the inherent risks involved in the use of products of human or animal origin, these guidelines require:[3]

(a) the assessment of viral safety in all products, based on the knowledge and adequate quality control of the starting material;

(b) the production process to incorporate viral inactivation or removal steps plus the validation of such steps; and

(c) control tests performed on the intermediates and/or final product.

Based on the public debate over 'mad cow disease', legislation is currently under way for the specific issue of transmissible spongiform encephalopathy (TSE). The current move is towards avoiding the use of ruminant material in pharmaceutical products.

THE MARKETING AUTHORIZATION APPLICATION REVIEW AND APPROVAL PROCESS

In 1995, two new procedures were put in place for marketing authorization in the EU, as outlined in the *Notice to Applicants*.[7] There are two ways in which a medicinal product may be marketed in the EU:

(a) Mutual Recognition Procedure, in which a marketing authorization is granted by the competent authority of a member state for its own territory (national authorization) and later recognized by the entire EU; and

(b) Centralized Procedure, in which a marketing authorization is granted by the European Commission for enforcement in the entire EU (a Community Authorization), and is under the control of the EMEA, situated in London.

In contrast to the USA (where an authorization is valid indefinitely provided the sponsor satisfies the obligations and is policed through inspections), a marketing authorization in the EU is valid for 5 years and must therefore be renewed; this is done by filing applications at least 3 months before the expiration date.

Also, unlike the structure of the FDA, there is no distinction between drugs and biologics in the European approval system, although specific guidelines exist for their development. A detailed discussion follows on the two procedures for the registration of medicinal products.

Mutual Recognition Procedure

The Mutual Recognition Procedure (see *Fig. 15.1*) is described in many articles and outlined in the *Notice to Applicants*.[7,8] This procedure relies on the competence of national authorities

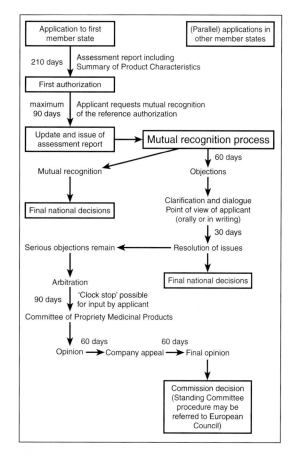

Fig. 15.1 Mutual recognition procedures.

(and not the EMEA) for the evaluation of medicinal products. The applicant files an MAA in one member state, indicating the desire for the MAA to be recognized in other member states. The member state is then referred to as the Reference Member State for the submission and is responsible for the initial assessment and approval of the MAA. The initial, 'national' portion of this procedure lasts 210 days.

Following approval in the Reference Member State, the file is updated to provide for responses to the Reference Member State's comments and questions. Once updated, a date is agreed for filing with other member states, known as Concerned Member States.

The subsequent phase is said to be bilateral and lasts for 90 days. In this phase, the Concerned Member States raises issues that can be discussed between them and the Reference Member State. National differences do exist and these need to be considered. For example, several authorities often request specific administrative documents in their own language. If a Concerned Member State raises a serious objection, which it considers a risk to public health and is not resolved during the discussion period, it would be possible for the discrepancy to go to arbitration by the CPMP. The CPMP would then evaluate the situation and give an opinion that leads to a binding decision for all affected member states. In practice, few companies go to arbitration, since this is often seen as being a too high-risk approach.

The Mutual Recognition Procedure has several advantages over the Centralized Procedure, as outlined in the *Notice to Applicants*.[7,9] It offers a possibility of a rapid review, the opportunity for the applicant to choose the Reference Member State, the ability to exclude any Concerned Member State in case of specific difficulties, and the option to withdraw applications when resolution cannot be reached. Marketing flexibility, with co-marketing agreements and the option of various trademarks in various countries, are also important advantages. The procedure does, however, require qualified knowledge at the local, national level and the appropriate local personnel to ensure smooth negotiations. The outcome of this procedure is the same as the following procedure: a harmonized Summary of Product Characteristics (SmPC) and package leaflet in the Concerned Member States. The SmPC contains the essential information of the product's properties and characteristics (equivalent to the USA package insert). Derived from the SmPC, the package leaflet is the information provided to patients and included in the product packaging.

Centralized Procedure

Council regulation EEC No 2309/93[10] created the EMEA on 1 January 1995. The primary responsibility of the EMEA is to oversee the Centralized Procedure for authorizing medicinal products (see *Fig. 15.2*). In the Centralized Procedure, there is a single application, a single evaluation, one fee, and a resultant single authorization issued by the European Commission allowing direct access to the entire EU market.[7]

The Centralized Procedure is compulsory for biotechnology products derived from recombinant deoxyribonucleic acid technology or from manipulation of genetic material, such as hybridoma and monoclonal antibody methods—the so-called 'List A' products. For new active substances and other innovative (as defined by legislation) medicinal products (such as new delivery systems that contribute a significant innovation (such as 'List B' products) the choice of authorization procedure is at the sponsor's option. The CPMP is the scientific committee that is responsible for formulating the EMEA's opinion on any question relating to the evaluation of human medicinal products, including the provision of scientific advice.

This procedure offers significant advantages because the one authorization automatically confers the same rights and obligations in all member states as if each member state had granted a national marketing authorization. As with the Mutual Recognition Procedure, one

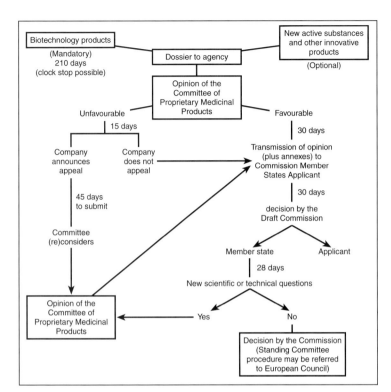

Fig. 15.2 Centralized procedure.

SmPC and one package leaflet is approved for use in all countries. Inconveniences of the system include the need for a single EU trademark (which often causes considerable practical problems), a single packaging look and, moreover, the possibility of a single rejection applicable to the whole EU, thus making it impossible to market the product in the EU without reapplying.

An expedited review by the Centralized Procedure has been granted to several products for life-threatening conditions (e.g. treatments for cancer and acquired immunodeficiency syndrome).[8] However, the procedure itself is already streamlined, with an overall timeline of 240 days, not including sponsor response time.

The SmPC package leaflet and package particulars must be submitted as part of the initial file in the 11 languages of the EU, plus Icelandic and Norwegian; however, the final 30 days of the 240 day procedure involves an intense amount of co-ordination with the EMEA to produce a final, correct translation for each of the languages.

Before a European license can take effect, the opinion of the CPMP must be made legally binding by the European Commission, in accordance with the Treaty of Rome. Only the European Commission and the European Council can make such decisions within the EU, and it is therefore the Commission that grants the Marketing Authorization. The CPMP's positive opinion is forwarded to the Commission, and a timeline of 90 days is fixed for the issuing of an approval. Hence, from submission to approval, the Centralized Procedure predicts a 310-day process, excluding company response time.

Since the EMEA seeks to increase public transparency in the process of a product approval, the European Public Assessment Report (EPAR) is released to the public within 3 months of the Commission decision. As with the 'Summary Basis of Approval' in the USA, the EPAR is a summary of the assessment report for products approved through the Centralized Procedure. There is no obligation for member states to release reports similar to EPARs for products approved through national procedures, although a move towards such reports is underway.

THE EUROPEAN DOSSIER

Regardless of which authorization procedure is used, the European dossier is made up of four parts:[7]

Part I: Summary of the Dossier
Part II: Chemical/Pharmaceutical/Biological
          Tests
Part III: Toxico-Pharmacological Tests
Part IV: Clinical Documentation

Part I summarizes the overall dossier and includes administrative details as well as the proposed SmPC and package leaflet. Both these documents, as well as the proposed outer and immediate packaging, must be provided in the 11 languages of the Community, plus Norwegian and Icelandic. Part I also includes three Expert Reports, which are critical reviews of each of the three remaining sections of the dossier. Each is written by an expert who has appropriate qualifications and who may be an employee of the sponsor. These reports serve as a high-level critique of the overall dossier, providing a balanced overview of the data presented, including its weaknesses. The

experts are required to provide justification for the statements proposed in the SmPC. The Expert Reports form a critical part of the MAA. In the EU, unlike the situation in the USA, the product review begins with a review of the summary-level documentation first (Expert Reports), with subsequent examination of the full data to establish that the summary conclusions are in fact supported. Therefore, well-written expert reports with a concise, interpretative approach are paramount to the successful review of any European dossier.

Parts II, III and IV contain the summary and the details of the experiments that have led the sponsor to motivate the application. With a few minor details, the amount of information required is similar in submissions in the USA, the EU and Japan, but the formats differ.

ORPHAN DRUGS

As of June 1999, orphan drug legislation was passed by the Council of Ministers in the EU, and finalization of the specifics are underway to establish a committee at the level of the EMEA.[11] This initiative takes into account the success of the orphan drug legislation in the USA, and its goal is to provide incentives for developing and marketing medicines intended to diagnose, prevent or treat rare diseases. The current text proposes a 10-year market exclusivity period, plus protocol development to applicants, guaranteed access to the Centralized Procedure, and a partial or total waiver of registration fees. The criteria for orphan drug designation will be for life-threatening or chronically debilitating diseases of an incidence of fewer than 5 in 10 000 people in the EU.[12]

PRICING AND REIMBURSEMENT

Although the authorization granted from the Centralized Procedure is immediately effective throughout the EU, there is still much progress to be made before a central approval in fact means simultaneous availability of the product in all the markets. Whether approved via the Centralized Procedure or the Mutual Recognition Procedure, reimbursement steps are necessary after approval. These are under the control of national legislation. In certain countries, such as Germany and the UK, the sponsor is able to determine the price and to sell immediately as soon as the MAA is obtained. In other member states, national procedures exist, varying in complexity and resulting in delays from approximately 2 weeks in Finland up to approximately 15 months in Belgium. In light of these national differences, which stem from differing health-care systems in member states, the overall goal of equal access throughout the EU is not being met.

France provides a good example of the potential negotiations (see *Fig. 15.3*). The French procedure has two steps: a technical dossier is first submitted to the Transparency Commission to justify that the drug adds therapeutic value, and then an economic file is submitted to the Economic Committee (Ministry of Social Security) to justify the proposed price and sales volume forecast. Despite legislation fixing the total procedure to 180 days, these negotiations can take up to 9–12 months.

MAINTAINING THE MARKETING AUTHORIZATION LICENSE

Once a medicinal product has been approved through either the Centralized Procedure or the Mutual Recognition Procedure, the Marketing

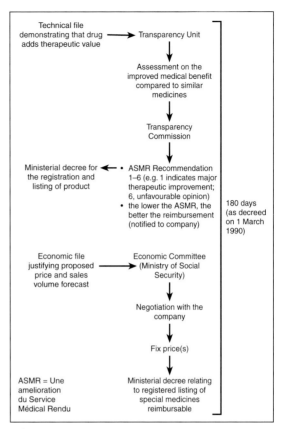

Fig. 15.3 Pricing and reimbursement procedures in France.

Authorization Holder (MAH) is responsible for a variety of post-approval activities, as discussed below.

Periodic Safety Update Reports

In addition to the specific requirements of 15-calendar day reporting for serious reactions,[5] Periodic Safety Update Reports must be submitted by the MAH every 6 months after approval for 2 years, then annually for 3 years, and then at the time of product license renewal every 5 years.

Post-approval commitments

Products that receive conditional approval from the Centralized Procedure are subject to annual assessment of the benefit:risk ratio. Data to be submitted as part of clinical obligations, which are legally binding, and pharmaceutical follow-up measures, which are not legally binding but often require world-wide specification changes, are fixed at the time of approval according to a set timeline. The annual reassessment involves summarizing the status of these data and continues until the MAH has fulfilled these obligations.

Variations

The MAH is responsible for taking into account technical and scientific progress and for making any amendments that may subsequently be required. They may also wish to alter or improve the product or to add additional safeguard measures for a variety of reasons. Specific requirements are in place to ensure that the MAH alerts the countries in which the product is approved of such amendments to the license, known as variations. These variations are divided into two categories in the EU: Type I and Type II variations (see *Figs. 15.4* and *15.5*). In general, Type I are 'minor' variations. A list of Type I variations is outlined in the Notice to Applicants, the majority being related to minor changes in the chemical, pharmaceutical, and biological documentation.[7] By definition, any change that does not fall within these defined categories, and does not require a new application, is regarded as a Type II variation. Type II variations typically involve changes to the SmPC or Package leaflet text.

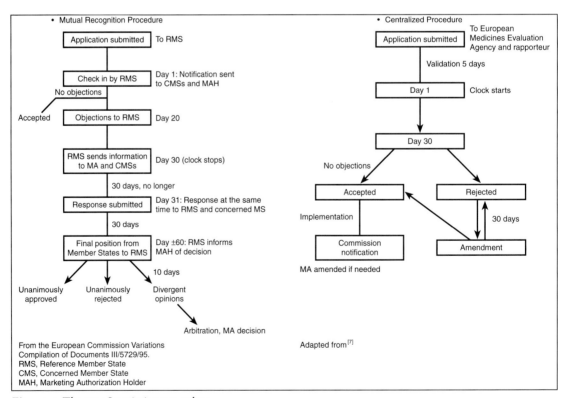

Fig. 15.4 *The type I variation procedure.*

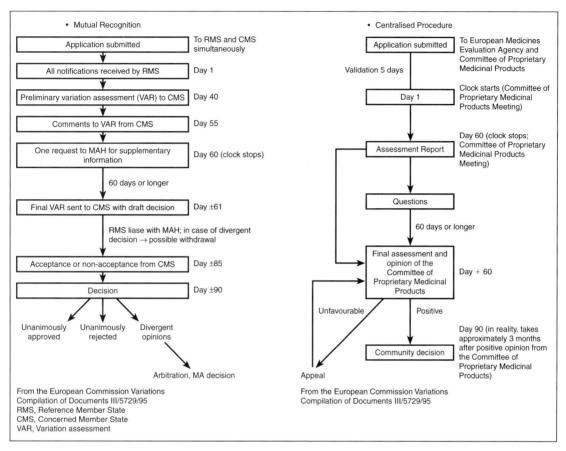

Fig. 15.5 The type II variation procedure.

Urgent Safety Restriction

Should the MAH receive information that is so important that it must be communicated immediately throughout the EU, a provision restriction (an Urgent Safety Restriction) can be implemented. Such cases usually arise around pharmacovigilance issues or when there is a concern about quality, perhaps requiring a batch recall.

CONCLUSIONS

The development of medicinal products for registration and marketing in Europe is relatively streamlined with the USA and Japanese requirements, thanks to the advent of the ICH process. The particularities of clinical trial performance are still governed at the national level at the moment. The registration procedures offered in Europe and the philosophy behind the role and mechanism of review of marketing authorizations differ from those in the USA and require European-based attention by the sponsor. For products of high therapeutic value that meet a clear unmet medical need, the outcome of the USA and EU processes is often quite similar, with a product indicated and approved for the relevant populations as supported by the pivotal trials in both the USA and Europe. Although advances have recently been made by the therapeutic availability of medicinal products that alleviate the symptoms of MS or even the progression of MS disability, MS can be considered a disease in which there is still a large unmet need to arrest or even cure it.

REFERENCES

1 Note for Preclinical Safety Evaluation of Biotechnology Derived Products (CPMP/ICH/302/95) (ICH 56). ICH website: http://www.ich.org/ All referenced guidelines are available in their most current form through the appropriate authority internet homepage (e.g. ICH, EMEA etc).

2 **European Medicines Evaluation Agency (EMEA).** EMEA Website. http://www.eudra.org/emea.html.

3 **Voisin Lestringant E.** Current issues in biotechnology. *Reg Affairs J* March 1998; 156–161.

4 **AFAR Working Group.** January 1999.

5 **Currie JC, Löfgren M.** New Drug Approval in the European Union: the EMEA. Waltham Massachusetts: PAREXEL International Corporation, June 1998: 1-882615-49-2.

6 *Good Clinical Practice: Consolidated Guidelines* (ICH). PMP/135/95/(ICH E6).

7 **European Medicines Evaluation Agency (EMEA).** *The Rules Governing Medicinal Products in the European Union. Notice to Applicants. Medicinal Products for Human Use,* volume 2A. 1998.

8 **McGettigan G.** Issues for biotechnology and innovative products. *Reg Affairs J* November 1998; 830–834.

9 **Lloyd K, McBain S, Swan J.** Experience of the mutual recognition procedure in the transitional phase. *Reg Affairs J* July 1998; 486–492.

10 **Council Regulation 2309/EEC.** *Official Journal of the European Communities* No. L 14/1; 1993.

11 *Official Journal of the European Communities* C276,7; 1998.

12 **Bogaert P.** EC Orphan medicines regulation formally proposed (editorial). *Reg Affairs J* November 1998.

16

Sponsors, monitoring committees, and investigators: the investigator's perspective

Fred D Lublin and Stephen C Reingold

The past decade has been a remarkably productive period for clinical trials in multiple sclerosis (MS). Not only have there been four new therapeutic agents, representing two different classes of drugs, approved for use throughout most of the world, but there have also been many earlier phase studies of promising new agents, some of which have moved to currently ongoing pivotal studies. Some preliminary studies, as well as some larger, pivotal trials, have failed, either because they have not achieved statistically significant outcomes or because the agents being tested have been proved to have unacceptable risk–benefit outcomes. Even those new agents that have been shown to be relatively safe and effective have only modest treatment benefit, and there is much need for new products, new dosing regimens of available products, and study of combinations of agents. All of this points to the ongoing importance of, and increasing attention to, randomized controlled clinical trials for new therapeutic agents in MS.

The majority of these studies have been, and will continue to be, performed by clinical investigators in partnership with industrial sponsors.[1] The 'pipeline' of innovative therapeutic modalities in pharmaceutical and biotechnological companies, coupled with the considerable expense of development of new agents from initial laboratory or animal testing through the pivotal trial phase, indicate the value and absolute necessity of such partnerships. Corporate sponsors may have the novel interventions and the financial capability of supporting the very complex and expensive infrastructure to undertake multicenter studies. Clinical investigators offer expertise in MS clinical trial design and conduct, and can provide the desired independence and objectivity that is necessary in undertaking a trial and in interpreting results.

Clinical investigators and representatives of biotechnology and pharmaceutical companies share an interest in finding safe and effective therapies for MS. However, the goals, needs, expectations, and priorities of clinical investigators, who may be academic physicians or private practitioners, differ at times from those of industrial sponsors. Although both groups are focused on finding the best (most efficacious and safest) possible therapies for the disease, clinical investigators tend to be less concerned about such pragmatic issues as the corporate source of any given agent, patent rights, profit potential, marketability, and internal corporate program prioritization. A commercial concern must, however, focus on such issues, since they relate to financial strength, corporate survival, and, often, the potential to continue pharmaceutical and biotechnological development in the future.

191

Although the joint interest of investigators and corporate sponsors in finding new MS treatments has led to successful synergies in recent times, it remains essential to recognize that these different perspectives can lead to difficulties in developing a consensus during the planning stages of trials, in activities during the conduct of trials, and in interpretation of, and access to, data after trials.

The potential for such problems can be avoided, at least in part, by formally establishing, before the start of a study, the elements of co-operation and interaction between corporate sponsors and clinical investigators. For large-scale, pivotal studies, this should include, among other details:

(a) The role of investigators in protocol design.

(b) The creation of an independent Advisory or Steering Committee, which will work with the sponsor and consultants to design the study protocol, advise the sponsor on any issues relating to the study before its initiation, during its conduct or after its conclusion, and serve during the study as a liaison between study investigators, other advisory groups and the sponsor. This Committee, as well as all other advisory groups and study investigators, should exclude from membership anyone with significant financial interest in the development of the new agent or any competing products. During the study, the Advisory or Steering Committee should regularly review the progress of the trial and the impact of new developments in the field. The Committee should consider protocol amendments if needed and assist the sponsor in issues of protocol adherence, in general or at specific centers.

(c) The creation of an independent Data and Safety Monitoring Committee (DSMC), which will primarily serve to ensure the pro-

tection of human subjects in the study. The authors believe that assessment of the protocol and its amendments and evaluation of the ongoing conduct of the study may have an impact on the risk–benefit evaluation for the study. As such, efforts to review and help to ensure the scientific validity and conduct of the study are also part of the responsibilities of the DSMB. For most trials the functions of ongoing monitoring of safety and efficacy data can be combined into a single monitoring group. Members of the DSMC should be independent of the study sponsor and of participating study sites and free of conflicts of interest. The DSMC should be composed of neurologists and others familiar with MS, others with expertise in monitoring adverse events and biostatisticians experienced in clinical trials. All members must be capable of understanding statistical, biological and medical arguments related to the trial and must be completely objective in their evaluations. Study investigators and employees of study sponsors should not participate in the DSMC's discussions, except as a resource to clarify the conduct of the study. A liaison officer (who may be an employee of the sponsor or a consultant) may be appointed to liaise among the DSMC, the Advisory or Steering Committee and the sponsor and so facilitate the communication of information among the interested groups. The DSMC should remain blinded throughout the study (if such is part of the trial design) but it must have the option to require additional analyses and even unblinding (of the DSMC members only) in the event of significant safety or efficacy concerns. On the basis of analyses of safety or efficacy data, or for ethical considerations, the DSMC may recommend early termination of the study to the Advisory or Steering Committee and to the sponsor. To perform their tasks, the DSMB must have complete and rapid access to study data. Before initiation of the study, the members of the DSMC must reach consensus among themselves, with the sponsor and with any associated contract research organization about their own function and operation, including details relating to blinding, form of data presentation, frequency and format of meetings, and criteria for early stopping of the study.

(d) Creation of a Publications Committee[2] to determine the manner of expeditiously reporting data analysis and to prepare manuscripts describing the study and its outcomes.

(e) Determining the role of investigators, advisory and monitoring committees, regulatory authorities and the sponsor(s) in evaluating need for any deviation in the original study plan or analysis. The maintenance of study design and integrity is of paramount importance.

(f) Deciding the nature and ensuring the independence of data analysis.

(g) Deciding 'ownership' of trial data, including guaranteed access to all collected data by study investigators, at the completion of the trial.

(h) Deciding the role of study investigators in interpretation and dissemination of data collected in 'extension' trials after the completion of the preplanned randomized trial.[3]

Patients who volunteer as study subjects do so, at least partly, out of a sense of duty to the greater good that may accrue to all with MS as a consequence of their participation. The interests of trial investigators and of study sponsors must, by necessity, be considered of secondary importance to the needs and interests of the patients involved in the study and of patients more broadly. However, a trial that is undertaken without proper recognition of the necessary contributions of both trial investigators and corporate sponsors and that does not include an advance plan to ensure that the interests of all parties are well served can diminish the contributions of the patient volunteers and compromise the ethics of everyone involved.

REFERENCES

1   Reingold SC. The new partnership in multiple sclerosis: relations with industry. *Multiple Sclerosis* 1995; **1**:141–142.

2   Lublin FD, Reingold SC. Guidelines for clinical trials of new therapeutic agents in multiple sclerosis: relations between study investigators, advisors and sponsors. *Neurology* 1997; **48**:572–574.

3   Goodkin DE, Reingold S, Sibley W et al. Guidelines for clinical trials of new therapeutic agents in multiple sclerosis: reporting extended results from phase III clinical trials. *Ann Neurol* 1999; in press.

17

Standardized reporting of randomized controlled multiple sclerosis clinical trials

Donald E Goodkin and Thomas A Lang

INTRODUCTION

A reader's confidence in the validity of reports of randomized controlled multiple sclerosis (MS) clinical trials and meta-analyses is largely determined by how thoroughly and clearly the authors describe the aim of the study, its aim, design, subjects, methods, procedures, findings, statistical analyses, results, and implications. Clinicians need this information to judge whether the conclusions reached are relevant to their practices, and meta-analysts need to know which trials have data that can be combined to yield reliable meta-analytic conclusions.

For this chapter, the authors accepted and proposed standards for reporting randomized controlled clinical trials (RCTs),[1,2] extension studies,[3] and meta-analyses.[2] Introductory comments and guidelines are provided in separate sections of this chapter for each of these studies. The authors believe that adherence to these standards will significantly improve a reader's ability to interpret the results and validity of scientific research.

GUIDELINES FOR REPORTING THE RESULTS OF RCTs

RCTs are ideally designed with clear-cut prospective outcomes, on which trial design and statistical power are based. The guidelines for reporting RCTs are contained in the *Consolidated Standards of Reporting Trials* (CONSORT). This statement includes a checklist of 21 points to be addressed when reporting the results of RCTs (*Table 17.1*).

Title of the RCT

Reports of RCTs should be identified as such in the title,[4] for example: 'Interferon-β 1b in treatment of secondary progressive multiple sclerosis: a placebo-controlled, multicenter randomized trial.' Declarative statements that state the conclusions of the study should be avoided.

Abstract

A structured abstract for RCTs should contain a description of the objectives of the study, its

195

Table 17.1 Headings, subheadings, and descriptors from the CONSORT statement

---

Title: Identify the study as a randomized trial

Abstract: Use a structured format

Introduction: State prospectively defined hypothesis, clinical objectives, and planned subgroup or covariate analyses

Methods

Protocol: Describe:

- planned study population, together with inclusion/exclusion criteria
- planned interventions and their timing
- primary and secondary outcome measure(s) and the minimum important difference(s); indicate how the target sample size was projected
- rationale and methods for statistical analyses, detailing main comparative analyses and whether they were completed on an intention-to-treat basis
- prospectively designed stopping rules (if warranted)

Assignment: Describe:

- unit of random assignment (e.g., individual, cluster geographic)
- method used to generate the allocation schedule
- method of allocation concealment and timing of assignment
- method used to separate the generator from the executor of assignment

Masking (blinding): Describe mechanism (e.g., capsules, tables); similarity of treatment characteristics (e.g., appearance, taste); allocation schedule control (location of code during trial and when broken); and evidence for successful blinding among participants, person doing the intervention, outcome assessors, and data analysts

Results

Participant flow and follow-up: Provide a trial profile (a figure) summarizing participant flow, numbers and timing of random assignment, interventions, and measurements for each randomly assigned group

Analysis:

- state estimated effect of intervention on primary and secondary outcomes measures, including a point estimate and measure of precision (confidence interval)
- state results in absolute numbers when feasible
- present summary data and appropriate descriptive and inferential statistics in sufficient detail to permit alternative analyses and replication
- describe prognostic variables by treatment group and any attempt to adjust for them
- describe protocol deviations from the study as planned, together with the reasons

Comment:

- state specific interpretation of the study findings, including sources of bias and impression (internal validity) and discussion of external validity, including appropriate quantitative measures when possible
- state general interpretations of the data in light of the totality of the available evidence

---

design, setting, patients, interventions, main outcome measures, main results, and conclusions as described by Haynes.[5] The results of planned primary and secondary outcome analyses adjusted for inequalities of demographic and clinical variables known to influence those outcomes should be summarized. Unless adequate justification is provided, exploratory subgroup analyses should not be reported in the abstract. Only conclusions directly supported by analyses of the planned primary and secondary outcomes should be stated. Equal emphasis must be given to positive and negative findings. The clinical relevance of such analyses should be noted, as should any requirement for additional study before the results can be applied in clinical settings.

Text

Introduction

The introduction for reports of RCTs should provide a summary of information justifying the trial and serving as the origin of the question considered or the hypothesis tested.[1]

Trial design and methods

DESIGN

Descriptions for the following aspects of RCTs should be provided:[1,2]

(a) type of trial;
(b) comparison groups;
(c) length of study periods;
(d) calendar time during which the study was conducted;
(e) type and test of masking procedures;
(f) methods for random assignment and allocation concealment; and
(g) the treatment effect, statistical power, and α-level assumed for the sample-size calculations.

SETTING

The following information should be provided for RCTs:[1,2] site identification and characterization as primary care, referral practice, secondary or tertiary care facility, ambulatory or hospital setting.

PATIENTS AND CONTROLS

The methods of selection, inclusion and exclusion criteria, management of dropouts, and informed consent procedures for entry into the Phase 3 RCT should be summarized.[1,2]

INTERVENTIONS

The generic names, doses, frequency and times, adjustments, and sources of interventions administered during the Phase 3 RCT should be reviewed[1,2] and reasons for change in those interventions during the study should be noted.[3]

OUTCOME MEASURES

The frequency and reliability of outcome measures and stopping criteria should be noted. Outcome measures for RCTs should be presented in the following order:

(a) Outcome measures planned before initiating data collection during the phase 3 RCT:
Primary endpoints
Secondary endpoints
Exploratory endpoints

(b) Outcome measures added after initiating data collection but before analysis of the planned outcomes for the phase 3 RCT. The rationale for change in any outcome measure from those originally planned should be provided.

(c) Exploratory analyses performed after analysis of the planned outcomes. The rationale for each exploratory analysis should be provided.

STATISTICAL METHODS AND DATA ANALYSIS

Statistical methods, including names and sources of software programs with references for non-standard methods, should be grouped under the previously listed headings for outcome measures. The principle of intention-to-treat should be applied to all analyses unless otherwise justified. Methods for selection of variables with a list of potential adjustment variables and their definitions should accompany the use of multivariate methods. Whether or not statistical adjustments for multiple comparisons were made should be explicitly stated. Procedures for monitoring, interim analyses and stopping rules should be provided. Methods for comparing proportions of withdrawals from treatment arms and methods for determining and adjusting for imbalances of relevant demographic and clinical variables between the treatment arms should be identified.[1,2]

Results

DEMOGRAPHIC AND CLINICAL CHARACTERISTICS OF PATIENTS

Baseline demographic characteristics should be provided by treatment group, as should the results of statistical tests for baseline imbalances.[2] An accounting of patients from onset to completion of the study should be sufficiently detailed to enable the reader to determine the number of patients at each stage of the study, from sample selection through to completion (*Fig. 17.1*). Thus, relevant data should be provided by treatment group for patients who completed the RCT and those who were lost to follow-up.

OUTCOME MEASURES

Deviations from the study protocol should be described, as should the reasons for any change

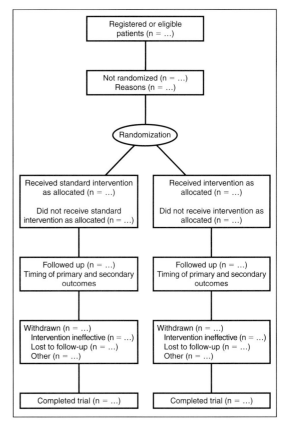

Fig. 17.1 *A standardized schematic summary for accounting for patients in RCTs and extension studies.*

in protocol. The results for all analyses of outcome data should be grouped under the headings noted above for groupings of outcome measures. The estimated effect of the intervention for all outcome measures should be stated in absolute numbers when feasible and accompanied by confidence intervals. As far as possible, summary data should be provided in sufficient detail to permit alternative analyses and replication. Prognostic variables should be identified, as should attempts to adjust for imbalances between treatment groups. The success of masking patients to treatment assignment should be explicitly stated.

ADVERSE EVENTS

All clinically important drug-related and non-drug-related adverse events during the phase 3 RCT should be compared across all study groups.

Discussion

The authors of the study report should recapitulate the main findings of the RCT and, if appropriate, discuss how the findings differ from and extend earlier findings. The effect of differences in relevant demographic and clinical variables across treatment groups entering and completing RCT on pre-planned analyses and rationale for all exploratory subgroup analyses and potential pitfalls of interpreting those analyses should be discussed. Unless it is adequately justified, a declaration of clinical efficacy should not be based on favorable results from exploratory subgroup analyses.

Supportive and contradictory data from other studies should be discussed, as should attempts to reconcile conflicting evidence.

Generalization of the main outcomes to clinical practice and implications for further studies and product development should be data-based.

GUIDELINES FOR REPORTING THE RESULTS OF EXTENSION STUDIES

As noted above, RCTs are ideally designed with clear-cut prospective outcomes, on which trial design and statistical power are based. In some cases, patients may continue to be studied in 'extension studies' after the original RCT is complete. In contrast to RCTs, extension studies are opportunistic, in that they aim to take advantage of data collected after the prescribed end of the trial for some or all patients originally enrolled. Extension studies thus provide a unique opportunity to collect efficacy and tolerability data and may help to generate hypotheses to be tested in subsequent properly designed and implemented prospective RCTs. Extension studies also provide an appealing mechanism to generate data for validating surrogate outcomes capable of predicting long-term change in clinically relevant measures of disability.

However, by their very nature, extension studies may be underpowered statistically and may involve patients in different demographic or clinical groups, and in different proportions, from the original RCT. Yet the tendency of the consumers—sponsors, clinicians, patients and third-party payers—is to view results from extension studies as being as powerful and meaningful as results from the original studies.

The following issues should be recognized and addressed in reports of extension studies:

(a) imbalance in relevant demographic and clinical variables between treatment groups at the beginning of an extension study resulting from informed censoring that occurred during the preceding Phase III RCT;

(b) imbalance in relevant demographic and clinical variables between treatment groups at the beginning of an extension study that reflect a study subject's choice not to participate in an extension study; and

(c) use and interpretation of exploratory subgroup analyses.

The proposed guidelines, developed as a result of recent experiences with extension studies that have followed phase 3 RCTs in MS, are intended to standardize the reports of such studies. These guidelines may also be useful when reporting extension studies for other diseases and will help ensure that issues that are relevant in reports of extension studies are adequately addressed. Adherence to these standards will improve the design of such studies and the reader's ability to interpret the results and validity of such reports.

Title of the report

The results of an extension study should be reported separately from its preceding RCT.[2] The title or subtitle should identify the report as an extension study. The title of extension studies should not contain a declarative sentence that is based on an exploratory subgroup analysis, favorable or unfavorable, in comparison with the pre-planned primary analyses of the preceding RCT.[3]

Abstract

The structured abstract for the extension study should state any aspect of the objective, design, setting, patients, interventions, main outcome measures, main results, and conclusions that differs from the preceding phase 3 trial.[3] The results of planned primary and secondary outcome analyses adjusted for inequalities of demographic and clinical variables known to influence those outcomes should be summarized. Unless adequate justification is provided, exploratory subgroup analyses should not be reported in the abstract. Only conclusions directly supported by analyses of the planned primary and secondary outcomes should be stated. Equal emphasis must be given to positive and negative findings. The clinical relevance of such analyses should be noted, as should any

requirement for additional study before the results can be applied in clinical settings.

Text

Introduction
The introduction for reports of extension studies should summarize the preceding phase 3 RCT and its results, including primary and secondary outcomes.[3] Hypotheses tested during RCTs and extension studies should be stated.

Trial design and method
DESIGN
The design of the phase 3 RCT should be recapitulated and any differences in design during the extension study should be noted.[3]

SETTING
Any changes and reason for changes in the sites participating in the extension study should be noted.[3]

PATIENTS AND CONTROLS
The methods of selection, inclusion and exclusion criteria, management of dropouts and informed consent procedures for entry into the phase 3 RCT should be recapitulated and reasons for change in those criteria for patients entered in the extension study, if any, should be noted.[1] The authors should indicate whether patients signed informed consent for the extension study.[3]

INTERVENTIONS
The generic names, doses, frequency and times, adjustments, and sources of interventions administered during the phase 3 RCT should be reviewed[1] and reasons for change in those interventions during the extension study should be noted.[3]

OUTCOME MEASURES

The frequency and reliability of outcome measures and stopping criteria for the RCT should be recapitulated. Outcome measures for extension studies should be explicitly stated and organized in the following order:

(a) Outcome measures planned before initiating data collection during the phase 3 RCT and continued in the extension phase:
    Primary endpoints
    Secondary endpoints
    Exploratory endpoints

(b) Outcome measures added after initiating data collection but before analysis of the pre-planned outcomes for the phase 3 RCT and continued during the extension study. The rationale for change in any outcome measure from those originally planned should be provided.

(c) Exploratory outcome analyses performed after analysis of the planned outcomes for the phase 3 RCT and continued during the extension study. The rationale for each exploratory analysis should be provided.

STATISTICAL METHODS AND DATA ANALYSIS

Statistical methods, including names and sources of software programs with references for non-standard methods, should be grouped under the previously listed headings for outcome measures. The principle of intention-to-treat should be applied to all analyses unless otherwise justified. Methods for selection of variables with a list of potential adjustment variables and their definitions should accompany the use of multivariate methods. Statistical adjustments for multiple comparisons should be explicitly stated. Procedures for monitoring and interim analyses should be described. Methods for comparing proportions of withdrawals from treatment arms and

methods for determining and adjusting for imbalances of relevant demographic and clinical variables between the treatment arms should be reported.

Results

DEMOGRAPHIC AND CLINICAL CHARACTERISTICS OF PATIENTS

Baseline demographic characteristics should be provided by treatment group and statistical imbalances should be tested for their effect on the outcomes. An accounting of patients from onset to completion of RCTs and through to completion of the extension study should be sufficiently detailed to enable the reader to determine the number of patients at each stage of the study, from sample selection through to completion. Thus, relevant data should be provided by treatment group for patients who completed the RCT or were lost to follow-up, patients who completed the RCT but declined to participate in the extension study, and patients who enrolled in the extension study, patients who were lost to follow-up, and patients who did and did not complete the extension study.

OUTCOME MEASURES

Deviations from the study protocol should be described, as should the reasons for any change in protocol. The results for all analyses of outcome data should be grouped under the headings noted above for groupings of outcome measures. The estimated effect of intervention for all outcome measures should be stated in absolute numbers when feasible and accompanied by confidence intervals. As far as extent possible, summary data should be provided in sufficient detail to permit alternative analyses and replication. Prognostic variables should be reported, as should attempts to adjust for imbalances between treatment groups. The success of masking patients to treatment assignment should be explicitly stated. Differences between the results of planned primary and secondary analyses and results of RCTs and their extension studies should be noted.

ADVERSE EVENTS

All clinically important drug-related and non-drug-related adverse events during the phase 3 RCT and extension studies should be compared across treatment groups.

Discussion

The authors of the study report should recapitulate the main findings of the RCT and extension study and, if appropriate, discuss how the findings of the extension study differ from and extend earlier findings. The effect of differences in relevant demographic and clinical variables across treatment groups entering and completing RCT and extension studies on planned analyses and the rationale for all exploratory subgroup analyses and potential pitfalls of interpreting those analyses should be discussed. Unless adequately justified, a declaration of clinical efficacy should not be based on favorable results from exploratory subgroup analyses.

Supportive and contradictory data from other studies should be discussed, as should attempts to reconcile conflicting evidence.

Generalization of the main outcomes to clinical practice and implications for further studies and product development should be data-based.

GUIDELINES FOR REPORTING THE RESULTS OF META-ANALYSES

Meta-analyses combine the results of several studies into a single outcome measure. By combining the samples from individual studies, a meta-analysis increases the overall sample size, which increases the statistical power of the analysis as well as the precision of the estimate of treatment effects. This approach is particularly appealing when several small studies suggest a treatment but no study by itself provides convincing evidence of efficacy. The following issues should be recognized and addressed when interpreting reports from meta-analyses:

(a) limitations imposed by combining results of studies with different populations, experimental designs and quality controls ('conceptual heterogeneity'); and

(b) potential bias resulting from a tendency towards preferentially incorporating studies with positive treatment effects ('publication bias').

The guidelines for reporting the results of meta-analyses address these issues.

Title of the report

The title or subtitle of meta-analysis studies should identify the report as a meta-analysis,[4] for example: 'Treatment of multiple sclerosis with azathioprine: a meta-analysis.' The title should not contain a declarative statement regarding efficacy.

Abstract

The abstract for meta-analyses should describe the study's objective, data sources, study selection, data extraction, data synthesis, and conclusions.[4]

Text

Introduction

The purpose(s) of the study, the relationship that was studied, and the reasons for studying it should be stated. The population(s) studied and to whom the results are to be generalized should be described.

Trial design and methods

The authors should state whether the research was guided by a written protocol. Written protocols reduce the potential for bias in judgements that must be made when conducting meta-analyses. Ideally, the protocol should address issues related to potential bias resulting from:

(a) methods used to search for studies included in the meta-analysis;

(b) inclusion and exclusion criteria for those studies;

(c) extracting data from the studies; and

(d) statistical analyses.

Operational definitions should be provided for explanatory and response variables. These definitions are particularly important because different definitions for the same variable in the studies included in the meta-analysis may not be suitable for combination.

The clinical results of the meta-analysis should be emphasized by defining the minimum clinically significant difference in the response variable.

The time period spanned by the studies included in the meta-analysis should be reported in order to place the results in the context of other medical developments and to allow replication.

Details should be provided for the information sources and search strategies used to find the studies that were analysed. Index terms used in searches of key words should be reported, as should the databases searched, dates covered by the search, and whether the search was conducted by a professional medical librarian.[2,4] Efforts made to supplement computer literature searches and to avoid inclusion of multiple publications by different authors from large trials should be described. This information can be used to determine the potential for selection bias.[6]

Measures taken to reduce and identify publication bias should be stated. (Publication bias refers to the fact that studies with statistically significant results are more likely to be published).[7]

The criteria for including and excluding studies from the meta-analysis should be reported. Inclusion and exclusion criteria should be as specific as possible so that only compatible, relevant studies of suitable quality are compared. Such studies should:

(a) test the same hypothesis and have the same outcome;[8,9]

(b) compare similar patients and similar interventions;[8,10] and

(c) meet a minimum standard of scientific quality.

The criteria used in extracting the data from the studies should be stated, as should a measure of inter-extractor reliability to establish consistent extraction.[6]

The specific statistical methods used to analyse the data should be described.[11] In particular, whether the analyses assume fixed effects or random effects should be stated.[2]

Results

The authors of the study should provide a summary measure with a confidence interval of the estimated size and direction of the effect of treatment.[10,12]

The results of the individual studies and of the meta-analysis should be summarized, usually in a graph or table; typically a graph of the meta-analysis consists of a plot of the odds ratio and its 95% confidence interval of each study included in the analysis.[3]

The statistical power of the analysis should be explicitly stated.

An assessment of the quality of each study included in the analysis should be provided.

All studies excluded from the meta-analysis should be listed, together with the reasons for their exclusion.

A sensitivity analysis to determine the impact of important choices and assumptions on the results of the meta-analysis should be reported. In sensitivity analysis, some studies are excluded to determine how their exclusion affects the results. If the effect is great, the studies may have a disproportionate impact on the results.

Discussion

The authors of the study should discuss the variability of the results of the individual trials ('statistical heterogeneity').[10] Homogeneous results are more easily interpreted than heterogenous results and the variation in results should be explained if possible.

The populations represented in the meta-analysis and the generalizability of the results of the meta-analysis to other populations should be discussed.

The implications of the results should be discussed. The discussion should integrate the strength of the evidence, the threshold at which the benefits exceed the risks of treatment, and the size of and precision of the estimated effect.[13]

REFERENCES

1 Begg C, Cho M, Eastwood S et al. Improving the quality of reporting of randomized controlled trials: The CONSORT statement. *JAMA* 1996; 276:637–639.

2 Lang T, Secic M. *How to Report Statistics in Medicine: Annotated Guidelines for Authors, Editors, and Reviewers.* Philadelphia: American College of Physicians, 1997.

3 Goodkin DE, Reingold DS, Sibley W et al. Guidelines for clinical trials of new therapeutic agents in multiple sclerosis: Reporting extended results from Phase III clinical trials, *Ann Neurol*; in press.

4 Iverson C, Flanagin A, Fontanarosa PB et al. *American Medical Association Manual of Style: a Guide for Authors and Editors.* 9th ed. Baltimore, MD: Williams and Wilkins, 1998.

5 Haynes RB, Mulrow CD, Huth EJ et al. More informative abstracts revisited. *Ann Intern Med* 1990; 113:69–76.

6 Felson DT. Bias in meta-analytic research. *J Clin Epidemiol* 1992; 45:885–892.

7 Dickersin K. The existence of publication bias and risk factors for its occurrence. *JAMA* 1990; 263:1385–1389.

8 West RR. A look at the statistical overview (or meta-analysis). *J R Coll Physicians Lond* 1993; 27:111–115.

9 Simes J. Meta-analysis: Its importance in cost-effectiveness studies. *Med J Aust* 1990; 153(suppl): S13–S16.

10 Wilson A, Henry DA. Meta-analysis. Part 2: Assessing the quality of published meta-analyses. *Med J Aust* 1992; 156:173–187.

11 Walter SD. Methods of reporting statistical results from medical research studies. *Am J Epidemiol* 1995; 141:896–906.

12 Laupacis A, Sackett DL, Roberts RS. An assessment of clinically useful measures of the consequences of treatment. *N Engl J Med* 1988; 318:1728–1733.

13 Guyatt GH, Sackett DL, Sinclair JC et al. User's guides to the medical literature. IX. A method for grading health care recommendations The Evidence-Based Medicine Group. *JAMA* 1995; 274:1800–1804.

18
The negative clinical trial: failure or opportunity?

Lael Stone and Richard A Rudick

INTRODUCTION

Reading the clinical trial literature in multiple sclerosis (MS), one notices the paucity of published negative trials. Recently, several large MS clinical trials have produced negative results or have been terminated because of unacceptable toxicities. Bias towards publication of clinical trials with positive results may prevent us from learning valuable lessons from negative trials. The purpose of this chapter is to discuss potential reasons for negative trials, to focus on one previously unpublished small negative trial on deoxyspergualin, to emphasize the important lessons that can be learned from failed clinical trials, and to encourage their publication.

WHAT ARE NEGATIVE CLINICAL TRIALS?

Negative clinical trials can be defined in various ways (*Table 18.1*), and there are lessons to be learned from each. A 'true negative' clinical trial is defined as a trial that is adequately powered to demonstrate efficacy, is fully enrolled, and reaches completion but finds no statistically significant difference between treatment and comparative groups. An example in this category is the sulfasalazine trial, which was a well-run and

Table 18.1 Categories of failed trials

True negative results—no differences in primary outcome measure between treatment groups

Mixed positive and negative results

False positive results

Trial terminated early

well-executed trial that showed no change in rate of progression between the treated and untreated groups. Theoretically, these data could result from a type 2 error (a false-negative result), or it could be a true negative result (i.e. there was no difference between the treatments). To the extent that a trial is well planned and appropriately executed, the latter is more likely.

A 'mixed result' clinical trial is defined as a trial that results in both negative and positive results. Mixed results may indicate an effect of the therapy on one of the outcome measures but not on another. In the several cladribine trials, the magnetic resonance imaging (MRI) data indicated a strong beneficial effect on MRI parameters, but the benefits on clinical measures were more modest and less consistent.

Another category of failed trials is those that

fail as a result of a type 1 error (trials with falsely positive results). This can result from technical problems, such as unblinding of subjects or examiners or inappropriate control groups. In some trials, explanations for a false-positive result are not evident, and a trial in this category may only be classified after a more definitive trial shows negative results. An example in this category is the initial oral myelin trial that showed improvement in a small subset of patients.[1] A subsequent multicenter trial showed no difference between treatment and control groups.[2]

Smaller trials (e.g. those with fewer than 250 patients) abound in the MS literature. These trials are particularly prone to false-negative or false-positive results. The difficulty is knowing, at trial completion, whether trial outcomes are false-positive or false-negative results. Only when a finding fails to be replicated can that be determined. An example might be the initial trial of glatiramer acetate in progressive MS patients, where the drug was beneficial in one center and not in the other,[3] whereas the larger multicenter trial led to FDA approval of the compound.[4] Another example might be the small trial of interferon-γ in MS, in which treated patients experienced a higher than anticipated number of relapses.[5] This interferon-γ trial is widely quoted as a rationale for the hypothesis that interferon-γ worsens MS, despite the fact that this was an extremely small trial. No one has tried to replicate the trial because of the concern of worsening patients' disease status.

Another type of failed clinical trial is one that is terminated before the anticipated end. Trials are most commonly terminated after an interim analysis by an Independent Review Board. A failed trial of this type could be stopped early because of unanticipated and unacceptable toxicity (e.g. the linomide trial). Although toxicity

data may be available in animals (or other patient groups) it is not always known whether the same type of problem will occur with human use (or in MS patients). For example, azathioprine causes a much higher rate of adverse effects, including cancer, when used in transplant patients, who are on many other potentially toxic agents, than when it is used in patients with rheumatologic disease, who tend to be on many fewer concombinant medications. Trials can also be terminated early because of interim analyses that reveal no potential for reaching a statistically significant difference between the groups by continuing the trial to its intended end-point, such as the National Institutes of Health deoxyspergualin trial, or the University of California at Los Angeles thalidomide trial.

It is not possible to reach an accurate estimation of the number of failed clinical trials, although *Table 18.2* provides a selected list of known negative trials. Dissemination of information is slower and less complete for negative trials. Often they are not published at all, and the only way of learning about the results is through 'the professional grapevine' at meetings and by other informal modes of communications. Therefore, those who are most heavily involved in MS research are most informed about negative trials, while those who are outside the 'inner circle' rely exclusively on published trials, putting them at a disadvantage when they design their own trials.

Some medical specialties may be more inclined than others to publish negative trials. In the literature about the acquired immune deficiency syndrome, a study was made of the publication rate for negative trials. It revealed that a significant number of negative trials were published, but whereas a positive trial would be published, on average, 4.7 years after enrollment began, a negative trial took, on average, 6.5 years from

Table 18.2 Contemporary clinical trials in MS with negative or mixed results

Oral Myelin

Sulfazalazine

Cladribine

Linomide

4–Aminopyridine

Thalidomide

Deoxyspergualin

Cyclophosphamide

Anti-tumor necrosis factor-α

Mitoxantrone

Ibuprofen

Azathioprine

Interferon-γ

Cyclosporine

Interleukin-10

Transforming growth factor-β

Interferon-α

Anti-CD4

Table 18.3 Reasons for negative clinical trials

Therapeutic agent not effective in MS or in the type of MS tested

Therapeutic agent not administered in correct dose or frequency or by the correct route to affect disease process

Unanticipated toxicities of therapeutic agent

Too short a time period to detect efficacy of therapeutic agent

Inappropriate outcome measure to detect effect

Technical problems, including unblinding of examiners or patients

Type 1 error

Type 2 error

initiation of enrollment to publication.[6] Needless to say, if a trial is not published or has delayed publication, it cannot be included in meta-analyses and it cannot affect clinical practice, contribute widely to our understanding of the disease process, or contribute to the design of future clinical trials.

REASONS FOR NEGATIVE TRIALS

Trials may be negative for a diverse group of reasons (*Table 18.3*). Many of these have to do with the therapeutic agent being tested. The pharmacokinetics of the agent may not have been fully appreciated before the trial was started, such that too high or too low a dose may be selected (e.g. as happened in the trials of deoxyspergualin and oral myelin). The recent oral myelin trial may have been negative because it used the wrong dose, because it used myelin from a non-human source, or because it used whole myelin instead of the most pertinent peptides. In addition, the route or frequency of administration may turn out to be wrong for the disease to be studied or remain controversial even after FDA approval of the medications (e.g. the β-interferons). The agent may turn out to have unanticipated toxicities, such as cladribine, which causes long-term bone-marrow suppression in some patients. The duration of treatment or the length of follow-up may have been too short. The optimum length for follow-up of a trial is still not known. Clinicians, patients, and pharmaceutical companies would like to use trial designs that are as short as possible; however, many of these designs use measures such as relapse rate or gadolinium-enhancing lesions on MRI, which may or may not predict disability progression.

There may be unanticipated design problems or problems with patient selection, particularly in a disease as heterogeneous as MS. Although the linomide trial was terminated early because of unanticipated toxicity of the agent, it appears that different centers were enrolling slightly different patients. After the trial was terminated, Wolinsky looked at the MRI characteristics of various centers who enrolled linomide patients and found remarkable differences between centers despite consistent application of clinical enrollment standards.[7] Enrollment may also be slowed, skewed or rendered less attractive by release of other FDA-approved agents during the course of the trial, such as occurred with the release of interferon-β 1b during the enrollment phase of the National Institutes of Health deoxyspergualin trial.

Unanticipated problems may occur with outcome measures. The primary clinical outcome measure may turn out to be not significantly changed whereas MRI parameters may be significantly affected, as occurred in some of the cladribine trials. The multi-center 4-aminopyridine trial showed no significant change in the primary outcome measure, the expanded disability status scale (EDSS) score. However, a significant therapeutic effect could be shown with another outcome measure, timed ambulation. Our expertise is growing in the choice of the most clinically relevant outcome measure, and in the use of composite measures such as the multiple sclerosis functional composite.

LESSONS TO BE LEARNED FROM NEGATIVE TRIALS

Table 18.4 lists lessons to be learned from clinical trials, with examples of each type. Performing a clinical trial may change our assumptions about the compound to be tested or hypotheses about the disease process. The example of interferon-γ has already been mentioned, but other examples include tumor necrosis factor (TNF)-α. Two patients with rapidly progressive MS were treated with intravenous infusion of a humanized mouse monoclonal anti-TNF-α antibody. No clinically significant neurologic changes were noted in the patients, but the number of gadolinium-enhancing lesions on MRI and the cells and immunoglobulin in the cerebrospinal fluid of each patient increased.[8] The researchers suggested that this treatment caused immune activation and increased disease activity.

Compounds may have unanticipated toxicities that are not related to the disease process, such as

Table 18.4 Lessons to be learned from clinical trials

Change in our assumptions about the mechanism of action of the proposed agent (e.g. oral myelin)

Change in our assumptions about the mechanism of pathophysiology of MS (e.g. interferon-γ)

Demonstration of the heterogeneity of MS (e.g. oral methotrexate)

Working through logistical problems (e.g. linomide MRI)

Testing of new outcome measures (e.g. IMPACT, interferon-β 1a in chronic progressive MS)

Testing of new trial designs (e.g. National Institutes of Health deoxyspergualin trial)

Examination of placebo effects (e.g. National Institutes of Health deoxyspergualin trial)

occurred with linomide. The linomide experience underscored the need for large phase 3 trial for safety, but also the difficulty of predicting toxicity from pre-clinical data. Although beagle dogs exhibited vasculitic changes, and cancer patients developed pericarditis, these complications were not anticipated in the MS population.

Several trials have illustrated the heterogeneity and the unpredictability of the disease process in MS. For example, the low-dose oral methotrexate trial showed beneficial effect of the agent in secondary progressive MS patients, but not in the primary progressive patients.[8] Several studies have illustrated the powerful placebo effect in MS patients, which makes it difficult to demonstrate a significant beneficial effect of the agent to be tested. This happened in the large-scale study of oral myelin. Both the treatment group and the control group did well in this trial.

Logistical problems can also be worked through in a trial that produces negative results, and the lessons learnt from setting up the trial can be applied to other similarly designed trials. For example, the linomide trial involved frequent MRI scanning with a proprietary MRI sequence, which was sent out and run on many scanners throughout the USA. Technical improvements, such as training examining physicians and technicians, and the use of new outcome measures can also add value to a clinical trial regardless of the efficacy of the therapeutic agent to be tested (e.g. the International Multiple sclerosis secondary Progressive Avonex Controlled Trial (IMPACT)).

THE NATIONAL INSTITUTES OF HEALTH DEOXYSPERGUALIN TRIAL

The rationale for the deoxyspergualin (DSG) trial grew out of the author's work at the National

Institutes of Health in the early 1990s on the natural history of contrast-enhancing lesions on MRI in early relapsing–remitting MS (RRMS) patients.[9,10] Although the significance of contrast-enhancing lesions is not fully understood, they were then, and remain in 1999, the only generally available non-invasive method of looking at the breakdown of the blood–brain barrier that is caused by inflammation. The inflammatory component of the disease process is felt to be particularly important in early RRMS. In the National Institutes of Health natural history study, MRI scans were performed on a group of RRMS patients on a monthly basis for 4 years. The statistician performed repeated sampling ('bootstrap analysis') of this monthly data in order to design trials using contrast-enhancing lesions on MRI as a primary outcome measure.

The major advantage of using contrast-enhancing lesions on MRI as a surrogate marker for disease activity and thus for trial design was that very small numbers of patients were required to do phase 2 trials to screen compounds for efficacy in MS. For a baseline versus treatment trial design, as few as 12 patients could be enrolled if the baseline was 6 months before a 6-month treatment period. The trial design is shown in *Fig. 18.1*. In order to use contrast-enhancing lesions as the outcome measure, the patients had to have a certain number of contrast-enhancing

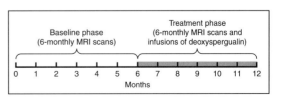

Figure 18.1   *Trial design of the National Institutes of Health deoxyspergualin trial*

Table 18.5 Results from the National Institute of Health deoxyspergualin trial

	EDSS	*Ambulation Index*	*Gadolinium-enhancing lesion count*	*Area of gadolinium enhancement (pixels)*
Baseline	4.2 (3.3, 5.1)	2.9 (2.2, 3.7)	7.9 (1.8, 13.9)	155 (46, 264)
Treatment	4.2 (3.0, 5.4)	2.7 (1.6, 3.9)	8.0 (0.9, 15.1)	145 (38, 253)

Parentheses indicate the range of values

lesions on MRIs during the baseline period. For this trial, the entry criterion was set at 0.5 lesions per month over a three-month enrollment period. Patients were thus followed on a monthly basis with contrast-enhanced MRI scans and clinical examinations to determine EDSS scores. During the treatment phase, patients were to receive 4 mg/kg of deoxyspergualin by infusion on monthly basis for 6 months. The primary outcome measure was comparison of monthly contrast-enhancing lesion frequency between the baseline and treatment periods.

Ten patients with RRMS were enrolled in the trial, with an enrollment goal of 14 patients. There was an unanticipated difficulty in enrollment owing to the FDA approval and commercial release of interferon-β 1b immediately before the enrollment period, although interferon-β 1b was not widely available initially and was at that time used with very narrow clinical indications. In this type of trial design, each patient effectively serves as his or her own control, and thus all personnel are unblinded to the treatment phase. An interim analysis was performed after 10 patients were enrolled, eight of who completed treatment. Results are shown in *Table 18.5*. There were no differences between the baseline and treatment phases in any of the patients. Unlike many trials in MS, no placebo effect was seen in clinical or MRI parameters. The trial was thus terminated before full enrollment, since it was determined

that, even if the remaining two patients were enrolled and turned out to show significant positive effects, the trial overall would still have a negative result. There were no toxicities or adverse effects of the treatment noted.

Lessons from the National Institutes of Health deoxyspergualin trial

Although this small trial was negative, as was the larger trial on deoxyspergualin carried out by Kappos and his colleagues in Europe (the results of which are also unpublished), several lessons can be learnt from the trial. The first is one of trial design. When this trial was performed, few if any trials had been undertaken with MRI parameters as the primary outcome measures. Owing to the minimum level of contrast-enhancing lesions required for entry, a significant amount of time and energy was needed to screen enough patients to meet the MRI criteria. Secondly, it was not thought that MRI parameters would show a placebo effect without clinical improvement, and indeed, there was no improvement in either clinical or MRI measures with the agent administered at this dose in this way. It is not known if patients in control or placebo groups who show improvement clinically would have improved MRI parameters as well. A third lesson was the unanticipated release of an FDA-approved compound for the treatment of MS. Approval of interferon-β 1b meant that the entry criteria had to be rewritten to exclude patients who were eligible for what was suddenly standard therapy in MS, even though they might have been the best candidates for deoxyspergualin. The fourth and fifth lessons are frequent in MS: results from animal studies in animal models may not correlate with future success in MS patients, and positive results from a few MS patients may not translate into positive results in an actual trial setting.

CONCLUSIONS AND RECOMMENDATIONS

A few of the most important conclusions from this discussion are as follows.

(a) There is a bias towards publishing positive over negative trials; many of the trials discussed in this chapter have not been, and may never be, published.

(b) Trials should be deliberately designed in such a way that useful information will come out of the trial, regardless of the efficacy results. For example, behavior of the control group, relationships between outcome measures, novel designs, biological effects of interventions, and the like may all be important contributions to the field of MS experimental therapeutics.

(c) Trial design and results should be published, whether or not the trial demonstrates efficacy.

ACKNOWLEDGMENT

Acknowledgment is made to John Noseworthy, MD for helpful discussion regarding these issues.

REFERENCES

1 Weiner HL, Mackin GA, Matsui M et al. Double-blind pilot trial of oral tolerization with myelin antigens in multiple sclerosis. *Science* 1993; **259**:1727–1730.

2 Bornstein MD, Miller A, Slagle S et al. A placebo-controlled, double blind, randomized, two-center, pilot trial of Cop 1 in chronic progressive multiple sclerosis. *Neurology* 1991; **41**:533–539.

3 Johnson JP, Brooks BR, Cohen JA et al. Copolymer 1 reduces relapse rate and improves disability in relapsing–remitting multiple sclerosis: results of a phase III multicenter, double-blind placebo-controlled trial. *Neurology* 1995; **45**:1268–1276.

4 Panich HS, Hirsch RL, Schindler J, Johnson KP. Treatment of multiple sclerosis with gamma interferon: exacerbations associated with activation of the immune system. *Neurology* 1987; **37**:1097–1102.

5 Ioannidis JPA. Effect of the statistical significance of results on the time to completion and publication of randomized efficacy trials. *JAMA* 1998; **279**:281–286.

6 Wolinsky J, Narayana, the MRI-AC for the North American Linomide Trialists. Prerandomization characteristics of relapsing and secondary progressive multiple sclerosis: subjects evaluated for the north american linomide trial by automated quantitative MRI. *Ann Neurol* 1997; **42**:458.

7 Van Ooston BW, Barkhof F, Truyen L et al. Increased MRI activity and immune activation in two multiple sclerosis patients treated with the monoclonal anti-tumor necrosis factor antibody cA2. *Neurology* 1996; **47**:531–534.

8 Goodkin DE, Rudick RA, Van der Brug Medendorp S et al. Low-dose (7.5 mg) oral methotrexate reduces the rate of progression in chronic progressive multiple sclerosis. *Ann Neurol* 1995; **37**:30–41.

9 McFarland HF, Stone LA, Calabresi PA et al. MRI studies of multiple sclerosis: implications of the natural history of the disease and on monitoring effectiveness of experimental therapies. *Multiple Sclerosis* 1996; **2**:198–205.

10 Smith ME, Stone LA, Albert PS et al. Clinical worsening in multiple sclerosis is associated with increased frequency and area of Gadopentatate Dimeglumine enhancing magnetic resonance imaging lesions. *Ann Neurol* 1993; **33**:480–489.

PART III

Clinical trials of disease modifying therapy

19

Emerging concepts of pathogenesis: relationship to multiple sclerosis therapies

Jorge R Oksenberg and Stephen L Hauser

A large body of immunologic, epidemiologic, and genetic data indicate that tissue injury in multiple sclerosis (MS) results from an abnormal (i.e. autoimmune) inflammatory response to one or more myelin antigens, a response that is probably triggered by an environmental exposure in a genetically susceptible host. The inflammatory changes that occur in MS may ultimately be shown to be secondary rather than primary, and only tentative assumptions of the nature of MS can be reasonably made at this time. Indeed, inflammation and selective destruction of central nervous system (CNS) elements may also occur in non-autoimmune conditions; such diseases of known etiology include genetic disorders (adrenoleukodystrophy, metachromatic leukodystrophy) and chronic virus infections with human T cell leukemia virus (HTLV)-1 and Theiler murine encephalomyelitis virus.

This said, recent data from multiple converging sources lend support to the classical concept that MS is mediated by a misguided cellular and humoral immune response directed against one or several myelin proteins. The autoimmune model of MS pathogenesis has set the tone for immunotherapy in this disease, first by general immunosuppresion using cytotoxic drugs, and more recently by selectively targeting a specific component of the immune response (*Table 19.1*).

The past few years has seen real progress in defining the molecular basis of MS, which has prepared the stage for new therapeutic approaches based on correction of specific underlying disease mechanisms. This chapter reviews the current understanding of the immunopathogenesis of MS and the nature of genetic susceptibility.

THE NATURE OF THE LESION IN MS

The pathological hallmark of MS is the plaque, a well-demarcated, gray or pink lesion that is characterized histologically by inflammation, demyelination, and gliosis (scarring) (*Fig. 19.1*).[1] MS plaques are multiple, generally asymmetric, and tend to concentrate in deep white matter near the lateral ventricles, the corpus callosum, the floor of the fourth ventricle, the deep periaqueductal region, the optic nerves and tracts, the corticomedullary junction, and the cervical spinal cord. It has been recently recognized that MS plaques are heterogeneous in their structural and immunopathological patterns. In Asian populations, one form of MS is characterized by disseminated CNS involvement and is associated with the human leukocyte antigen (HLA)-DR2

Table 19.1 Experimental strategies for selective immunosuppressive therapy

Monoclonal antibodies to:

    T-cell sub populations (CD4)[a]

    T-cell receptors[b]

    Adhesion molecules[b]

    Accessory molecules (CD40, CD80)[c]

    MHC class II molecules[c]

    Cytokine receptors[c]

    Activation markers (B7, CD52)[c]

    Macrophages[c]

    Cytokines[c]

T-cell vaccination[a]

TCR peptide vaccination[a]

Immunomodulation by Linomide[a]

Oral induced tolerance[a]

Inhalation induced tolerance[c]

Cytokine receptor analogs and antagonists[a]

Cytokines (TGF-b[b], IL-4[c], IL-10[c])

Antigen-induced programmed T-cell death (apoptosis)[c]

Antigen peptides TCR analogs and antagonists[c]

Blocking co-stimulation pathway (anergy)[c]

Blocking co-stimulation pathway (Th1/Th2 commitment)[c]

MHC class II-peptides complexes[b]

Anti-IgD peptide conjugates[c]

Superantigen modulation[c]

Metalloprotease inhibitors[b]

Blocking-signal transduction pathways[c]

cAMP-phosphodiesterase inhibitors[c]

Complement inhibitors[c]

Regulation of MHC gene expression[c]

---

[a] clinical trials completed with disappointing to inconclusive results
[b] Pre-clinical trial stage
[c] Experimental stage

genotype ('Western-type MS'), whereas more restricted forms of disease in which optic nerve and or spinal cord involvement predominate are not associated with DR2; lesions in the non-DR2 associated condition ('Asian-type' MS) are fre-

quently more severe and necrotizing than in the disseminated form.[2]

A significant perivascular and parenchymal infiltration by mononuclear cells, both thymus-derived (T) cells and macrophages, is characteristic of the acute MS lesion (see *Fig. 19.1c*). Although fewer in number, B cells and plasma cells also contribute to the inflammatory response to some extent.[3,4] T cells in the parenchyma and in the perivascular cuffs consist of variable numbers of CD4+ and CD8+ cells.[5,6] Although the vast majority of these bear the common form of the antigen cell receptor (i.e. the α–β heterodimer), T cells carrying the other form of the T-cell receptor, the γ–δ heterodimer, have been also identified in significant numbers in MS lesions.[7,8] The selective accumulation and compartmentalization of activated T cells during certain stages of the plaque cycle indicate a specific pattern in the homing of T cells to the lesion, and suggests an immune response to discrete antigenic complexes.[9–14]

Controversy still surrounds the nature of the initial pathologic event in MS. The earliest detectable event in plaque development is an increase in permeability of the blood–brain barrier (BBB) associated with inflammation.[15] Following the breach in the BBB, myelin appears to be the primary target of the pathogenic immune reaction.[6,16] Myelin breakdown appears to be mediated by Fc-receptor and complement-receptor-mediated phagocytosis, leukocyte stripping, or vesicular disruption of myelin sheaths. Vesicular disruption of the myelin membrane is an early pathologic feature (see *Fig. 19.1d*), a finding that can be simulated in vitro by the application of cytokines, autoantibodies, or calcium ionophores. As lesions evolve, axons traversing the plaque show marked irregular beading, proliferation of astrocytes occurs, and

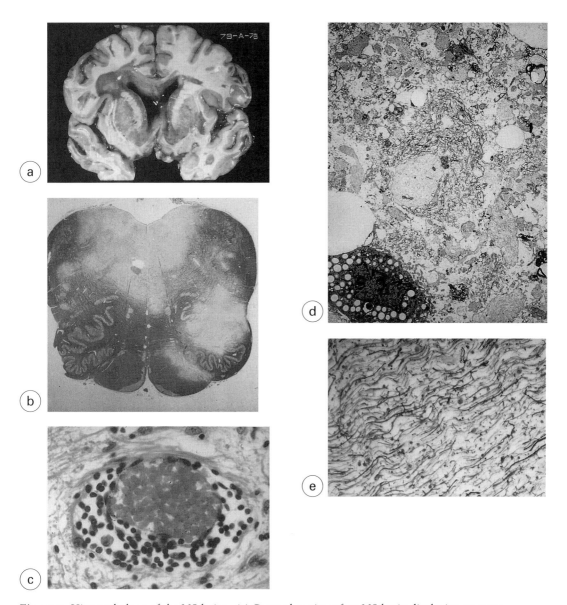

Fig. 19.1 Histopathology of the MS lesion. (a) Coronal section of an MS brain displaying an acute periventricular area of demyelination and edema in the left temporal white matter and a smaller, linear plaque in a mirror position. The older plaque is less edematous and therefore better demarcated. (b) Low power horizontal section through the medulla at the level of the inferior olives illustrating multiple asymmetric sharply outlined areas of myelin loss which appear clear (luxol fast blue). (c) Microscopic section of a recent lesion, in which lymphocytes and macrophages appear as black, rounded nuclei surrounding a blood vessel. Some inflammatory cells have migrated farther into the brain parenchyma. (d) Electron micrograph of MS myelin pathology on a biopsy of subcortical white matter. Desintegrating myelin membranes around the axon (center) have been transformed into a vesicular network. Fibrous astroglial processes, naked axons and a reactive ameboid microglial cell (lower left corner) can also be identified. (Courtesy of Dr Cedric Raine, Albert Einstein College of Medicine, NY.) (e) Relative preservation of axons within a plaque.

lipid-laden macrophages that contain myelin debris are prominent. Progressive fibrillary gliosis ensues and mononuclear cells gradually disappear. In some MS lesions, but not in others, proliferation of oligodendrocytes appears to be present initially, but these cells are apparently destroyed as the gliosis progresses. In chronic MS lesions, complete or nearly complete demyelination, dense gliosis (more severe than in most other neuropathologic conditions), and loss of oligodendroglia are found. In some chronic active MS lesions, gradations in the histologic findings from the center to the lesion edge suggest that lesions expand by concentric outward growth.

Preservation of oligodendrocytes and axon cylinders in the presence of demyelination is characteristic (see *Fig. 19.1e*), although this finding is relative rather than absolute; in approximately 10% of lesions there is significant axonal destruction and, in rare cases, complete destruction of the neuropil and cavitation occur. Ozawa, Lassman and colleagues found that oligodendrocytes were preserved in early lesions of relapsing MS but were destroyed in chronic lesions.[17] Brueck and colleagues observed preservation of oligodendrocytes in some patients but significant loss in others.[18] This seemed to correlate more with the individual patient rather than the disease stage, suggesting heterogeneity in the pathogenesis of demyelination.[3] A pathological pattern characterized by alterations in the most distal extension of the oligodendrocyte process, the periaxonal region, has been reported in virus and toxic models of demyelination and in the study of stereotaxic brain lesion biopsy specimens.[19,20] Morphological features included early and uniform widening of inner myelin lamellae (biphasic myelinopathy) and degeneration of inner glial loops ('dying-back' oligodendrogliopathy); these features preceded complete destruction of myelin sheaths. Because the oligodendrocytes were morphologically preserved in this early stage, it was proposed that the initial event in MS is the functional interference with the myelinating capacity of these cells. Subsequently, degeneration of both the inner myelin lamellae and the inner oligodendroglial loop occur. As a consequence of this injury, novel or aberrant antigens may be exposed, triggering the infiltration of inflammatory cells.

What are the clinical consequences of axonal loss? Based on a 30-month longitudinal magnetic resonance spectroscopy study of 29 patients who had either a relapsing or secondary progressive clinical course, indices of axonal damage or loss, such as brain *N*-acetyl aspartate (a chemical component of CNS axons involved in energy store), provided a pathological marker that correlates with disability.[21] Furthermore, abundant transected and dystrophic axons have been detected in sites of active inflammation.[22,23] Hence, loss of axons may be a cause of tissue atrophy in some MS patients and consequent neurological disability.

Recent attention has focused on the mechanisms of oligodendrocyte damage. Some studies,[24] but not all,[25] have shown that in some MS lesions, but not in all, cells with oligodendroglial morphology are apoptotic. Necrosis of oligodendrocytes has been observed as well. In any single lesion, oligodendrocyte destruction may occur via either apoptosis or necrosis, but not both.[3] It is still unclear if oligodendrocyte destruction is immunologically mediated or if it results from loss of trophic support from myelin and exposure to a toxic inflammatory microenvironment. It is interesting to speculate that the extent of remyelination correlates with the degree of oligodendrocyte preservation in the lesions. As the inflammation proceeds, oligodendrocytes at the periphery of the plaque, as well as astrocytes, proliferate under the influence of factors released into the microenvironment. These oligodendrocytes, which appear to continue to function as myelinating cells, may be derived from surviving or progenitor cells.[26,27] When inflammation decreases, the edema disappears and conduction is restored, possibly as a result of the expansion of sodium channels into the demyelinated axon.[15] Remyelination is not essential to remission.

Up-regulation of major histocompatibility complex (MHC) molecules has been proposed as a marker of plaque activity.[28,29] Class I MHC antigens have been identified in plaque tissue on endothelial cells, infiltrating lymphocytes, and astroglia, whereas class II determinants have been reported in various studies as being expressed on endothelial cells, macrophages, microglia, and astroglia. On the other hand, a study by Bo and colleagues[30] provided compelling evidence that the only cells in the active lesions expressing class II antigens are macrophages and microglia. The high expression of MHC class II molecules in MS brains suggests that the local microenvironment may be enriched in MHC-activating factors such as interferon (IFN)-γ, and that antigen is possibly presented to T cells.[31]

Because the level of cell surface expression of MHC class II molecules directly affects the nature and magnitude of the immune response, the study of the mechanisms involved in the regulation of class II expression in the MS plaque is essential for understanding the inflammatory response in the affected brain. The class II transcriptional transactivator (CIITA), is a key intermediate that is responsible for constitutive and IFN-γ-inducible class II expression.[32] CIITA also directs expression of the invariant chain and HLA-DM, two molecules involved in class II biosynthesis and antigen processing.[33] Soos and

colleagues recently reported that astrocytes express CIITA, Ii, DM, and the costimulatory molecule B7-1, suggesting that non-professional CNS antigen-presenting cells participate in the processing and presentation of autoantigens as well as in T-cell activation.[34,35] It has also been observed that the regulatory cytokines transforming growth factor (TGF)-β and IFN-β suppress class II expression by interfering with IFN-γ-inducible CIITA transcription and activity.[36,37] Hence, regulation of CIITA expression or function may offer an important therapeutic opportunity for MS.

It is important to note, however, that in many silent plaques devoid of T-cell infiltrates, class II MHC may be expressed at high levels on reactive microglia. In addition, up-regulation of MHC class II antigens is not unique to MS tissue, since it has also been detected in neurodegenerative diseases and after trauma. One school of thought proposes that glial MHC class II expression is necessary but not sufficient for effective antigen presentation to encephalitogenic CD4+ T cells.[38] In this view, in vitro studies do not support a primary immune response leading to T-cell proliferation and aggression, but rather show that microglia may protect the CNS from autoreactive T cells by inducing their apoptosis. Although intercellular adhesion molecule (ICAM-I) and B7, which are co-stimulatory molecules, have been identified on microglia from humans and mice, the case for an effective antigen presentation in the brain requires further experimentation. Other molecules that are up-regulated in the MS lesion include a variety of cytokines, adhesion molecules, fibronectin, urokinase plasmin activator receptor, and stress proteins.[39–42]

MS AS AN AUTOIMMUNE DISEASE

Support for the notion that MS is an autoimmune disease comes from study of the neuropathology of the MS brain, the genetic association with the MHC locus, and the extensive work with laboratory models of demyelination. An essential prerequisite to defining the molecular basis of an autoimmune disease is knowledge of the responsible autoantigen or autoantigens (*Table 19.2*). The role of individual autoantigens as inducers of demyelination has proved difficult to investigate in humans; therefore, investigators have turned to animal models. Beginning in the 1930s, Rivers and others defined the experimental autoimmune disease experimental allergic (or autoimmune) encephalomyelitis (EAE) (*Fig. 19.2*).[43] EAE can be induced in a variety of animal species, including non-human primates, by immunization with myelin proteins or their peptide derivatives. When studied in genetically susceptible animals, immunization induces brain inflammation accompanied by varied signs of neurologic disease. EAE and MS share common clinical, histologic, immunologic and genetic features; hence EAE is widely considered to be a relevant model for the human disease. Demonstration in the early 1960s that EAE could be adoptively transferred by myelin-sensitized T cells[44] inaugurated the era of T-cell immunology in MS research, an approach that in many respects dominates the field to this day.

The two quantitatively major myelin proteins, myelin basic protein (MBP) and proteolipid protein (PLP), make up about 30% and 50% of myelin proteins by weight respectively (*Fig. 19.3*). They can each effectively induce EAE and have received the most attention as potential T-cell autoantigens in MS. Both are thought to participate in myelin compaction—MBP between intracytoplasmic surfaces (the major dense line on electron microscopy) and PLP between adjacent myelin lamellae (the intraperiod line on electron microscopy). The major immune response detected in the laboratory in MS patients is directed against MBP[45,46]. Several studies have shown that human MBP-specific T cells preferentially recognize epitopes located in the center and in the C-terminal part of the MBP molecule, around residues 84–102 and 143–168. Although anti-myelin T-cell responses can be detected in the peripheral blood of healthy people, in MS patients MBP-reactive T cells undergo chronic stimulation in the peripheral blood[47–49] and appear to migrate selectively to the CNS, where they are detected in MS lesions[12] and CSF.[50,51] Furthermore, it was recently shown that 84% of MBP-reactive T cells isolated from subjects with MS were recovered from the CD45RO+ memory T cell compartment.[52] By contrast, MBP-specific T cells isolated from control subjects were predominantly CD45RA+ naïve T cells, indicating the predominant involvement of activated MBP-specific T cells in the pathogenesis of MS. A similar conclusion could be drawn from the data of Scholz and colleagues, who demonstrated in a series of elegant experiments that only MS-derived MBP-specific CD4+ T cells could be expanded in vitro in the absence of the costimulatory molecule B7.[53]

The importance of MBP-reactive cells in autoimmunity was also demonstrated in healthy, unimmunized *Callithrix jacchus* marmosets (common marmosets). In this species, MBP-reactive T-cell clones isolated from the peripheral blood of unimmunized animals, efficiently induced CNS inflammatory disease when transferred into naïve sibs.[54,55] (The common marmoset is a small New World monkey that is characterized by a natural chimerism of bone

Table 19.2 Putative autoantigens in MS

Myelin basic protein (MBP)

Proteolipid protein (PLP)

Myelin oligodendrocyte glycoprotein (MOG)

Myelin associated glycoprotein (MAG)

Heat shock proteins

β-arrestin and arrestin

Glial fibrillary acidic protein (GFAP)

2',3'-cyclic nucleotide 3' phosphodiesterase

Astrocyte-derived calcium-binding protein (S1000β)

Transaldolase

Sodium channels

Oligodendrocyte *Alu*-peptide

marrow elements between siblings; this allowed the adoptive transfer of cells between individuals across histocompatibility barriers.)

In addition to T cells, it is also possible that a humoral immune response to MBP plays an important role in MS. In most MS patients, an elevated level of intrathecally synthesized immunoglobulins can be detected in the CNS. Although the specificity of these antibodies is mostly unknown, anti-MBP specificities have been detected.[56] Warren and colleagues reported that 111 of 116 chronic progressive MS patients had anti-MBP antibodies in the cerebrospinal fluid (CSF).[57] Most patients who had no anti-MBP antibody in the CSF did have antibodies to PLP. The epitope for the antibody response to human MBP fits precisely the minimal T-cell epitope PVVHFFKNTVTP for HLA-DRB1*1501-restricted T lymphocytes. This antibody response may be directed to a processed fragment of MBP presented on B cells with anti-MBP specificity, which is thus able to trigger T cells that are reactive to the same epitope. In this

way, the antibody need not be directed to MBP in its native conformation in the myelin membrane, but rather it may be directed to a processed epitope of MBP or to a microbe sharing homology with the MBP epitope (e.g. molecular mimicry).

Because MBP is located not only in the CNS but also in the peripheral nervous system, it is difficult to explain the specificity of MS for the CNS on the basis of autoimmunity to MBP. PLP was until recently thought to be expressed exclusively in the CNS, but is now known to be expressed in the peripheral nervous system as well.[58] The most promising candidate as MS autoantigen that has been identified recently is myelin oligodendrocyte glycoprotein (MOG). MOG is CNS-specific, and has been shown to be a potent autoantigen in rodent and primate EAE models[59–61]. When immunized against MOG, *C. jacchus* marmosets develop a chronic relapsing form of EAE that is unique in that the histologic lesions are identical to those of MS.[62] T cells that recognize MBP, MOG, or both enter the CNS and disrupt the BBB; they cause inflammation but not demyelination. Demyelination requires the presence of antibodies against MOG, which gain access to the CNS across the disrupted barrier. This model has clarified the immune components of an MS-like lesion and demonstrated that the demyelinating lesion is not exclusively T-cell mediated; rather a synergistic T-cell and antibody response is required to produce demyelination (*Table 19.3*). The finding that MS-like demyelination occurs only in the presence of autoantibodies against MOG explains to a great extent why typical EAE in rodents, mediated exclusively by T cells, is an inflammatory but not a demyelinating disease.

The MOG gene is located on chromosome 6p21 within the MHC locus, and encodes a

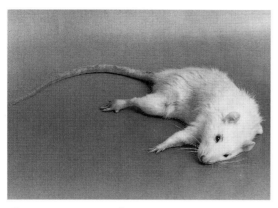

Fig. 19.2 Experimental autoimmune encephalomyelitis (EAE) is a prototypic experimental model for autoimmune inflammatory disease of the CNS; it can be induced in a variety of animal species, including non-human primates, by injection of myelin proteins or their peptide derivatives, as well as by adoptive transfer of CD4+-activated T cells specific for MBP or PLP. When injected into 'susceptible' animals, these reagents induce brain inflammation and cause ataxia and paralysis, first of the tail and hind limbs and then progressing to the forelimbs. Death eventually results. (Figure courtesy of Professor Claude CA Bernard.)

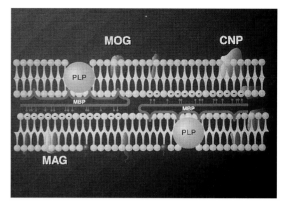

Fig. 19.3 Schematic representation of the molecular architecture of the central myelin sheath. Myelin is formed by a membrane extension of oligodendrocytes. This membrane extension wraps around the axon. Central myelin consists of about 75–80% lipids and 20–25% proteins. PLP accounts for about 50% of total myelin protein and MBP another 30%. Myelin-associated glycoprotein (MAG) and MOG each constitute about 3% of whole myelin protein. PLP is integrated in the myelin membrane. MBP is a cytosolic protein. MAG is located in the periaxonal space of the myelin sheath. MOG is located at the surface and so it is the myelin protein most exposed to humoral and cellular immune responses. PLP, MBP, and MOG are encephalitogenic in sensitive animals. (Figure courtesy of Professor Claude CA Bernard, La Trobe University, Melbourne, Australia). Adapted from Crang AJ, Rumsby MGR. Molecular organization in central nerve myelin. In: Palo J, ed. Advances in Experimental Medicine and Biology, vol. 100. Myelination and Demyelination. New York and London: Plenum Press, 1978, 235.

protein of molecular mass 26–28 kDa. This protein is a member of the immunoglobulin superfamily and it may form dimers of about 58 kDa. MOG may function to terminate myelin synthesis.[63] The extracellular N-terminal domain contains many conserved consensus residues that are also present in immunoglobulin variable region folds, suggesting a primordial receptor function. MOG is a quantitatively minor protein constituting 0.05% of CNS myelin pro-teins (see *Fig. 19.3*), and it is located exclusively on CNS oligodendrocyte surfaces and on the out-ermost lamellae of the myelin sheath. This makes it readily accessible to an immune attack, and in particular to attack by an autoantibody. The

Table 19.3 Cellular components in MS pathogenesis

MS as a T-cell mediated disease

- T-cells express gelatinases for blood-brain-barrier extravasation
- Significant T-cell infiltration in the acute lesion
- Peripheral myelin-specific T cells are in an *in vivo* activated state
- T-cell derived cytokines (either pathogenic or protective) are expressed in the lesion
- TCR rearrangements from MS brain lesions encode CDR3 regions identical to those found in T-cells recognizing MBP
- T-cell receptor genes linked to disease susceptibility (MS and EAE)
- MHC class I restricted CD8+ T cells can lyse oligodendrocytes and axons *in vitro*
- EAE can be transferred by myelin sensitized T cells in rodents and in *C. jacchus*
- T-cell inactivation prevents and cures EAE
- Apoptosis of T cells may correlate with EAE resolution

MS as a B-cell mediated disease

- Elevated level of restricted intrathecally synthesized immunoglobulins
- Plasma immunoglobulins from MS patients induce *in vitro* myelinolysis
- CNS immunoglobulins from MS patients induce *in vitro* myelinolysis
- Clonally expanded B cells detected in the CNS
- Anti-MBP antibodies in the brain and CSF
- Anti-MOG antibodies bound to the disintegrating myelin in *C. jacchus* EAE and MS
- Anti-MOG antibodies induce *in vitro* myelinolysis
- Requirement for anti-MOG antibodies to induce demyelination in EAE
- Complement deposition at the edge of lesions
- Immunoglobulin deposition on macrophages contacting myelin
- Immunoglobulin RFLPs associated to diseases susceptibility

MS as a macrophage/microglia mediated disease

- Significant macrophage infiltration in the acute lesion
- Expression and release of molecules necessary for antigen presentation and inflammation
- Secretion of mediators of myelin destruction
- Secretion of factors toxic to oligodendrocytes
- Macrophage depletion prevents EAE

---

recently published molecular model of the extracellular domain of MOG predicts the accessibility and conformation of the main encephalitogenic EAE epitope p35–55.[64] Other minor components of myelin as well as other antigens, including heat shock proteins, ion channels, β-arrestin and arrestin, glial fibrillary acidic protein (GFAP), oligodendrocyte Alu-peptides, and astrocyte-derived calcium-binding protein (S1000β) have also been proposed as candidate antigens in

MS (see *Table 19.2*).[65] It is also possible that the autoimmune response is initially directed against a single epitope but that there is a subsequent diversification of T-cell and B-cell responses to other epitopes of the same antigen, and even other antigens present at the site of inflammation.[66] This concept has been termed 'determinant spreading' or 'epitope spreading'.

In summary, it appears likely that a multifaceted cellular and humoral immune response against multiple different proteins underlies autoimmunity in MS. In both healthy people and those with MS, T-cell and B-cell repertoires against autoantigens may share similar or even identical specificities. Peripheral regulatory mechanisms are then necessary to keep such cells under control in order to prevent their activation and the development of spontaneous autoimmune responses. CD8+ T cells have been suggested as active regulators or suppressors of the response of encephalitogenic CD4+ T cells after recognition of either their T-cell receptor idiotype or activation markers.[67–70] In recent experiments with different knock-out and transgenic lines of mice, the existence of subsets of α/β CD4+ T cells with the capability of controlling MBP-specific or self-reactive T cells was firmly demonstrated as well.[71,72]

Triggering an MS attack

Magnetic resonance imaging (MRI) studies have provided invaluable contributions to our understanding of the dynamics of the MS disease process. MRI measurements of the breakdown of the BBB, a marker of inflammation in MS, indicate that very frequent 'bursts' of inflammation occur in patients with active disease. These bursts are often multifocal and appear approximately monthly, or between seven and 10 times more frequently than clinical attacks of MS; thus most bursts are clinically silent.

What is it that triggers these bursts of multifocal inflammation in MS? The most plausible theories propose that recurrent exposures to exogenous pathogens activate encephalitogenic T cells in peripheral blood. This could occur by bacterial or viral-mediated non-specific polyclonal activation of T cells and B cells, by molecular mimicry, by an innocent bystander mechanism, or by superantigens. Molecular mimicry refers to induction of an autoimmune response because of a structural homology between a self-protein and a protein in a viral or bacterial pathogen. MBP shares extensive amino acid homologies with proteins of measles, influenza, and adenovirus. For example, residues 91–101 of MBP (a region known to be commonly recognized by human MBP-reactive T cells) share identical stretches of between four and six amino acids with adenovirus. Homology may be necessary at only a few amino acids for efficient T-cell recognition to occur.[73,74] Thus, microbial peptides that contain the *HFFK* motif (e.g. Epstein–Barr virus, papillomavirus variants, adenovirus type 12, influenza virus type A) have acquired sufficient homology to permit HLA-DR2 binding and MBP-specific T-cell interaction. In MS patients, antibodies and T cells that recognize the MBP epitope PVV*HFFK*NTVTP will also recognize these microbial sequences. In addition, amino acid identity may not even be required for cross-reactivity to occur between the autoantigen and the mimic as long as they share chemical properties at critical residues that allow anchoring to HLA and interaction with the T-cell receptor.[75–77]

The innocent bystander hypothesis proposes that activation of autoimmune T cells occurs as a consequence of viral infections of the CNS; such infections may be asymptomatic. As examples, immune responses against MBP are generated during measles encephalitis[78] and HTLV-1 infection in humans,[79] and coronavirus infection in rodents.[80] Thus, a neurotrophic virus may infect the nervous system, and in so doing stimulate an immune response not only to the virus but also to normal nervous system proteins.[81] This may occur via release of cytokines that amplify autoreactive T-cell responses or via an increase in the efficiency of presentation of autoantigens by local antigen-presenting cells.[82]

Another potential mechanism implicates superantigens in the etiology of autoimmunity. The term 'superantigen' defines antigens that (at very low concentrations—in the picomolar range) can stimulate subsets of T cells. Superantigens bind with high affinity to class II MHC molecules outside the antigen-binding groove. They interact with the variable region of the β-chain of the TCR in the region of the β-pleated sheet, away from the antigen binding site (the CDR3 region). In a non-MHC restricted manner, without need for antigen processing, the class II superantigen complexes trigger proliferation of T cells expressing particular TCR-Vβ chains. A notable feature of superantigenic stimulation is that the responding T cells initially mount a vigorous response but are then deleted or lose the ability to respond to antigen (i.e. they become anergic). Exogenous superantigens include the toxins of many common bacteria and possibly the components of certain viruses. Superantigens are associated with numerous human diseases, including food poisoning, toxic-shock syndrome, and scalded skin syndrome. Brocke and colleagues found that superantigens can also trigger relapses of paralysis in the EAE model.[83] In one study,[84] the ability of staphylococcal toxins to stimulate human T cells specific to MBP or PLP was examined; all myelin-specific T cells responded in proliferation studies to at least one superantigen. In some experiments, the superantigenic toxins were more than 10^5-fold more potent in stimulating the T cells than were the myelin antigens to which the T cells were initially sensitized. Hence superantigen stimulation accompanying gastrointestinal or upper respiratory infections has the clear potential to activate pre-existing myelin-specific T cells and perhaps to induce exacerbations.

A model for MS immunopathogenesis

Because the likely role of an undefined environmental exposure, our partial knowledge of the full set of genes involved in conferring susceptibility, and the clinical heterogeneity of the disease, it has been difficult to formulate a unifying mechanism that explains the pathogenesis of MS. Nevertheless, it is likely that lymphocytes activated in the periphery home into the CNS, become attached to receptors on endothelial cells, and then proceed to pass across the BBB, through the endothelium and the subendothelial basal lamina and directly into the interstitial matrix. Interestingly, in EAE, this process has been shown to be dependent on the activation state of the T cells, but it is independent of their antigen specificity. Thus, MBP-reactive T cells cross the BBB with no greater efficiency than, for example, insulin-reactive T cells.

After traversing the BBB, pathogenic T cells are reactivated by fragments of myelin antigens presented in the framework of MHC class II molecules on the surface of antigen-presenting cells (macrophages, microglia, and perhaps astrocytes). It is possible that enhanced or dysregulated MHC class II expression by antigen-presenting cells within the CNS predisposes to autoimmunity in MS, as is the case in EAE. Reactivation induces release of pro-inflammatory cytokines that further open the BBB and stimulate chemotaxis, resulting in a second, larger wave of inflammatory cell recruitment and leakage of antibody and other plasma proteins into the CNS. Pathogenic T cells may not be capable of producing or inducing tissue injury in the absence of this secondary leukocyte recruitment. For example, in EAE that is mediated by adoptive transfer of MBP-reactive encephalitogenic T lymphocytes, these cells are among the first to infiltrate the CNS, but they constitute only a minor component of the total infiltrate in the full-blown lesion.

A second class of molecule involved in leukocyte extravasation comprises a family of soluble chemoattractants named chemokines. Chemokines are members of a growing family of small serum proteins of 7–16 kDa. They are primarily involved in selective trafficking and homing of leukocytes to sites of infection and inflammation, leukocyte maturation in the bone marrow, tissue repair and vascularization, and hemopoiesis and renewal of circulating leukocytes.[85,86] The aberrant secretion of chemokines has been detected in a wide variety of inflammatory and infectious diseases, and their role in MS susceptibility and pathogenesis is under intense investigation.[87]

The present view of MS pathogenesis is markedly 'CD4-centric.' However, whereas the role of T cells as initiators and regulators of the CNS inflammatory response is well established, their role as direct effectors of myelin injury is uncertain. The most convincing mechanisms of myelin damage involve antibody binding, complement activation, and macrophage and microglia activation followed by myelin phagocytosis and release of toxic factors (see below).

Nevertheless, potential T-cell-mediated mechanisms of myelin damage have been shown in vitro; TNF-α kills myelinating cells in culture,[88,89] and anti-MBP CD4+ T cells can display cytolytic functions.[90] Activated T cells constitute the major subset of apoptotic cells in experimental acute lesions, a phenomenon possibly associated with resolution of EAE.[91] Other mechanisms such as lymphocyte CNS exit and T-cell anergy have also been postulated to explain EAE recovery. The hypothesis that a genetically determined failure of activation-induced apoptosis of autoreactive T cells in the CNS plays a significant role in the initiation or perpetuation of the inflammatory response in MS needs to be tested.[92]

The resident microglia, which lie within the parenchyma, also become activated as a result of locally released cytokines.[93] Microglia act as scavengers that remove debris and as antigen-presenting cells that present processed antigens to T cells, thereby contributing to their local clonal expansion. Mutual interactions between T cells and macrophages induce proliferation of both cell types through mediation of such molecules as interleukin (IL)-2 and colony stimulating factors. Furthermore, endothelia and T cells provide colony stimulating factors that maintain macrophage activation and prevent apoptosis and cell death. Microglia are also likely to induce myelin damage directly through the release of mediators such as free radicals (nitric oxide and superoxide anion), vasoactive amines, complement, proteases, cytokines (IL-1, TNF-α), and eicosanoids.[94,95]

As discussed above, B-cell activation and antibody responses are necessary for the full development of demyelination, both in human and experimental disease. For example, little or no demyelination is usually observed in EAE induced in Lewis rats by injection of purified MBP or by passive transfer of MBP-reactive lymphocytes.[96] Extensive demyelination can be induced in these animals by intravenous injection of anti-MOG monoclonal antibodies when the BBB is breached.[97] More recently, Genain and colleagues used immunogold-labeled peptides of myelin antigens and high-resolution microscopy to detect MOG-specific autoantibodies bound in situ to the disintegrating myelin in lesions of *C. jacchus* EAE and in acute human MS.[62] Myelin-specific infiltrating B cells have been detected in the MS brain, and in MS CSF there is a high frequency of clonally expanded B cells that have properties of post-germinal center memory or antibody-forming lymphocytes.[98] Antibodies may participate in myelin destruction through different mechanisms, such as by the facilitation of macrophage phagocytosis through myelin opsonization or by complement fixation.[99] CNS immunoglobulins may also induce myelinolysis through activation of a calcium-dependent, myelin-associated protease acting on MBP.[100] Interestingly, in the Theiler virus model, a natural antibody with specificity for a unique CNS component promotes remyelination. Hence, a pathogenic as well as reparative role for the humoral immune response could be postulated.[101] Recent results showing the ability of MBP and MOG-specific T-cell lines, as well as B cells and monocytes to produce brain-derived neurotrophic factor provide additional support for the hypothesis that the inflammatory infiltrate in MS brain may, in certain circumstances, have a neuroprotective effect.[102] These observation are significant for the design of selective and non-selective immunotherapies.

This model of MS pathogenesis provides a useful conceptual framework for understanding the mechanisms of action of existing therapies for this disorder, as well as the rationale behind drugs that are currently under development. Interference with one or several steps in the disease process—activation of T cells in the periphery, adhesion to brain vasculature, migration across endothelia, antigen recognition and reactivation within the CNS, opening of the BBB, and tissue damage mediated by T-helper 1 cytokines or antibody—is the goal of all MS therapies. Most experimental therapies focus on interference with antigen presentation to encephalitogenic T cells (altered peptide ligand, intravenous antigen), induction of a T-helper 2 (Th_2) response (oral tolerance), blockade of adhesion molecules (anti-VLA4 antibody), administration of anti-inflammatory cytokines (IL-10, TGF-β) or neutralization of proinflammatory cytokines (anti-TNF antibody, soluble TNF receptor). β-Interferons most likely have pleiotropic effects and appear to act by antagonizing the IFN-γ-mediated MHC up-regulation of antigen-presenting cells, altering the pattern of cytokine response to a Th_2 pattern, and blocking migration across endothelia. Copolymer 1 (a synthetic protein designed as an analog of MBP) may induce active T-cell suppression against MBP, and saturate MHC molecules on antigen-presenting cells, thereby preventing presentation of autoantigens. Glucocorticoids are potent inhibitors of antigen-presenting cell function. The chemotherapeutic drug cyclophosphamide is lympholytic and stimulates production of Th_2 cytokines.

One exciting approach to experimental therapy targets proteases that are expressed by activated T cells and are responsible for lysis of the dense subendothelial basal lamina by T cells as they migrate across the BBB to reach the CNS parenchyma. The clinical relevance of metalloproteinases is underlined by the observation that some proteases are present in the CSF of patients with MS but not in the CSF of normal controls.[103] Although macrophages are a rich source of enzymes that will disrupt the endothelium and allow traffic into the subendothelial basal lamina, T cells may have their own arsenal of proteases. The authors recently demonstrated that highly purified normal peripheral blood T lymphocytes express two matrix metalloproteinases, gelatinase A (72 kDa) and gelatinase B (92 kDa).[104] Functionally, the secretion of gelatinases by T cells correlates with the migratory and cytotoxic capacity of the cells. Both gelatinases are structurally related and share the proteolytic selectivity for basal lamina collagens. Remarkably, the sequence in the putative cleavage of the TNF-α precursor reveals homologies with peptide sequences known to be cleaved by metalloproteinase-like enzymes.[105,106] Thus, metalloproteinases may act not only as mediators of cell traffic across the BBB but they may also increase the inflammatory and homing reactions through TNF processing. Inhibition of gelatinases by enzyme inhibitors results in suppression of cell migration across a model brain endothelium in vitro and in amelioration of clinical signs in a rodent EAE model of MS.[107]

MULTIPLE SCLEROSIS AS A GENETIC DISEASE

An underlying genetic susceptibility plays a clear role in the etiology of MS (*Table 19.4*). A genetic component in MS pathogenesis is suggested by familial clustering and the frequent occurrence of MS in some ethnic populations (particularly those of northern European origin) compared with others (e.g. African and Asian groups), irrespective of geographic location.[108,109] High incidence rates for this disorder are found in Scandinavia, Iceland, the British Isles and the countries settled by the inhabitants of these areas and their descendants.[110,111] For example, in the USA, Canada, Australia and New Zealand the prevalence of MS is higher among Caucasians (about 100 per 100 000) than in other racial groups. The highest reported prevalence of MS, estimated at 250 cases per 100 000 population, occurs in the Orkney Islands, north of mainland Scotland. MS is uncommon in Japan (2 per 100 000) and other Asian nations, sub-Saharan Africa, the Indian subcontinent, and the native populations of Oceania and the Americas. The observation of resistant ethnic groups residing in high-risk regions, as for example Gypsies in Hungary, suggests that the relatively low risk in some ethnic groups results from genetic resistance rather than environmental factors.

Familial aggregation in MS, recognized by Charcot before the turn of the century, is well documented.[108,109] One measure of aggregation is the λs statistic, defined as the ratio of the lifetime risk to siblings of affected individuals (Ks) versus the population prevalence (K) of the disease (λs = Ks/K). For MS, the total λs is between 20 (0.02/0.001) and 40 (0.04/0.001),[108,112] a value similar to or greater than that for insulin-dependent diabetes mellitus. Half-sibling[113] and adoption[114] studies indicate that genetic factors, not environmental factors, are responsible for familial aggregation. In addition, twin studies from different populations consistently indicate that a monozygotic twin of an MS patient is at higher risk (25–30% concordance) of MS than is a dizygotic twin (2–5%),[115] providing additional evidence for a complex genetic etiology to MS.

Table 19.4 MS as a genetic disease

Radical clustering of MS cases. Resistant ethnic groups residing in high risk regions

Familial aggregation of MS cases. Increased relative risk to siblings ($\lambda_s = 20–40$)

High disease concordance in monozygotic twins (25–30%) compared with dizygotic twins and non-twin siblings (3–5%)

No detectable effect of shared environment on MS susceptibility in first-degree non-biological relatives (spouses, adoptees)

Suggestive correlations between certain polymorphic loci and disease susceptibility

Gene identification in MS

Genetic studies in EAE have been very informative in defining the complex interplay of multiple genes that can result in brain inflammation and demyelination.[116] These studies have also been useful in validating EAE as an MS disease model. The best-characterized EAE susceptibility gene resides within the MHC on murine chromosome 17.[117,118] Induction and full clinical manifestations of EAE are strongly influenced by inherited differences (polymorphisms) of MHC class II region genes; certain MHC haplotypes are permissive for EAE, whereas others are resistant. However, the concept of susceptibility vs resistance in EAE is relative, rather than absolute as evidence demonstrates that modifications of the experimental protocol will induce detectable disease in 'resistant strains'. The use of classic genetics and whole-genome screening has identified several additional genetic regions that participate in conferring EAE susceptibility, including loci on chromosomes 3, 6 (TCR-β gene chains (TCRB)), 7, 15, 17 (MHC), 17 (distal to MHC) and X. Other regions, including segments on chromosomes 1–5, 7–12, and 14–18, have been implicated as containing disease-modifying genes.[116] These studies provide compelling evidence for the hypothesis that susceptibility to autoimmune demyelination is largely genetically determined. A multiple-locus model is applicable; each locus may contribute to a specific stage of EAE pathology, although some loci are probably involved in several steps of the autoimmune process.[116] However, no locus seems to be an absolute requirement for the susceptible phenotype (i.e. a susceptible EAE phenotype can be achieved in different crosses by different combinations of genotypes). As the roster of genes that contribute to EAE is completed, such genes will represent strong 'candidates' for testing in MS.[119]

Case-control study designs versus family-based study designs

Several confounding factors, such as genetic heterogeneity and phenocopies, as well as gene–gene and gene–environment interaction, must be considered in the analysis of a complex disease (*Table 19.5*). The genetic analysis of MS has

Table 19.5 Confounding factors in genetic studies of MS

Etiologic heterogeneity
- Identical genes, different phenotypes

Genetic heterogeneity
- Different genes, identical phenotypes

Unknown genetic parameters
- Single vs multiple genes
- Mode of inheritance
- Incomplete penetrance

Gene – gene interactions (additive or multiplicative)

Unidentified non-heritable and environmental factors

Publication bias

traditionally focused on association studies of candidate genes, in which the frequencies of marker alleles in groups of patients and healthy controls are compared and the difference is subjected to statistical analysis (*Table 19.6*). The association is often expressed as the relative risk that a person will develop the disorder if he or she carries the particular allele or marker, compared to a person who does not carry the allele or marker. Candidate genes are defined as genes that are logical possibilities as playing a role in a disease; for MS, candidate genes might encode cytokines, immune receptors, and proteins involved in viral clearance. With the notable exception of the MHC locus, case–control-association studies have met with only modest success in identifying disease-causing genes in MS, in part because of the difficulty in selecting from among the many candidate gene possibilities and because of the likely modest effect of any single MS susceptibility gene. An additional limi-

tation is imposed by the difficulty in identifying a perfectly matched control group, increasing the possibility that a potentially positive association is biologically irrelevant because of population admixture. Furthermore, even when cases and controls are adequately matched, most study designs involve relatively small sample sizes, which lack the statistical power to detect small or moderate gene effects.

Family-based studies, on the other hand, allow the identification of unambiguous haplotypes and are amenable to more informative genetic analyses using multiple statistical approaches. The theoretical foundation and methodology for testing are currently available to examine family data in a variety of ways based on the structure of pedigrees in a given study.[120] For example, family collections may consist of extended multigenerational pedigrees, affected sib pairs, alone or with parents and other affected siblings, affected individuals with parents and/or unaffected siblings, or in some cases, a combination of any of these types. Depending on the sample collection strategy, family studies can provide evidence for or against linkage and association to a particular marker, which is not possible using a case–control design. As the human gene map improves, family-based studies of candidate genes will probably become an increasingly valuable approach for the analysis of MS susceptibility (*Table 19.7*).

The MHC and human demyelination

The genetic association between MS susceptibility and the MHC locus has been known for more than 20 years. Despite great progress in understanding the immunobiology of the MHC, much remains to be learned about the underlying mech-

Table 19.6 Case–control studies of candidate genes in MS

Chromosome 1	*Chromosome 14*
Interleukin 10 (1q31-q32)	T-cell antigen receptor (TCR) A/D (14q11.2)
Transforming growth factor (TGFβ) 2 (1q31)	Immunoglobulin (Ig) genes (14q32)
HRES-1 retro-element (1q32-q42)	Alpha-1 antitrypsin (14q24)
Transforming growth factor (TGFβ) 3R (11p32-p33)	*Chromosome 16*
Rhesus blood group (1p36.2-p34)	Interleukin 4 receptor (16p12.1-p11.2)
Chromosome 2	*Chromosome 17*
Interleukin 1 receptor antagonist/interleukin 1B	2'3'-cyclic nucleotide 3'-phosphodiesterase (17q21)
(IL-1ra/IL-1B) (2q14.2)	Myeloperoxidase (17q23.1)
Chromosome 3	Oligodendrocyte myelin glycoprotein
Chemokine receptor 5 (CCR5) (3p21)	(OMGP) (17q11.2)
Chromosome 4	Ecotropic viral integration 2 (17q11)
Interleukin 2 (4q26-q27)	*Chromosome 18*
Chromosome 5	Myelin basic protein (MBP) (18q22)
Interleukin 4 (5q23-q31)	*Chromosome 19*
Chromosome 6	Third component of complement (19p13)
Pc 1 Duarte (6p21)	Apolipoprotein E (APOE) (19q13)
HLA DR, DQ, DP, DM (6p21.3)	Intracellular adhesion molecule-1 (ICAM-1)
Tumor necrosis factor (6p21.3)	(19p13.3-p13.2)
Transporters associated with antigen processing	Transforming growth factor 1 (TGFβ) (19q13)
(6p21.3)	Myelin associated glycoprotein (MAG) (19q13.1)
Myelin oligodendrocyte glycoprotein (MOG) (6p21.3)	*Chromosome 22*
Heat shock protein 70 (HSP 70) (6p21.3)	CYP2D6 (22q13)
Chromosome 7	*Chromosome X*
T-cell antigen receptor (TCR) B (5q35)	Gamma-aminobutyric acid A3 receptor
ER V3 retro-element	(GABRA3) (Xq22-q28)
Chromosome 10	Proteolipid protein (Xq22)
Fas Apo-1 antigen (10q24.1)	
Chromosome 12	
Interferon γ (12q14-q15)	*Mitochondrial sequences*

anism responsible for its genetic association to many autoimmune disease states. MHC class I and class II molecules are highly polymorphic cell surface glycoproteins whose primary role in an immune response is to display and present short antigenic peptide fragments to antigen-specific T cells. The importance of MHC compatibility in clinical transplantation stimulated the development of reagents and methods aimed at allowing full comprehension of the degree of genetic variability in the system. As a result, an impressive body of knowledge has accumulated on the func-

Table 19.7 Family-based studies of candidate genes in MS

Chromosome 1	*Chromosome 12*
Interleukin 10 (1q31-q32)	Neurotrophin 3 (12p13)
Transforming growth factor B2 (1q31)	Erb-B3 (12p)
Transforming growth factor BR3 (1p32-p33)	Interferon gamma (12q14-q15)
Chromosome 2	Insulin-like growth factor 1 (12q23)
Interleukin 1 receptor antagonist/	*Chromosome 14*
interleukin 1B (IL-1ra/IL-1B) (2q14.2)	T-cell receptor (TCR) A/D (14q11.2)
Chromosome 3	Transforming growth factor B3 (14q24)
Transforming growth factor BR3 (3p22)	Immunoglobulin (Ig) gene (14q24)
Chromosome 4	*Chromosome 15*
Fibroblast growth factor (FGF) R (4p16.3)	Insulin growth factor (IGF) 1R (15q25)
Platelet-derived growth factor (PDGF) Rα (4q11-q12)	TRK-C (15q24-q25)
Fibroblast growth factor (FGF) 2 (4q25)	*Chromosome 16*
Interleukin 2 (4q26-q27)	Interleukin 4 receptor (16p12.1-p11.2)
Chromosome 5	*Chromosome 17*
Interleukin 4 (5q23-q31)	2'3'-cyclic nucleotide 3'-phosphodiesterase (17q21)
Fibroblast growth factor 1 (5q31.1-q33.2)	Oligodendrocyte myelin glycoprotein (OMGP) (17q11.2)
Chromosome 6	*Chromosome 18*
HLA-DR/DQ (6p21.3)	Myelin basic protein (MBP) (18q22)
Myelin oligodendrocyte glycoprotein (MOG) (6p21.3)	Golli-MBP (18q22)
Chromosome 7	*Chromosome 19*
Erb-B (7p12)	Apolipoprotein E (APOE) (19q13)
Platelet-derived growth factor (PDGF) α (7p22)	Transforming growth factor 1 (19q13)
T-cell receptor (TCR) B (7q35)	Myelin associated glycoprotein (MAG) (19q13.1)
Chromosome 8	*Chromosome 22*
Fibroblast growth factor (8p12)	Platelet-derived growth factor (PDGF) B (22q12.3-q31)
Glial growth factor (GGF) (8p21)	*Chromosome X*
Chromosome 10	Proteolipid protein (PLP) (Xq22)
Fibroblast growth factor BR2 (10q25)	

tion and population genetics of the human MHC (the HLA system) (*Fig. 19.4*). The ability to respond to an antigen, whether foreign or self, and the nature of that response, is partly determined by the unique amino acid sequences of MHC alleles, an observation that provided the rationale for focusing on associations between HLA genotypes and susceptibility to autoimmune disease.[121]

The majority of MHC association studies in MS have focused on Caucasians of northern European descent, where predisposition to disease has been consistently associated with the class II HLA-DRB1*1501–DQA1*0102–

DQB1*0602 haplotype (the molecular designation for the serologically defined 'DR2' haplotype).[122] Attempts to localize further a susceptibility gene within the DR or DQ region of the HLA have not provided consensus. When the effect of DRB1*1501 is removed form the DR2 haplotype, evidence against[123] and in favor[124] of a primary role for the DQA1*0102–B1*0602 heterodimer have been reported.

The mechanism(s) underlying linkage and association of HLA-DRB1*1501–DQA1*0102–DQB1*0602 with MS are not yet fully understood. These MHC molecules may fail to negatively select (delete) autoreactive T cells within the embryonic thymic microenvironment. Alternatively, HLA-DRB1*1501 genes, DQA1*0102–DQB1*0602 genes, or both may encode a class II recognition molecule with a propensity to bind peptide antigens of myelin and to stimulate encephalitogenic T cells. As previously discussed, it is known that DRB1*1501 bind with high affinity to the 89–98 MBP

peptide. X-ray crystallography of the DR2–MBP peptide complex reveals that the peptide binding domain of DRB1*1501 has a large hydrophobic pocket created by an alanine at position 71 of the β chain, into which the glutamic acid at position 93 of MBP is bound, anchoring the MBP–DR2 complex.[125] It is likely that tyrosine residues in copolymer 1 also binds to this hydrophobic pocket of DR2, thereby interfering with presentation of this key MBP peptide to pathogenic T cells.

For some closely located genes, certain combinations of alleles (alternative variants of a single gene, each with a unique DNA sequence) preferentially occur together on the same chromosome.[126] The recombination rate between HLA-A and HLA-B for example, is 0.31%, much smaller than expected for a physical distance of 1.4 Mbp. Such genes are said to be in linkage disequilibrium (LD), and the combination of alleles is referred to as a haplotype. LD refers, then, to the presence of alleles at different loci occurring together more frequently than would be expected

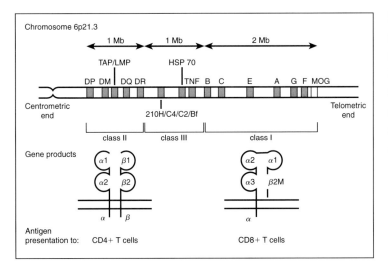

Fig. 19.4 Genetic organization of the MHC. The diagram shows the relative positions of the major MHC class I and class II loci involved in antigen presentation, as well as other examples of the more than 250 genes encoded within this complex of 3×10^6 base pairs.

by independent segregation. It is also interesting to note that some regions with a high level of a LD may encompass loci that are in complete equilibrium with each other. It is relevant to MS that the 1501 allele of the HLA-DRB1* gene preferentially occurs with the 0602 form of the DQB1* gene. The strong LD across the entire MHC region, and the fact that DRB1*1501 and DQB1*0602 are found on this haplotype predominantly in northern Europeans, has prevented a clear resolution of the relative contribution of each MHC gene to MS pathogenesis. It is plausible that the classical HLA genes do not themselves predispose to MS but are located close to another unidentified gene, which actually confers susceptibility. More than 240 genes have been mapped in this region, including proteins that control antigen processing and transport, the complement proteins C2, factors B and C4, heat shock protein 70, steroid 21-hydroxylase, the gene for hemochromatosis, and genes for the cytokine TNF, and the myelin protein MOG.

Because the patterns of genomic disequilibrium are shaped by the population history (founding size, bottlenecks, expansions), the combinations of particular DRB1, DQA1 and DQB1 alleles within a given population can be unique. For example, in Caucasians DRB1*0405 is coupled to DQA1*0301 and DQB1*0302, but in Japanese it is coupled to DQA1*0301 and DQB1*0401, in Africans to DQA1*0301 and DQB1*0201, and in Filipinos to DQA1*0101 and DQB1*0503. By conducting association studies in various ethnic groups with different haplotypic combinations, the different contribution of individual genes can be discerned. Family-based studies will permit differentiation between *cis* and *trans* effects of specific allelic interactions between different genes in the region.

Scanning the entire genome

An alternative strategy to the analysis of individual candidate genes merges the basic principles of Mendelian genetics with the increasing power of molecular biology. This approach, which has become known as positional cloning or locational cloning, involves first determining the chromosomal region of the genomic defect by genetic linkage analysis and then isolating the disease gene without any prior knowledge of the protein product and function. Positional cloning is greatly facilitated by the presence of chromosomal abnormalities, such as deletions or translocations, which will indicate the location of the gene responsible for the phenotype under investigation. In MS, no gross chromosomal abnormalities have been identified, and hence gene localization requires the collection of pedigrees with more than one affected member and the establishment of linkage by tracking the inheritance of discrete chromosomal segments that co-segregate with the disease.

In contrast to monogenic diseases, for complex disorders such as MS linkage analysis must be performed on an extremely large group of people if small genetic effects are to be detected or if genetic heterogeneity is present. The smaller the genetic contribution, the larger is the required screen and the more stringent is the required inclusion criteria to minimize effects of genetic heterogeneity. A multiple-stage whole-genome screen in multiplex MS families collected in the USA according to rigorous clinical criteria was completed in 1996.[127,128] The study used 443 markers on all chromosomes with an average spacing of 9.6 centimorgans (cM), and genotyped 471 people belonging to families with between two and eight affected members with MS. The data was analysed with a combination of parametric (model-based) and non-parametric (model-free) statistical methods. This multianalytical strategy identified 19 possible susceptibility regions (defined as 'regions of interest'), including 5q13–23, 7q21–22, 19q13, and the MHC on 6p21. Parallel efforts in the UK,[129] Canada[130] and Finland[131] identified additional potential MS loci. Follow-up screenings in larger, confirmatory datasets of multiplex families are in progress.

It is not surprising that these studies generated considerable interest in the neurology and immunology communities, nor is it surprising that the data were received with certain discouragement. Some critics emphasized the absence of total or even predominant replication between the different genomic screens. It should be noted, however, that because each study used a somewhat overlapping but different set of genetic markers and different inclusion clinical criteria, the direct comparison of results is not straightforward. Nevertheless, the careful analysis of the composite data indicates common regions of interest between the different studies (*Table 19.8*). More interestingly, a recent meta-analysis of the published data singled out discrete overlapping susceptibility chromosomal regions at chromosomes 5, 6, 17 and 19.[132] In this regard, follow-up screens in a confirmatory USA data set provided additional support for susceptibility loci at 6p21 in the MHC region and at 19q13 near the Apo E locus. Other potential candidate genes in this interval are TGF-β1 and IL-11.

A second type of meta-analysis attempted to cluster autoimmune-susceptibility loci from a comparison of the linkage results from 23 human and experimental immune-mediated diseases.[133] Overlapping of susceptibility loci was detected, suggesting that in some cases, part of the pathophysiology of clinically distinct autoimmune disorders may be controlled by a common set of genes. Undoubtedly, these common regions will be the focus of intensive investigation with dense batteries of genetic markers and the direct analysis of candidate genes mapped to these regions.

Genome searches underscore a role for the MHC

In the USA genome scan, the MHC locus at chromosome 6p21 was one of 19 regions identified as suggestive of harboring a susceptibility gene for MS. Follow-up analysis of the MHC locus in 98 multiplex families confirmed the significant genetic linkage to this region (lod score of 4.60), and the specific association with the HLA-DRB1*1501 allele ($p < 0.001$), demonstrating that sporadic and familial MS share common genetic components (*Table 19.9*).[134] Interestingly, 25% of the families, most of them HLA-DRB1*1501-negative, showed no linkage to the MHC locus, most likely indicating the presence of genetic heterogeneity among familial MS in Caucasians.

It is noteworthy that the MHC region was identified as 'of interest' in a second-tier data set from the UK but not in the Canadian population. Failure to identify linkage to the MHC region in the Canadian data set and in the first-tier UK data set could have resulted from the use of different sets of markers for screening, the inclusion of primary progressive MS patients (more than one-third of the Canadian multiplex population) and other differences in the UK and Canadian data sets compared with the USA data set. Indeed, it is likely that MS encompasses more than one fundamental phenotype. Whether the genotype dictates different forms of MS in response to a common causative agent or trigger,

Table 19.8 Regions of overlap between whole genome scans in MS

US	UK	Canada	Finland
	1p36-p33	1p36-p33	
2p23	2p23-p21	2p23-21	
	3p14-p13	3p14-p13	
3q22-q24		3q22-q24	
4q31-qter	4q31-qter		
		5p14-p12	5p14-22
5q13-q23	5q12-q13	5q12-q13	
6p21	6p21		6p21
6q27	6q22-27		
7q11-q22		7q21-q22	
	17q22		17q22-24
18p11		18p11	
19q13	19q12-13	19q13	

Table 19.9 Linkage results split by HLA-DR2 status

Marker	SimIBD P value		Sibpair MLS		Lod Score Aut Dom		Lod Score Aut Rec	
	DR2+	DR2−	DR2+	DR2−	DR2+	DR2−	DR2+	DR2−
HLA-DR	0.12	0.24	2.41	0.00	5.10	0.00	4.25	0.00
TNFβ	0.19	0.22	0.80	0.01	1.54	0.00	1.06	0.05
D6S273	0.05	0.29	1.00	0.06	2.15	0.01	1.48	0.02

or whether the genotype reflects different diseases with different environmental causes, is not known. Clearly, however, clinical and paraclinical (e.g. MRI) variables will assume increasing importance as stratifying elements for future genetic studies of MS.

A model of inheritance for MS

Taken together, the available data is compatible with a complex multifactorial etiology in MS, including both genetic and environmental factors. A simple model of inheritance for all MS is unlikely and cannot account for the non-linear decrease in disease risk in families with increasing genetic distance from the MS proband. Recurrence risk estimates in first-, second-, and third-degree relatives, combined with twin data, predict that the MS-prone genotype results from multiple independent or interacting genes, each of small or moderate effect. Thus, MS is a polygenic disorder. It is also possible that genetic heterogeneity exists, meaning that different genes influence susceptibility in some people but not in others. Recent data highlight the importance of the MHC region in conferring genetic susceptibility to MS. Susceptibility may be mediated by the class II genes themselves (DR, DQ or both), related to the known function of these molecules in the normal immune response (e.g. antigen binding and presentation and T-cell repertoire determination). The possibility that other genes in the MHC or the telomeric region of the MHC are responsible for the observed genetic effect cannot be excluded. The data also show that, although the MHC region plays a significant role in MS susceptibility, much of the genetic effect in MS remains to be explained. By analogy with emerging data on the genetic basis of EAE, it will be of particular interest to identify whether some loci are involved in the initial pathogenic events while others influence the development and progression of the disease. Their characterization will help to define the basic etiology of the disease, improve risk assessment and influence therapeutics. The development of new molecular tools to define the immune response in MS and to characterize its genetic basis are opening a window into the intricacies of genetic and environmental interactions that take place in this disorder.

REFERENCES

1 Hauser SL, Goodkin SL. Multiple sclerosis and other semyelinating siseases. In: Fauci AD, Braunwald E, Isselbacher JD et al. *Harrison's Principle of Internal Medicine* 14th edn. New York: McGraw Hill, 1998, 2409–2418.

2 Kira J, Kanai T, Nishimura Y et al. Western versus Asian types of multiple sclerosis: two immunogenetically and clinically distinct patient groups. *Ann Neurol* 1996; 40:569–574.

3 Lucchinetti CF, Brueck W, Rodriguez M, Lassmann H. Multiple sclerosis: lessons from neuropathology. *Semin Neurol* 1998; 18:337–349.

4 Lassman H, Suchanek G, Ozawa K. Histopathology and the blood–cerebrospinal fluid barrier in multiple sclerosis. *Ann Neurol* 1994; 36:S42–S46.

5 Hauser SL, Bhan AK, Gilles F et al. Immunocytochemical analysis of the cellular infiltrates in multiple sclerosis lesions. *Ann Neurol* 1986; 19:578–587.

6 Raine CS. The Dale E McFarlin memorial lecture: the immunology of the multiple sclerosis lesion. *Ann Neurol* 1994; 36:S61–S72.

7 Selmaj K, Brosnan CF, Raine CS. Colocalization of TCR γδ lymphocytes and hsp65+ oligodendrocytes in multiple sclerosis. *Proc Natl Acad Sci U S A* 1991; 88:6452–6456.

8 Hvas J, Oksenberg JR, Fernando R et al. Gamma/delta T-cell receptor repertoire in brain lesions of patients with multiple sclerosis. *J Neuroimmunol* 1993; 46:225–234.

9 Oksenberg JR, Stuart S, Begovich AB et al. Limited heterogeneity of rearranged T-cell receptor V alpha transcripts in brains of multiple sclerosis patients. *Nature* 1990; 345:344–346.

10 Lee SJ, Wucherpfennig KW, Brod SA, Benjamin D. Common T cell receptor V beta usage in oligoclonal T lymphocytes derived from cerebrospinal fluid and blood of patients with multiple sclerosis. *Ann Neurol* 1991; 29:33–40.

11 Usuku K, Joshi N, Hatem CJ et al. T-cell receptor expression by cerebro-spinal fluid cells in multiple sclerosis. *Neurology* 1992; 42 (suppl 3):187a.

12 Oksenberg JR, Panzara MA, Begovich AB et al. Selection for T-cell receptor Vβ-Dβ-Jβ gene rearrangements with specificity for a myelin basic protein peptide in brain lesions of multiple sclerosis. *Nature* 1993; 362:68–70.

13 Allegretta M, Albertini RJ, Howell MD et al.

Homologies between T cell receptor junctional sequences unique to multiple sclerosis and T cells mediating experimental allergic encephalomyelitis. *J Clin Invest* 1994; **94**:105–109.

14 Renno T, Zeine R, Girard JM et al. Selective enrichment of Th1 CD45RB low CD4+ T cells in autoimmune infiltrates in experimental allergic encephalomyelitis. *Int Immunol* 1994; **6**:347–354.

15 McDonald WI. The pathological and clinical dynamics of multiple sclerosis. *J Neuropathol Exp Neurol* 1994; **53**:338–343.

16 Kermode AG. Breakdown of the blood–brain barrier precedes symptoms and other MRI signs of new lesions in multiple sclerosis. *Brain* 1990; **113**:1477–1489.

17 Ozawa K, Suchanek G, Breitschopf H et al. Patterns of oligodendroglia pathology in multiple sclerosis. *Brain* 1994; **117**:1311–1322.

18 Brueck W, Schmied M, Suchanek G et al. Oligodendrocytes in the early course of multiple sclerosis. *Ann Neurol* 1994; **35**:65–73.

19 Ludwin SK, Johnson ES. Evidence of a 'dying-back' gliopathy in demyelinating disease. *Ann Neurol* 1981; **9**:301–305.

20 Rodriguez M, Scheithauer BW, Forbes G, Kelly PJ. Oligodendrocyte injury is an early event in lesios of multiple sclerosis. *Mayo Clin Proc* 1993; **68**:627–636.

21 De Stefano N, Matthews PM, Fu L et al. Axonal damage correlates with disability in patients with relapsing–remitting multiple sclerosis. Results of a longitudinal magnetic resonance spectroscopy study. *Brain* 1998; **121**:1469–1477.

22 Trapp BD, Peterson J, Ranshoff RM et al. Axonal transection in the lesions of multiple sclerosis. *N Engl J Med* 1998; **338**:278–285.

23 Sorensen TL, Ransohoff R. Etiology and pathogenesis of multiple sclerosis. *Semin Neurol* 1998; **18**:287–294.

24 Dowling P, Husar W, Menonna J et al. Cell death and birth in multiple sclerosis brain. *J Neurol Sci* 1997; **149**:1–11.

25 Bonetti B, Raine CS. Multiple sclerosis: oligodendrocytes display cell-death related molecules in situ but do not undergo apoptosis. *Ann Neurol* 1997; **42**:74–84.

26 Wu E, Raine CS. Multiple sclerosis: interactions between oligodendrocytes and hypertrophic astrocytes and their ocurrence in other, non-demyelinating conditions. *Lab Invest* 1992;

67:88–99.

27 Prineas JW, Barnard RO, Kwon EE et al. Multiple sclerosis. Remyelination of nascent lesions. *Ann Neurol* 1993; **33**:137–151.

28 Traugott U. Relevance of class I and class II MHC-expressing cells to lesion development. *J Neuroimmunol* 1987; **15**:283.

29 Sanders V, Conrad AJ, Tourtellote WW. On classification of post-mortem multiple sclerosis plaques for neuroscientists. *J Neuroimmunol* 1993; **46**:207–216.

30 Bo L, Mark S, Kong P et al. Detection of MHC class II antigens on macrophages and microglia, but not astrocytes and endothelia in active MS lesions. *J Neuroimmunol* 1994; **51**:135–146.

31 Traugott U, Reinherz E, Raine CS. Multiple sclerosis: Distribution of T cell subsets within active lesions. *Science* 1983; **219**:308–310.

32 Mach B, Steimle V, Martinez-Soria E, Reith W. Regulation of MHC class II genes: lessons from a disease. *Annu Rev Immunol* 1996; **14**:301–331.

33 Wolf PR, Ploegh HL. How MHC class II molecules acquire peptide cargo: biosynthesis and trafficking through the endocytic pathway. *Annu Rev Immunol* 1995; **11**:267–306.

34 Soos JM, Morrow J, Ashley TA et al. Astrocytes express elements of the class II endocytic pathway and process central nervous system autoantigens for presentation to encephalitogenic T cells. *J Immunol* 1998, **161**:5959–5966.

35 Soos JM, Ashley TA, Morrow J et al. Differential B7 costimulatory molecule expression by astrocytes correlates with T cell activation and cytokine production. *Int Immunol* 1999; in press.

36 Lee YJ, Han Y, Lu HT et al. TGF beta suppresses IFN gamma induction of class II MHC gene expression by inhibiting class II transactivator messenger RNA expression. *J Immunol* 1997; **158**:2065–2075.

37 Lu HT, Riley JL, Babcock GT et al. Interferon (IFN)β acts downstream of IFN-γ-induced class II transactivator messenger RNA accumulation to block major histocompatibility complex class II gene expression and requires the 48-kD DNA-binding protein, ISGF3-γ. *J Exp Med* 1995; **182**:1517–1525.

38 Perry VH. A revised view of the central nervous system microenvironment and major histocompatibility complex class II antigen presentation. *J Neuroimmunol* 1998; **90**:113–121.

39 Sobel RA, Mitchell ME, Fondren G. Intercellular adhesion molecule-1 (ICAM-1) in cellular immune reactions in the human central nervous system. *Am J Pathol* 1990; **136**:1309–1316.

40 Raine CS, Canella B. Adhesion molecules and central nervous system inflammation. *Semin Neurosci* 1992; 4:201–211.

41 Raine CS. Multiple sclerosis: immune system molecule expression in the central nervous system. *J Neuropathol Exp Neurol* 1994; **53**:328–337.

42 Cannella B, Raine C. The adhesion molecule and cytokine profile of multiple sclerosis lesions. *Ann Neurol* 1995; **37**:424–435.

43 Rivers TM, Sprunt DH, Berry GP. Observations on attempts to produce acute disseminated encephalomyelitis in monkeys. *J Exp Med* 1933; **58**:39–53.

44 Paterson PY. Transfer of allergic encephalomyelitis in rats by means of lymph node cells. *J Exp Med* 1960; 3:119–135.

45 Olsson T, Baig S, Hojeberg B, Link H. Antimyelin basic protein and antimyelin antibody-producing cells in MS. *Ann Neurol* 1990; **27**:132–136.

46 Steinman L. Specific motifs in T cell receptor VβDβJβ gene sequences in multiple sclerosis lesions in brain. *Behring Inst Mitt* 1994; **94**:148–157.

47 Allegretta M, Nicklas JA, Sriram S, Albertini RJ. T cells responsive to myelin basic protein in patients with multiple sclerosis. *Science* 1990; **247**:718–721.

48 Lodge PA, Johnson C, Sriram S. Frequency of MBP and MBP peptide reactive T cells in the HPRT mutant T-cell population of MS patients. *Neurology* 1996; **46**:1410–1415.

49 Illes Z, Kondo T, Yokoyama K et al. Identification of autoimmune T cells among in vivo expanded CD25+ T cells in multiple sclerosis. *J Immunol* 1999; **162**:1811–1817.

50 Hafler DA, Duby AD, Lee SJ et al. Oligoclonal T lymphocytes in the cerebrospinal fluid of patients with multiple sclerosis. *J Exp Med* 1988; **167**:1313–1322.

51 Soderstrom M, Link H, Sim JB et al. T cells recognizing multiple peptides of myelin basic protein are found in the blood and enriched in the cerebrospinal fluid in optic neuritis and multiple sclerosis. *Scand J Immunol* 1993; **37**:355–368.

52 Burns J, Bartholomew B, Lobo S. Isolation of myelin basic protein-specific T cells predominantly from the memory T-cell compartment in multiple sclerosis. *Ann Neurol* 1998; **45**:33–39.

53 Scholz C, Paton KT, Anderson DE et al. Expansion of autoreactive T cells in multiple sclerosis is independent of exogenous B7 costimulation. *J Immunol* 1998; **160**:1532–1538.

54 Massacesi L, Genain CP, Lee-Parritz D et al. Active and passively induced experimental autoimmune encephalomyelitis in common marmosets: a new model for multiple sclerosis. *Ann Neurol* 1995; **37**:519–530.

55 Genain CP, Lee-Paritz D, Nguyen MH et al. In healthy primates, circulating autoreactive T cells mediate autoimmune disease. *J Clin Invest* 1994; **94**:1339–1345.

56 Bernard CCA, Randell VB, Horvath L et al. Antibody to myelin basic protein in extracts of multiple sclerosis brain. *Immunology* 1981; **43**:447–457.

57 Warren KG, Catz I, Johnson E, Mielke B. Anti-myelin basic protein and anti-proteolipid protein specific forms of multiple sclerosis. *Ann Neurol* 1994; **35**:280–289.

58 Garbern JY, Cambi F, Tang XM et al. Proteolipid protein is necessary in peripheral as well as central myelin. *Neuron* 1997; **19**:205–218.

59 Johns TG, Kerlero de Rosbo N, Menon KK et al. Myelin oligodendrocyte glycoprotein induces a demyelinating encephalomyelitis resembling multiple sclerosis. *J Immunol* 1995; **154**: 5536–5541.

60 Genain CP, Abel K, Belmar N et al. Late complications of immune deviation therapy in a nonhuman primate. *Science* 1996; **274**:2054–2056.

61 Bernard CCA, Johns TG, Slavin A et al. Myelin oligodendrocyte glycoprotien: a novel candidate autoantigen in multiple sclerosis. *J Mol Med* 1997; **75**:77–88.

62 Genain CP, Cannella B, Hausr SL, Raine CS. Identification of autoantibodies associated with myelin damage in multiple sclerosis. *Nature Med* 1999; 5:1–6.

63 Brunner C, Lassmann H, Waehneldet TV et al. Differential ultrastructural localization of myelin basic protein, myelin oligodendroglia glycoprotein, and 2′,3′-cyclic nucleotide 3′-phosphodiesterase in the CNS of adult rats. *J Neurochem* 1989; 52:296–304.

64 Hjelmstrom P, Penzotti JE, Henne RM, Lybrand TP. A molecular model of myelin oligodendrocyte glycoprotein. *J Neurochem* 1998; **71**:1742–1749.

65 Oksenberg JR, Hauser SL. Pathogenesis of multiple

sclerosis: relationship to therapeutic strategies. In: Goodkin D, Rudick R, eds. *Treatment of Multiple Sclerosis*. London: Springer, 1996, 17–46.

66 Miller SD, Vanderlugt CL, Begolka WS et al. Persitstent infection with Theiler's virus leads to CNS autoimmunity via epitope spreading. *Nature Med* 1997; 3:1133–1136.

67 Lider O, Santos LMB, Lee CSY et al. Suppression of experimental allergic encephalomyelitis by oral administration of myelin basic protein. II. Suppression of disease and in vitro immune responses is mediated by antigen-specific CD8+ T lymphocytes. *J Immunol* 1989; 142:748–752.

68 Jiang H, Zhang SL, Pernis B. Role of CD8+ T cells in murine experimental allergic encephalomyelitis. *Science* 1992; 256:1213–1215.

69 Koh DR, Fung-Leung WP, Ho A et al. Less mortality but more relapses in experimental allergic encephalomyelitis in CD8-/- mice. *Science* 1992; 256:1210–1213.

70 Correale J, Rojany M, Weiner LP. Human CD8+ TCR-αβ+ and TCR-γδ+ cells modulate autologous autoreactive neuroantigen-specific CD4+ T-cells by different mechanisms. *J Neuroimmunol* 1997; 80:47–64.

71 Olivarez-Villagomez D, Wang Y, Lafaille JJ. Regulatory CD4+ T cells expressing endogenous T cell receptor chains protect MBP-specific transgenic mice from spontaneous autoimmune encephalomyelitis. *J Exp Med* 1998; 188:1883–1894.

72 Van de Keere F, Tonegawa S. CD4+ T cells prevent spontaneous EAE in anty-myelin basic protein T cell receptor transgenic mice. *J Exp Med* 1998; 188:1875–1882.

73 Gautam A, Pearson C, Smilek D et al. A polyalanine peptide containing only five native basic protein residues induces autoimmune encephalomyelitis. *J Exp Med* 1992; 176:605–609.

74 Steinman L. Escape from 'horror autotoxicuss': pathogenesis and treatment of autoimmune disease. *Cell* 1995; 80:7–10.

75 Wucherpfennig WW, Strominger JL. Molecular mimicry in T cell-mediated autoimmunity: viral peptides activate human T cell clones specific for myelin basic protein. *Cell* 1995; 80:695–705.

76 Hemmer B, Fleckenstein BT, Vergelli M et al. Identification of high potency microbial and self ligands for a human autoreactive class II-restricted T cells clone. *J Exp Med* 1997; 185:1651–1659.

77 Karpuj MA, Steinamn L, Oksenberg JR. Multiple

sclerosis: a polygenic disease involving epistatic interactions, germline rearrangements and environmental effects. *Neurogenetics* 1997; 1:21–28.

78 Johnson RT, Griffin RE, Hirsch RL et al. Measles encephalomyelitis: clinical and immunological studies. *N Engl J Med* 1984; 310:137–141.

79 Hara H, Morita M, Iwaki T et al. Detection of HTLV-I proviral DNA and analysis of TCR V beta CDR3 sequences in spinal cord of HAM/TSP. *J Exp Med* 1994; 180:831–839.

80 Watanabe R, Wege H, ter Meujlen V. Adoptive transfer of EAE-like lesions from rats with corona virus-induced demyelination and encephalomyelitis. *Nature* 1983; 305:50–53.

81 Evans CF, Horwitz MS, Hoobs MV, Oldstone MBA. Viral infection of transgenic mice espressing a viral protein in oligodendrocytes leads to chronic central nervous system autoimmune disease. *J Exp Med* 1996; 184:2371–2384.

82 Tough DF, Borrow P, Sprent J. Induction of T cell proliferation by viruses and type I interferon in vivo. *Science* 1996; 272:1947–1950.

83 Brocke S, Gaur A, Piercy C et al. Induction of relapsing paralysis in EAE by bacterial superantigen. *Nature* 1993; 365:642–645.

84 Burns J, Littlefield K, Gill J, Trotter JL. Bacterial toxin superantigens activate human T lymphocytes reactive with myelin autoantigens. *Eur J Immunol* 1992; 32:352–357.

85 Premack BA, Schall TJ. Chemokine receptors: gateways to inflammation and infection. *Nature Med* 1996; 2:1174–1178.

86 Baggiolini M. Chemokines and leukocyte traffic. *Nature* 1998; 392:565–568.

87 Hvas J, McLean C, Justesen J et al. Perivascular T cells express the pro-inflammatory chemokine RANTES mRNA in multiple sclerosis lesions. *Scand J Immunol* 1997; 46:195–203.

88 D'Souza S, Alinauskas K, McCrea E et al. Differential susceptibility of human CNS-derived cell populations to TNF-dependent and independent-mediated injury. *J Neurosci* 1995; 15:1513–1618.

89 Brosnan CF, Raine CS. Mechanisms of immune injury in multiple sclerosis. *Brain Pathol* 1996; 6:243–257.

90 Vergelli M, Hemmer B, Muraro PA et al. Human autoreactive CD4+ T cell clones use perforin- or Fas/Fas ligand-mediated pathways of target cell lysis. *J Immunol* 1997; 158:2756–2761.

91 Gold R, Hartung HP, Lassman H. T cell apoptosis in

autoimmune diseases: termination of inflammation in the nervous system and other sites with specialized immune-defense mechanisms. *Trends Neurosci* 1997; 20:339–404.

92 Pender MP. Genetically determined failure of activation-induced apoptosis of autoreactive T cells as a cause of multiple sclerosis. *Lancet* 1998; 351:978–981.

93 Sriram S, Rodriguez M. Indictment of the microglia as the villain in multiple sclerosis. *Neurology* 1997; 48:464.

94 Merrill JE, Benveniste EN. Cytokines in inflammatory brain lesions: helpful and harmful. *Trends Neurosci* 1996; 19:331–338.

95 Brenner T, Brocke S, Szafer F et al. Inhibition of nitric oxide synthase for treatmetn of experimental autoimmune encephalomyelitis. *J Immunol* 1997; 158:2940–2946.

96 Bernard CCA, Kerlero de Rosbo N. Multiple sclerosis: an autoimmune disease of multifactorial etiology. *Curr Opin Immunol* 1992; 4:760–765.

97 Schluesener HJ, Sobel RA, Linington C, Weiner HL. Monoclonal antibodies against a myelin oligodendrocyte glycoprotein induces relapses and demyelination in central nervous system autoimmune disease. *J Immunol* 1987; 139:4016–4021.

98 Qin Y, Duquette P, Zhang Y et al. Clonal expansion and somatic hypermutation of VH genes of B cells from cerebrospinal fluid in multiple sclerosis. *J Clin Invest* 1998; 102:1045–1050.

99 Roddy J, Clark I, Hazelman BC et al. Cerebrospinal fluid concentrations of the complement MAC inhibitor CD59 in multiple sclerosis patients and in patients with other neurological disorders. *J Neurol* 1994; 241:557–560.

100 Kerlero de Rosbo N, Bernard CCA. Multiple sclerosis brain immunoglobulins stimulate myelin basic protein degradation in human myelin: a new cause of demyelination. *J Neurochem* 1989; 53:513–518.

101 Asakura K, Rodriguez M. A unique population of circulating autoantibodies promotes central nervous system remyelination. *Multiple Sclerosis* 1998; 4:217–221.

102 Kerschensteiner M, Gallmeier L, Behrens L et al. Activated human T cells, B cells, and monocytes produce brain-derived neurotrophic factor in vitro and in inflammatory brain lesions: a neuroprotective role of inflammation? *J Exp Med* 1999; 189: 865–870.

103 Leppert D, Ford J, Stabler G et al. Matrix metalloproteinase-9 (gelatinase B) is selectively elevated in CSF during relapses and stable phases of multiple sclerosis. *Brain* 1998; 121:2327–2334.

104 Leppert D, Waubant E, Galardi R et al. T-cell gelatinases mediate basement membrane transmigration in vitro. *J Immunol* 1995; 154:3479–4389.

105 Gearing AJH, Beckett P, Christodoulou M. Processing of tumor necrosis factor-alpha precursor by metalloproteinases. *Nature* 1994; 370: 555–557.

106 McGeehan GM, Becherer JD, Bast RC et al. Regulation of tumor necrosis factor-alpha processing by a metalloproteinase inhibitor. *Nature* 1994; 370:558–561.

107 Gijbels K, Galarady RE, Steinman L. Reversal of experimental allergic encephalomyelitis with hydroxamate inhibitor of matrix metalloproteases. *J Clin Invest* 1994; 94:2177–2182.

108 Ebers GC, Sadovnick AD. The role of genetic factors in multiple sclerosis susceptibility. *J Neuroimmunol* 1994; 54:1–17.

109 Oksenberg JR, Seboun E, Hauser SL. Genetics of demyelinating diseases. *Brain Pathol* 1996; 6:289–302.

110 Poser CM. Viking voyages: the origin of multiple sclerosis? An essay in medical history. *Acta Neurol Scand Suppl* 1995; 161:11–22.

111 Compston A. Genetic epidemiology of multiple sclerosis. *J Neurol Neurosurg Psychiatry* 1997; 62:553–561.

112 Risch N. Corrections to linkage strategies for genetically complex traits. III. The effect of marker polymorphism on anlaysis of affected relative pairs. *Am J Hum Genet* 1992; 51: 673–675.

113 Sadovnick AD, Ebers GC, Dyment DA et al. Evidence for genetic basis of multiple sclerosis. *Lancet* 1996; 347:1728–1730.

114 Ebers GC, Sadovnick AD, Risch NJ. A genetic basis for familial aggregation in MS. Canadian Collaborative Study Group. *Nature* 1995; 377: 150–151.

115 Sadovnick AD, Armstrong H, Rice GPA et al. A population-based study of multiple sclerosis in twins: update. *Ann Neurol* 1993; 33:281–285.

116 Seboun E, Oksenberg JR, Hauser SL. Molecular and genetic aspects of multiple sclerosis. In: Rosenberg RG, Prusiner SB, DiMauro S, Barchi RL, eds. *The*

Molecular and Genetic Basis of Neurological Disease 2nd edn. Boston: Butterworth–Heinemann, 1996: 631–660.

117 Blankenhorn EP, Stranford SA. Genetic factors in demyelinating diseases: genes that control demyelination due to experimental allergic encephalomyelitis and Theiler's murine encephalitis virus. *Reg Immunol* 1992; **4**:331–343.

118 Encinas JA, Weiner HL, Kuchroo VK. Inheritance of susceptibility to experimental autoimmune encephalomyelitis. *J Neurosci Res* 1996; **45**:655–669.

119 Kuokkanen S, Sundvall M, Terwilliger P et al. A putative vulnerability locus to multiple sclerosis maps to 5p14-p12 in a region syntenic to the murine locus EAE2. *Nature Genet* 1996; **13**:477–480.

120 Haines JL, Pericak-Vance MA. *Approaches to Gene Mapping in Complex Human Diseases*. New York: Wiley-Liss, 1998.

121 Nepom G, Erlich HA. MHC-class II molecules and autoimmunity. *Annu Rev Immunol* 1991; **9**:493–525.

122 Olerup O, Hillert J. HLA class II-associated genetic susceptibility in multiple sclerosis: a critical evaluation. *Tissue Antigens* 1991; **38**:1–15.

123 Allen M, Sandberg-Wollheim M, Sjogren K et al. Association of susceptibility to multiple sclerosis in Sweden with HLA class II DRB1 and DQB1 alleles. *Hum Immunol* 1994; **39**:41–48.

124 Spurkland A, Ronningen K, Vandvik B et al. HLA-DQA1 and HLA-DQB1 genes may jointly determine susceptibility to develop multiple sclerosis. *Hum Immunol* 1991; **30**:69–75.

125 Smith KJ, Pyrdol J, Gauthier L et al. Crystal structure of HLA-DR2 (DRA*0101, DRB1*1501) complexed with a peptide from human myelin basic protein. *J*

Exp Med 1998; **188**:1511–1520.

126 Begovich AB, McKlure GR, Suraj V et al. Polymorphism, recombination and linkage disequilibrium within the HLA class II region. *J Immunol* 1992; **148**:249–258.

127 The Multiple Sclerosis Genetics Group. A complete genomic screen for multiple sclerosis underscores a role for the major histocompatibility complex. *Nature Genet* 1996; **13**:469–471.

128 The Multiple Sclerosis Genetics Group. Clinical demographics of multiplex families with multiple sclerosis. *Ann Neurol* 1998; **43**:530–534.

129 Sawcer S, Jones HB, Feakes R et al. A genome screen in multiple sclerosis reveals susceptibility loci on chromosome 6p21 and 17q22. *Nature Genet* 1996; **13**:464–468.

130 Ebers GC, Kukay K, Bulman DE et al. A full genome search in multiple sclerosis. *Nature Genet* 1996; **13**:472–476.

131 Kuokkanen S, Gschwend M, Rioux JD et al. Genomewide scan of multiple sclerosis in Finnish multiplex families. *Am J Hum Genet* 1997; **61**:1379–1387.

132 Lewis CM, Wise LH, Lanchbury JS. Meta-analysis of genome search results. *Am J Hum Genet* 1998; **63**:A1351.

133 Becker KG, Simon RM, Bailey-Wilson JE et al. Clustering of non-major histocompatibility complex susceptibility candidate loci in human autoimmune diseases. *Proc Natl Acad Sci U S A* 1998; **95**:9979–9984.

134 The Multiple Sclerosis Genetics Group. Linkage of the MHC to familial multiple sclerosis suggests genetic heterogeneity. *Hum Molec Genet* 1998; **7**:1229–1234.

20
Interferons

Chris H Polman, Robert M Herndon and Carlo Pozzilli

BACKGROUND

Overview of interferons

Interferons (IFNs), first recognized because of their anti-viral properties,[1] are a key defense mechanism involved in control of virus infections. They are small proteins secreted by nucleated cells in response to viral infection or other stimulation. IFNs act principally in a paracrine fashion on other cells in their immediate vicinity. They have strong immunomodulatory effects as well as anti-viral properties. On the basis of their cellular source they were initially classified as leukocyte, fibroblast or immune IFN. IFNs are now known to consist of a family of more than 20 different proteins, categorized as type I IFN (leukocyte and fibroblast IFN) and type II IFN (immune IFN) (*Table 20.1*). In humans, three distinct varieties of type I IFN (IFN-α, IFN-β, and IFN-ω) and a single type II IFN (IFN-γ) have been described to date. Current nomenclature is based on sequence analysis of the IFN genes, type I IFN genes being located on the short arm of chromosome 9 and type II on chromosome 12. There are more than 10 different IFN-α subtypes, and at least 25 allelic variants. All type I IFNs are very similar in chemical structure. IFN-α subtypes have 70% amino acid homology (i.e. 70% of the 165 or 166 amino acids are the same). IFN-β (166 amino acids) has about 30% amino acids homology with IFN-α. IFN-ω is more closely related to IFN-α. IFN-γ is a glycoprotein that contains 143 amino acids; it forms a homodimer.

IFNs exert effects through binding to high-

Table 20.1 Classification of interferons

Interferon type	Cellular source	Chromosome location	Molecular size (kDa)
Type I			
α,ω	Leucocytes	9	16–27.5
β	Fibroblasts	9	20–23
Type II			
γ	CD4+ Th$_1$ lymphocytes	12	40–70 (20–25 monomeric)

affinity cell surface receptors. There is one receptor for all type I IFNs and a separate receptor for IFN-γ. The type I receptor consists of at least two components, each of which has extracellular, transmembrane and cytoplasmic domains. These two receptor components become linked when type I IFN binds to the receptor subunits; two associated protein kinases are brought together, initiating a cascade of reactions that leads to transcription of the IFN-responsive genes. There is some evidence that there may be differences in the way some type I IFN subtypes bind, presumably reflecting differences in their three-dimensional conformation. Such differences could trigger subtype-specific responses, perhaps through the use of separate intracellular signaling pathways. Therefore, it is likely that type I IFN subtypes differ with respect to their individual activities; at present it is not clear whether these differences are mainly quantitative.[2]

History of interferon treatment in multiple sclerosis

As elegantly reviewed by Jacobs and Johnson,[3] who can be considered pioneers in this field, the rationale for initial tests of IFNs in patients with multiple sclerosis (MS) was based on the belief that the disease might be caused by a persistent or latent viral central nervous system (CNS) infection in persons with altered immune systems, and on the observed anti-viral and immunomodulatory activities of the IFNs.

During the late 1970s natural IFN-α and IFN-β were employed in phase I clinical trials. Because of limited availability of natural IFN, only small numbers of patients were included in these studies. No clear benefits were observed in these pilot studies, but natural IFN-α and IFN-β

were both well tolerated. In some of the studies IFNs were administered intrathecally because it was believed that IFN administered systemically did not effectively cross the blood–brain barrier (BBB).

The earliest trial of natural IFN-β that suggested efficacy was conducted by Jacobs and colleagues.[4] Natural IFN-β (1 MIU), was injected intrathecally twice weekly for 4 weeks, and then monthly for 5 months in 10 MS patients. Ten MS patients who did not have serial lumbar punctures were used as controls. There were significantly fewer relapses in IFN-β recipients compared with both pre-treatment rates and rates in the untreated controls. Later, Jacobs and colleagues[5] reported a larger multicenter trial that used comparable methods and doses but that also included concurrent blinded controls. The results again indicated reduction in relapse rates in treated patients compared to controls.

Because there was some evidence for decreased IFN-γ levels in the cerebrospinal fluid (CSF) of MS patients, a pilot study was performed by Panitch and colleagues[6] to assess safety and efficacy of systemic IFN-γ. This trial was terminated early because of an unexpected increase in the number of relapses during treatment. It was suggested that induction of human leukocyte antigen (HLA)-DR surface antigen on peripheral blood monocytes (indicating class II up-regulation) may have contributed to the increased relapse rate. The results of this trial raised the possibility that endogenous IFN-γ might play a role in the induction of MS relapses. Subsequent studies have focused on type 1 IFNs because it was recognized that they had a number of immunomodulatory effects that were different from IFN-γ.

Despite these early studies, it was felt that intrathecal administration of IFN-β was not likely to become an accepted mode of MS therapy because of the need for multiple lumbar punctures, with the associated inconvenience and concerns about adverse side effects (e.g., arachnoiditis). Therefore, studies were initated using intravenous, intramuscular or subcutaneous administration.These studies were feasible because of the ready availability of highly purified recombinant IFN-β. Natural IFN was abandoned.

Major efforts to evaluate the safety and efficacy of systemic recombinant IFN-β in MS were started in the US by Jacobs and by Johnson. These research programs, which started about a decade ago, have resulted in regulatory approval in the USA, Europe, or both, of three commercially available preparations of IFN-β. These are (in alphabetical order) Avonex® (IFN-β 1a, produced by Biogen), Betaseron/Betaferon® (IFN-β 1b, produced by Berlex–Schering) and Rebif® (IFN-β 1a produced by Ares-Serono).

It is important to realize that accurate comparisons of the various preparations as used in the different studies are difficult. The specific activity of the preparations differs and is higher for IFN-β 1a than for IFN-β 1b, which might be related to increased tendency in the latter for aggregate formation.[7] In addition, there is considerable controversy about the effects of different routes of administration and different dosage schedules on the biological effects of IFN-β.[8,9]

The clinical evidence leading to regulatory approval, and the scientific debate that has surrounded this approval are reviewed here. Evidence for the IFN preparations currently available is given in the order of regulatory approval.

EVIDENCE TO SUPPORT THE EFFICACY OF IFN-β IN MS

An overview of characteristics of commercially available IFN-β products and results obtained in phase 3 clinical trials is given in *Tables 20.2* and *20.3*.

Interferon-β 1b

IFN-β 1b (Betaseron® in the USA, Betaferon® in Europe) is a non-glycosylated recombinant IFN-β preparation produced by *Escherichia coli* in which serine is substituted for cysteine at position 17.

Pilot studies

Initial studies were performed by Johnson and colleagues,[10] who reported positive findings from a pilot study treating a small group of MS patients with varying doses of IFN-β 1b. Patients tolerated IFN-β 1b at dosages up to 8 MIU (according to other reference standards used at that time, the initial publications described a dosage of 45 MIU) every other day.

Phase 3 trial in relapsing–remitting MS

A phase 3 trial in relapsing–remitting MS (RRMS)[11] was conducted in seven American and four Canadian centers. It involved 372 patients with RRMS and mild-to-moderate disability (expanded disability status scale (EDSS) scores up to 5.5, mean 2.9). Treatment consisted of 8 MIU (250 μg) IFN-β 1b, 1.6 MIU (50 μg) IFN-β 1b, or placebo given by subcutaneous injection every other day. The trial was designed to last for 2 years, but patients were given the option to continue for an additional year at the end of years 2, 3, and 4. The primary outcome

Table 20.2 Characteristics of commercially available IFN-β preparations

	Recombinant IFN-β 1b	*Recombinant IFN-β 1a*	*Recombinant IFN-β 1a*
Brand name	Betaseron®, Betaferon®	Avonex®	Rebif®
Produced by	Berlex, Schering AG	Biogen	Ares-Serono
Production system	Bacteria: *Escherichia coli*	Mammalian cells: hamster CHO cells	Mammalian cells: hamster CHO cells
Chemical structure	165 amino acids Serine at 17 Lacks methionine at 1	166 amino acids Cysteine at 17 Methionine at 1	166 amino acids Cysteine at 17 Methionine at 1
Glycosylation	No	Yes	Yes
Molecular weight (kDa)	18.5	22–24	22–24
Specific activity	32 MIU/mg	> 300 MIU/mg	> 300 MIU/mg
Recommended route of administration	Subcutaneous	Intramuscular	Subcutaneous
Recommended dosage	8 MIU (250 μg) every other day	6 MIU (30 μg) once weekly	6 MIU (22 μg) three times weekly

CHO = Chinese hamster ovary

measures were the difference in relapse rates and the proportion of patients remaining free of relapses. Additional outcome measures were the severity of relapses as documented with the neurologic rating scale (NRS), the effect on disability as measured by the number of patients for whom there was a worsening of at least 1.0 EDSS point (confirmed at 3 months), and the T2-weighted lesion load on annual magnetic resonance imaging (MRI) scans. After the first 3 years the results of 2- and 3-year data were analysed and presented; patients were followed to the point of drop-out and all data derived to that point were included in the analysis. Data were also analysed separately for drop-outs, to evaluate any systematic bias this might have introduced.

The annual relapse rate after 2 years was 1.27 for patients receiving placebo, 1.17 for patients receiveing 1.6 MIU IFN-β, and 0.84 for patients receiving 8 MIU IFN-β (8 MIU versus placebo, $p = 0.0001$). The results suggested a dose response to IFN-β. Compared with placebo, treatment with the higher dose reduced the relapse rate by 31%, increased the time to first relapse and the proportion of patients who were free of relapses, and reduced by about 50% the number of patients who had moderate and severe relapses. EDSS scores changed little from baseline in both the placebo and the treatment arms.

Yearly brain MRI analyses were presented for 327 of the total 372 patients in the study. The patients in the placebo group had a mean

Table 20.3 Overview of results of phase 3 clinical trials

Interferon-β 1b (Betaseron®, Betaferon®)

Inclusion criteria

Disease type	Relapsing–remitting	Secondary progressive
Definition of activity	Two exacerbations in the previous 2 years	Two exacerbations or 1.0 (0.5) EDSS progression in the previous 2 years
EDSS range	0–5.5 (mean 2.9)	3.0–6.5 (mean 5.1)
Treatment dosage	Low dose (1.6 MIU), high dose (8.0 MIU), subcutaneously every other day	8 MIU subcutaneously every other day
Primary endpoint	Annual exacerbation rate	Confirmed EDSS progression—1.0 (5.5 or lower) or 0.5 (6.0 or higher) point
Number of patients	372	718
Planned duration	2 years	3 years
Effective duration	Extensions up to 5 years	Terminated after 2.5 years (mean)

Results

Primary endpoint	Reduction in relapse rate (30%)	Increase in time to EDSS progression (9–12 months)
Secondary endpoints		
Clinical	Increase in patients who are free of exacerbations; reduced exacerbation severity; no effect on disability	Increase in time to EDSS 7.0 (wheelchair-bound); reduced relapse rate (31%)
MRI	Significant effect on progression of total (T2) lesion load; reduced number new lesions (T2)	Significant effect on progression of total (T2) lesion load; reduced number of new lesions (T1 enhanced and T2)

Interferon-β 1a (Avonex®)

Inclusion criteria

Disease type	Relapsing
Definition of activity	Two exacerbations in the previous 3 years
EDSS range	1–3.5
Treatment dosage	30 μg intramuscularly once weekly
Primary endpoint	Confirmed (6 months) EDSS progression of 1.0 point
Number of patients	301
Planned duration	2 years
Effective duration	Median 1.5 years (range 0.5–2.3 years)

Results

Primary endpoint	Increase in time to EDSS progression
Secondary endpoints	
Clinical	Reduction in relapse rate (18–32%)
MRI	Reduced number and volume gadolinium-enhancing lesions; reduced number new T2 lesions; no significant effect on T2 lesion load

Interferon-β 1a (Rebif®)

Inclusion criteria

Disease type	Relapsing–remitting
Definition of activity	Two exacerbations in the previous 2 years
EDSS range	0–5 (mean 2.5)
Treatment dosage	Low dose (22 μg), high dose (44 μg), subcutaneously three times weekly
Primary endpoint	Annual exacerbation rate
Number of patients	560
Planned duration	2 years
Effective duration	2 years, extension ongoing

Results

Primary endpoint	Reduction in relapse rate (30%)
Secondary endpoints	
Clinical	Increase in patients who are free of exacerbations; reduced exacerbation severity; increase in time to EDSS progression
MRI	Significant effect on progression total (T2) lesion load; reduced number of new active lesions (T1 enhanced and T2)

increase of 17% in total lesion load at 3 years, compared with a mean decrease of 6% in those on high-dose IFN-β 1b. In addition, there also was a significant reduction in disease activity as measured by new or active lesions on annual MRI scans. The median number of enlarging lesions was reduced compared to placebo patients in the 8 MIU group from 3.0 to 0.5; the median number of new lesions was reduced from 2.0 to 0.5. Many of the MRI analyses also suggested a dose response, with a greater benefit from the higher dose of IFN-β 1b. Additional analyses were performed on a cohort of 52 patients at the Vancouver site, who had MRI scans every 6 weeks. This analysis also documented that IFN-β 1b reduced the accumulation of new lesions.

In general, IFN-β 1b was well tolerated. Flu-like symptoms were seen in the majority of patients in the first few months of the trial, but thereafter these symptoms gradually subsided. The other main side effect was swelling and redness at the injection site, which continued to occur after most injections. The most severe form of injection type reaction, injection site necrosis, occurred at some time in 5% of patients. Laboratory abnormalities included mild leukopenia and lymphopenia and increased liver enzymes. These typically subsided after some months. Depression and suicide attempts tended to be more frequent in IFN-β 1b recipients.

The extended study results, reported in 1995, included a median follow-up of almost 4 years. Compared with placebo, IFN-β had persistent beneficial effects on relapse rate in the 8 MIU treatment arm in each of 5 years. The difference was highly significant for the first 2 years of the study but lost statistical significance thereafter. Loss of a significant benefit on relapse rate beyond the second year could be due to fewer relapses observed during the study because of a natural decline of relapse rate observed in all arms of the study, to fewer patients remaining in the study with time (with reduced statistical power to observe an effect), to loss of efficacy, or to some combination of these factors. Of the original cohort, 217 patients had a fourth-year or fifth-year MRI scan. For these patients all scans were reanalysed at the same point in time. There was no significant progression of lesion load in the 8 MIU arm (after 5 years, increase of 3%), whereas there was a highly significant increase in lesion load over time in the placebo arm ($p = 0.0001$). Confirmed EDSS progression occurred in fewer IFN-treated patients than controls, but the difference did not reach statistical significance ($p = 0.096$).

This study provided convincing evidence that IFN-β 1b had a favorable impact on the disease as documented by the primary clinical outcome measures and confirmed with MRI parameters. However, some experts raised concerns about some of the conclusions, because it was not clear how often and at what point in time relapses were verified by neurological examination, or how this may have influenced the analysis, and because an intention-to-treat analysis was planned but not truly accomplished.[12] The latter might have introduced a systemic bias, since there was a high drop-out rate after the end of the second and third year. Because of this concern, data on drop-outs were analysed and compared with results in the patients who completed the study. Patients with more severe MS tended to drop out of all the treatment arms, but this was especially true in the placebo group, as evidenced by higher relapse rates, greater annual increases in EDSS, and higher new annual lesion burden in drop-outs. This pattern of more severe cases withdrawing from the placebo group would have the effect of lessening the apparent efficacy, however, and would not lead to false-positive results. Therefore, it seems likely that the results of the trial were valid, and the therapeutic effects may have been underestimated.

Phase 3 trial in secondary progressive MS

A second multicenter trial of IFN-β 1b was started in Europe in 1994[13], to determine the efficacy of IFN-β 1b in preventing disability in patients with secondary progressive MS (SPMS). It enrolled 718 patients with SPMS (EDSS between 3.0 and 6.5) who had been clinically active, which was defined as two relapses or a deterioration of at least 1.0 EDSS point in the 2 years preceding the study. Treatment consisted of 8 MIU of IFN-β 1b or placebo subcutaneously on alternate days. The primary outcome was the time to confirmed neurological deterioration, defined as a 1.0 point increase on EDSS sustained for at least 3 months. Worsening of 0.5 points from baseline EDSS scores of 6.0 or higher were considered to be equal to 1.0 worsening for baseline EDSS scores lower than 6.0. Pre-defined secondary outcome variables were the time to becoming wheelchair bound (EDSS 7.0), annual relapse rate, T2 lesion volume on annually performed MRI scans, and the number of newly active MRI lesions in a cohort of 125 patients who had monthly contrast-enhanced MRI scans during months 1–6 and 19–24. The study was designed for 3 years of treatment in all patients, but an interim efficacy analysis was prospectively planned to take place after all patients completed at least 24 months of treatment. An alpha level of 0.0133 was predetermined for the intention-to-treat analysis of the primary end-point as the minimum criterion to terminate the trial early.

Based on the planned interim analysis showing a highly significant difference in favor of IFN-β

1b on the primary end-point ($p = 0.0008$), the independent advisory board recommended stopping the study and switching placebo patients to active drug. At the time the study was terminated, 85% of all EDSS values to be collected in the 3-year study were available, and the mean time on study was 795 days for 358 placebo patients and 807 days for 360 IFN-β 1b patients. The delay of disability progression became apparent after 9 months of treatment and was significant until the end of the study. By comparing the survival rates for the various time periods in the study, the delay of progression ranged from 9 to 12 months. The proportion of patients with disability progression was about 50% in the placebo group and about 39% in the IFN-β 1b group ($p = 0.0048$). The beneficial effect on disability progression was present in patients with and without superimposed relapses before or during the study, and was consistent across all baseline EDSS levels studied. The time to becoming wheelchair restricted was significantly prolonged ($p = 0.0133$), and the proportion of patients becoming wheelchair restricted was 24.6% in the placebo group and 16.7% in the IFN-β 1b group ($p = 0.0277$). The relapse rate was significantly reduced by 31% over the entire study period. The number of corticosteroid courses given and the number of hospitalizations related to MS were also significantly reduced in the IFN-β 1b group. During the study, 57 patients were lost to follow-up; these included 31 placebo patients and 26 IFN-β 1b recipients. All other patients were followed until the end of study and were included in data analysis (intention-to-treat analysis) irrespective of whether they continued study drug treatment.

Treatment with IFN-β 1b resulted in a significant difference in the changes in MRI T2 lesion load measured annually in those patients of whom evaluable MRI scans were available (n = 690 at baseline, n = 607 at month 24). The mean T2 lesion volume increased in the placebo group by about 8% at 2 years, while the mean T2 lesion volume decreased by about 5% in the IFN-β 1b group. In 125 patients who had monthly MRI scans during months 1–6 and 19–24, a marked and significant reduction of new T2 and gadolinium-enhancing lesions was demonstrated. The mean cumulative number of new lesions on the monthly scans at 6 months was 10.24 in the placebo group and 3.57 in the IFN-β 1b group. At 24 months, the mean cumulative number of new lesions on all monthly scans was 7.19 in the placebo group and 1.53 in the IFN-β 1b group. The difference between the groups were significant at the first MRI scan and thereafter.

In addition to the known adverse events of IFN-β 1b treatment, other adverse events associated with IFN-β 1b treatment included hypertension (4% versus 1%, $p = 0.0117$) and muscle hypertonia (38% versus 27%, $p = 0.0032$). Symptomatic hypertonia was not accompanied by objective findings on the neurological examination. Enhanced spasticity with IFN-β 1b treatment has also been reported in patients with primary progressive MS (PPMS) by Bramanti and colleagues.[14] No increased depression was observed in the study, as assessed by adverse event documentation, a standardized depression scale (Montgomery Asberg Depression Rating Scale), or suicide attempts.

This study was the first to provide clear evidence that treatment with IFN-β 1b delays the development of sustained disability progression in patients with active SPMS.

Additional clinical studies

A number of studies have been performed at the National Institutes of Health (NIH) to characterize the MRI response to treatment with IFN-β 1b, using a baseline-versus-treatment design.[15,16] In a group of 29 RRMS patients with at least six pre-treatment monthly MRI scans and six on-treatment MRI scans, the mean frequency of gadolinium-enhancing lesions decreased significantly from 7.26 per month to 0.66 per month. The patients in this study all had very high MRI activity as measured by gadolinium-enhancing lesions. The patients showed a surprisingly homogeneous response, in that almost all patients exhibited decreases in contrast-enhancing lesions. Based on the degree of response, patients were classified as responders, partial responders, or non-responders. No differences could be identified between responders and non-responders in age at MS onset, EDSS, or number of gadolinium-enhancing lesions on the initial MRI study. The sample size was relatively small, so differences based on these parameters cannot be excluded.

Some studies have investigated the effect of IFN-β 1b on measures of neuropsychological function (see Chapter 3). Pliskin and colleagues[17] studied visual reproduction in 30 patients who participated in the multicentre study in RRMS. A significant improvement in Wechsler Memory Scale Visual Reproduction-Delayed Recall scores was found in subjects receiving 8 MIU IFN-β 1b. These results need to be interpreted cautiously because the neuropsychological studies were not instituted before initiating study drug (i.e. there were no baseline neuropsychological studies). Effects on verbal memory functioning were examined in 167 patients with RRMS and 112 matched normal controls by Selby and colleagues.[18] Subjects treated with IFN-β 1b (n = 73) did not perform significantly better than those not receiving the drug (n = 94), although the mean performance of treated subjects tended to be higher across all 10 verbal memory tests applied. A beneficial effect of IFN-β 1b in this study could have been obscured by the process of patient selection, since patients were not randomized for treatment, or by the fact that neuropsychological function was relatively preserved in this patient sample.

Post-marketing experience in thousands of patients has confirmed that flu-like symptoms are transient and persist indefinitely in only about 4% of patients, and that they can be treated effectively with ibuprofen before and during the 8–24 hours after injection. Injection site necrosis occurs at some time in 4–5% of patients, but only rarely after each injection or at multiple sites. In some patients, poor injection technique or unintentional intravascular injection may be a contributing factor. Necrotizing cutaneous lesions caused by IFN-β 1b injections have been investigated by a number of groups.[19,20,21] Biopsy specimens show a mixed perivascular infiltrate, focal capillary or venous thrombosis, and a localized vasculitis in some patients. A more systematic biopsy study involved 10 patients with various types of cutaneous lesions at the injection sites, including subtle non-inflamed sclerotic dermal plaques, erythematous plaques, and cutaneous ulcers. There was a spectrum of histological findings including fibrosis and vascular thrombosis.[22]

Currently, a large phase 3, double-masked, placebo-controlled study evaluating two doses of IFN-β 1b (8 MIU every other day or 5 MIU/m^2 every other day) in SPMS is ongoing in the USA. The primary end-point, and the entry criteria were essentially the same as in the European SPMS study. Additional end-points focus on relapse rate, MRI, cognition, quality of life, corticosteroid use, and hospitalizations.

Interferon-β 1a (Avonex®)

IFN-β 1a (Avonex®) is a glycosylated recombinant IFN-β preparation that is obtained from Chinese hamster ovary (CHO) cells. It is identical to the native molecule at the biochemical and molecular level. It has been administered clinically by the intramuscular route.

Pilot studies

Pilot studies relevant to the phase 3 trial were mainly those with intrathecal administration of natural IFN-β reviewed earlier.[4,23] Several factors led to the decision to proceed with a trial of IFN-β 1a using intramuscular injections:

(a) the risks of intrathecal therapy were felt to be unsatisfactory for routine use in MS patients;

(b) patient acceptance of intrathecal therapy was expected to be limited;

(c) several lines of evidence suggested that systemically administered IFN might be effective, including evidence for inducible IFN activity in the brain after systemic administration, even with an intact BBB;

(d) it was thought that an effect on circulating lymphocytes could have an effect on the CNS; and

(e) the development of recombinant DNA technology meant that the use of higher doses had become feasible.

Phase 3 trial in relapsing MS

Design factors

The IFN-β 1a phase 3 trial was planned and a research proposal submitted to the NIH. The initial plan included intrathecal and systemic arms. It was extensively modified in consultation with and on the recommendations of the NIH review committee, leading to the final design. In the process, the intrathecal arm of the study was dropped.[24] Several important design features that directly affected the study results deserve comment.

A decision was made to not use relapses as the primary outcome measure based in part on the risk of unblinding. Patients must report relapses to the neurologist. It was thought that reporting of relapses by unblinded patients might be biases. That was considered unacceptable for the primary study outcome measure. This concern also affected the dose chosen for the trial. That decision was based on a pilot trial, which showed that 30 μg was the highest dose that could be effectively masked, along with the observation that markers of the IFN response were elevated for about 1 week after each dose. A blinding analysis carried out after completion of the study demonstrated that blinding was effective.

There was discussion regarding the use of more than one dose, but no systemic IFN had been shown to be effective at the time, and the study was planned as a phase 2 trial. Therefore, a single dose was felt to be adequate to establish an effect of therapy. A second dose would have increased the cost of the trial by about 50%, which was a significant issue for an NIH-sponsored trial. It was only after the trial was funded and a pharmaceutical company became involved that the study was converted to a phase 3 trial. Based on these factors, treatment consisted of 30 μg IFN-β 1a or placebo given once weekly via the intramuscular route.

The trial was designed to last 2 years. Inclusion criteria included definite MS with disease duration at least 1 year, EDSS of 1.0–3.5, at least two relapses in the previous 3 years documented in the medical record, and no relapses for at least

2 months at study entry. The primary outcome variable was time to disability progression of at least 1.0 point on the EDSS present on at least two consecutive scheduled study visits (i.e. lasting at least 6 months). The decision to use disability as the primary end-point and to use survival analysis rather than a fixed period of treatment was done in collaboration between the investigator group and the NIH review committee. This had several important consequences, which were both good and bad. First, it largely eliminated the potential effect of unblinding on the primary outcome measure. With the use of a blinded examining physician to determine the EDSS score, there was little risk of bias based on unblinding, even if patients were able to guess whether they were on IFN-β 1a or placebo. Secondly, survival analysis, rarely used in MS trials previously, is a highly efficient method of capturing information on the primary end-point. This results in a lower required sample size. Thirdly, survival trials are commonly terminated when the prospectively determined statistical goals are met, adding to the efficiency of the method. Fourthly, this type of analysis has the disadvantage that there are relatively few patients at later time points, so that data may be inadequate to establish statistical significance for some important secondary end-points. Fifthly, this type of study focuses efficacy analysis on shorter treatment times, so it can be difficult to detect a delayed treatment effect. This problem can be exaggerated if there are significant recruiting delays.

The decision to require a 1.0 point worsening on the EDSS sustained for 6 months was based on a pilot trial demonstrating that a 1.0 point change in the EDSS could be reliably detected.[25] The investigator group decided by consensus that a 1.0 point worsening, sustained for 6 months, was clinically meaningful. A 2.0 point change sustained at 6 months may have been a less controversial primary end-point.[26] As indicated, sustained worsening of at least 1.0 point as measured by a blinded examining physician (separate from the treating physician) was introduced to minimize the unblinding that can occur when relapses are used as the primary outcome. Unfortunately, even with the EDSS outcome, the examining physician may be able to surmise that a patient has reported a relapse if a special study visit is scheduled outside the regularly scheduled interval visits. It may be preferable in future trials to have the treating physician assess relapses and to restrict the contact with the examining physician to fixed intervals.

Results of the trial

A total of 301 patients with relapsing MS were enrolled at four clinical centers. Treatment with IFN-β 1a resulted in significant delay by 37% in the time to sustained EDSS progression ($p = 0.02$).[27] The Kaplan–Meier estimate of the proportion of patients progressing by the end of 104 weeks was 34.9% in the placebo group and 21.9% in the IFN-β 1a group. Post hoc analyses using more stringent end-points was completed to explore further the effect of IFN-β 1a treatment on EDSS scores.[28] When disability progression was defined as a 1.0 point worsening or greater sustained for 1 year (as opposed to 6 months), the Kaplan–Meier estimates of the proportion of patients progressing by week 104 was 29.8% in the placebo group and 11.5% in the IFN-β 1a group ($p = 0.002$). When disability progression was defined as requiring at least a 2.0 point worsening (as opposed to a 1.0 point worsening) sustained for 6 months, the Kaplan–Meier estimate of the proportion of patients progressing by the end of 104 weeks was 18.3% in the placebo group and 6.1% in the

IFN-β 1a group ($p = 0.028$). The percentage with sustained worsening to at least an EDSS of 4 was 14% in the placebo group and 5% in the IFN-β 1a group ($p = 0.014$). The percentage with sustained worsening to an EDSS of 6 (unilateral assistance needed to walk) was 7% in the placebo group and 1% in the IFN-β 1a group ($p = 0.028$). The time to sustained EDSS 4.0 was increased in the IFN-β 1a group by 65%, and the time to sustained EDSS 6 was increased in the IFN-β 1a group by 86%. These analyses indicate that IFN-β 1a treatment markedly reduced large amounts of worsening on the EDSS scale observed in some placebo-treated patients. The results should be interpreted with some caution, because they are based on a relatively small sample and because the follow-up period was rather short.

The treatment effect of IFN-β 1a on EDSS was further supported by a statistically significant difference in favor of IFN-β 1a using a composite score based on timed measures of neurologic function. The combination of the timed 10 m walk, nine-hole peg test, and box and blocks test was as sensitive as the EDSS in detecting efficacy.[28]

The effect on relapses in this trial has been the subject of controversy. For all study participants, regardless of the time on study, there was an 18% reduction in the annualized relapse rate in the IFN-β 1a group ($p = 0.03$). For only those study participants who were entered into the trial early enough to complete two years or more, there was a 32% reduction in the annualized relapse rate in the IFN-β 1a group ($p = 0.002$). It is important to emphasize that patients were in the study for less than 2 years because of the study design, which called for variable periods of follow-up, and not because they dropped out of the study. Nevertheless, there are a number of possible explanations for the observed difference between reduction in relapse rates in the 2-year cohort compared with the entire study cohort. One explanation would be that the treatment effect on relapses increased over time. Another contributing factor may have been that the inclusion of patients with very little time on the study decreased the relapse rate in the placebo cases because more patients had no relapses. This would result in a lower annualized relapse rate in the comparative group and an apparent decrease in the treatment effect. Another possibility is that patients who were more active were entered into the trial in the early months of recruitment, with patients who were less active entering the trial towards the end. This would have the effect of lowering the relapse rate in those patients on the study for less time.

Patients treated with IFN-β 1a had significantly lower number and volume of gadolinium-enhanced brain lesions on MRI scans (*p* values ranging between 0.02 and 0.05). Active treatment resulted in a significant decrease in the number of new, enlarging, and new plus enlarging T2 lesions over 2 years.[29] The median increase in T2 lesion volume at 1 year was 455 mm^3 in placebo patients and 152 mm^3 in IFN-β 1a patients; at 2 years, the corresponding figures were 1410 mm^3 and 628 mm^3. The treatment group differences did not reach statistical significance at 2 years.

Treatment with IFN-β 1a was well tolerated and caused no substantial toxicity. More than 90% of patients completed treatment as planned. Flu-like symptoms were reported more frequently in IFN-β 1a recipients, but these symptoms were mild and transient. All patients had weekly injections given either at the study sites or by a designated health-care professional, so that there was good ascertainment of injection site reactions.

There was no inflammation or pain at injection sites, and study nurses who injected the medication weekly were unable to identify which patients were receiving IFN-β 1a.

One criticism of this trial has been that the placebo group did worse than natural history control groups. However, natural history control groups are probably not an appropriate comparison, and progression rates in the IFN-β 1a study were comparable to relapsing–remitting cohorts in the sulfasalazine trial and the IFN-β 1a (Rebif®) trial.[30,31]

Additional clinical studies

A phase 4 safety extension study using IFN-β 1a was started about 1 year after the initial trial was completed. The IFN-β 1a product used for the extension study and for clinical use was made in a new manufacturing facility that incorporated additional purification steps instituted to reduce aggregate formation. The extension study is continuing. As of August 1998, the median duration of treatment was 128 weeks. Seventy-five percent of the patients had received drug for more than 2 years at this time and 37% had received drug for over 2.5 years. No new adverse events or risks have been identified. The number of courses of intravenous corticosteroids were used as a surrogate for relapses. Patients who had received placebo in the initial trial had a decrease in annual intravenous corticosteroid courses from 0.83 to 0.44 (*p* = 0.001). The rate in patients who had received IFN-β 1a in the initial trial decreased from 0.59 to 0.48, although this change was not statistically significant (*p* = 0.10). This study, which is continuing, suggests that the safety and effectiveness of the drug is sustained.

Additional ongoing clinical trials include a placebo-controlled trial of 30 μg IFN-β 1a intramuscularly once weekly in patients with a first episode suggestive of inflammatory demyelinating disease. The primary outcome measure for this study is the time to new clinical relapse. A dose-ranging study is comparing 30 μg and 60 μg IFN-β 1a once-weekly intramuscular administration in patients with RRMS. The primary outcome measure is the time to confirmed EDSS progression. A placebo-controlled trial of 60 μg IFN-β 1a once weekly intramuscularly is being conducted in patients with SPMS. The primary outcome measure is a change in the MS functional composite, which consists of quantitative tests of walking speed, arm function, and cognitive function (see Chapter 2).

Interferon-β 1a (Rebif®)

IFN-β 1a (Rebif®) is another glycosylated recombinant IFN-β preparation obtained in Chinese hamster ovary cells. It is identical to the native molecule at both the biochemical and the molecular level. It has been clinically applied so far via the subcutaneous route.

Pilot studies

The first promising results with this form of recombinant IFN-β 1a were obtained in a trial in RRMS designed to investigate effects on MRI.[32] After a 6-month pre-treatment period, 68 patients were randomly assigned to receive either 3 MIU (11 μg) or 9 MIU (33 μg) of IFN-β 1a by subcutaneous injection three times per week for an initial period of 6 months. All patients were examined by gadolinium-enhanced MRI every month during both pre-treatment and treatment phases. The trial used the mean number and volume of gadolinium-enhancing lesions seen on monthly T1-weighted MRI as the primary end-point.

Analysis of data from the first 12 months of the study showed that the mean number and volume of gadolinium-enhancing lesions per patient per scan were significantly lower during treatment with IFN-β 1a than during the pre-treatment period. The number of lesions was reduced by 49% with the 11 μg dose and by 64% with the 33 μg dose, while lesion volume was reduced by 61% with the 11 μg dose and by 73% with the 33 μg dose. The initial findings were confirmed by results obtained from the same group of patients after 2 years of treatment.[33] The difference in efficacy between the low dose and the high dose became significant only in the second year of treatment, suggesting that this dose effect increases with time.

Phase 3 trial in RRMS

The PRISMS (Prevention of Relapses and disability by Interferon beta-1a Subcutaneously in MS) trial involved 560 patients with RRMS from 22 centres in Europe, Canada, and Australia.[31] All patients had at least two relapses during the 2 years before the study and an EDSS score of 0–5.0 at the time of entry into the study. They were randomly assigned to receive 6 MIU (22 μg) or 12 MIU (44 μg) of IFN-β 1a or placebo three times weekly by subcutaneous injection for 2 years. The primary outcome measure was the number of relapses over the course of the study. Secondary efficacy end-points were the time to the first and second relapse, the proportion of relapse-free patients, progression in disability (defined as an increase in EDSS of at least 1.0 point sustained over at least 3 months), the need for corticosteroid therapy and hospital admission, and disease activity and burden of disease (as measured by MRI). A further efficacy end-point used in this trial was the Integrated Disability Status Scale (IDSS), a new measure that is calculated from the area under a curve generated by plotting the EDSS score against time.[34] This is intended to measure the overall change in EDSS over time. An intention-to-treat analysis was conducted on all outcome measures. Of the 560 patients randomized, 502 (90%) completed 2 years of treatment. Because roughly half of the patients who stopped therapy early were followed clinically, 2 years of data were available for 533 (95%) patients.

The mean number of relapses during the 2 years of the study was significantly lower in both IFN-β 1a groups than in the placebo group ($p < 0.005$). The percentage reduction was 27% with the 22 μg dose and 33% with the 44 μg dose. The mean number of moderate or severe relapses and the mean number of corticosteroid courses were significantly decreased in patients receiving IFN-β 1a (at both doses) and the mean number of hospital admissions for MS was significantly reduced in patients receiving the higher dose (significant differences from placebo for both doses; no significant differences between doses).

Both doses of IFN-β 1a delayed progression in disability and decreased accumulated disability as measured by the IDSS. There were no significant differences between the two doses of IFN in the time to disability progression or in the proportion of patients with disability progression, however. A dose effect in favor of the higher dose was evident in some of the MRI findings, particularly the number of new lesions seen on T2-weighted and gadolinium-enhanced T1-weighted images.[35] The burden of disease measured with proton density or T2 MRI showed an accumulation of 10.9% in the placebo-treated patients and a decrease of 1.2% and 3.4% in the 22 μg and 44 μg groups, respectively ($p < 0.0001$ compared with placebo for both doses). The number of T2-active lesions on the twice-yearly MRI scans was also significantly lower in the low-dose and high-dose groups than in the placebo group (difference 67% and 78%, $p < 0.0001$), and there was a dose effect in favor of the 44 μg dose over the 22 μg dose ($p = 0.0003$).

Both doses of IFN-β 1a were well tolerated. The most common events were headache, fever, and myalgia. The only significant difference between patients treated with IFN-β 1a and placebo recipients was the occurrence of injection site reactions, which were equally common with both doses of IFN-β 1a. The incidence of depression was similar in the three groups. Significant, though asymptomatic, decreases in white cells and neutrophil counts and significant increases in aminotransferases were seen in patients treated with IFN-β 1a. The changes were more pronounced in patients receiving the higher dose. There were 17 (3%) adverse events that resulted in drop-out from the study: two in the placebo group, six in the 22 μg group and nine in the 44 μg group.

Despite the claim by the authors of the study that there was a dose-response effect for most of the clinical outcome measures and especially so for the MRI outcomes, the accompanying editorial commented that the evidence for a clinically relevant dose-related treatment effect was not convincing.[36] On the one hand, the use of the higher dose of IFN-β 1a in this trial did not lead to a proportional increase in clinical benefits, suggesting a plateau of the therapeutic effects at higher doses. On the other hand, the dose effects seen on some of the MRI end-points raises the possibility that clinical differences between the two doses may not be adequately reflected by the clinical parameters, or may be delayed beyond the 2-year follow-up. Studies with longer follow-up and studies aimed at evaluating the effects of an increased dose in the individual patient may clarify this issue.

Additional clinical studies

In the OWIMS (Once Weekly Interferon beta-1a in MS) study, 293 patients with RRMS were randomized to receive 6 MIU (22 µg) or 12 MIU (44 µg) of IFN-β 1a or placebo by subcutaneous injection once weekly for 48 weeks. The primary outcome measure was disease activity measured by monthly cranial MRI scans that included analysis of both T2 lesions and gadolinium-enhancing lesions. Preliminary reports of the study results showed that the number of active lesions was reduced in a dose-dependent fashion by IFN-β 1a.[37] Over the first 24 weeks of treatment, the median reduction in the number of active (new T2 and gadolinium-enhancing) lesions on monthly scans compared with placebo was 29.6% (not significant) with the lower dose and 53.5% ($p < 0.01$) with the higher dose. In addition, active treatment had a beneficial effect on several secondary outcome measures, including the percentage of MRI scans showing active lesions, total T2 lesion load, and relapse rate. These results confirm previous data showing that the number of active lesions seen on MRI represents the most sensitive tool to demonstrate the dose effect of IFN-β 1a.[35,38]

The ability of IFN-β 1a to delay the onset of clinically definite MS after a first attack is at present under investigation in a multicentre, randomized, double-blind, placebo-controlled, phase 3 clinical trial named ETOMS (Early Treatment of MS).[39] The primary objective of the study is to evaluate the efficacy of IFN-β 1a, administered subcutaneously in a dosage of 22 µg once a week for 2 years, in reducing the rate of conversion to clinically definite MS as defined by the occurrence of a second relapse after a first attack sug-

gestive of MS. Secondary end-points are the time to the second relapse, the duration and the severity of the second relapse, and the disease activity and burden of disease as measured by annual MRI. The baseline characteristics of the 311 patients who entered the study have recently been reported.[40] The most common symptoms at presentation were, in decreasing order of frequency, sensory, motor, visual, and oculomotor. A multifocal clinical presentation was observed in 14% of the patients and was associated with a higher MRI disease burden. The results of ETOMS will be available by the end of 1999.

Another multicentre, randomized, double-blind, placebo-controlled, phase 3 trial including more than 600 patients is ongoing in the treatment of secondary progressive MS.[41] In this trial, patients were randomized to receive 6 MIU (22 µg) or 12 MIU (44 µg) of IFN-β 1a or placebo, three times a week by subcutaneous injection for 3 years. The primary aim of the trial is to investigate the effects of therapy on the deterioration of disability, as defined as the time to an increase by 1.0 point on the EDSS scale (or by 0.5 point in patients with baseline scores above 5.5). Secondary objectives are the number of relapses, the duration and severity of relapses, the disease activity and lesion burden as measured by MRI, and safety and tolerability. The results of this trial are expected to be available by the end of 1999.

MECHANISM OF ACTION OF IFN-β IN MS

An overview of the biological effects of IFN-β is shown in *Table 20.4*.

This chapter is written in the assumption that the mechanism of action of all licensed IFN-β

Table 20.4 Overview of relevant biological effects of IFN-β

Effects of IFN-β on cytokine production
    Suppression of production of IFN-γ
    Increased production of IL-10
    More generalized shift from production of pro-inflammatory to anti-inflammatory cytokines

Effects of IFN-β on permeability of BBB
    Effects on adhesion molecules, chemokines, and matrix metalloproteinases

Effects of IFN-β on glial cells

Other potential targets for the therapeutic action of IFN-β
    Down-regulation of activation markers on immunocompetent cells
    Down-regulation of antigen presentation
    Antiproliferative effects on T lymphocytes
    Reinstatement of deficient suppressor cell function
    Effects on T-lymphocyte apoptosis
    Anti-viral effects

preparations is essentially the same, and therefore no distinction is made here between studies performed with IFN-β 1b and those with IFN-β 1a. In addition to the information presented here, the reader may find authoritative reviews on the mechanisms of action of IFN-β in MS by Weinstock-Guttman and colleagues,[42] Arnason and colleagues,[43] and Yong and colleagues.[44]

Knowledge on the mechanism of action of IFN-β is far from complete and research in this field has been significantly hampered by the fact that the pharmacokinetics of IFN-β in MS patients is only partially understood. Biological markers have often been used as a means of indirectly quantifying the effects of IFN-β because the methods of quantifying IFN-β in the blood are biological and time consuming and require the handling of infectious agents. These methods have tended to yield either very low or no measurable levels of IFN-β after subcutaneous or intramuscular administration. It is hoped that enzyme-linked immunosorbent assays that have recently become available will be helpful in the future in that they will allow to study the relation between dosage of IFN-β, serum levels, clinical effects and observed immunologic effects.[45,46]

Pan and colleagues[47] have performed radioactive labeling experiments to examine the permeability of the mouse (BBB) and blood–spinal cord barrier for various cytokines, including type I IFN (IFN-α) and IFN-γ. They found that, although there were regional differences, IFNs had access to the CNS. The cervical and lumbosacral spinal cord had higher permeability than the thoracic spinal cord and brain. Although important, these studies may or may not be relevant to the therapeutic effects in MS, because it is not clear whether IFN-β directly exerts therapeutic effects in the CNS. It might well be that it induces its effects in the periphery and that these effects involve cell-mediated transfer of activity. Some evidence for this can be derived from experiments by Fleischman and colleagues,[48] who found that at least part of the biological effect of IFN could be passively transferred to other laboratory animals by injection of blood cells and not plasma.

Among the many mechanisms that have been suggested as being responsible for the beneficial effects of IFN-β (which probably should be classified as mainly anti-inflammatory), two have been especially highlighted. These are the effects on cytokine production by various inflammatory cell types and those on the permeability of the BBB to inflammatory cells.

Effects of IFN-β on cytokine production

Based on studies in murine models, activated CD4+ T lymphocytes can be subdivided into T-helper 1 (Th$_1$) and T-helper 2 (Th$_2$) cells on the basis of the profile of cytokines that they produce. Th$_1$ cells secrete IL-2, tumor necrosis factor (TNF)-β, and IFN-γ, which regulate pro-inflammatory effector mechanisms involved in cell-mediated immunity. The Th$_2$ subset produces IL-4, IL-5, IL-6, IL-10, and IL-13, up-regulates humoral immunity, and down-regulates inflammatory effector mechanisms in cell-mediated immunity. There is some experimental evidence to suggest that Th$_1$ cytokines may propagate inflammation in MS whereas Th$_2$ cytokines may inhibit the disease process. Of cautionary note, however, is the fact that the Th$_1$ versus Th$_2$ paradigm represents an extreme oversimplification, that many cells secrete combinations of Th$_1$ and Th$_2$ cytokines, and that an immune shift in the direction of the anti-inflammatory Th$_2$ phenotype might also have an unfavorable effect on the MS, probably by an increase in antibody-mediated tissue damage. This has already been clearly demonstrated for a primate model of MS. Recent neuropathological studies, which demonstrate the pathological heterogeneity of MS and re-emphasize the important role of antibody-mediated demyelination in some subforms of disease, have again alerted us to this possibility.[49,50] Even though there are some conflicting results, most studies suggest that IFN-β causes a shift of cytokine production from that of a Th$_1$-like to a Th$_2$-like phenotype.

The rationale of giving IFN-β in MS was partly based on antagonistic effects on IFN-γ-induced immunologic reactions and, indeed, a number of studies have documented that IFN-β reduces the number of IFN-γ-producing cells and the production of IFN-γ.[51,52] Remarkably, it has been reported, however, that the number of IFN-γ-secreting cells in the blood rises in more than 50% of MS patients in the first 2 months after onset of IFN-β therapy and then fall back into the normal range after 3 months.[53] The down-regulating effect on IFN-γ might be significant because IFN-γ is a pro-inflammatory cytokine with many functions, including the activation of cells of the monocyte lineage, and the up-regulation of several adhesion molecules on endothelial cells that regulate the passage of inflammatory cells through the BBB (see below). In humans, IFN-γ has been demonstrated to worsen the symptoms of MS (see above). The mechanism by which IFN-β can counteract the effect of IFN-γ is by blocking antigen presentation, because induction of MHC class II expression on many cell types is a prominent feature of IFN-γ. Indeed, this has been demonstrated for a number of antigen-presenting cells by Jiang and colleagues.[54] In their experiments, treatment of human fetal astrocytes, microglial cells, or B lymphocytes with IFN-β resulted in a reduction in the IFN-γ-enhanced alloantigen-induced T-cell responses. This reduction ranged between 50% and 80% and was associated with a significant reduction in HLA class II (DR) expression. The mechanism by which IFN-β inhibits IFN-γ-enhanced class II expression might be dependent on the cell type.[55,56]

Another cytokine that has been implicated as being affected by treatment with IFN-β is IL-10. In vitro studies have demonstrated that IFN-β significantly stimulates IL-10 secretion by monocytes[57] and T lymphocytes[58] after brief incubation. Subsequently it was demonstrated that treatment with IFN-β also causes in vivo increases in plasma IL-10 levels, in vivo responses in individual patients being closely related to in vitro responses.[59] Both in vitro and in vivo effects of IFN-β were also studied by Rudick and colleagues.[60] They demonstrated that IFN-β induced accumulation of IL-10 messenger RNA (mRNA) and protein secretion by cultured peripheral blood mononuclear cells and that intramuscular injections of IFN-β increased serum levels of IL-10. This increase was dose-dependent and relatively specific in that it was not observed for TGF-β, another anti-inflammatory cytokine.

Two recent studies have strengthened the importance of the relationship between IL-10 induction by IFN-β treatment and clinical efficacy. Porrini and colleagues[61] studied a number of in vitro immunomodulatory effects of IFN-β (Concanavalin A (ConA)-induced suppressor cell function and IFN-γ production) and found that these effects could be substantially blocked by the administration of an anti-IL-10 monoclonal antibody. Rudick and colleagues[62] studied in vivo immunologic effects of IFN-β treatment and their relationship to clinical efficacy. Cytokines were measured in blood and CSF and it was found that single intramuscular injections of IFN-β were associated with significant up-regulation of IL-10 and IL-4 but not of IFN-γ mRNA in peripheral blood mononuclear cells. Serum IL-10 levels increased after injection and significantly increased concentrations of CSF IL-10 were shown in those patients who had received IFN-β 1a in a clinical trial for about 2 years. Remarkably, this increase correlated with a favorable therapeutic response.

Other effects on cytokine production that have been observed, although less consistently, during treatment with IFN-β include a decrease in TNF-α production, an increase in IL-6 production, inhibition of IL-1β production, an increase in the production of the natural IL-1 antagonist IL-1 receptor antagonist, and an increase in the pro-duction of TGF-β and its receptor.[63–66] Although most of these studies point in the same direction (that of a shift from a pro- to an anti-inflammatory cytokine profile), it is important to realize that other studies that have been published do not suggest that IFN-β has an effect on the cytokine secretion of mononuclear cells in MS.[67,68] It is not at all clear whether these conflicting results are due to different laboratory techniques being employed, to differences between the in vitro and the in vivo situation, to heterogeneity in patients studied or to the fact that the response to IFN-β seems to show marked fluctuations over time.[69]

Effects of IFN-β on permeability of the BBB

One of the most dramatic effects observed in clinical studies with IFN-β is the pronounced reduction in gadolinium-enhancing lesions on contrast-enhanced MRI that occurs almost immediately after onset of treatment (described earlier). Since gadolinium enhancement is merely a reflection of unphysiologic BBB permeability, a therapeutic effect at this level seems most likely. The infiltration of T cells through the BBB into the CNS is considered a key event in the pathogenesis of MS.[70] Only activated T cells penetrate an intact BBB, whose first and strongest component is the endothelial lining. A cascade of sequentially interacting pairs of adhesion molecules seems to be responsible for the transendothelial migration of T cells into the target organ. First, T cells establish a loose and reversible contact with endothelial cells via selectins and their ligands. This initial selectin-mediated rolling is followed by a firm irreversible adhesion mediated by integrins and members of the immunoglobulin superfamily, such as very late antigen (VLA)-4 binding to vascular cell adhesion molecule (VCAM)-1 and leukocyte function-associated molecule (LFA)-1 binding to ICAM-1. The subsequent transendothelial migration is thought to be mediated mainly by VLA-4–VCAM-1 interaction. Some of these adhesion molecules, such as ICAM-1, VCAM-1 and selectins, are shed from the surface of endothelial cells and T cells after their interaction and can be measured as circulating forms in the serum; according to some studies the levels of these circulating forms increase with the severity of pathology. Following these events, the production of proteases (especially matrix metalloproteinases) by T cells is important because, after migration across endothelial cells, the basement membrane has to be degraded in order for cells to extravasate into the CNS parenchyma.

Many different in vitro experiments, both on endothelium and peripheral blood mononuclear cells, have investigated the effects of IFN-β on adhesion phenomena and adhesion molecules. Effects of IFN-β on expression of ICAM-1, VCAM-1, VLA-4, or E-selectin were small and inconsistent.[71–73] Remarkably, the counteractive effect of IFN-β on IFN-γ-induced expression of MHC class II molecules was a very consistent finding in these studies. In vivo experiments, using sera and blood mononuclear cells from MS patients treated with IFN-β were performed by Calabresi and colleagues[74] and by Corsini and colleagues.[75] Calabresi[74] determined levels of soluble VCAM-1, ICAM-1, E-selectin, L-selectin, and TNF receptor (60 kDa) in monthly serum samples from 11 patients with MS before and during treatment with IFN-β 1b and correlated the levels with the number of newly enhancing lesions on monthly contrast-enhanced MRI scans. The only significant change during treatment was the increase in soluble VCAM-1, which

correlated with a decrease in the number of contrast-enhancing lesions on MRI. An initial increase in soluble VCAM was followed by a subsequent decrease, which was explained by reduced expression over time following initial shedding into the bloodstream. Interpretation of these data of course is complicated by the fact that it is impossible to determine the origin of soluble adhesion molecules in the serum: are measured differences related to processes at the level of the BBB or do they represent altered adhesion molecule expression at the level of other target organs, for example lymphoid organs? Corsini[75] found that monocytes and lymphocytes isolated from MS patients during treatment with IFN-β adhered less well to human endothelial cells than did cells obtained before treatment.

Two groups have independently demonstrated that the therapeutic mechanism of IFN-β might be based on a diminished capacity of T lymphocytes to migrate through the BBB owing to the decreased activity of a neutral proteinase, gelatinase B (matrix metalloprotienase (MMP)-9).[76,77]

Effects of IFN-β on glial cells

The effects of IFN-β in the CNS are poorly understood and highly speculative, since it is not known whether IFN-β as administered in the clinical context reaches the CNS compartment in a biologically active form and in significant concentrations. The effects of IFN-β on a number of glial cells have been studied and the results seem to depend on the cell type studied and on the state of maturation and differentiation. IFN-β has been shown to be capable of antagonizing IFN-γ-mediated class II expression on cultured human astrocytes, an astrocytoma cell line and neonatal rodent microglia, whereas this effect could not be demonstrated for fetal astrocytes and adult microglia.[56] It also is a critical regulator of IL-1 receptor antagonist and IL-1 expression in human microglia.[78]

Now that recent evidence from both neuropathological and MRI studies strongly suggests that neuronal loss can appear early in MS, and can even, although clinically silent, be a very important prognostic factor for the development of permanent disability, it is important to focus research on the direct and indirect effects that IFN-β might have on neurons.[79] So far only limited research has been performed, but initial studies suggest that IFN-β is capable of decreasing induced nitric oxide production by a human astrocytoma cell line, and that pre-treatment of astrocytes with type I IFN impairs IFN-γ-induced production of nitric oxide synthase as well as neuronal mitochondrial respiratory chain damage.[80–82] Other studies have demonstrated that IFN-β can limit astrocyte proliferation in vitro, which has been suggested to be an important factor limiting neuronal repair in MS lesions, and that it can promote production of nerve growth factor by astrocytes.[83,84] It has to be re-emphasized that these results can so far only be interpreted as preliminary and that therefore it is impossible to determine whether these effects of IFN-β really occur in vivo and whether they play any role in limiting damage to neuronal cells or promoting neuronal repair.

Other targets for the therapeutic action of IFN-β in MS

This review does not claim to give a complete discussion of mechanisms that might play a role in mediating the therapeutic action of IFN-β.

Mechanisms that are not discussed here include down-regulation of activation markers on immunocompetent cells, anti-proliferative effects on T lymphocytes, and reinstatement of the deficient suppressor cell function in MS patients.[68,85,86]

Preliminary evidence suggests that IFN-β has an effect on serum levels of soluble CD95 (APO-1/Fas).[59,87] CD95-mediated apoptosis has been recognized as one of the mechanisms for regulating the survival of activated T cells. Elimination of inflammatory T cells by apoptosis appears to play an important role in the down-regulation of inflammation in the CNS.[88]

Of course, the possibility that the main beneficial effect of IFN-β in MS is related to its antiviral effects cannot be completely excluded. The fact that herpesviruses are present in many MS plaques and that these viruses are activated by other viral infections that activate MS raises the possibility that they are an aggravating factor that might be favorably influenced by IFNs. The observation that in patients who participated in the phase 3 trial for IFN-β 1b in RRMS (see above) there was no difference in the number of viral illnesses between IFN-β and placebo recipients does, however, make this option less likely.[89]

Unfortunately, animal research has not been very helpful in elaborating the effects of IFN-β and its underlying mechanisms in MS. Initial studies in the animal model experimental allergic encephalomyelitis (EAE) could even be considered as misleading because they gave variable results in relation to administration of IFN-β and suggested that (as opposed to findings in MS) administration of exogenous IFN-γ might provide protection against subsequent relapses.[90] Recent observations that the length of treatment determines whether IFN-β prevents or aggravates EAE and that discontinuation of treatment with IFN-β leads to very severe relapses of EAE also do not have an obvious clinical correlate in MS.[91,92]

ANTIBODIES INDUCED BY TREATMENT WITH IFN-β

Neutralizing antibodies

One concern related to treatment with IFN-β may be the occurrence of neutralizing antibodies. Although some immunologic studies have provided evidence that certain neutralizing antibodies can have a positive effect by prolonging the biologic half-life of a cytokine, in most diseases the development of neutralizing antibodies to an externally administered agent has been associated with loss of efficacy. For example, if neutralizing antibodies to insulin develop in a person with insulin-dependent diabetes mellitus, the effect of the therapy is lessened and insulin dosage may have to be adjusted upwards. For IFN-α it is also well established in various conditions that development of therapy-induced neutralizing antibodies is associated with a loss of clinical response. The frequency of patients developing neutralizing anti-IFN-α antibodies is highly variable, this being partly explained by heterogenous treatment regimens and study designs and by different preparations of IFN-α having different immunogenic potential. It is important to recognize that not all antibodies that develop during IFN treatment are neutralizing; many of the antibodies that have the capacity to bind to IFN in immunoassays do not have neutralizing effects as measured by biological assays.

The concern about the potentially unfavorable effects of neutralizing antibodies on the impact of IFN-β on disease activity in MS was raised by the final report of the North American multicenter trial of IFN-β 1b in RRMS.[93] Evidence of diminution of therapeutic efficacy in 35% of MS patients treated with IFN-β 1b who developed neutralizing antibodies was further documented in a subsequent publication.[94] In those who became positive, usually in the first year of treatment, the relapse rates after 18 months resembled rates in placebo patients, the numbers of enlarging MRI lesions were significantly increased and there was increased new lesion formation on the MRI compared with those who remained neutralizing antibody-negative. There was some evidence that neutralizing antibodies might also be associated with a reduction in the frequency of some IFN-β-associated side effects.

Data available so far indicate that the frequency with which MS patients develop neutralizing antibodies against IFN-β is lower with IFN-β 1a therapy than with IFN-β 1b therapy. In the phase 3 trials with IFN-β 1a, neutralizing antibodies developed in 20% of patients treated with Avonex® and in 23.8% (low dose) and 12.5% (high dose) of patients during treatment with Rebif®. Rudick and colleagues[95] performed detailed analyses of the clinical and biological significance of neutralizing antibodies to IFN-β 1a (Avonex®). For patients in the phase 3 study, a trend towards reduced benefit as measured by MRI activity was observed in neutralizing antibody-positive patients compared with neutralizing antibody-negative patients. These patients and patients participating in a phase 4 safety extension study (where only 5% developed neutralizing antibodies) demonstrated that development of neutralizing antibodies resulted in titer-dependent reduction in the in vivo induction of IFN-inducible molecules neopterin and β-2 microglobulin.

The straightforward conclusion that development

of neutralizing antibody positivity is associated with reduced efficacy of therapy is, however, challenged by a number of observations. Petkau and White[96] criticized the initial analyses on neutralizing antibody positivity in the large North American study with IFN-β 1b; these analyses were based on a comparison of disease activity between patients who became neutralizing antibody-positive and those who remained neutralizing antibody-negative. They argued that such cross-sectional analyses do not directly address the question of whether the change from neutralizing antibody-negative to neutralizing antibody-positive status is associated with diminished effectiveness of IFN-β in these patients. They therefore re-analysed the 5 years of data on relapse rates, EDSS scores, and MRI lesion burdens for patients who changed from neutralizing antibody-negative to neutralizing antibody-positive status using longitudinal data analysis, correcting for possible time trends over the course of the trial. This analysis did not support un unequivocal conclusion that the change to neutralizing antibody positivity is associated with reduced efficacy.

Some studies suggest that those MS patients who go on to develop neutralizing antibodies may be predisposed to becoming antibody-positive and may have had more disease activity already before the initiation of IFN therapy. One study suggested that those MS patients who had a high IgG secretion in vivo following pokeweed mitogen stimulation were more likely to develop neutralizing antibodies to IFN-β 1b.[97] In an Italian study in which patients with RRMS were monitored with frequent gadolinium-enhanced MRI before and during treatment with IFN-β 1a (Rebif®), it was found that relapse rate, baseline disability, and the volume of lesions on T2-weighted MRI were significantly higher during

the 6-month baseline period before the start of treatment in patients who developed neutralizing antibody during treatment.[98]

Although additional data sets are needed to resolve all questions on the relevance of neutralizing antibodies, some preliminary conclusions and guidelines can be justified on the basis of the data that have been presented so far.[99]

It is likely that change from neutralizing antibody-negative to neutralizing antibody-positive status is associated with some reduction of efficacy of IFN-β. It must also be remembered that at present it is not clear what titers should be considered high and that the antibody response to IFN-β may fluctuate over time, in that even those with very high titers can become neutralizing antibody-negative during continued treatment.

Development of neutralizing antibodies seems to be more frequent in patients being treated with IFN-β 1b than in those on IFN-β 1a (28–37% and 5–24% respectively). Although this difference can easily be interpreted as representing the reduced immunogenicity of IFN-β 1a because it structurally resembles the natural human protein and has less tendency to form aggregates, it cannot be excluded that differences in frequencies reported are also related to differences in assays applied in the various studies. Measurement of antibody should always state not only the value achieved but also the technique used.[100] There are four major ways in which anti-IFN-β antibodies are currently measured: enzyme-linked immunosorbent assay, immunoblotting, neutralization of IFN-β inhibition of virally mediated cell lysis, and neutralization of IFN-β induction of the MxA protein. Although the enzyme-linked immunosorbent assay is most likely to measure total binding antibody (and not only neutralizing antibody), it is not known at this time which assay correlates best with decreased bioactivity of administered IFN-β.

The detection of neutralizing antibodies at any titer should not be the sole reason to discontinue treatment with IFN-β. The patient's disease status is of paramount importance. There is clear evidence that treatment continues to be effective in some of the patients who have high levels of neutralizing antibodies. Therefore, at present there is not enough information regarding the interpretation of the results of existing IFN-β assays to warrant routine testing outside the research setting. In the context of treatment failure on clinical grounds, however, knowledge of the neutralizing antibody status can be helpful for making a decision regarding stopping the drug.[101,102]

The need for further studies to investigate the effects of anti-IFN-β antibodies cannot be stressed enough, especially since at least some of these antibodies have been shown to cross-react with natural IFN-β, which is likely to play an important role in the natural defense against a number of diseases.

Induction of autoantibodies or autoimmune disease by IFN-β

A few reports have suggested that IFN-β treatment may induce autoantibody production or overt autoimmune diseases such as lupus erythematosus, dysthyroidism, myasthenia gravis, or autoimmune hepatitis.[103–106] So far these autoimmune phenomena have mainly been reported for IFN-β 1b, although it is likely that this is related to the fact that this preparation has been available longer rather than to intrinsic differences between the various products. The question whether IFN-β treatment may induce

autoimmune phenomena in MS patients needs to be addressed because long-term experience with IFN-α has clearly shown that this type I IFN does induce autoimmune disease and because IFN-β is presumed to cause a shift from a Th_1 to a Th_2 cytokine production profile, which then could lead to enhanced B-cell mediated autoimmunity.[107] That this phenomenon has the potential to occur was recently demonstrated in a phase 1 study in which MS patients were treated with a humanized antilymphocyte antibody Campath-1H, which induced prolonged T-lymphocyte suppression in combination with a significant rise in B-lymphocyte counts, which led to the unexpected development of autoimmune thyroid disease in one third of treated patients.[108] So far, however, reported incidence of autoimmune disease in patients treated with IFN-β 1b does not exceed the frequency that can be expected.[109] Remarkably, in two studies that followed MS patients longitudinally during treatment with IFN-β, there was no evidence of increased frequency of autoantibodies during a mean follow-up of 9 months.[110,111] Further follow-up is needed to confirm these findings during long-term treatment.

HOW CAN THE EFFICACY OF IFN-β BE IMPROVED?

Given the observation that there is an obvious dose–response relationship in most IFN-β clinical trials in which variable dosages have been used, the most obvious suggestion of how to improve the efficacy of IFN-β would be to increase the dosage. A dosage of IFN-β 1a (Avonex®) that is twice the officially licensed dosage is presently being tested in a large European study and the ongoing US secondary progressive MS study with

IFN-β 1b includes one arm in which the dosage of IFN-β is titrated in relation to body surface, resulting in a higher dosage administered for those with large body surface. One has to recognize, however, that it is unknown whether the dose–response relationship continues to persist beyond those dosages that have been tested so far, and that at higher dosages toxicity may increasingly be encountered as a limiting factor.

There might be ways of limiting IFN-β-associated toxicity. Weber and colleagues[112] have shown that patients receiving IFN-β 1b in combination with oral pentoxifylline report fewer side effects during the first 3 months of treatment than those receiving IFN-β 1b alone. They also found that patients treated with IFN-β 1b alone had up-regulated TNF-α as well as IFN-γ mRNA expression during the first month, findings that were not detected in patients receiving both drugs. Several groups have suggested that early side effects of IFN-β can be reduced by low-dose oral corticosteroid use at the onset of treatment (for example 30 mg IFN-β daily for 2 weeks, followed by gradual tapering over the next 2 weeks).[53,113] This has been attributed to suppression of the increase in the number of IFN-γ-producing cells and to a decrease in IL-6 induction that occurs during the first months of treatment.[114] Recently, the initial results were reported of an open-labeled tolerability study of increasing dosages of IFN-β 1a (Avonex®) (30 μg, 60 μg, and 90 μg) in moderately disabled MS patients. In this study, all patients received 650 mg acetaminophen 1 hour before administration of IFN-β 1a and then every 6 hours for a total of three doses. These patients were also randomized into one of four groups: no additional treatment, oral prednisone (60 mg for 6 days), intravenous methylprednisolone (1000 mg for 3 days), and pentoxifylline (400 mg orally twice daily for 3

days). The lower dose of IFN-β 1a was tolerated well, with a suggestion that pentoxifylline in particular may be of benefit in reducing side effects.[115]

Oral administration of IFN-β would be another possible way of reducing side effects. At present, experts disagree about the potential for oral IFN-β to be effective in MS, but preliminary observations have shown that oral administration of type I IFN may have immunomodulatory effects that could be beneficial in the treatment of MS.[116]

Another way of increasing efficacy of IFN-β 1b would be to combine it with other drugs that are likely to have a favorable impact on the course of the disease under the assumption that they can provide synergistic or additive benefit. Candidate drugs would include corticosteroids, glatiramer acetate, intravenous immunoglobulin, methotrexate, and azathioprine among others. Before applying combination therapies in daily practice, well-designed clinical trials should be performed, as pointed out by Lublin and Reingold[117] for the US National MS Society Task Force on Combination Treatments, because additive effects have to be demonstrated and because it can not be excluded in advance that combination therapy may be less effective than either agent alone. At this time, combination therapies of IFN-β with glatiramer acetate, azathioprine, and all-*trans* retinoic acid are subject of various clinical studies.[118] A combination that has already been proved safe and that may also have a synergistic effect is that of IFN-β with intravenous methylprednisolone. Gasperini and colleagues,[119] using longitudinal MRI data, found that treatment with IFN-β in comparison to placebo prolongs the reduction in the number and volume of enhancing lesions as induced by treatment with intravenous methylprednisolone.

DISEASE MANAGEMENT WITH IFN-β

Who should be treated with interferon-β?

The question of who should be treated with IFN-β is also covered in Chapters 30, 31, and 32.

In the report of the Quality Standards Subcommittee of the American Academy of Neurology that was issued in 1994[120] it was recommended that IFN-β should be prescribed to patients who have definite MS, who have active relapsing–remitting disease (at least two acute relapses during the previous 2 years), are ambulatory (EDSS of 5.5 or lower) and are aged between 18 and 50 years. Class I evidence (evidence from randomized, controlled clinical trials) exists for these patients and expert consensus suggested that IFN-β may be helpful. These criteria have subsequently been adopted in many other countries, minor adaptations being made especially regarding the age limits, which are being judged to be derived from standard clinical trial procedures rather than to represent meaningful biological differences. Since 1994, additional evidence to support the efficacy of IFN-β in this patient group has become available (see above), even somewhat loosening the criterion that requires at least two relapses in the previous 2 years, since in the study with IFN-β 1a (Avonex®) patients with two relapses in 3 years were also included.[27]

Recently, class I evidence has also become available for patients with active secondary progressive MS (at least two relapses during the previous year or progression of at least 1.0 EDSS point) and EDSS scores up to and including 6.5. Based on the assumption that the results of ongoing clinical trials with IFN-β 1a will be confirmatory, it is obvious that the treatment recommendations should be expanded to include this population of MS patients. At present it is not clear whether treatment should be advocated for patients who have EDSS scores higher than 6.5 (experts have not so far reached consensus as to whether the likelihood of causing more pronounced side effects should be considered as a treatment-limiting factor in this disabled population) or to patients with primary progressive MS (there are ongoing clinical trials in this population, which clearly represents a different biological entity in the spectrum of MS; Thompson and colleagues[121] and Bramanti and colleagues[14] have reviewed this area). An overview of treatment recommendations for patients in various disease phases is shown in *Table 20.5*.

A very important question to address is how early treatment with IFN-β should be initiated. For patients with a single demyelinating episode who have a high likelihood of progressing to definite MS there will be class I evidence available within the next few years since two large, multicenter trials are under way to determine whether treatment of such mono-symptomatic patients with IFN-β 1a is associated with lower conversion rates to clinically definite MS. Class I evidence, however, will not be available in the next few years for the large population of patients who have definite MS but who do not at present show clinical signs of disease activity. On the one hand, approximately 20% of patients have relatively benign disease, and they most likely do not require disease-modifying therapy. On the other hand, one should not postpone treatment untill after persistent neurological deficits have occurred, since none of the currently available therapies for MS reverses fixed deficits. At present there is no consensus as to whether MRI can play a role in selecting patients for IFN-β treatment. Serial MRI studies have demonstrated disease activity (manifested as new lesions) in the

Table 20.5 Recommendations for treatment initiation with IFN-β

Patient category	Recommendation
Active relapsing–remitting (Two relapses in the previous 2–3 yrs)	Treatment indicated, based on randomized, controlled clinical trials
Active secondary progressive (Two relapses or 1.0 EDSS progression in the previous 2 years)	Treatment indicated, based on one randomized, controlled clinical trial
Relapsing–remitting or secondary progressive disease not meeting the criteria for activity	No direct data available, treatment may be helpful for those who have subclinical disease
Primary progressive	Await results of randomized, controlled clinical trials
Monophasic syndrome	Await results of randomized, controlled clinical trials
Patients with EDSS of 7.0 or higher	No direct data available, fear for worsened pattern of side effects

brain even in early clinical stages and during periods when the disease is clinically quiescent. More recently, attention has also been focused on measures of cerebral atrophy that can develop early in the disease and that might be sensitive indicators of subclinical disease activity. Atrophy seems to be associated with axonal loss, which is increasingly being recognized as the most important feature leading to irreversible deficit.[50,79,122] Recently, Rudick (1998; personal communication) reported on post hoc analyses of MRI data of a subgroup of the patients in the original IFN-β 1a (Avonex®) clinical trial.[27] In this trial, 48 patients were treated with IFN-β 1a and 46 with placebo, the groups being well balanced for relevant demographic factors. Although these patients had a mean EDSS score of only 2.3, they had considerable brain atrophy (significantly reduced brain parenchymal fraction) in comparison with controls. During the trial, a drug treatment effect as measured with this brain parenchymal fraction was observed: the treatment group had significantly less cerebral atrophy than the placebo patients ($p = 0.03$ at 2 years). Although these data are very important in that they reflect a treatment effect on a relevant measure of subclinical disease activity in patients with early disease, one has to remember that these patients were included in the clinical trial because of clinical disease activity and therefore cannot be used to directly answer the question whether patients with only subclinical disease activity should be treated (i.e. whether side effects in these patients are being outweighed by long-term benefits).

Subgroups of patients: responders and non-responders

The question of whether we can identify subgroups of patients who are likely to respond better than others can at present only be answered with a 'no.' MRI data from studies where frequent scanning was used were analysed for this purpose, but clear conclusions could not be drawn.[15] Koudriavtseva and colleagues[38] used linear regression analysis to analyse determinants of therapeutical response and (disappointingly) found that clinical parameters rather than MRI parameters had the strongest predictive value. In their study they found that the effect of IFN-β 1a on MRI disease activity depends slightly on relapse rate (the patients with the lower number of relapses showing greater response) and level of disability before treatment (the patients with the lower baseline EDSS showing greater response). Collection of data addressing the issue of responders versus non-responders would be extremely relevant because it could facilitate a more efficient and more cost-effective prescription pattern for this very expensive treatment.

Initiating therapy with IFN-β

The key issues to be addressed at an education session that should take place at least once before initiating treatment are good injection proce-

dures, management of side effects and counseling about realistic expectations. Training is given for drug preparation and administration; some side effects can be dealt with quite easily. Giving IFN-β in the evening allows the patient to sleep through the flu-like symptoms that are frequently associated with initiation. Paracetamol or ibuprofen are recommended at the time of injection and the following day for minimizing these side effects, and dose escalation can be helpful in the initial stages. Side effects suffered by patients who receive IFN-β subcutaneously include injection-site reactions. These can be dealt with using good injection technique and site rotation. Patients experiencing discomfort with injection should be recommended to inject only after the drug to be administered has warmed to room temperature, or to use ice on the area before and after injection. For patients with severe skin reactions, switching to treatment with intramuscular IFN-β 1a (Avonex®) should be recommended. Now that more patients with higher disability will be started on treatment it is important to make patients aware of the potential danger of a temporary worsening of neurological symptoms, including spasticity.

After beginning therapy, adverse effects, effectiveness, and compliance with the injection technique should be monitored every 3 months. Complete blood counts and liver enzyme levels should be done every 3 months. Education remains an important factor in maintaining compliance through the early phases of therapy. This is especially true for patients with fatigue, fatigue–depression interaction and a progressive course of the disease, since initial studies have shown that these factors are significantly associated with early treatment discontinuation.[123] Initial experiences suggest that increasing depression occurring shortly after initiating treatment with IFN-β should be rigorously treated to increase adherence to treatment.[124]

Discontinuing treatment with IFN-β

Present evidence suggests that IFN-β remains effective as long as it is administered. Kaplan–Meier curves as they are presented on the primary outcome of large phase 3 clinical trials do not always allow a conclusion with regard to the question whether the treatment efficacy increases, remains constant, or decreases over time. In the studies with IFN-β, various analyses of secondary clinical end-points clearly suggest persistence of effect during treatment; MRI data from the cohort that was frequently scanned in the European phase 3 trial in secondary progressive multiple sclerosis[125] show that the suppression of new lesion development is equally strong or even stronger during months 19–24 than during months 1–6. On the basis of these observations, it should be recommended that therapy should be continued indefinitely unless there is clear lack of benefit, severe toxicity, or intention to become pregnant. The Quality Standards Subcommittee of the American Academy of Neurology[120] defined clear lack of benefit as either continuous deterioration for more than 6 months or three relapses requiring corticosteroid therapy during a 1-year period. It is obvious that these criteria should be revised now IFN-β is also indicated for patients with active secondary progressive disease. Severe toxicity associated with treatment with IFN-β has been reported, although extremely infrequently.[126,127]

IFN-α

Based on the similarities of both type I IFNs (IFN-α and IFN-β) and on the fact that they bind to the same receptor, it can be assumed that IFN-α might also have a favorable impact on the course of MS. This indeed was demonstrated by Durelli and colleagues,[106] who tested the effects of high dose (9 MIU intramuscularly every other day) systemic recombinant IFN-α in RRMS. This dosage was used because previous studies using lower doses of IFN-α had failed to demonstrate clinical efficacy and because this dosage had been associated with acceptable side effects in patients with other diseases. Twenty MS patients (with at least two clearly defined relapses in the 2 years before the study and an EDSS of 6.0 or lower) were randomized to receive IFN-α or placebo for 6 months. Clinical relapses or new or enlarging lesions on serial MRI occurred in two of 12 patients treated with interferon-α-2a (rIFN-α) (Roferon®) and in seven of eight placebo-treated patients ($p < 0.005$). There was only one enlarging MRI lesion in the rIFN-α group, whereas 27 new or enlarging lesions were present in the placebo group ($p < 0.01$). The treatment with rIFN-α did not result in serious side effects, but fever, malaise, and fatigue occurred frequently. Immunological analyses suggested that the beneficial effect might be mediated by a down-regulation of the production of pro-inflammatory cytokines IFN-γ and TNF-α.[128] Subsequently, these authors reported that disease activity resumed after discontinuation of treatment. The reduction of both clinical and MRI signs of disease activity, the immunological effects, and the side effects were temporary and restricted to the period of rIFN-α administration.[129] More prolonged and larger trials are warranted to come to a balanced conclusion on the important issues of long-term efficacy and tolerance of IFN-α therapy in MS.

CONCLUSION

The goal of therapy in patients with MS is to prevent relapses and progressive worsening of the disease, which most likely translates into more time to participate in social and physical activities, and an improved quality of life. Even though it is obvious that IFN-β does not represent a cure for MS, it is the only drug that has so far been proved to be capable of reducing the frequency of relapses and slowing the accumulation of disability. Therefore, treatment with IFN-β should now be considered early in the disease course for patients with active disease. Because efficacy data are quite robust and because IFN-β has been shown to suppress the development of new lesions as well as brain atrophy on MRI in the early stages of disease, it is tempting to hypothesize that prevention of long term clinical deterioration can be achieved by early treatment in as many patients as possible. One must be aware, however, that direct evidence to support this hypothesis is still lacking and that, therefore, decisions to initiate treatment should be based on open communications with patients in which both benefits and side effects are explained in as much detail as desired.

REFERENCES

1 Isaacs A, Lindenmann J. Virus interference: I. The interferon. *Proc R Soc Lond [Biol]* 1957; **147**:258–267.

2 Foster GR, Finter NB. Are all type I human interferons equivalent? *J Viral Hep* 1998; **5**:143–152.

3 Jacobs L, Johnson KP. A brief history of the use of interferons as treatment of multiple sclerosis. *Arch Neurol* 1994; **51**:1245–1252.

4 Jacobs L, O'Malley J, Freeman A, Ekes R. Intrathecal interferon reduces exacerbations of multiple sclerosis. *Science* 1981; **214**:1026–1028.

5 Jacobs L, Salazar AM, Herndon R et al. Multicentre double-blind study of effect of intrathecally administered natural human fibroblast interferon on exacerbations of multiple sclerosis. *Lancet* 1986; ii:1411–1413.

6 Panitch HS, Hirch RL, Schindler J, Johnson KP. Treatment of multiple sclerosis with gamma interferon: exacerbations associated with activation of the immune system. *Neurology* 1987; **37**:1097–1120.

7 Runkel L, Meier W, Pepinsky RB et al. Structural and functional differences between glycosylated and non-glycosylated forms of human interferon beta. *Pharmacol Res* 1998; **15**:641–649.

8 Alam J, McAllister A, Scaramucci J et al. Pharmacokinetics and pharmacodynamics of interferon-beta-1a in healthy volunteers after intravenous, subcutaneous or intramuscular administration. *Clin Drug Invest* 1997; **14**:35–42.

9 Munafo A, Spertini F, Rothuisen L et al. Pharmacodynamic responses to r-hIFN-β-1a administered subcutaneously once a week or three times a week over one month. *Multiple Sclerosis* 1997; **3**:343(P22).

10 Johnson KP, Knobler RL, Greenstein JI et al. Recombinant interferon beta treatment of relapsing remitting multiple sclerosis: pilot study results (abstract). *Neurology* 1990; **40 (suppl 1)**:261.

11 The IFNB Multiple Sclerosis Study Group. Interferon beta-1b is effective in relapsing–remitting multiple sclerosis. I. Clinical results. *Neurology* 1993; **43**:655–661.

12 Goodkin DE. Interferon beta-1b. *Lancet* 1994; **344**:1057–1060.

13 Polman CH, Dahlke F, Thompson AJ et al. Interferon beta-1b in secondary progressive multiple sclerosis: outline of the clinical trial. *Multiple Sclerosis* 1995; **1 (suppl)**:51–54.

14 Bramanti P, Sessa E, Rifici C et al. Enhanced spasticity in primary progressive MS patients treated with interferon beta-1b. *Neurology* 1988; **51**:1720–1723.

15 Stone LA, Frank JA, Albert PS et al. The effect of interferon beta on blood brain barrier disruptions demonstrated by contrast-enhanced magnetic resonance imaging in relapsing remitting multiple sclerosis. *Ann Neurol* 1995; **37**:611–619.

16 Stone LA, Frank JA, Albert PS et al. Characterization of MRI response to treatment with interferon beta-1b: contrast-enhancing MRI lesion frequency as a

primary outcome measure. *Neurology* 1997;
49:862–869.

17 Pliskin NH, Hamer DP, Goldstein DS et al. Improved delayed visual reproduction test performance in multiple sclerosis patients receiving interferon β-1b. *Neurology* 1996; 47:1463–1468.

18 Selby MJ, Ling N, Williams JM, Dawson A. Interferon beta 1-b in verbal memory functioning of patients with relapsing remitting multiple sclerosis. *Percept Motor Skills* 1998; 86:1099–1106.

19 Sheremata WA, Taylor JR, Elgart GW. Severe necrotizing cutaneous lesions complicating treatment with interferon beta-1b. *N Engl J Med* 1995; 122:105–107.

20 Webster GF, Knobler RL, Lublin FD et al. Cutaneous ulcerations and pustular psoriasis flare caused by recombinant interferon beta injections in patients with multiple sclerosis. *J Am Acad Dermatol* 1996; 34:365–367.

21 Feldmann R, Low-Weiser H, Duschet P, Gschnait F. Necrotizing lesions caused by interferon beta injections in a patient with multiple sclerosis. *Dermatology* 1997; 195:52–53.

22 Elgart GW, Sheremata W, Ahn YS. Cutaneous reactions to recombinant human interferon beta-1b: The clinical and histologic spectrum. *J Am Acad Dermatol* 1997; 37:553–558.

23 Jacobs L, Salazar AM, Herndon R et al. Intrathecally administered natural human fibroblast interferon reduces exacerbations of multiple sclerosis. *Arch Neurol* 1987; 44:589–595.

24 Jacobs L, Cookfair DL, Rudick RA, Herndon RM. A Phase III trial of intramuscular recombinant interferon beta for exacerbating remitting multiple sclerosis: design and conduct of study; baseline characteristics of patients. *Multiple Sclerosis* 1995; 1:118–135.

25 Goodkin DE, Cookfair D, Wende K et al. Inter- and intra-rater scoring agreement using grade 1.0 to 3.5 of the Kurtzke Expanded Disability Status Scale (EDSS). *Neurology* 1992; 42:859–863.

26 Rudick RA, Goodkin DE, Jacobs LD et al. The impact of Interferon beta-1a on neurologic disability in multiple sclerosis. *Neurology* 1997; 49:358–363.

27 Jacobs LD, Cookfair DL, Rudick RA et al. Intramuscular interferon beta-1a for disease progression in relapsing multiple sclerosis. *Ann Neurol* 1996; 39:285–294.

28 Goodkin DE, Priore R, Wende K et al. Non-physician based continuous measures of manual dexterity and ambulation can be used to improve the ability of the EDSS to detect clinical worsening in an MS clinical trial. *Ann Neurol* 1997; 42:268.

29 Simon JH, Jacobs LD, Campion M et al. Magnetic resonance studies of intramuscular Interferon β-1a for relapsing multiple sclerosis. *Ann Neurol* 1998; 43:79–87.

30 Noseworthy JH, O'Brien P, Erickson BJ et al. The Mayo Clinic–Canadian Cooperative trial of sulfasalazine in active multiple sclerosis. *Neurology* 1998; 51:1342–1352.

31 PRISMS Study Group. Randomised double-blind placebo-controlled study of interferon β-1a in relapsing/remitting multiple sclerosis. *Lancet* 1998; 352:1498–1504.

32 Pozzilli C, Bastianello S, Koudriatseva T et al. Magnetic resonance imaging changes with recombinant human interferon-β-1a: a short term study in relapsing–remitting multiple sclerosis. *J Neurol Neurosurg Psychiatry* 1996; 61:251–258.

33 Pozzilli C, Bastianello S, Koudriatseva T et al. An open randomized trial with two different doses of recombinant human interferon beta 1-a in relapsing–remitting multiple sclerosis: clinical and MRI results at 24 months. *J Neurol* 1997; 244 (suppl 3):25.

34 Lui C, Li Wan Po A, Blumhardt LD. Summary measure statistic for assessing outcome of treatments trials in relapsing and remitting multiple sclerosis. *J Neurol Neurosurg Psychiatry* 1998; 64:726–729.

35 Li D, Zhao G, Hyde R et al. Comparison of proton density/T2 and gadolinium-enhanced T1 MRI in demonstrating a treatment effect and dose difference in PRISMS trial of interferon β-1a. *J Neurol* 1998; 245:457.

36 Goodkin DE. Commentary. Interferon β therapy for multiple sclerosis. *Lancet* 1998; 352:1486–1487.

37 Freedman MS for the OWIMS Study Group. Dose-dependent clinical and magnetic resonance imaging efficacy of IFN beta-1a (R/Rebif) in multiple sclerosis. *Ann Neurol* 1998; 44:992.

38 Koudriavtseva T, Pozzilli C, Fiorelli M et al. Determinants of Gd-enhanced MRI response to IFN-β-1a treatment in relapsing-remitting multiple sclerosis. *Multiple Sclerosis* 1998; 4:403–407.

39 Comi G, Barkhof F, Durelli L et al. Early treatment of multiple sclerosis with Rebif (recombinant human interferon beta): design of the study. *Multiple Sclerosis* 1995; 1:24–27.

40 Comi G, Filippi M, Barkhof F et al. ETOMS study:

baseline characteristics of the included population. *J Neurol* 1998, 245:P314.

41 Sandberg-Wolheim M, Hommes OR, Hughes RA et al. Recombinant human interferon beta in the treatment of relapsing–remitting and secondary progressive multiple sclerosis. *Multiple Sclerosis* 1995; **1**:48–50.

42 Weinstock-Guttman B, Ransohoff RM, Kinkel RP, Rudick RA. The interferons: biological effects, mechanisms of action, and use in multiple sclerosis. *Ann Neurol* 1995; **37**:7–15.

43 Arnason BGW, Dayal A, Qu ZX et al. Mechanisms of action of interferon-β in multiple sclerosis. *Springer Semin Immunopathol* 1996; **18**:125–148.

44 Yong VW, Chabot S, Stuve O, Williams G. Interferon beta in the treatment of multiple sclerosis. *Neurology* 1998; **51**:682–689.

45 Khan OA, Xia Q, Bever CT et al. Interferon beta-1b serum levels in multiple sclerosis patients following subcutaneous administration. *Neurology* 1996; **46**:1639–1643.

46 Khan OA, Dhib Jalbut SS. Serum interferon β-1a (Avonex) levels following intramuscular injection in relapsing-remitting MS patients. *Neurology* 1998; **51**:738–742.

47 Pan W, Banks WA, Kastin AJ. Permeability of the blood–brain and blood–spinal cord barriers to interferons. *J Neuroimmunol* 1997; **76**:105–111.

48 Fleischmann RW, Koeren S, Fleischmann CM. Orally administered interferons exert white blood cell suppressive effects via a novel mechanism. *Proc Soc Exp Biol Med* 1992; **201**:200–207.

49 Genain CP, Abel K, Belmar N et al. Late complications of immune deviation therapy in a nonhuman primate. *Science* 1996; **274**:2054–2057.

50 Lassmann H. Neuropathology in multiple sclerosis: new concepts. *Multiple Sclerosis* 1998; **4**:93–98.

51 Noronha A, Toscas A, Jensen MA. Interferon β decreases T cell activation and interferon γ production in multiple sclerosis. *J Neuroimmunol* 1993; **46**:145–154.

52 Petereit HF, Bamborschke S, Esse AD, Heiss WD. Interferon gamma producing blood lymphocytes are decreased by interferon beta therapy in patients with multiple sclerosis. *Multiple Sclerosis* 1997; **3**:180–183.

53 Dayal AS, Jensen MA, Lledo A, Arnason BGW. Interferon-gamma-secreting cells in multiple sclerosis patients treated with interferon beta-1b. *Neurology* 1995; **45**:2173–2177.

54 Jiang H, Milo R, Swoveland et al. Interferon β-1b

reduces IFN-γ-induced antigen presenting capacity of human glial cells and B cells. *J Neuroimmunol* 1995; **61**:17–25.

55 Lu HT, Riley JL, Babcock GT et al. Interferon beta acts downstream of IFN-γ induced class II transactivator mRNA accumulation to block MHC class II gene expression. *J Exp Med* 1995; **182**:1517–1525.

56 Hall GL, Compston A, Scolding NJ. Beta-interferon and multiple sclerosis. *Trends Neurosci* 1997; **20**:63–67.

57 Porrini AM, Gambi D, Reder AT. Interferon effects on interleukin-10 secretion. *J Neuroimmunol* 1995; **61**:27–34.

58 Rep MHG, Hintzen RQ, Polman CH, van Lier RAW. Recombinant interferon-β blocks proliferation but enhances interleukin-10 secretion by activated human T cells. *J Neuroimmunol* 1996; **67**:111–118.

59 Rep MHG, Schrijver HM, van Lopik TH et al. Interferon(IFN)-β treatment enhances CD95 and interleukin-10 expression but reduces interferon-γ producing T cells in MS patients. *J Neuroimmunol* 1999; **96**:92–100.

60 Rudick RA, Ransohoff RM, Peppler R et al. Interferon beta induces interleukin-10 expression: relevance to multiple sclerosis. *Ann Neurol* 1996; **40**:618–627.

61 Porrini AM, DeLuca G, Gambi D, Reder AT. Effects of an anti-IL-10 monoclonal antibody on rIFNβ-1b-mediated immune modulation. *J Neuroimmunol* 1998; **81**:109–115.

62 Rudick RA, Ransohoff RM, Lee JC et al. In vivo effects of interferon beta-1a on immunosuppressive cytokines in multiple sclerosis. *Neurology* 1998; **50**:1294–1300.

63 Brod SA, Marshall GD, Henninger EM et al. Interferon β-1b treatment decreases tumor necrosis factor-α and increases interleukin-6 production in multiple sclerosis. *Neurology* 1996; **46**:1633–1638.

64 Coclet-Ninin J, Dayer JM, Burger D. Interferon beta not only inhibits interleukin-1 beta and tumor necrosis factor-alpha but stimulates interleukin-1 receptor antagonist production in human peripheral blood mononuclear cells. *Eur Cytokine Netw* 1997; **8**:345–349.

65 Nicoletti F, Di Marco R, Patti F et al. Blood levels of TGF-beta 1 are elevated in both relapsing remitting and chronic progressive MS patients and are further augmented by treatment with interferon-beta 1b. *Clin Exp Immunol* 1998; **113**:96–99.

66 Ossege LM, Sindern E, Patzold F, Malin JP.

Immunomodulatory effects of interferon β-1b in vivo: induction of the expression of transforming growth factor-β1 and its receptor type II. *J Neuroimmunol* 1998; **91**:73–81.

67 Byskosh PV, Reder AT. Interferon β-1b effects on cytokine mRNA in peripheral mononuclear cells in multiple sclerosis. *Multiple Sclerosis* 1996; **1**:262–269.

68 Pette M, Pette DF, Muraro PA et al. Interferon-β interferes with the proliferation but not with the cytokine secretion of myelin basic protein-specific, T-helper type 1 lymphocytes. *Neurology* 1997; **49**:385–392.

69 Ferrarini AM, Sivieri S, Bulian P et al. Time-course of interleukin-2 receptor expression in interferon beta-treated multiple sclerosis patients. *J Neuroimmunol* 1998; **84**:213–217.

70 Archelos JJ, Hartung HP. The role of adhesion molecules in multiple sclerosis: biology, pathogenesis and therapeutic implications. *Mol Med Today* 1997; **14**:310–321.

71 Huynh HK, Oger J, Dorovini-Zis K. Interferon-β downregulates interferon-γ-induced class II MHC molecule expression and morphological changes in primary cultures of human brain microvessel endothelial cells. *J Neuroimmunol* 1995; **60**:63–73.

72 Dhib-Jalbut S, Jiang H, Williams GJ. The effect of interferon β-1b on lymphocyte–endothelial cell adhesion. *J Neuroimmunol* 1996; **71**:215–222.

73 Miller A, Lanir N, Shapiro S et al. Immunoregulatory effects of interferon-β and interacting cytokines on human vascular endothelial cells. *J Neuroimmunol* 1996; **64**:151–161.

74 Calabresi PA, Tranquill LR, Dambrosia JM et al. Increases in soluble VCAM-1 correlate with a decrease in MRI lesions in multiple sclerosis treated with IFN-β-1b. *Ann Neurol* 1997; **41**:669–674.

75 Corsini E, Gelati M, Dufour A et al. Effects of β-IFN-1b treatment in MS patients on adhesion between PBMNCs, HUVECs and MS-HBECs: an in vivo and in vitro study. *J Neuroimmunol* 1997; **79**:76–83.

76 Leppert D, Waubant E, Burk MR et al. Interferon beta-1b inhibits gelatinase secretion and in vitro migration of human T cells. *Ann Neurol* 1996; **40**:846–852.

77 Stuve O, Dooley NP, Uhm JH et al. Interferon β-1b decreases the migration of T lymphocytes in vitro: effects on matrix metalloproteinase-9. *Ann Neurol* 1996; **40**:853–863.

78 Liu JSH, Amaral TD, Brosnan CF, Lee SC. IFNs are critical regulators of IL-1 receptor antagonist and IL-1 expression in human microglia. *J Immunol* 1998; **161**:1989–1996.

79 Trapp BD, Peterson J, Ransohoff RM et al. Axonal transection in the lesions of multiple sclerosis. *N Engl J Med* 1998; **338**:278–285.

80 Guthikonda P, Baker J, Mattson DH. Interferon-beta-1b decreases induced nitric oxide production by a human astrocytoma cell line. *J Neuroimmunol* 1998; **82**:133–139.

81 Stewart VC, Giovannoni G, Land JM et al. Pretreatment of astrocytes with Interferon-α/β impairs interferon-γ induction of nitric oxide synthase. *J Neurochem* 1997; **68**:2547–2551.

82 Stewart VC, Land JM, Clark JB, Heales SJR. Pretreatment of astrocytes with Interferon-α/β prevents neuronal mitochondrial respiratory chain damage. *J Neurochem* 1998; **70**:432–434.

83 Boutros T, Croze E, Yong VW. Interferon-β is a potent promoter of nerve growth factor production by astrocytes. *J Neurochem* 1997; **69**:939–946.

84 Malik O, Compston DAS, Scolding NJ. Interferon beta inhibits mitogen induced astrocyte proliferation in vitro. *J Neuroimmunol* 1998; **86**:155–162.

85 Arnason BGW. Short analytical review. Interferon beta in multiple sclerosis. *Clin Immunol Immunopathol* 1996; **81**:1–11.

86 Genc K, Dona DL, Reder AT. Increased CD80+ B cells in active multiple sclerosis and reversal by interferon β-1b therapy. *J Clin Invest* 1997; **99**:2664–2671.

87 Zipp F, Weller M, Calabresi PA et al. Increased serum levels of soluble CD95 (APO-1/Fas) in relapsing remitting multiple sclerosis. *Ann Neurol* 1998; **43**:116–120.

88 Bauer J, Bradl M, Hickey WF et al. T-cell apoptosis in inflammatory brain lesions. *Am J Pathol* 1998; **153**:715–724

89 Panitch HS, Bever CT, Katz E, Johnson KP. Upper respiratory tract infections trigger attacks of multiple sclerosis in patients treated with interferon-β (abstract). *J Neuroimmunol* 1991; **35 (suppl 1)**:125.

90 Heremans H, Dillen C, Groenen M et al. Chronic relapsing experimental autoimmune encephalomyelitis (CREAE) in mice: enhancement by monoclonal antibodies against interferon-γ. *Eur J Immunol* 1996; **26**:2393–2398.

91 Ruuls SR, de Labie MCDC, Weber KS et al. The length of treatment determines whether IFN-β

prevents or aggravates EAE in Lewis rats. *J Immunol* 1996; 157:5721–5731.

92 van der Meide PH, de Labie MCDC, Ruuls SR et al. Discontinuation of treatment with IFN-β leads to exacerbation of EAE in Lewis rats. *J Neuroimmunol* 1998; 84:14–23.

93 The IFNB Multiple Sclerosis Study Group, the UBC MS/MRI Analysis Group. Interferon beta-1b in the treatment of multiple sclerosis: final outcome of the randomized controlled trial. *Neurology* 1995; 45:1277–1285.

94 The IFNB Multiple Sclerosis Study Group, the University of British Columbia MS/MRI Analysis Group. Neutralizing antibodies during treatment of multiple sclerosis with interferon beta-1b: experience during the first three years. *Neurology* 1996; 47:889–894.

95 Rudick RA, Simonian NA, Alam JA et al. Incidence and significance of neutralizing antibodies to interferon beta-1a in multiple sclerosis. *Neurology* 1998; 50:1266–1272.

96 Petkau J, White R. Neutralizing antibodies and the efficacy of interferon beta 1b in relapsing–remitting multiple sclerosis. *Multiple Sclerosis* 1997; 3:402.

97 Oger J, Vorobeychick G, Paty DW. IgG secretion in vitro in relation with antibody status in MS patients treated with interferon beta 1b. *Multiple Sclerosis* 1997; 3:406.

98 Antonelli G, Bagnato F, Pozzilli C et al. Development of neutralizing antibodies in patients with relapsing–remitting multiple sclerosis treated with IFN-β1a. *J Interferon Cytokine Res* 1998; 18:345–350.

99 Paty DW, Goodkin D, Thompson A, Rice G. Guidelines for physicians with patients on IFNβ-1b: the use of an assay for neutralising antibodies. *Neurology* 1996; 47:865–866.

100 Pachner AR. Anticytokine antibodies in beta interferon-treated MS patients and the need for testing: plight of the practicing neurologist. *Neurology* 1997; 49:647–650.

101 Paty DW, Li DKB, the UBC MS/MRI Study Group, the IFNB Multiple Sclerosis Study Group. Interferon beta-1b is effective in relapsing–remitting multiple sclerosis. II. MRI analysis. *Neurology* 1993; 43:662–667.

102 Cross AH, Antel JP. Antibodies to beta-interferons in multiple sclerosis. Can we neutralize the controversy? *Neurology* 1998; 50:1206–1208.

103 Neau JP, Guilhot F, Boinot C et al. Development of

chorea with lupus anticoagulant after interferon therapy. *Eur Neurol* 1996; 36:235–236.

104 Schwid SR, Goodman AD, Mattson DH. Autoimmune dysthyroidism in patients with multiple sclerosis treated with interferon beta-1b. *Arch Neurol* 1997; 57:1169–1170.

105 Blake G, Murphy S. Onset of myasthenia gravis in a patient with multiple sclerosis during interferon beta-1b treatment. *Neurology* 1997; 49:1747–1748.

106 Durelli L, Bongioanni MR, Cavallo R et al. Chronic systemic high-dose recombinant interferon alpha-2a reduces relapse rate, MRI signs of disease activity, and lymphocyte interferon gamma production in relapsing remitting multiple sclerosis. *Neurology* 1994; 44:406–413.

107 Yoshikawa M, Fukui H, Tsujii T. Immunological adverse effects of interferon treatment. *Clin Immunother* 1995; 4:361–375.

108 Coles AJ, Paolillo A, Molyneux P et al. Monoclonal antibody treatment exposes three mechanisms underlying the clinical course of multiple sclerosis. *Ann Neurol* 1998; 44:464.

109 Wynn DR, Rodriguez M, O'Fallon WM, Kurland LT. A reappraisal of the epidemiology of multiple sclerosis in Olmsted City, Minnesota. *Neurology* 1990; 40:780–785.

110 Colosimo C, Pozzilli C, Frontoni M et al. No increase of serum autoantibodies during therapy with recombinant human interferon-β-1a in relapsing–remitting multiple sclerosis. *Acta Neurol Scand* 1997; 96:372–374.

111 Kivisakk P, Lundahl J, von Heigl Z, Frederikson S. No evidence for increased frequency of autoantibodies during interferon-β-1b treatment of multiple sclerosis. *Acta Neurol Scand* 1998; 97:320–323.

112 Weber F, Polak TH, Gunther A et al. Synergistic immunomodulatory effects of Interferon-β-1b and the phophodiesterase inhibitor pentoxifylline in patients with relapsing remitting multiple sclerosis. *Ann Neurol* 1998; 44:27–34.

113 Rio J, Nos C, Marzo ME et al. Low-dose steroids reduce flu-like symptoms at the initiation of IFN-β-1b in relapsing–remitting MS. *Neurology* 1998; 50:1910–1912.

114 Martinez-Caceres EM, Rio J, Barrau M et al. Amelioration of flulike symptoms at the onset of interferon-β-1b therapy in multiple sclerosis by low-dose steroids is related to a decrease in interleukin-6 induction. *Ann Neurol* 1998; 44:682–685.

115 Simonian N, Goodman A, Guarnaccia et al. An open-label tolerability study of Interferon β-1a in combination with steroids and pentoxifylline in patients with moderate to severe multiple sclerosis. *Ann Neurol* 1998; **44**:504.

116 Brod SA, Kerman RJ, Nelson LD et al. Ingested IFN-alpha has biological effects in humans with relapsing–remitting multiple sclerosis. *Multiple Sclerosis* 1997; **3**:1–7.

117 Lublin FD, Reingold SC. Combination therapy for treatment of multiple sclerosis. *Ann Neurol* 1998; **44**:7–9.

118 Qu ZX, Dayal A, Jensen MA, Arnason BGW. All-trans retinoic acid potentiates the ability of interferon beta-1b to augment suppressor cell function in multiple sclerosis. *Arch Neurol* 1998; **55**:315–321.

119 Gasperini C, Pozzilli C, Bastianello S et al. Effect of steroids on Gd-enhancing lesions before and during recombinant beta interferon 1a treatment in relapsing remitting multiple sclerosis. *Neurology* 1998; **50**:403–406.

120 Quality Standards Subcommittee of the American Academy of Neurology. Practice advisory on selection of patients with multiple sclerosis for treatment with Betaseron. *Neurology* 1994; **44**:1537–1540.

121 Thompson AJ, Polman CH, Miller DH et al. Primary progressive multiple sclerosis. *Brain* 1997; **120**:1085–1096.

122 Scolding N, Franklin R. Axon loss in multiple sclerosis. *Lancet* 1998; **352**:340–341.

123 Neilley LK, Goodin DS, Goodkin DE, Hauser SL. Side effect profile of interferon beta-1b in MS: results of an open label trial. *Neurology* 1996; **46**:552–554.

124 Mohr DC, Goodkin DE, Likosky W et al. Treatment of depression improves adherence to interferon beta-1b therapy for multiple sclerosis. *Arch Neurol* 1997; **54**:531–533.

125 European Study Group on interferon β-1b in secondary progressive MS. Placebo-controlled multicentre randomised trial of interferon β-1b in treatment of secondary progressive multiple sclerosis. *Lancet* 1998; **352**:1491–1497.

126 Durelli L, Bongioanni MR, Ferrero B et al. Interferon treatment for multiple sclerosis: autoimmune complications may be lethal. *Neurology* 1998; **50**:570–571.

127 Linden D. Severe Raynaud's phenomenon associated with interferon-β treatment for multiple sclerosis. *Lancet* 1998; **352**:878–879.

128 Bongioanni MR, Durelli L, Ferrero B et al. Systemic high-dose recombinant-alpha-2a-interferon therapy modulates lymphokine production in multiple sclerosis. *J Neurol Sci* 1996; **143**:91–99.

129 Durelli L, Bongioanni MR, Ferrero B et al. Interferon alpha-2a treatment of relapsing remitting multiple sclerosis: disease activity resumes after stopping treatment. *Neurology* 1996; **47**:123–129.

21
Glatiramer acetate

Corey C Ford

INTRODUCTION

Multiple sclerosis (MS) is a disease of the central nervous system (CNS) that is characterized by multifocal, immune-mediated inflammation and myelin damage. The exact etiologic factors or agents that cause MS remain a mystery, although polygenic determinants that require exposure to an unknown environmental trigger are probable. One class of potential environmental triggers is an antigen of viral, bacterial or other origin. Small peptide fragments of viral protein components, with amino acid sequences similar to antigenic segments of myelin proteins, could induce a cross-reactive autoimmune attack by a process of molecular mimicry.[1]

Important insights into the mechanisms of immune-mediated myelin damage have come from animal models. For example, immunizing an animal to antigenic myelin components or peptide fragments can trigger experimental allergic encephalomyelitis (EAE), a form of CNS demyelination. Effective antigens in EAE induction include the major myelin proteins, myelin basic protein (MBP), proteolipid protein (PLP), and myelin oligodendrocyte glycoprotein (MOG). In fact, it is known that patients with MS, as well as normal persons, have potentially autoreactive T-cells specific to these myelin antigens in their peripheral circulation.[2–7]

The possibility that MS is driven at certain stages by similar immune mechanisms has led to extensive studies of antigen-specific immune-modulating strategies. Knowledge that axonal injury and axonal transection occurs early in MS and may correlate with permanent neurological deficits has provided additional motivation to find more effective treatments to slow or halt the inflammatory disease process.[8]

The synthetic copolymer drug glatiramer acetate (Copaxone®) has been studied extensively as a therapeutic agent for MS. After a small open label study and pilot trials, data from a large phase 3 study led to approval of glatiramer acetate by the Food and Drug Administration (FDA) in the USA for relapsing–remitting MS (RRMS) in 1997. Additional information from a 6-month extension of this trial confirmed the efficacy and tolerability of glatiramer acetate as a treatment for RRMS. Most recently, 5-year data acquired in an ongoing, open-label study of patients originally enrolled in the phase 3 trial, showed sustained benefit in terms of relapse rate reduction and apparent slowing of the progression of disability. When the FDA approved copolymer 1 for use in MS, the generic name, glatiramer acetate, was applied. The trademark name of the drug is Copaxone®, and all three names are used in different parts of this review.

HISTORY OF COPOLYMER 1

The discovery and development of copolymer 1 (glatiramer acetate) is a fascinating story of scientific ingenuity and serendipity. As an immune-mediated disease of the CNS, MS presents inherent barriers for human research. The development of animal models of demyelination has been an important step in unraveling the immune mechanisms that underlie MS. EAE is a T-cell-mediated disease that can be induced in susceptible animals by inoculating them with CNS tissue in complete Freund's adjuvant. Certain purified protein components of myelin, such as MBP, can also be encephalitogenic or capable of producing EAE when injected into a susceptible animal.[9,10] Three decades ago, Ruth Arnon and her colleagues at the Weitzmann Institute in Israel were interested in the structural mechanisms of EAE induction by such protein antigens, and they synthesized a family of 11 different copolymers (copolymer 1 up to copolymer 11) as potential encephalitogens. The copolymers were synthesized with amino acid compositions chosen to be similar to myelin basic protein. None of the copolymers proved capable of inducing EAE, but several had the property of preventing the development of EAE or reducing disease severity in animals inoculated with MBP. Copolymer 1, which is composed of L-glutamate, L-lysine, L-alanine and L-tyrosine, was the most potent of these, and it reduced the incidence of EAE in MBP-challenged guinea pigs from 75% to 20%.[11,12]

Cross-reactivity of copolymer 1 and MBP was shown at both the T-cell and B-cell levels. The degree of cross-reactivity of copolymer 1 with MBP in assays of lymphocyte transformation and delayed hypersensitivity and by monoclonal antibody binding studies correlated well with the ability of copolymer 1 to suppress EAE.[13] Furthermore, the immune-modulating effect of copolymer 1 seemed to be restricted to a response induced by myelin antigens and was not due to general immunosuppressive properties.[14] The D-amino acid isomer of copolymer 1 did not have immunologic cross-reactivity with MBP and had no effect in suppressing the development of EAE.[15]

An important series of experiments showed that copolymer 1 could suppress the development or reduce the severity of EAE in a variety of animals, including mice, rats, guinea pigs, rabbits, and primates.[16–20] Studies in primates were of particular relevance to the treatment of MS in humans. It was known that Rhesus monkeys and baboons were very sensitive to MBP-induced EAE and typically died of the disease within 2 weeks of the onset of symptoms. Treatment with copolymer 1 was found to reverse EAE in these animals after the appearance of symptoms. This was an important result in considering testing in humans with MS. Toxicity testing in animals did not reveal mutagenic or other serious side effects, and the stage was set for copolymer 1 to enter clinical testing in humans.

CLINICAL TRIAL DATA

Initial trial in human subjects—1977

Copolymer 1 was used first in three patients with acute disseminated encephalomyelitis (ADE) and four in the terminal stages of MS.[21] ADE is similar to EAE in its disease course and immunopathology. The ADE patients received 2 mg of copolymer 1 by intramuscular injection every day for 2 weeks, and the MS patients received 2–3 mg every 2–3 days for 3 weeks. The

MS patients continued to receive weekly injections of 2–3 mg for an additional period of 2–5 months. The ADE patients treated with copolymer 1 all recovered completely within 3 weeks, as did one control ADE patient treated with corticosteroids. A second control ADE patient treated with corticosteroids had neurological sequelae. The MS patients, all of whom had severe levels of disability, were apparently stable during treatment. Copolymer 1 was well tolerated by both patient groups. No side effects or toxicities were obvious in this small study, supporting the toxicology data that had been obtained in animals. Despite a lack of a clear benefit in this restricted group of patients, the tolerability and apparent safety of copolymer 1 led to further clinical studies in patients with MS.

Preliminary efficacy trial—1982

A small, phase 1 clinical trial was conducted by Bornstein and colleagues[22] at the Einstein College of Medicine to begin assessing the efficacy of copolymer 1 in MS and to further study toxicity and safety. In this trial, 16 patients with MS were enrolled, 12 with chronic progressive disease and four with RRMS. The study used open-label copolymer 1 and both the examining neurologists and the patients knew they were receiving the drug. The protocol utilized a dose of 20 mg copolymer 1 injected intramuscularly five times weekly for 3 weeks, three times weekly for 3 weeks, twice weekly for 3 weeks, and then once weekly for the remainder of the 6-month trial.

At the end of the study, two of the four patients with RRMS and three of the 12 patients with progressive disease were assessed as being better and showed reduced numbers of relapses or slowed progression. It was not possible to determine whether the apparent beneficial responses represented an effect of treatment or a placebo effect. As in previous animal and human studies, copolymer 1 was well tolerated, and no significant toxicities or undesirable effects were noted.

Pilot trial of copolymer 1 in RRMS—1987

The first randomized, double-blind study of copolymer 1 in MS was also conducted by Bornstein and colleagues at the Albert Einstein College of Medicine.[23] The primary end-point of the pilot trial was to determine the proportion of relapse-free patients on copolymer 1 treatment compared to placebo, as well as to characterize any toxicities or significant side-effects.

The study enrolled 48 patients in 24 pairs matched for age, sex and disability and stratified in three ranges on the Disability Status Scale (DSS), 0–2, 3–4, and 5–6. The DSS is an instrument for rating neurologic disability caused by MS on a scale of 1 to 10.[24] Two additional unmatched patients were also enrolled. The random assignment of one member of a pair to placebo or copolymer 1 placed the second member in the other treatment group. All patients had active MS, defined as exacerbations in the previous 2 years, and all were between 20 and 35 years of age. The 50 patients were selected from a pool of 140 patients who were screened for the study. Each patient was assessed every 3 months after an initial visit for a total period of 2 years. Neurological examinations were performed at each visit by a neurologist, who was blinded to the patient's treatment group. Patients were seen at other times for suspected exacerbations, defined as new or worsening neurological symptoms persisting for at least 48 hours or more and producing objective changes on examination leading to a 1-point

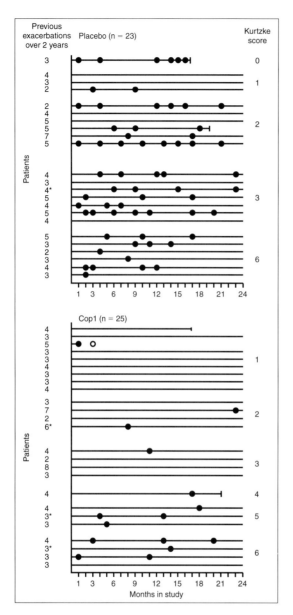

Fig. 21.1 *Relapses occurring during the 2 years of the pilot RRMS trial. Each line represents a patient and each circle an exacerbation. Patients are grouped according to their Kurtzke EDSS score on entry to the trial. The numbers of pre-trial exacerbations are indicated to the left. Discontinued lines represent patients who withdrew before completion. The open circle indicates an exacerbation that occurred after withdrawal but that was included as a study event. Patients who were not included in the matched-pair analyses are indicated by an asterisk. (Reprinted by permission of the New England Journal of Medicine, Bornstein et al, Vol. 317, 408–414. © 1987 Massachusetts Medical Society. All rights reserved.)*[23]

increase in their DSS. Subjective symptoms alone, such as sensory changes, were not considered as exacerbations. About 75% of exacerbations in both placebo and treatment groups were treated with corticosteroids. Samples for routine complete blood counts and blood chemistry as well as urine specimens were collected at the 3-monthly visits.

Seven patients did not complete the full 2 years of the trial. Two of these patients were in the placebo group and were excluded from the final analysis. Partial data available from the other five drop-outs was included in the analyses.

Twenty-two patient pairs (44 patients) were included in a matched analysis of the primary end-point. Four other patients were included in an unmatched analysis. Discordant pairs were those in which one patient had exacerbations on copolymer 1 or placebo when the matched patient in the other treatment group had none. There were 12 discordant pairs, 10 on copolymer 1 who had no exacerbations while their placebo matches did and two on placebo who had exacerbations while their copolymer 1 matches did not. Statistical analysis showed a significant difference in discordant pairs in favor of fewer relapses in those treated with copolymer 1 compared to the placebo treatment group ($p = 0.039$). The unmatched analysis also reached statistical significance for the occurrence of fewer exacerbations on copolymer 1 ($p = 0.045$).

There was a total of 16 exacerbations in the 25 patients on copolymer 1 and 62 in the 23 receiving placebo (*Fig. 21.1*). Data stratified by entry DSS showed that patients in the lower disability ranges who received copolymer 1 tended to have fewer relapses than patients with higher DSS at entry. More patients on copolymer 1 completed the trial relapse-free, and patients receiving placebo were more likely to have had three or more relapses. Each of these study results reached statistical significance. Survival curves showed a significant ($p = 0.05$) slowing of progression of disability at the end of 24 months as measured by an increase of 1 full point on the DSS sustained for 3 months (*Fig. 21.2*).

No abnormalities were noted in any laboratory measures during the study. Two patients had an unusual, transient post-injection reaction to copolymer 1. This reaction consisted of flushing, chest tightness, sweating, dyspnea and anxiety. The symptoms resolved in 5–30 minutes without sequelae. One of the patients with these symptoms developed uncomfortable urticaria and pruritus after restarting the medication and was

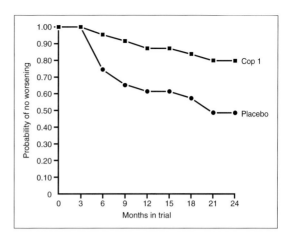

Fig. 21.2 *Curves represent the probability of no worsening from the baseline Kurtzke EDSS score in the pilot RRMS trial. Worsening was determined when first observed but was counted only if it continued for 3 months. (Reprinted by permission of the* New England Journal of Medicine, *Bornstein et al, Vol. 317, 408–414. © 1987 Massachusetts Medical Society. All rights reserved.)*[23]

treated with epinephrine (adrenaline) and corticosteroids.

Trial in chronic-progressive MS—1991

A single clinical trial of copolymer 1 has been completed for patients with chronic progressive MS.[25] This double-blind, placebo-controlled trial was conducted at two study centers in the USA, the Albert Einstein College of Medicine in New York and the Baylor College of Medicine in Houston, Texas. Inclusion criteria for the study demanded that patients had evidence of a progressive disease course for at least 18 months with no more than two relapses in the preceding 24 months. A total of 169 patients from a screened pool of over 2000 patients was found to be eligible for a pre-trial observation period to document progression of disability. Entry disability ranged from 2.0 to 6.5 on the Kurtzke

Expanded Disability Status Scale (EDSS).[26] The EDSS is a disability rating instrument for MS; it is similar to the DSS but it has half-point increments in the scale from 1 to 10. The EDSS is based on assessment of Functional System Scales (FSS) of neurological functions, including pyramidal, sensory, cerebellar, bowel and bladder, brainstem, mental, and visual functions. Progression for study entry was defined in one of the following ways:

(a) a 1.0 point worsening on the EDSS;

(b) a 2.0 point worsening in one of the functional systems scores of the EDSS;

(c) a 1.0 point worsening in each of two unrelated functional systems; or

(d) a 2.0 point worsening on the Ambulation Index.

Patients were required to have documented progression of disability by at least one of these measures persisting for at least 3 months. Of the 169 patients followed for 6–15 months, 106 showed progression and were entered into the study. A retrospective analysis of data from this clinical trial suggested that 30 out of the 106 patients enrolled probably had primary progressive MS and the remaining 76 had secondary progressive MS.

The primary study end-point was the time to confirmed progression persisting for at least 3 months, defined in one of the following ways:

(a) a 1.0 point worsening on the EDSS for patients with baseline EDSS ≥ 5.0; or

(b) a 1.5 point worsening on the EDSS for patients with entry EDSS < 5.0.

Secondary end-points included time to unconfirmed progression, time to progression of 0.5 points on EDSS, EDSS change from study entry, and a neurologist's impression of the patient's overall clinical status.

Fifty-five patients were enrolled at the Albert

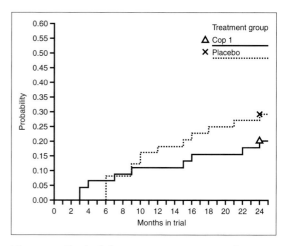

Fig. 21.3 *Trial of glatiramer acetate in secondary progressive MS. Probability of progressing to confirmed progression. (Reproduced from Bornstein et al. Neurology 1991; 41: 533–539 with permission.)*[25]

Einstein College and 51 at the Baylor College. Ten patients on copolymer 1 and 10 on placebo withdrew from the study; 86 patients completed the 2-year trial. Of the withdrawals, three were counted as reaching confirmed progression, two from the copolymer 1 group and one from the placebo group. The other 17 withdrawals were not included in the analysis for primary end-point. Survival curves for the probability of progression in each treatment arm are shown in *Fig. 21.3*. There was a trend for less progression in the groups receiving copolymer 1 compared to the groups receiving placebo (17.6% versus 25.5%), but this did not reach statistical significance. When the data was analysed separately by center, there was a statistically significant decrease in confirmed progression at the Einstein site, 21.4% for copolymer 1 compared to 38.5% for placebo (*p* = 0.041). Confirmed progression for patients receiving copolymer 1 was similar at the two centers, whereas the placebo group was more than twice as likely to progress at the

Einstein site than at Baylor. Categorical analysis of change in EDSS from baseline by study group showed a trend in favor of copolymer 1, but this did not reach statistical significance (*Fig. 21.4*). Overall, 56.9% of patients receiving copolymer 1 were stable or improved during the trial, compared to 49.1% of patients receiving placebo.

There were 12 patients who experienced the transient, self-limited injection reaction and more patients receiving copolymer 1 than patients receiving placebo reported soreness (83% vs 47%), itching (61% vs 17%), swelling (80% vs 23%), or redness (85% vs 30%).

Phase 3 double-blind, placebo-controlled trial—1995

After publication of the positive pilot study of copolymer 1 in RRMS, there was great interest in confirming safety and efficacy of the drug in a larger, phase 3 trial. The further development and testing of copolymer 1 was assumed by Teva Pharmaceuticals Ltd of Petah Tikva, Israel, and considerable effort was put into standardizing manufacturing methods to provide the kilogram quantities of drug needed to conduct such a trial. The final product was approved in the USA by the FDA and consisted of random, synthetic polypeptide chains ranging in molecular weight from 4 to 13 kDa. The four amino acids L-alanine, L-glutamate, L-lysine, and L-tyrosine were combined in a molar ratio of 4.2, 1.4, 3.4, to 1.0, respectively. A dose of 20 mg administered subcutaneously by daily injection for 24 months was selected as the study dose in this double-blind, placebo-controlled trial.

The trial began in October 1991 at 11 university-based MS centers in the USA. The primary end-point of the study was the mean number of MS relapses in subjects receiving copolymer 1

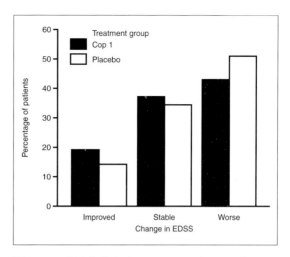

Fig. 21.4 *Trial of glatiramer acetate in secondary progressive MS. Changes in EDSS score from baseline by treatment group. (Reproduced from Bornstein et al. Neurology 1991; 41: 533–539 with permission.)*[25]

compared to those receiving placebo. Relapses were defined as the appearance or reappearance of one or more neurological abnormalities persisting for at least 48 hours. A relapse was not confirmed unless the patient was stable or improving for the previous 30 days. Prospectively defined secondary end-points included:

(a) the proportion of relapse-free patients;

(b) the time to first relapse after initiation of therapy;

(c) the mean change in EDSS and Ambulation Index from baseline to study completion; and

(d) the proportion of patients with sustained progression, defined as an increase of 1 full point on the EDSS persisting for at least 3 months.

Patients were given a 30-day supply of copolymer 1 at monthly visits and they were instructed to report adverse events, changes in their condition, or the use of concomitant medications. Every 3 months, each patient underwent a detailed assessment by two neurologists. One neurologist was a blinded examiner, who performed the EDSS evaluation and other objective assessments without information pertaining to symptoms or adverse events. The second neurologist acted as a treatment physician, assessing symptoms and adverse events and making decisions whether to treat relapses with corticosteroids. A nurse co-ordinator at each site performed nursing assessments and collected blood and urine samples for laboratory analysis. All patients and study personnel, including the neurologists and co-ordinators, were blinded to the individual study drug assignment.

A total of 284 patients were screened for the trial, and 251 were randomized to copolymer 1 or placebo. The two groups were well matched for age, sex, duration of disease, mean relapse rate in the preceding 2 years, EDSS, and Ambulation Index. The mean age of the subjects was 34 years and 73% were women. All had clinically definite or laboratory supported MS with EDSS scores ranging from 0 to 5.0. The proportion of patients in different EDSS ranges is shown in *Table 21.1*.

Patients were not enrolled in the study unless they were clinically stable, without corticosteroids, for the preceding 30 days. No patient had previously received copolymer 1, immunosuppressive therapy or total lymphoid irradiation. Other exclusion criteria included pregnancy, positive serology for human immunodeficiency virus or human T cell leukemia virus-1, insulin-dependent diabetes mellitus or chronic need for aspirin or non-steroidal anti-inflammatory drugs. Women of childbearing potential were required to use an appropriate method of contraception.

There were 161 confirmed relapses in the group receiving copolymer 1 and 210 in the group receiving placebo. Relapse confirmation required that symptoms be accompanied by

Table 21.1 Pivotal trial of Copaxone® in RRMS. Entry EDSS ranges for patients randomized to study drug or placebo. (Adapted from Johnson.[27])

EDSS Range	Copolymer 1	Placebo	Total Fraction (N = 251)
0 to 2.0	20%	27%	47%
>2.0 to 4	23%	18%	41%
>4.0 to 5.0	7%	5%	12%
			100%

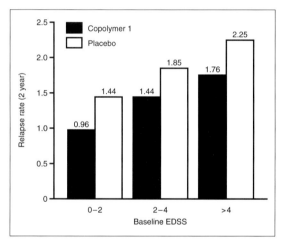

Fig. 21.5 Changes in relapse rate observed over 2 years, by baseline EDSS score in the phase 3 trial of glatiramer acetate. The numbers above each bar represent the mean 2-year relapse rate for each group. (Reproduced from Johnson et al. Neurology 1995; 45: 1269–1276 with permission.)[27]

objective abnormalities on neurological examination resulting in a minimum of one half step increase in the EDSS, a 2 point increase on one of seven FSS, or a one point change on two or more FSS. The mean annualized relapse rate was 0.59 per year for the patients receiving copolymer 1 and 0.84 per year for the group receiving

Table 21.2 Disability experience measured by EDSS and Ambulation Index of Copaxone® and placebo groups (secondary end-points) in the pivotal trial in RRMS. (Reproduced from Johnson et al. *Neurology* 1995; 45: 1268–1276 with permission.)[27]

	Copolymer 1	*Placebo*	p *Value*
Proportion of patients with a change in disability between baseline and conclusion			
Improved (EDSS decrease ≥1)	24.8%	15.2%	
No change	54.4%	56.0%	0.037*
Worse (EDSS increase ≥1)	20.8%	28.8%	
EDSS change from baseline (mean ± SD)	−0.05 ± 1.13	0.21 ± 0.99	0.023†
Proportion of progression-free patients	78.4%	75.4%	NS
Ambulation index (mean ± SD)	0.27 ± 0.94	0.28 ± 0.93	NS

EDSS Expanded Disability Status Scale.
NS Not significantly different.
* Categorical repeated measures.
† Repeated-measures analysis of covariance.

placebo, a 29% reduction ($p = 0.007$). The effects of copolymer 1 on relapse rate reduction reached 33% in the group of patients with lowest EDSS scores (between 0 and 2) at study entry (*Fig. 21.5*).

Several of the secondary end-points of the trial were designed to evaluate the effects of copolymer 1 on progression of neurological disability. The results of analyses for these end-points are shown in *Table 21.2*. Mean EDSS change from baseline was significantly lower for the treatment group than the placebo group ($p = 0.023$). Changes in Ambulation Index and the number of progression-free patients, defined as an increase

of 1 or more steps on the EDSS sustained for 3 months, showed little difference between groups. A categorical analysis of patients who were the same, better, or worse during the trial showed a statistical benefit for copolymer 1 (see *Table 21.2* and *Fig. 21.6*).

Treatment with copolymer 1 was not associated with any hematologic, metabolic, urinary or cardiac abnormalities. Mild erythema, stinging and induration at injection sites were the most common adverse events reported. The transient post-injection reaction first observed in the pilot trial occurred more often in patients receiving copolymer 1 than in patients receiving placebo.

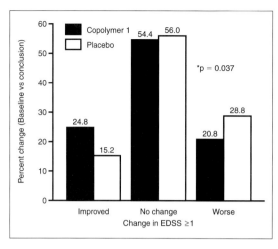

Fig. 21.6 *The percentage of patients who improved, were unchanged, or were worse by 1 or more EDSS steps between baseline and the last (24-month) measurement (repeated measures analysis of covariance (ANCOVA)) in the phase 3 trial of glatiramer acetate. The numbers above the bars represent the percentage of patients in the respective glatiramer acetate or placebo group. (Reproduced from Johnson et al.* Neurology *1995;* **45:** *1268–1276 with permission.)*[27]

This random, unpredictable reaction occurred in 15% of patients receiving copolymer 1; it usually occurred within seconds or minutes of an injection. Variable combinations of flushing, chest tightness, a sense of shortness of breath, palpitations, and anxiety characterized the reaction. Typical reactions lasted between 30 seconds and 30 minutes and no patients experienced serious sequelae. Four patients in the copolymer 1 group and one in the placebo group discontinued therapy because of this reaction. Three women became pregnant while enrolled in the trial and all were taking active drug. One had a therapeutic abortion and the other two discontinued treatment and delivered normal infants.

This 2-year pivotal trial confirmed that daily, subcutaneous injections of copolymer 1 were effective in reducing the relapse rate in patients with RRMS.[27] By several secondary end-point analyses, copolymer 1 showed benefit in slowing the progression of disability. On the basis of the 24-month core trial data, the FDA approved copolymer 1 (Copaxone®) in December 1997 for use in RRMS. Glatiramer acetate was selected as the generic name for Copaxone®.

Extension period of the phase 3 trial—1998

Early in the course of the phase 3 trial, a decision was made to continue all patients on blinded study medication until the last patient enrolled in the trial completed 24 months. Some patients were on blinded medication for up to 35 months, and there was an average of 5.5 months of additional double-blind study data. The blinding and protocol conditions of the extension period of the study were unchanged. The 24-month core study data and the extension phase data were combined in a second report of the safety and efficacy of Copaxone®.[28]

The characteristics of the patients continuing in the double-blind extension period of the trial are shown in *Table 21.3*. Approximately equal numbers of patients in the Copaxone (n = 19) and placebo (n = 17) arms of the 24 month core study dropped out after nearly equal periods of time. A total of 215 patients completed 24 months of the core study and these patients were eligible to continue in the extension phase. Of these, 203 (94.4%) elected to enter the extension phase. Near the end of the 24-month core study period, interferon-β 1b (Betaseron®) became the first drug approved by the FDA for the treatment of RRMS. All patients in the Copaxone® trial were notified of this development and signed a new informed consent to continue in the trial. The availability of interferon-β 1b for their

Table 21.3 Characteristics of patients in the initial and extended glatiramer acetate study. (Reproduced from Johnson et al. *Neurology* 1998; 50: 701–708 with permission.)[28]

| | Initial 24-month study | | | | | | Extension study | | | |
| | Randomized (n = 251) | | Completed 24 months (n = 215) | | Dropouts (n = 36) | | Entered (n = 203) | | Completed (n = 194) | |
	Glatiramer acetate (n = 125)	Placebo (n = 126)	Glatiramer acetate (n = 106)	Placebo (n = 109)	Glatiramer acetate (n = 19)	Placebo (n = 17)	Glatiramer acetate (n = 99)	Placebo (n = 104)	Glatiramer acetate (n = 97)	Placebo (n = 97)
Age (y)	34.58 ± 5.97	34.33 ± 6.49	34.80 ± 5.87	34.03 ± 6.55	33.37 ± 6.53	36.29 ± 5.87	34.68 ± 5.81	34.03 ± 6.63	34.71 ± 6.04	34.25 ± 6.58
Duration of disease (y)	7.25 ± 4.85	6.64 ± 5.09	7.46 ± 4.89	6.82 ± 5.20	6.10 ± 4.56	5.54 ± 4.28	7.39 ± 4.91	6.82 ± 5.24	7.30 ± 4.91	6.62 ± 5.21
Prior 2-year relapse rate	2.91 ± 1.26	2.93 ± 1.13	2.96 ± 1.30	2.94 ± 1.11	2.63 ± 1.01	2.82 ± 1.29	3.00 ± 1.32	2.93 ± 1.13	2.97 ± 1.33	2.94 ± 1.10
Baseline EDSS	2.82 ± 1.19	2.42 ± 1.28	2.77 ± 1.19	2.42 ± 1.28	3.08 ± 1.18	2.41 ± 1.34	2.77 ± 1.21	2.42 ± 1.30	2.77 ± 1.19	2.36 ± 1.29

EDSS = Expanded Disability Status Score.

disease was the most common reason patients gave for dropping out of the core study and not continuing in the extension phase. There was no evidence that any bias was introduced into the extension phase data by the subgroup of patients opting not to continue, and their characteristics are also summarized in *Table 21.3*.

The mean MS relapse rate was the primary end-point of both the core and extension phases of the trial. The combined data from the core period and the extension period showed that the annualized mean relapse rate was 0.67 per year for the Copaxone®-treated cohort and 0.99 per year for the placebo group, a reduction of 32% ($p = 0.002$). This result compared well with the 29% reduction in relapse rate observed in the core trial period. At the end of the extension phase of the trial, 24.6% of the placebo group and 33.6% of the Copaxone® group were free of relapses from study initiation ($p = 0.035$). The numbers of patients having no relapses, one or two relapses or three or more relapses during the

Table 21.4 MS relapse experience (24-month core period and extended trial periods). (Reproduced from Johnson et al. *Neurology* 1998; 50: 701–708 with permission.)[28]

	Glatiramer acetate	Placebo	p Value
Core study (24 mo)			
Number of relapses per patient			
0	42	34	
1–2	60	55	0.023
≥3	23	37	
Core and extension			
Number of relapses per patient			
0	42	31	
1–2	53	51	0.008
≥3	30	44	

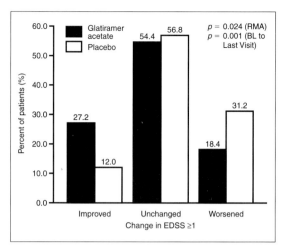

Fig. 21.7 *The percentage of patients who improved, were unchanged, or were worse by 1 or more EDSS steps between baseline and the last measurement in the extension period of the phase 3 trial. Repeated measures analysis (RMA) and baseline (BL) to last visit observations are shown. The RMA and the p value of 0.024 refer to a repeated measures analysis of the proportion of patients in each of the three categories (improved, no change, or worsened) at each time point (every 3 months). As shown by the numbers above the bars, 27.2% of patients treated with glatiramer acetate and 12% of patients receiving placebo showed an improvement at study termination. The p value of 0.001 is derived from the Cochran–Mantel–Haenszel test on the 2 × 3 contingency table (two treatment groups by the three categorical changes of improved, no change, or worsened). (Reproduced from Johnson et al. Neurology 1998; 50: 701–708 with permission.)[28]*

study are shown in *Table 21.4*. Patients receiving placebo were more likely to have had multiple relapses ($p = 0.008$).

Compared to the 24 month core trial data, more of the secondary measures of progression of disability showed significant benefit with Copaxone® treatment. A simple categorical analysis demonstrated that more Copaxone®-treated patients improved by one or more EDSS steps than placebo patients, who were more likely to worsen (*p* = 0.001) (*Fig. 21.7*). Time to worsening by 1.5 or more steps on the EDSS was evaluated using a Kaplan–Meier approach. In order to eliminate bias resulting from higher EDSS scores during relapses, the period of time from the onset of each relapse to stable recovery or plateau of disability for 30 days was determined. All EDSS data from these relapse intervals were removed before performing the survival analysis. Only 21.6% of Copaxone®-treated patients worsened by 1.5 or more EDSS steps while not in a relapse, compared to 41.6% of the placebo patients (*Fig. 21.8*). This was a significant difference of almost 50% (*p* = 0.001). At the end of the extended trial, 25 of the 125 placebo patients and 16 of 125 of the Copaxone®-treated patients were worse by ≥ 1.5 points on the EDSS. This result differs from the Kaplan–Meier analysis, in which patients who reach the progression end-point of ≥ 1.5 EDSS steps are, by definition, excluded from further analysis. Some patients who reached this end-point in the Kaplan–Meier data improved at later times, resulting in fewer patients showing this level of progression at the end of the extended study than reaching the end-point at any time during the study. This finding is common to clinical trials in RRMS and can be a source of confusion.

Safety and tolerability of Copaxone® was confirmed in the extension period. There were no laboratory abnormalities associated with Copaxone® use. Mild injection reactions of erythema and pain occurred in approximately two thirds of patients injecting Copaxone® and one third of patients injecting placebo. By the end of the extension phase, 19 patients had had at least one transient, self-limited injection reaction. One

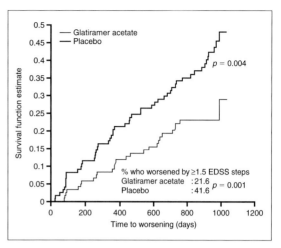

Fig. 21.8 *Time to increased disability determined by ≥ 1.5 EDSS steps (Kaplan–Meier analysis) in the extension period of the phase 3 trial. In the placebo group, 41.6% of patients worsened by ≥ 1.5 EDSS steps during the extended trial, whereas only 21.6% of those receiving glatiramer acetate worsened (p = 0.001; χ² test). EDSS scores that were determined during the period of recovery after each relapse (the relapse–remission interval) were excluded from the analysis. (Reproduced from Johnson et al. Neurology 1998; 50: 701–708 with permission.)[28]*

patient experienced a total of seven such reactions in 30 months, yet continued on treatment. Overall, this unusual reaction occurred about 1 in every 840 daily injections.

Long-term open-label use of glatiramer acetate in MS

At the end of the extension period of the phase 3 trial of Copaxone® in RRMS, patients still in the study were given the opportunity of continuing treatment in an open-label study. Patients who had been receiving glatiramer acetate or placebo

Table 21.5 Comparison of the baseline characteristics in the double-blind trial of patients who were or were not in the group completing 5 years on open-label glatiramer acetate.

Characteristic	Glatiramer acetate group		Placebo group	
	Not included	Included	Not included	Included
n	40	85	41	85
Sex (% female)	70.0%	70.6%	80.5%	74.1%
Age first symptom appeared (mean)	26.90	27.81	27.51	27.89
No. of relapses during 2 years prior to entry (mean)	2.73	3.0	3.1	2.85
Baseline EDSS score (mean)	2.75	2.85	2.35	2.45

for 2–3 years were placed on open-label drug. Of the total of 251 patients enrolled in the original double-blind trial, 170 completed 5 years in the open label study, 85 from the Copaxone®-treatment group and 85 from the placebo group. Baseline characteristics of the patients completing 5 years of open label Copaxone® are shown in *Table 21.5*. These patients were followed at 6-month intervals and they reported to the study centers for evaluations of relapses and problems as they did in the phase 3 trial (*Fig. 21.9*). Neurological assessments for EDSS were recorded at each visit along with safety and adverse event information.

At completion of the pivotal double-blind trial, this cohort of 170 patients had a relapse rate of 0.77 per year in the placebo group and 0.56 per year in the glatiramer acetate-treated group. Both groups together had an annual relapse rate of 0.24 up to and including year 5 of the open label study (*Fig. 21.10*).[29] The patients who were on glatiramer acetate from study outset showed a steady yearly decline in relapse rate. By the end of the fifth year, the relapse rate

for this subgroup of 85 patients was 0.16 (*Fig. 21.11*). This rate corresponds to one attack every five to six years. During this same 5-year period, the mean EDSS for the glatiramer acetate treated cohort remained stable (*Fig. 21.12*). The open-label glatiramer acetate data supports the opinion that this drug provides continued benefit and tolerability in the treatment of RRMS, with two thirds of the patients enrolled in the pivotal trial continuing to use the drug for up to 8 years.

There are inherent limitations to measuring efficacy in open-label studies. The absence of a placebo arm for comparison is important; however, there is no ethical way to obtain long-term efficacy data using a placebo group when effective treatments for a disease are available. Comparisons can be made to natural history data or to placebo groups from other clinical trials, but such comparisons are hazardous because studies are conducted differently, enroll diverse types of patients, and the outcome measures can be difficult to compare across trials. Additionally, patients who drop out of open label studies may introduce a bias, especially if the reason is disease

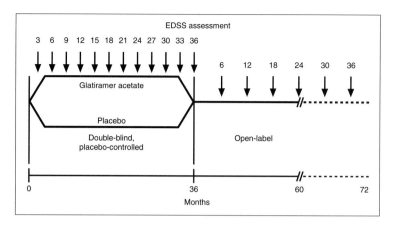

Fig. 21.9 *Design of USA pivotal trial of Copaxone® in RRMS. Both double-blind and open-label phases are shown.*

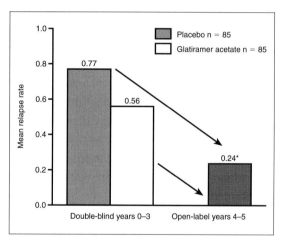

Fig. 21.10 *Open-label glatiramer acetate study. Relapse rate in the double-blind and open-label phases up to and including year 5. The year 4 and 5 data include patients who were initially on glatiramer acetate and those who switched from placebo to active drug.*

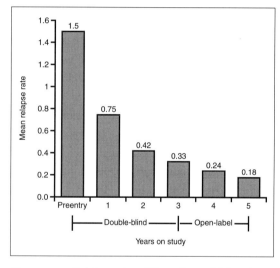

Fig. 21.11 *Relapse rates of the cohort of 85 patients who initially received glatiramer acetate in the double-blind study and who completed 5 years in the open-label phase.*

activity and progression of disability. Despite these difficulties, open-label studies remain the best alternative to placebo-controlled trials for obtaining long-term safety and efficacy data. Open-label extensions of phase 3 clinical trials can enhance the confidence of patients and clinicians in their choice of therapy. It would be sensible for future phase 3 trials in MS to plan for ongoing open-label studies after the initial double-blind study is completed.

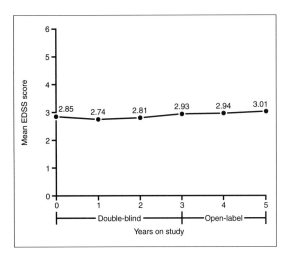

Fig. 21.12 *Mean EDSS scores of the cohort of 85 patients who initially received glatiramer acetate in the double-blind study and who completed 5 years in the open-label phase.*

Data from magnetic resonance imaging in support of the efficacy of glatiramer acetate

The phase 3 trial of Copaxone® did not include center-wide, serial magnetic resonance imaging (MRI) data as secondary end-points of efficacy. Twenty-seven patients in the study at the University of Pennsylvania site underwent frequent MRI scans. Analysis of the number of gadolinium-enhancing lesions suggested a trend in favor of Copaxone®-treated patients, but the small number of patients scanned did not allow for statistical confirmation of benefit.

A more recent study followed monthly MRI changes in a group of 10 patients with RRMS.[30] The patients received monthly gadolinium-enhanced MRI scans for a period of 9–27 months before receiving therapy with glatiramer acetate. Six of the subjects had scans for 25–27 months before initiation of treatment. Each patient then received monthly MRI for 10–14 additional months while on glatiramer acetate. The incidence of new gadolinium-enhancing lesions was decreased in the patients receiving glatiramer acetate (0.92 per month) compared to their pre-treatment scans (2.20 per month). This represented a 57% reduction but was significant only at the 0.1 level by Wilcoxon signed rank test. If the occurrence of new gadolinium-enhancing lesions per month was stratified into observations of 0, 1, 2, . . . n lesions in the pre- and post-treatment period, the difference was significant by a Mantel–Haenszel test ($p = 0.003$). The six patients with the longest pre-treatment scan period showed a significant decrease in the percentage change in lesion load area during the treatment phase ($p = 0.05$).

In 1997, a large, randomized, double-blind, placebo-controlled MRI trial was initiated at 29 centers in Canada and five European countries. Patients were randomized to glatiramer acetate or placebo for 9 months followed by an open-label phase for an additional 9 months. MRI scans were performed monthly for the first 9 months and every 3 months for the remaining 9 months. The design of this study to investigate the effects of glatiramer acetate on MRI lesion load and new lesion formation is shown in *Fig. 21.13*. Patients were required to have a diagnosis of RRMS with at least one or more relapses in the 2 years preceding entry into the trial and at least one gadolinium-enhancing lesion on a screening MRI scan. A total of 485 patients were screened and 239 were enrolled in the study. There were no significant demographic or MRI differences in the placebo and treatment groups at study entry.

The primary outcome measure was the number of gadolinium-enhancing lesions on T1-weighted images. There were several secondary end-points, including:

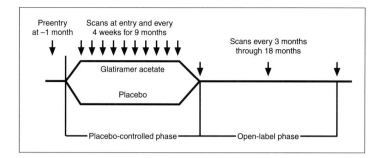

Fig. 21.13 Design of randomized double-blind, placebo-controlled MRI trial of Copaxone.

(a) The proportion of patients with gadolinium-enhancing lesions;

(b) gadolinium-enhancing lesion volume;

(c) Number of new gadolinium-enhancing lesions;

(d) Total number of lesions on T2-weighted images;

(e) The number of new lesions on T2-weighted images; and

(f) Hypointense lesion ('black holes') volume on T1-weighted images.

A preliminary analysis of the study was provided by Dr G Comi (personal communication). The 9-month double blind data showed a 35% reduction in the total number of gadolinium-enhancing lesions in the group receiving glatiramer acetate compared to placebo ($p = 0.0007$). The change in volume of gadolinium-enhancing lesions from baseline in the treated cohort was less than in the placebo group ($p = 0.0098$). The mean number of new gadolinium-enhancing lesions and the mean number of new T2-weighted image lesions in the treated group were both reduced by 35% ($p = 0.001$ for both). Change in total T2-weighted image lesion volume from baseline was lower for the treated patients ($p = 0.0245$). The reduction in relapse rate was 33% ($p = 0.0117$), consistent with the pivotal phase 3 trial core plus extension data. These results complement the clinical data for efficacy of glatiramer acetate and provide further data on safety and tolerability.

IMMUNOLOGY AND MECHANISM OF ACTION

It is probable that the mechanism of action of glatiramer acetate is very different from that of the β-interferons (see Chapter 20). The possibility that the immune pathology in MS could be driven in part by specific T-cell responses to myelin antigens has been long considered (see Chapter 20). Putative myelin autoantigens in MS include MBP, MOG, and PLP.[31] Evidence from animal models for a potential role of these antigenic proteins in demyelinating diseases such as MS derives from their use as encephalitogens in the induction of EAE. In fact, the initial interest in glatiramer acetate was related to its ability to suppress the induction of EAE by MBP, PLP and MOG.[32–34] Glatiramer acetate clearly inhibits cell-mediated immune responses to MBP and cross-reacts with MBP at both the cellular and humoral levels.[13,15,35,36] The avid binding of glatiramer acetate to MHC class II (major histocompatibility) sites on antigen-presenting cells interferes with antigen presentation to T-cells.[37,38] In order to bind to MHC class II molecules, many antigens require pre-processing by proteolytic enzymes secreted by the antigen-presenting cells. Such pre-processing is not needed for glatiramer acetate binding, and protease inhibitors do not interfere with glatiramer acetate binding to MHC class II sites on various antigen-presenting cells, including monocytes, splenic macrophages, and B cells transformed by Epstein–Barr virus.[39] The binding of glatiramer acetate to MHC class II sites blocks interactions with not only MBP but also other myelin antigens such as PLP and MOG.[34,40]

Glatiramer acetate suppression of EAE triggered by MBP might also be prevented by the induction of MBP specific T-suppressor cells.[41] T-helper cell lines induced by MBP secrete cytokines of the pro-inflammatory T-helper 1 (Th_1) profile (IL-2, IFN-γ) or both Th_1 and anti-inflammatory T-helper Th_2 profiles (IL-4, IL-6, and IL-10). Glatiramer acetate-induced T cell lines progressively shift to a Th_2 secretion profile.[36] In these studies glatiramer acetate-induced T cells exposed to MBP also responded by secreting Th_2 cytokines (IL-4, IL-6, and IL-10). Adoptive transfer of these glatiramer acetate-specific T cells suppressed the development of EAE induced by whole mouse spinal cord homogenate (MSCH). Since MSCH-induced EAE involves MBP as a major encephalitogenic antigen, it was possible that the amelioration of disease by glatiramer acetate was related more to suppression of the MBP antigen responses than to other antigenic components of myelin. A follow-up study demonstrated that glatiramer acetate-specific T cells secreting Th_2 cytokines suppressed EAE that was induced by antigens to which the cells did not cross-react. EAE that was induced by PLP and PLP epitopes p139–151 (relapsing–remitting EAE) and p178–191

(chronic progressive EAE) were both improved by adoptive transfer of glatiramer acetate-specific T cells.[42] These experiments suggested that bystander suppression by glatiramer acetate-induced T cells is an important mechanism of action, since cross-reactivity to the inducing antigen was not required. Activated T cells specific to any antigen are capable of crossing the blood–brain barrier.[43] If glatiramer acetate-specific T cells are able to migrate across the blood–brain barrier and are reactivated by MBP presented by in situ antigen-presenting cells they would secrete cytokines of the suppressor, Th_2 profile. By this mechanism, glatiramer acetate could suppress the immune response associated with myelin damage regardless of the primary inducing antigen or initial triggering event.

The picture emerges that glatiramer acetate copolymers bind efficiently to MHC class II molecules on peripheral antigen-presenting cells and displace other potential myelin antigens. Subsequent interaction with T cells and their specific receptors in a tri-molecular complex leads to induction of glatiramer acetate-specific T cells. These T cells are suppressor in nature and cross the blood–brain barrier where they are reactivated in situ by the cross-reacting antigens originating from MBP. The reactivated Th_2 cells secrete suppressor cytokines, thereby producing bystander suppression of the immune response directed against myelin. Whereas MBP-specific T suppressor cells either maintain some Th_1 properties or can shift back to a Th_1 profile when reactivated in vivo, glatiramer acetate-specific Th_2 cells appear to be confined to their suppressor profile. This mechanism may be critical in diseases such as EAE and MS, in which epitope spreading has been demonstrated.[31,44]

All studies of glatiramer acetate in the treatment of MS have shown that patients develop binding antibodies to the drug. The antibody levels reach a maximum after 3–6 months and then decline. Clinical data suggest that these antibodies are not neutralizing antibodies, and there is no evidence that drug efficacy is compromised by their development.[27,45,46]

SUMMARY

Glatiramer acetate is a novel preparation of synthetic copolymers with proven therapeutic benefit in MS. It is perhaps the only drug currently available for use in MS that has truly been derived from studies of the more than 100 compounds shown to prevent or ameliorate EAE.

Patients with MS have a life-long disease for which no cure is currently available. Treatments are needed that have sustained efficacy, slowing progression of disability and reducing the frequency of relapses. Patient tolerability is an important aspect of any treatment for a chronic illness. Although the β-interferons are generally well tolerated, a significant proportion of patients have problems with flu-like side effects such as malaise, low grade fever, chills, and myalgias. Glatiramer acetate has no flu-like side effects. It is regarded as the most tolerable of the available MS treatments, a characteristic that is important for patients who may require therapy for years or even decades. Transient post-injection reactions occur infrequently and have never been associated with serious sequelae. Injection-site reactions are typically minor and rarely a cause for discontinuing therapy. Since the mechanism of action of glatiramer acetate is different from that of the β-interferons, patients and their physicians have the option of using a different drug when lack of efficacy or side effects of one agent mandate a change. Reduction in relapse rate and slowed progression of disability make glatiramer

acetate a legitimate first-line drug for the treatment of relapsing forms of MS.

Since the recognition that both glatiramer acetate and the interferons are effective in the treatment of MS, the thought of combining the two drugs for potential synergy has been considered (see Chapter 29). To date no controlled trials of combined therapy have been performed, leaving the clinician with little objective evidence to support such an approach. A small in vitro study found that mitogen-induced T-cell activation was suppressed better by glatiramer acetate and interferon-β 1b together than by either drug alone.[47] However, in a recent study, CSJL/J F1 or SJL/J mice were given glatiramer acetate or saline before induction of EAE, and then treated with murine interferon-β. Mice receiving glatiramer acetate or interferon-β alone showed amelioration of EAE severity. Those receiving both agents developed EAE with a severity similar to untreated animals. The beneficial effects of each drug alone were compromised in combination and, although the results may not extend to MS, the authors emphasized the need for caution in trials of combined therapy in humans (Staley Brod; personal communication). Until scientific data from a carefully designed study are available, combination therapy lacks a scientific basis and is not the practice in most active centers specializing in the treatment of MS.

The development of glatiramer acetate and the β-interferons as treatments for MS represents a critical milestone in the care of patients with this disabling disease. Clinicians and patients now have proven therapeutic options, which clearly modify the disease course and offer the realistic hope of delaying progression. Most patients with clinically definite MS and a history of relapses should be considered for treatment with one of these agents while the search for better agents and a cure continues.

REFERENCES

1 Ewing C, Bernard CCA. Insights into the etiology and pathogenesis of multiple-sclerosis. *Immunol Cell Biol* 1998; **76**:47–54.

2 Allegretta M, Nicklas JA, Sriram S, Albertini RJ. T cells responsive to myelin basic protein in patients with multiple sclerosis. *Science* 1990; **247**:718–721.

3 Chou YK, Bourdette DN, Offner H et al. Frequency of T cells specific for myelin basic protein and myelin proteolipid protein in blood and cerebrospinal fluid in multiple sclerosis. *J Neuroimmunol* 1992; **38**:105–14.

4 Hohlfeld R, Meinl E, Wever F et al. The role of autoimmune T lymphocytes in the pathogenesis of multiple sclerosis. *Neurology* 1995; **45**:S33–S38.

5 Jingwu Z, Medaer R, Hashim GA et al. Myelin basic protein-specific T lymphocytes in multiple sclerosis and controls: precursor frequency, fine specificity, and cytotoxicity. *Ann Neurol* 1992; **32**:330–338.

6 Ota K, Matsui M, Milford EL et al. T-cell recognition of an immunodominant myelin basic protein epitope in multiple sclerosis. *Nature* 1990; **346**:183–187.

7 Steinman L, Waisman A, Altmann D. Major T-cell responses in multiple sclerosis. *Molec Med Today* 1995; **1**:79–83.

8 Trapp BD, Peterson J, Ransohoff RM et al. Axonal transection in the lesions of multiple sclerosis. *N Engl J Med* 1998; **338**:278–285.

9 Bernard CCA, Mandel TE, MacKay IR. Experimental models of human autoimmune disease: overview and prototypes. In: Rose NR, MacKay IR, eds. *The Autoimmune Diseases II*. San Diego, California: Academic Press, 1992, 47–106.

10 Kerlero de Rosbo N, Mendel I, Ben-Nun A. Chronic relapsing experimental autoimmune encephalomyelitis with a delayed onset and an atypical clinical course, induced in PL/J mice by myelin oligodendrocyte glycoprotein (MOG)-derived peptide: preliminary analysis of MOG T cell epitopes. *Eur J Immunol* 1995; **25**:985–993.

11 Teitelbaum D, Meshorer A, Hirshfeld T et al. Suppression of experimental allergic encephalomyelitis by a synthetic polypeptide. *Eur J Immunol* 1971; **1**:242–248.

12 Arnon R. The development of Cop 1 (Copaxone®), an innovative drug for the treatment of multiple sclerosis: personal reflections. *Immunol Lett* 1996; **50**:1–15.

13 Teitelbaum D, Aharoni R, Sela M, Arnon R. Cross-reactions and specificities of monoclonal antibodies against myelin basic protein and against the synthetic copolymer 1. *Proc Natl Acad Sci U S A* 1991; **88**:9528–9532.

14 Einstein ER, Chao LP, Csejtey J, Kibler RF. Species specificity in response to tryptophan modified encephalitogen. *Immunochemistry* 1972; **9**:73–84.

15 Webb C, Teitelbaum D, Herz A, Arnon R. Molecular requirements involved in suppression of EAE by synthetic basic copolymers of amino acids. *Immunochemistry* 1976; **13**:333–337.

16 Teitelbaum D, Meshorer A, Arnon R. Suppression of experimental allergic encephalomyelitis in baboons by Cop 1. *Isr J Med Sci* 1977; **13**:1038.

17 Teitelbaum D, Webb C, Bree M et al. Suppression of experimental allergic encephalomyelitis in rhesus monkeys by a synthetic basic copolymer. *Clin Immunol Immunopathol* 1974; **3**:256–262.

18 Lando Z, Teitelbaum D, Arnon R. Genetic-control of susceptibility to experimental allergic encephalomyelitis in mice. *Immunogenetics* 1979; **9**:435–442.

19 Teitelbaum D, Webb C, Meshorer A et al. Suppression by several synthetic polypeptides of experimental allergic encephalomyelitis induced in guinea pigs and rabbits with bovine and human basic encephalitogen. *Eur J Immunol* 1973; **3**:273–279.

20 Webb C, Teitelbaum D, Abramsky O et al. Suppression of experimental allergic encephalomyelitis in Rhesus monkeys by a synthetic basic copolymer (abstract). *Isr J Med Sci* 1975; **11**:1388.

21 Abramsky O, Teitelbaum D, Arnon R. Effect of a synthetic polypeptide (Cop 1) on patients with multiple sclerosis and with acute disseminated encephalomyelitis. *J Neurol Sci* 1977; **31**:433–438.

22 Bornstein MB, Miller AI, Teitelbaum D et al. Multiple sclerosis: trial of a synthetic polypeptide. *Ann Neurol* 1982; **11**:317–319.

23 Bornstein MB, Miller AI, Slagle S et al. A pilot trial of Cop 1 in exacerbating–remitting multiple sclerosis. *N Engl J Med* 1987; **317**:408–414.

24 Kurtzke JF. On the evaluation of disability in multiple sclerosis. *Neurology* 1961; **11**:686–694.

25 Bornstein MB, Miller AI, Slagle S. A placebo-controlled, double-blind, randomized, two-center, pilot trial of Cop 1 in chronic progressive multiple sclerosis. *Neurology* 1991; **41**:533–539.

26 Kurtzke JF. Rating neurological impairment in multiple sclerosis: an expanded disability status scale (EDSS). *Neurology* 1983; **33**:1444–1452.

27 Johnson KP, Brooks BR, Cohen JA, the Copolymer 1 Multiple Sclerosis Research Group. Copolymer 1

reduces relapse rate and improves disability in relapsing-remitting multiple sclerosis: results of a phase III multicenter, double-blind, placebo-controlled trial. *Neurology* 1995; **45**:1268–1276.

28 **Johnson KP, Brooks BR, Cohen JA, the Copolymer 1 Multiple Sclerosis Research Group.** Extended use of glatiramer acetate (Copaxone®) is well tolerated and maintains its clinical effect on multiple sclerosis relapse rate and degree of disability. *Neurology* 1998; **50**:701–708.

29 **Ford CC, Brooks BR, Cohen JA, the Copolymer 1 Multiple Sclerosis Research Group.** Sustained efficacy of glatiramer acetate for injection in a 5+ year trial of relapsing remitting MS. *Multiple Sclerosis* 1998; **6**:521.

30 **Mancardi GL, Sardanelli F, Parodi RC.** Effect of copolymer-1 on serial gadolinium-enhanced MRI in relapsing remitting multiple sclerosis. *Neurology* 1998; **50**:1127–1133.

31 **Bernard CCA, Kerlero de Rosbo N.** Multiple sclerosis: an autoimmune disease of multifunctional etiology. *Curr Opin Immunol* 1992; **4**:760–765.

32 **Teitelbaum D, Aharoni R, Arnon R, Sela M.** Specific inhibition of the T-cell response to myelin basic protein by the synthetic copolymer Cop 1. *Proc Natl Acad Sci U S A* 1988; **85**:9724–9728.

33 **Kerlero de Rosbo N, Mendel N, Milo R et al.** The autoimmune response to myelin oligodendrocyte glycoprotein (MOG) in multiple sclerosis and MOG-induced experimental autoimmune encephalomyelitis: effect of copolymer-1. *Eur J Neurol* 1996; **3 (suppl 4)**:57–58.

34 **Teitelbaum D, Fridkis-Hareli M, Arnon R, Sela M.** Copolymer 1 inhibits chronic relapsing experimental allergic encephalomyelitis induced by proteolipid protein (PLP) peptides in mice and interferes with PLP-specific T cell responses. *Neuroimmunology* 1996; **64**:209–217.

35 **Arnon R, Sela M, Teitelbaum D.** New insights into the mechanism of action of copolymer-1 in experimental allergic encephalomyelitis and multiple-sclerosis. *J Neurol* 1996; **243 (suppl 1)**:S8–S13.

36 **Aharoni R, Teitelbaum D, Sela M, Arnon R.** Copolymer 1 induces T cells of the T helper type 2 that cross react with myelin basic protein and suppress experimental autoimmune encephalomyelitis. *Proc Natl Acad Sci U S A* 1997; **94**:10821–10826.

37 **Racke MK, Martin R, McFarland H, Fritz RB.** Copolymer-1 induced inhibition of antigen-specific T cell activation: interference with antigen presentation. *Neuroimmunology* 1992; **37**:75–84.

38 **Fridkis-Hareli M, Teitelbaum D, Gurevich E et al.** Direct binding of myelin basic-protein and synthetic copolymer-1 to class-II major histocompatibility complex-molecules on living antigen-presenting cells: specificity and promiscuity. *Proc Natl Acad Sci U S A* 1994; **91**:4872–4876.

39 **Fridkis-Hareli M, Teitelbaum D, Arnon R, Sela M.** Synthetic copolymer 1 and myelin basic protein do not require processing prior to binding to class II major histocompatibility complex molecules on living antigen-presenting cells. *Cell Immunol* 1995; **163**:229–236.

40 **Fridkis-Hareli M, Teitelbaum D, Rosbo K et al.** Synthetic copolymer 1 inhibits the binding of MBP, PLP and MOG peptides to class II major histocompatibility complex molecules on antigen-presenting cells. *J Neurochem* 1994; **63 (suppl 1)**:S61–S61.

41 **Aharoni R, Teitelbaum D, Arnon R.** T suppressor hybridomas and interleukin-2 dependent lines induced by copolymer 1 or by spinal cord homogenate down-regulate experimental allergic encephalomyelitis. *Eur J Immunol* 1993; **23**:17–25.

42 **Aharoni R, Teitelbaum D, Sela M, Arnon R.** Bystander suppression of experimental autoimmune encephalomyelitis by T-cell lines and clones of the Th$_2$ type induced by copolymer-1. *J Neuroimmunol* 1998; **91**:135–146.

43 **Wekerle H, Linington C, Lassmann H, Meyermann R.** Cellular immune reactivity within the CNS. *Trend Neurosci* 1986; **9**:271–277.

44 **McRae BL, Vanderlugt CL, Dal Canto MC, Miller SD.** Functional evidence for epitope spreading in the relapsing pathology of experimental autoimmune encephalomyelitis. *J Exp Med* 1995; **182**:75–85.

45 **Brenner T, Meiner Z, Abramsky O et al.** Humoral responses to copolymer-1 in multiple-sclerosis patients: preferential production of IgG1 over IgG2. *Ann Neurol* 1996; **40**:111.

46 **Teitelbaum D, Brenner T, Sela M, Arnon R.** Antibodies to copolymer 1 do not interfere with its therapeutic effect (abstract). *Eur J Neurol* 1996; **3**:134.

47 **Milo R, Panitch HS.** Additive effects of copolymer-1 and interferon beta-1b on the immune responses to myelin basic protein. *J Neuroimmunol* 1995; **61**:185–193.

22
Cladribine

George Rice

BACKGROUND

Cladribine (2-chlorodeoxyadenosine, 2-CDA, Leustatin™) was developed as a highly specific lymphocytotoxic agent.[1] This purine nucleoside is resistant to the action of adenosine deaminase and accumulates in resting and dividing lymphocytes, inducing apoptosis. The resulting immune deficiency mimics that of adenosine deaminase deficiency.

The presumed mechanism of action is a selective and sustained depletion of lymphocytes. Cladribine treatment induces a four-fold decrease in the CD4+ T cell to CD8+ T cell ('helper:suppressor') ratio, which lasts for many months. By comparison, treatment with cyclophosphamide[2] or chlorambucil[3] produces a transient, two-fold decline in this ratio. Cladribine has become the drug of choice for hairy cell leukemia[4] and is used widely in lymphoid malignancies.[5]

These features led to its first trials in multiple sclerosis (MS), at the Scripps Clinic La Jolla CA, USA, and to a subsequent, multicenter phase 3 trial. These trials are reviewed in detail below.

THE SCRIPPS TRIAL OF CLADRIBINE IN SECONDARY PROGRESSIVE MS

The study design

A pilot study of cladribine in four patients with secondary progressive multiple sclerosis (SPMS) suggested a clinical effect and reasonable tolerability. This led to a randomized, placebo-controlled trial, with a cross-over planned after 1 year.

Patients were selected on the basis of disease progression, the magnitude of which was not specified. Though not indicated in the papers,[6,7] all but one of the patients had SPMS (Sipe J; personal communication). Patients were excluded if they had received corticosteroids or cytotoxic chemotherapy during the previous 6 months. A central venous line was inserted in all patients to facilitate administration of the drug. This was abandoned in subsequent studies, when it was learned that the drug could be given safely by the subcutaneous route.

Patients were matched according to age, sex, and disease severity. One member from each pair was assigned randomly to receive cladribine. A 'treating' physician had access to the hematological data but disability scores were derived by a second, blinded evaluator.

Statistical considerations

The primary outcome measure was the proportion of patients who improved neurologically (by 15%) on the Scripps disability scale (SNRS). The proportions that had improved were compared and a Kaplan–Meier analysis was performed. The magnetic resonance imaging (MRI) analysis was intended as a secondary outcome measure. The difference in the total T2 lesion volume at 6 and 12 months was compared to the disease burden at baseline. The change in gadolinium enhancement was compared between members in each of the treatment pairs.

It was intended to stop the trial if the Scripps scale was significantly different (at the 0.01 level after 1 year). Because efficacy was demonstrated after 1 year, the trial was analysed as a conventional randomized parallel group study. The authors claim that an intent-to-treat analysis was performed on all patients, with similar results to that seen in the 24 'evaluable' pairs (data not shown).

Results

The study as conducted

Three cladribine-treated patients dropped out before 1 year (one death due to hepatitis B, one patient with a hip fracture, and one with presumed worsening of MS). Two of these were replaced with new subjects to maintain the match. One placebo-assigned patient dropped out after 4 months because of worsening of MS and was not replaced. The final analysis was based on the 24 remaining pairs (data were carried forward on the placebo patent who did not complete 12 months on study).

A significant result was claimed after the first year. After this, patients were rolled over to the alternate treatment. In the second year, the dose was lowered to 1.2 mg/kg because of unexpected thrombocytopenia at the original dose of 2.8 mg/kg. The blind was maintained, but the entire investigative group was aware that cladribine had been effective.

Study outcomes

The disability data were presented[6] as the means of two different scales, the Scripps and the Kurtzke (EDSS) scales, measured at 6 and 12 months. The means of the differences in these scores between the matched pairs were plotted for the first year, and the differences were significant. Many have commented on the substantial differences (measuring 1.3 Kurtzke points) between the patients receiving placebo- and the cladribine-treated patients after 1 year. This is rather unusual worsening in a control group of SPMS patients.

The proportion of patients worse by 1 or more Kurtzke points was compared at the 12 month mark. This was not a 'confirmed' disability definition. One of the 24 cladribine-treated patients was worse compared to seven of the 23 placebo patients. The statistical significance in the difference between these proportions was less robust (P = 0.02).

The T2 MRI data were analysed similarly, in that differences between treatment pairs at 6 and 12 months were compared to baseline. These differences were significant. The data on gadolinium enhancement were dichotomized. More of the patients receiving cladribine had improved gadolinium scans, and this was statistically significant.

A formal blinding questionnaire was not administered after the first and second years and was probably unnecessary, given the general difficulty with such questionnaires and the virtual absence of side effects in the cladribine-treated patients. One patient succumbed to fatal hepatitis B in the second month on protocol. This was not attributed to treatment, although there are some concerns about this. Marrow suppression was serious in one patient who was taking phenytoin concurrently. It occurred in several others as well. Cladribine was highly effective in the induction of a durable lymphocytopenia. Herpes zoster occurred in two of the 24 cladribine-treated patients.

Limitations

Because clinical efficacy was not shown in the subsequent phase 3 trial[8] (see below), it is necessary to scrutinize the Scripps study for type I errors (false-positive results). Sources of concern include the following issues.

(a) The replacement of cladribine dropouts is troublesome in a small cross-over trial. An intent-to-treat analysis, which would have included data from these patients, is mentioned reassuringly, but not reported in detail.

(b) The disability scores upon which efficacy was determined were not 'confirmed' by a definition of sustained worsening over the standard 3–6 month period used in other trials.

(c) The use of means of ordinal scores (e.g. the Kurtzke scale) as an outcome measure is problematic.

(d) In the second year of the study, five of the 24 patients destined to receive placebo in the cross-over limb actually received one dose of cladribine.

(e) Rapid worsening of the placebo group pre-saged the ultimate failure of the trial's reproducibility. This kind of placebo-group worsening has been the Achilles' heel of many previous studies.

(f) The late (month 27–30) worsening of patients who received cladribine initially, although perhaps contaminated by small numbers and examiner unblinding (which should have mitigated the crash), suggested that the early treatment effect was not durable.[7]

(g) Although the significance of the marrow suppression was downplayed in the original paper,[4] it was the subject of a full paper that was published later.[9]

Conclusions

Most investigators were intrigued by the durability of the lymphopenia, which has remained a fashionable treatment objective in SPMS. The persistent suppression in gadolinium enhancement was attractive, as was the suppression in the T2 burden of disease. Most observers have been troubled by the disability claim, because of the unusual behavior in the placebo group, and there have been lingering concerns about the marrow suppression, especially at the higher dose.

THE SCRIPPS TRIAL IN RELAPSING–REMITTING MS

The study design

The Scripps trial was an 18-month, randomized, placebo-controlled, double-blind study of patients with clinically definite, relapsing-remitting MS

(RRMS) of at least 1 year's duration. All patients had a history of two or more relapses in the previous 2 years, with Kurtzke Expanded Disability Status Score (EDSS) ≤ 6.5 at study entry. The key exclusion criteria were treatment with an immunosuppressive drug within the previous three months, previous total lymphoid irradiation, or previous extensive myelosuppressive chemotherapy.

Clinical neurological exams, plus the Scripps Neurologic Rating Scale (SNRS) and EDSS rating scales, were to be performed at baseline and repeated by the same blinded neurologist every month for the first year and every 3 months for the second year. MRI was to be performed for each patient at baseline, and then monthly in the first year, and every 6 months in the second year.

The drug was given subcutaneously because this was found to produce the same bioavailability as the intravenous route and had greater ease of administration.[10] Each patient received a course of five consecutive daily subcutaneous injections of cladribine, 0.07 mg/kg per day, or an equivalent volume of saline placebo, fractionated into two or three injection sites, and given monthly for 6 months for a total cumulative dose of 2.1 mg/kg of cladribine.

Statistical considerations

The primary outcome measures were the joint frequency and severity of clinical relapses as judged by neurological examination and the number of gadolinium-enhancing lesions on MRI brain scans. These outcomes were assessed at 1 year. A sample size of 25 patients per group was estimated to ascertain a decline in the annual rate of exacerbations, from 1.0 in the placebo group to 0.5 in the cladribine group, with a two-sided alpha of 0.05.

It was estimated that the rate of enhancing lesions in the placebo group would remain at 50% throughout the course of this study, whereas the frequency of enhancing lesions in the cladribine-treated group would decline from 50% to less than 10% at 1 year. A sample size of 25 patients per treatment group would be sufficient to detect a difference of 50% versus 10% with a power of 0.90, using a two-sided alpha of 0.05. An intent-to-treat analysis of the 12-month data was intended.

Results

The study as conducted

After completion of screening evaluations, 52 patients were stratified according to sex, age (10-year intervals), and degree of disability (as measured by SNRS, in 10-point intervals). The stratified groups were randomized in blocks of four to receive either the placebo or cladribine. Twenty-seven patients were randomized to the cladribine arm and 25 to placebo. Each group lost one patient: one placebo-treated patient had a confounding conversion disorder and one cladribine-treated patient who moved away. All remaining patients received standard treatment interventions without deviations, as specified in the protocol, leaving 26 cladribine patients and 24 placebo patients who were evaluable at 12 months. During the period from 12 to 18 months, five placebo-treated patients withdrew: two patients moved, two withdrew for unspecified reasons, and one withdrew because of worsening MS. One cladribine-treated patient withdrew because of worsening MS. Thus, 25 cladribine patients and 19 placebo patients were evaluable over the entire 18-month period.

Between 12 and 18 months, the blinding was

removed from two cladribine patients and two placebo patients for unspecified reasons. Because of potential bias, the information concerning their exacerbations, subsequent to the point of unblinding, was not used in the analysis.

The two groups were similar in terms of baseline clinical characteristics, although more patients in the placebo group had experienced only one exacerbation in the year before the study.

Study outcomes

There was a statistically significant reduction in the frequency and severity of exacerbations in the cladribine-treated group compared to the placebo group from months 7–12. In this period, the relapse rate in the cladribine-treated group was 0.77 per year, compared to 1.67 per year in the placebo group. Regression analysis identified that cladribine treatment and two baseline covariates, lower baseline EDSS and fewer baseline exacerbations, were predictive of reduced exacerbations during the trial.

In secondary analyses the effect was sustained until 18 months, but this observation must be tempered by a drop-out rate of 25% among the placebo patients and the unblinding of two additional patients in each group.

Cladribine treatment completely suppressed gadolinium-enhancing lesions on MRI after study month 6 in the cladribine group, whereas lesion enhancement persisted in the placebo group. The effect was evident at month 6 and persisted until the end.

Mild segmental herpes zoster occurred in two cladribine-treated patients and in one placebo patient. Cladribine-treated patients experienced no side effects that might have led to unblinding of patients or the examining neurologists.

Limitations

The primary outcome measure (frequency of attacks at month 12) was not reported.[11] The significant effect occurred in the second and third semesters of treatment. This appears to be a post hoc subset analysis. The most robust effect occurred in the last third of the study, when there was the fewest number of patients and controls. The dropout of 25% of the placebo patients in the last semester is of some concern, as is the absence of a statement for the reasons for unblinding in two patients from each group. The statistical analysis does not appear to have considered either multiple comparisons or repeated measures.

It is uncertain whether the intention-to-treat analysis of the data was rigorously conducted. There was substantial discussion that the MRI effect was preserved if the drop-outs were excluded. The data for the intention-to-treat analysis and the evaluable groups are not compared side by side.

Although attacks were suppressed and their severity mitigated, the reader is not given information about the effect of cladribine on the use of corticosteroids or the prevention of hospitalizations. No information is provided about the time to the next exacerbation or the number of cladribine-treated patients in each group who shared the benefit. Although these were not predetermined outcome measures, they have become industry standards in other trials. When these data are missing, it raises the possibility that they were not supportive of a treatment effect.

Baseline covariates were examined. It was shown that a lower attack rate in the year before treatment was associated with fewer attacks on study. The two groups were not well matched in this regard, but in a manner that would have made it potentially more difficult to show a treatment effect. Based on the coavariate analysis, the placebo group appeared to be destined to have fewer exacerbations.

Conclusions

Because of the limitations in the statistical analysis, the significance of the clinical outcomes would not be considered strong. The impermanent duration of effect of cladribine means that retreatment will be necessary if cladribine is to become a practical long-term therapy for MS. The suppression of MRI-enhancing lesions with cladribine was robust. Cladribine given subcutaneously at a total dosage of 2.1 mg/kg was safe and well tolerated.

THE PHASE 3 TRIAL OF CLADRIBINE IN SPMS

The study design

This trial was a randomized, double-blind, parallel-group, placebo-controlled, multicenter study to evaluate the safety and efficacy of cladribine in patients with primary progressive MS or SPMS.[8] Patients ranged in age from 21 to 65 years, with EDSS scores from 3.0 to 6.5. Progression was defined by clinical worsening over the previous 12 months. No restrictions were applied to the extent of this progression before the study. Patients were excluded if they had been treated with corticosteroids, other immunosuppressive agents, or β-interferon within the 3 months before randomization.

Patients were to be randomized to receive one of the following regimens:

(a) six courses of cladribine 0.07 mg/kg per day (plus two courses of placebo)—cumulative target dose: 2.1 mg/kg;

(b) two courses of cladribine 0.07 mg/kg per day (plus six courses of placebo)—cumulative target dose: 0.7 mg/kg; or

(c) eight courses of placebo (0.5% albumin).

The patients received subcutaneous injections of the assigned dose for 5 consecutive days. The lower dose was chosen to minimize marrow toxicity. The extra placebo injections given to cladribine-treated patients were designed to facilitate any unexpected problems with marrow suppression, in which case a dose of cladribine could be withheld and placebo given.

Statistical considerations

The primary clinical efficacy assessment was a comparison of the change in mean EDSS at 12 months relative to baseline (means of ordinals). In addition, treatment failure (proportions) and time to treatment failure (Kaplan–Meier) were analysed. For patients with a baseline EDSS score of 3.0–5.0, a confirmed increase of 1.0 point on the EDSS constituted the definition of treatment failure. For patients with a baseline EDSS score of 5.5–6.5, this definition was met by a confirmed increase of 0.5 points on the EDSS. Neurological assessments were performed every 2 months.

The MRI outcome measures included the number and volume of gadolinium-enhancing lesions and the change in the T2 burden of disease. Scans were performed at baseline, 6 months and 12 months.

The sample size of 50 in each treatment group was predicted with the assumption, based on the experience from the previous study in SPMS, that there would be a mean difference of 1.0 EDSS point between the placebo and cladribine groups at the end of the study.

Results

The study as executed

A total of 159 patients were randomized into three study groups, which were not significantly different in age, sex, duration of disease, and baseline disability, as defined by the EDSS or Scripps scales. Approximately 30% of each group was made up of patients with primary progressive disease. All patients were followed for a minimum of 15 months. Drop-outs were negligible and deviations from scheduled dosing were negligible.

Study outcomes

The mean disability did not change significantly over time among the three groups, as assessed either by mean EDSS or the SNRS scores. The outcomes were similar in patients with primary progressive MS and SPMS. Time to treatment failure was studied with the Kaplan–Meier analysis. Significant differences were not detected among the three groups. Exacerbation rates and corticosteroid interventions were unaffected by treatment.

Approximately 30% of patients in each group had gadolinium enhancement on the baseline MRI scan. Cladribine, given in either dose, had a remarkable effect on the suppression of gadolinium enhancement. The number and volume of enhancing lesions decreased significantly in cladribine groups relative to the placebo group. At 12 months, mean enhancing volume was essentially eliminated in both cladribine groups ($p = 0.003$ for 0.7 mg/kg cladribine versus placebo; $p = 0.0005$ for 2.1 mg/kg cladribine versus placebo). At 12 months, there was a 94%, 87%, and 50% reduction in enhancing lesions in patients who had baseline enhancing lesions in the 2.1 mg/kg cladribine group, the 0.7 mg/kg cladribine group, and the placebo group, respectively. Categorical analysis of the volume of the gadolinium-enhancing lesions (absent/present) revealed a significant reduction in both dosage groups when compared with placebo ($p = 0.012$ for the 0.7 mg/kg cladribine versus placebo; $p = 0.002$ for 2.1 mg/kg cladribine versus placebo). At 12 months, there was a dose-related trend toward decreasing T2 volumes in the cladribine groups relative to the placebo group.[12]

Cladribine was well tolerated. No serious complications of marrow suppression were identified. Two outbreaks of herpes zoster occurred in each of the three treatment groups.

Treatment with cladribine produced a dose-dependent reduction in the counts of neutrophils, platelets, and lymphocytes. Intermediate effects were identified with the lower dose. The lymphocyte suppression was durable. The differences were apparent after the first cycle of treatment, and they persisted for the duration of the study, long after the drug was discontinued.

Limitations

The study was probably underpowered. A problem in the original power calculation was the unexpected constitution of the phase 3 study by MS patients with more advanced disability and with primary progressive MS. The mean EDSS score in this study was 5.6, compared to 4.6 in the Scripps study. Placebo-treated patients with this baseline disability are less likely to progress in a clinical trial.[13] The trial was too short. It is conceivable that the true benefit from cladribine treatment might take several years, as appears to be the case with other agents such as azathioprine or interferon-β 1b.[14]

The dose might have been too low. In the current study, the doses were chosen to minimize marrow toxicity of the drug. The lower dose (2.1 mg/kg) used in this study suppressed the mean lymphocyte count by 60%; this compares with 70% in the Scripps study (in which the dose of cladribine was 2.8 mg/kg). The intensity of the dosing schedule differed in the two trials, and this may account for the lack of clinical efficacy in the larger study. More patients in the Scripps study encountered complications of iatrogenic immunosuppression, and 10% of patients in that study developed herpes zoster, compared to 4% in the phase 3 study.

The MRI study afforded very convincing support for an effect on gadolinium enhancement. However, limiting the scanning to every 6 months made it impossible to ascertain an effect on new or enlarging T2 lesions.

Cladribine might not work in progressive MS, even though it appears to suppress gadolinium enhancement. Preliminary studies suggest that clinical and radiological worsening can be predicted by gadolinium enhancement and by new T2 lesions.[15] This observation suggests that the favorable MRI outcomes might have translated into a clinically meaningful effect in a more highly powered study. This needs to be explored further.

Serial MRI scanning has been positioned as a surrogate marker for disease activity in MS clinical trials in progressive MS. The use of MRI to screen new treatments in MS has been thrown into the spotlight by this experiment. These three studies have corroborated the robust effect of cladribine on the MRI, which is more convincing than the clinical efficacy. In clinical trials in which clinical and MRI outcomes go in the same direction, each observation bolsters the other. MRI efficacy in the absence of clinical efficacy poses a difficult conundrum for the USA Federal Drug Administration (FDA) and for insurance payers.

Conclusions

Treatment with cladribine was not shown to alter the course of disease progression significantly, as assessed by the primary outcome measures (change in mean EDSS; time to treatment failure). The MRI findings were compelling. Gadolinium enhancement was virtually eliminated by treatment with cladribine. The T2 burden of disease did not change in the cladribine-treated patients and worsened in the placebo patients. Treatment was safe and well tolerated, and the persistent, dose-dependent lymphopenia was remarkable.

CLADRIBINE AND OTHER AUTOIMMUNE DISORDERS

Cladribine has not been studied extensively in other autoimmune diseases. It is currently being studied in rheumatoid arthritis and lupus nephritis. Experience in chronic immune thrombocytopenic purpura has been disappointing.[16] There is not enough experience in other autoimmune disorders for a consensus statement, but reports of paradoxical immunological activation are of some concern.[17]

WHERE DO WE GO FROM HERE?

The tantalizing effect of cladribine on MRI outcome measures in MS and its impressive tolerability (at the dosage of 2.1 mg/kg) compared to other myelosuppressive agents, deserve further study, and it is hoped that further trials, designed with adequate power, will be undertaken.

The drug is not at present approved by the FDA for use, nor has it been approved by the Health Protection Branch of Canada (HPB). Its use outside the research setting cannot be advocated at present.

REFERENCES

1 Carson DA, Wasson DB, Beutler E. Antileukemic and immunosuppressive activity of 2-chloro, 2-deoxyadenosine. *Proc Nat Acad Sci U S A* 1984; **81**:2232–2236.

2 Moody DJ, Fahey JL, Grable E et al. Administration of monthly pulses of cyclophosphamide in multiple sclerosis patients. *J Neuroimmunol* 1987; **14**:175–182.

3 Chiapelli F, Myers L, Ellison GW et al. Preferential reductions in lymphocyte subpopulations induced by monthly pulses of chlorambucil: studies in patients with chronic progressive multiple sclerosis. *Int J Immunopharmacol* 1991; **13**:455–461.

4 Beutler E. Cladribine (2-chlorodeoxyadenosine). *Lancet* 1992; **340**:952–956.

5 Piro LD. 2 Chlorodeoxyadenosine treatment of lymphoid malignancies. *Blood* 1992; **79**:843–845.

6 Sipe JC, Romine JS, Koziol JA et al. Cladribine in treatment of chronic progressive multiple sclerosis. *Lancet* 1994; **344**:9–13.

7 Beutler E, Sipe JC, Romine JS, Koziol JA, McMillan R, Zyroff J. The treatment of chronic progressive multiple sclerosis with cladribine. *Proc Natl Acad Sci U S A* 1996; **93**:1716–1720.

8 Rice GPA, Cladribine Study Group. Cladribine and chronic progressive multiple sclerosis: The results of a multicenter trial. *Neurology* 1997; **48**:1730.

9 Beutler E, Koziol J, McMillan R et al. Marrow suppression produced by repeated doses of cladribine. *Acta Haematol* 1994; **91**:10–15.

10 Liliemark J, Albertioni F, Hassan M et al. On the bioavailability of oral and subcutaneous 2-chloro-2'-deoxyadenosine in humans: alternative routes of administration. *J Clin Oncol* 1992; **10**:1514–1518.

11 Romine JS, Sipe JC, Koziol JA et al. A double-blind, placebo-controlled trial of cladribine in relapsing remitting MS. *Proc Assoc American Physicians* 1999; **111**:35–44.

12 Rice G, Cladribine Study Group. The effect of cladribine on MRI findings in progressive multiple sclerosis: final results of a placebo-controlled trial. *Ann Neurol* 1998; **44**:504.

13 Weinshenker BG, Issa M, Baskerville J. Meta-analysis of the placebo-treated groups in the clinical trials of progressive multiple sclerosis. *Neurology* 1996; **46**:1613–1619.

14 European Study Group on interferon β 1b in secondary progressive MS. Placebo-controlled multi-centre randomised trial on interferon β 1b in treatment of secondary progressive multiple sclerosis. *Lancet* 1998; **352**:1491–1497.

15 Molyneux PD, Filippi M, Barkhof F et al. Correlations between monthly enhanced MRI lesion rate and changes in T2 lesion volume in multiple sclerosis. *Ann Neurol* 1998; **43**:332–339.

16 Figueroa M, McMillan R. 2-chlorodeoxyadenosine in the treatment of chronic refractory immune thrombocytopenic purpura. *Blood* 1993; **1**:3484–3485.

17 Houssiau FA, Delannoy A, Devogelaer JP. Paradoxical immunologic effects of 2DCA therapy. *Arthritics Rheum* 1998; **41**:1704–1705.

23
Intravenous immunoglobulin

Franz Fazekas, Siegrid Strasser-Fuchs, Ralf Gold and Hans-Peter Hartung

INTRODUCTION

Over the past few years, intravenous immunoglobulin (IVIG) has become an important treatment option for various autoimmune-related neurological diseases.[1–3] Efficacy equalling that of plasmapheresis has been convincingly documented in Guillain–Barré syndrome and in chronic inflammatory demyelinating polyneuropathy.[3–5] Although myasthenia gravis has been less extensively studied, some have similar views in regard to treating a myasthenic crisis,[6] and in multifocal motor neuropathy, the benefits of IVIG (although limited) have to be weighed against quite aggressive therapies such as cyclophosphamide.[7] In all these examples, the ease of administration, good tolerability and a reasonable safety profile are factors that are cited in favour of IVIG. These possible advantages over alternative immunomodulating therapies may also be of interest for patients suffering from other neurological autoimmune disorders such as multiple sclerosis (MS).

This chapter begins with a short outline of the potential mechanisms of the action of IVIG in MS and then carefully reviews published randomized placebo-controlled clinical trials of IVIG in MS. On the basis of these results, the authors have tried to determine the present role of IVIG in MS and to outline future directions of research in order to clarify unresolved questions.

IMMUNOLOGICAL PROPERTIES AND SAFETY OF IVIG PREPARATIONS

Immunoglobulins are the carriers of humoral immunity and are able to recognize a broad spectrum of immunogenic structures. The immense variation in their antibody-binding specificities is produced by the contribution of germ-line diversity and of somatic mutation.[8] A prototypic immunoglobulin molecule is composed of four polypeptide chains—two identical heavy and two identical light chains—which are joined into a macromolecular complex by disulphide bonds. There exist two functional domains—the Fab-fragment contains the antigen-binding site of the molecule and bears the recognition function and the Fc-part is responsible for biological effector functions such as complement fixation or binding to respective Fc receptors on immunoinflammatory cells.[9]

Commercially available IVIG preparations are derived from pools of 3000 to 10 000 donors.[10,11] The product is purified by enzymatic

309

treatment at low pH, which is followed by fractionation and chromatography. The purified immunoglobulin is stabilized with glucose, maltose, glycine, sucrose, mannitol or albumin. The final product contains more than 95% IgG, less than 2.5% IgA and a negligible amount of IgM. Although in principle the subclass contribution of IVIG corresponds to that of normal human serum, there is some variation between manufacturers according to the size and composition of the donor pools used.[11] To minimize the possibility of transmission of infectious diseases by IVIG, regulations require that only selected donors should be accepted, and the purification process includes various steps to eliminate infectious agents; these techniques are constantly updated and improved[12,13] (e.g. by the recent introduction of ultrafiltration in the purification procedure).

Kinetics

The overall half-life of most IgG subclasses contained in IVIG after administration is approximately 18–32 days, which is similar to that of native immunoglobulin. After intravenous infusion of high doses of IVIG (2 g/kg body weight), serum IgG levels have been shown to increase five-fold and then to decline by 50% in 72 hours.[14] These rapid shifts of IgG serum concentration within the first 3 days are a consequence of extravascular redistribution, but they may also reflect increased catabolism.[15] Pre-treatment serum levels are reached after 2–4 weeks.[14] High-dose IVIG infusions also lead to an increase of as much as two-fold in the concentration of IgG in the cerebrospinal fluid (CSF) within 48 hours.[14] However, it takes only 1 week for IgG levels in the CSF to return to normal.

Mechanisms of action

In recent years, multiple immunomodulatory effects of IVIG have been documented. These have been extensively described in numerous reviews.[2,10,11,16,17] However, it has not so far been possible to identify one single mode of action as the crucial mechanism. It is conceivable that various immunoregulatory effects of IVIG act in concert to equilibrate the disturbed immune network.

Healthy people generate IgG antibodies against a wide spectrum of normal human proteins, including so-called anti-idiotypic antibodies, which attach to the antigen-binding region of the F(ab) part of another immunoglobulin. As a consequence, IVIG that is derived from a large pool of human donors may include anti-idiotypic antibodies that bind to and neutralize pathogenic autoantibodies and prevent interaction with their autoantigen.[18–20] It has also been suggested that binding of the anti-idiotypic antibodies to antigenic determinants and the surface IgM or IgG on B cells would result in a down-regulation of antibody production.[21] With these actions in mind, it certainly must be considered that the efficacy of IVIG preparations could vary with the selection and size of the donor pool. However, such speculations have not yet been substantiated experimentally or clinically.

The Fc portion of immunoglobulins interacts with many phagocytic cells of the reticuloendothelial system that express Fc receptors on their cell surface. These Fc receptors link cellular and humoral immunity by serving as a bridge between antibody specificity and effector cell function.[9] Pathogenic antibodies can bind to the Fc receptor and thereby target macrophages. Access amounts of immunoglobulins may compete with this binding and block or at least reduce the damaging effects of inflammatory effector cells.[22] There is corroborating evidence from experimentally induced inflammatory neuropathy in rats that intact human IVIG can reduce disease severity.[23] In addition to the mere blockade of Fc receptors, immunoglobulins and complexes derived from them can cross-link Fc receptors and thus mediate apoptosis of B cells.[15,24]

Clinical studies have also shown changes in the cytokine profile of patients treated with IVIG. This appears to be due to a modulation of the production and secretion of cytokines by lymphocytes or monocytes.[25,26] Up-regulation of interleukin (IL)-1-receptor antagonists and IL-8 secretion have been induced by IVIG. In addition, IVIG preparations may also influence the cytokine network since they contain traces of interferon (IFN)-γ and transforming growth factor (TGF)-β in varying amounts as well as neutralizing antibodies against IL-1α, IL-6 and the class I interferons (INF-β).[27–28]

Immunoglobulins can also bind complement components with their constant domain (Fc) and thus prevent tissue damage caused by the complement activation cascade. Direct evidence of the functionality of this mechanism in humans has been demonstrated in dermatomyositis.[29] Recent experimental data also suggest an enhanced physiological cleavage of C3b-containing complexes by IgG,[30] which is dependent on the presence of factors I and H. These properties may act in concert and may also prevent binding to the oligodendrocyte surface and myelin proteins.[31]

Apart from the impact on the humoral immune system, IVIG has also been shown to act on T lymphocytes. Changes in both CD8$^+$ suppresser–cytotoxic T cells and CD4$^+$ helper T cells have been demonstrated after IVIG treatment.[32,33] Antibodies directed against several T-cell surface molecules are present in IVIG; these include antibodies against the T-cell receptor,[34]

CD4 and major histocompatibility complex (MHC) molecules.[35] IVIG also contains neutralizing antibodies against bacterial and viral superantigens that stimulate T cells non-specifically.[36] Furthermore, soluble CD4 or CD4-like activity and soluble human leukocyte antigen (HLA) molecules are found in trace amounts in IVIG.[37] Induction of T-cell apoptosis by components of the Fas–FasL system[38] or soluble HLA class 1 molecules[39] included in therapeutic preparations of IVIG may also exert a regulatory role on T-cell function by eliminating effector cells.

Finally, experimental evidence suggests that IVIG may have the capacity to promote remyelination. Following the observation that polyclonal immunoglobulins against spinal cord homogenate were able to enhance remyelination in the inflammatory model of Theiler's virus encephalitis,[40] further studies showed that more specific antibodies that react with myelin basic protein also have the capacity to promote remyelination in this model.[41] Studies have identified a monoclonal IgM antibody that can facilitate remyelination and suppress inflammation and that also has some effect in a toxic model of demyelination.[42,43] This monoclonal antibody was shown to be polyreactive, recognizing antigens present on the surface and in the cytoplasm of oligodendrocytes and other glial cells.[44] Assuming that the remyelination-promoting properties of these antibodies relate to the oligodendrocyte surface activity, IVIG that contains such autoantibodies could exert a beneficial effect.

RANDOMIZED PLACEBO-CONTROLLED TRIALS OF IVIG IN MS

Earlier observations on the potential efficacy of IVIG in MS have been reviewed previously.[45,46]

Table 23.1 Randomized, double-blind, placebo-controlled trials on IVIG in RRMS

Study	AIMS[47]	Achiron et al[48]	Sørensen et al[49]
Number of patients	148	40	26
Study design	Parallel	Parallel	Cross-over
Duration of study	2 years	2 years	2 × 6 months
Primary end-point	Disability	Relapses	MRI activity
IVIG dosage	0.15–0.2 g/kg per month	0.4 g/kg daily for 5 days then 0.4 g/kg every 2 months	2 g/kg per month

More recently, this potential efficacy has been tested in three prospective, randomized placebo-controlled studies.[47–49] All three studies focused on patients with relapsing–remitting MS (RRMS) but they took different approaches to determine the potential benefit of IVIG on the course of the disease (*Table 23.1*). These trials are summarized in more detail below.[50]

The Austrian Immunoglobulin in MS Trial

The Austrian Immunoglobulin in MS (AIMS) Trial randomized 150 patients with RRMS to receive either IVIG at a dosage of 0.15–0.2 g/kg body weight or physiological saline every month over a period of 2 years.[47] Inclusion criteria were a clinically definite diagnosis of RRMS with complete and incomplete remissions, a baseline Kurtzke's Expanded Disability Status Scale (EDSS) score of between 1.0 (minor neurological signs without disability) and 6.0 (ambulatory with assistance), and a history of at least two clearly identified and documented relapses during the previous 2 years. Patients had to have stopped any immunosuppressive or immunomodulatory therapy at least 3 months before enrolment and were excluded if they had taken corticosteroids within 2 weeks of study entry. A centralized, computer-generated randomization schedule stratified patients by centre, age, sex and progression rate (i.e. the actual EDSS score divided by the duration of the diseases in years). Patients were seen and cared for each month in their centre by the treating physician. Study assessments were performed by a second neurologist, who was unaware of treatment allocation, at scheduled intervals (baseline and every 6 months) or in the event of a possible relapse.

Primary outcome measures were the differences between the groups in the absolute change of the EDSS score and in the proportion of patients who improved, remained stable, or worsened in disability, as defined by an increase or a decrease of at least 1 point on the EDSS score by the end of the study. Secondary outcome measures were the number of relapses, the annual relapse rate, the proportion of relapse-free patients, and the time until first relapse during the study period. A relapse was defined as the appearance or re-appearance of one or more neurological abnormalities that resulted in an objective change of at least 1 point in one of the functional scores and that was present for at least 24 hours after a stable or improving neurological state of at least 30 days. Further analyses examined the course of disability and relapse rates in both groups over the study period and examined the impact of baseline variables on treatment efficacy.[51] Demographic variables and disease characteristics were well balanced between both groups. A total of 64 patients in the IVIG group and 56 in the placebo group completed 2 years of treatment.

Intention-to-treat analysis showed mild improvement in the IVIG-treated patients over the study period from a baseline EDSS of 3.33 (95% CI: 3.01–3.65) to a final mean EDSS of 3.09 (95% CI: 2.72–3.46). In contrast, the placebo group deteriorated slightly from a baseline EDSS of 3.37 (95% CI: 2.96–2.76) to 3.49 (95% CI: 3.06–3.92). This change in EDSS scores (IVIG −0.23, placebo 0.12) was significantly different ($p = 0.008$). A similar and significant difference was maintained when only those patients who completed the study were analysed. There was an improvement of 1 point or more on the EDSS score in 23 (31%) of the IVIG-treated patients, compared with 10 (14%) of the placebo group. In contrast, deterioration of disability occurred in 12 (16%) of the IVIG-treated patients and in 17 (23%) of the placebo group ($p = 0.041$). Overall, 24% of patients did better on IVIG than on placebo when the differences in the rates of improvement (17%) and prevention of deterioration (7%) between IVIG and placebo treated groups were added.

The number of relapses in the IVIG-treated patients was about half of that in the placebo group (62 versus 116). This resulted in a significantly higher proportion of relapse-free patients who were receiving IVIG (53% versus 26%; $p = 0.03$). IVIG treatment reduced the annual relapse rate from a pre-study rate of 1.3 (95% CI: 1.09–1.51) to a mean of 0.52 (95% CI: 0.32–0.72) during the study period. In placebo-

treated patients, the annual relapse rate was 1.41 (95% CI: 1.21–1.61) before participating in the study and 1.26 (95% CI: 0.75–1.77) during the study. Hence, IVIG treatment was associated with a 59% reduction in the annual relapse rate compared to placebo ($p = 0.0037$).

The drop in relapse rate following IVIG was noticeable within the first 6 months of treatment.[51] Over the study period, the relapse rate also continuously decreased in the placebo group; however, monthly relapse rates of IVIG-treated patients were always significantly lower than those of the placebo patients. The mean EDSS score of the IVIG group improved in parallel, and significantly, from 3.33 ± 1.38 to 3.05 ± 1.73 within the first 6 months of the study ($p = 0.002$). After this, it remained fairly stable. Placebo treatment was associated with a slight, gradual increase in the EDSS as described above.

Side effects were rarely observed in the AIMS trial; they consisted of a transient rash that developed a few days after infusion in two IVIG patients and a worsening of depression in another patient in the IVIG group, which finally led him to terminate the study.

Study on the effects of IVIG on relapses

A study by Archiron et al[48] followed 40 patients with a 2-year history of clinically definite RRMS confirmed by magnetic resonance imaging (MRI) studies. Further inclusion criteria were an average annual exacerbation rate of 0.5 to 3.0 in the 2 years preceding the study and an EDSS score of 0.0 to 6.0. Patients were assigned to treatment groups by block-stratified randomization that took into account annual exacerbation rate, age, and disease duration. Twenty patients received IVIG at a loading dose of 0.4 g/kg body

313

weight per day for 5 consecutive days. Subsequent booster doses of IVIG in a dosage of 0.4 g/kg body weight once daily were administered every 2 months. Physiological saline served as placebo. Patients were examined at baseline and monthly thereafter by two independent neurologists. A relapse was defined as the rapid appearance, re-appearance or worsening of one or more neurological abnormalities persisting for at least 48 hours after a stable or improving neurological state of at least 30 days. Objective changes on neurological examination by a neurologist who was blind to the patient's treatment was required, and deterioration accompanied by fever was not considered. The severity of the exacerbation was graded according to the Kurtzke EDSS. MRI of the brain was performed on a 0.5 Tesla magnet. Primary end-points of the study were the annual exacerbation rate, the proportion of exacerbation-free patients and the time until first exacerbation. Secondary outcome measures were exacerbation severity, neurological disability (as measured by EDSS and distribution of cumulative disability over time), and annual brain MRI score.

The annual exacerbation rate in the IVIG-treated patients dropped from 1.85 ± 0.26 in the pre-study period to 0.75 ± 0.16 in the first year and 0.42 ± 0.14 in the second year ($p < 0.05$ compared with baseline). Annual exacerbation rate of the placebo group was 1.55 ± 0.17 before the study, 1.8 ± 0.2 in the first year and 1.42 ± 0.23 in the second year of the trial. Hence, in both years of the study the annual exacerbation rate of the group receiving IVIG was significantly lower than that of the placebo group ($p = 0.0006$). The number of exacerbation-free patients was also significantly higher following medication with IVIG during both years and the total study period.

There was a trend towards reduced neurological disability in the IVIG group (baseline EDSS: 2.9 ± 0.43; study completion EDSS: 2.6 ± 2.2) whereas a minor increase occurred in the placebo group (baseline EDSS: 2.8 ± 0.37; study completion EDSS: 2.97 ± 1.47). Distribution of the change in disability over time was significantly in favour of IVIG treatment. The proportion of patients who improved by at least 1 point on the EDSS was 23.5% following IVIG compared with 10.8% in the placebo group. The proportion of patients who worsened by at least 1 point was 13.7% and 17.1%, respectively ($p = 0.03$). The mean annual severity of exacerbations in the IVIG group versus the placebo group was not significantly different during either study year.

MRI examinations were analysed by generating an MRI score based on the number and diameter of demyelinating plaques. Mean MRI scores were not significantly different between the treatment groups. However, by the end of the second year the number of patients examined had fallen to 30.

The incidence of notable side effects was low. Out of 630 infusions administered throughout the trial, there were 12 of 316 (3.8%) events recorded in the IVIG group and 7 of 314 (2.2%) in the placebo group ($p < 0.05$). Side effects in both groups included fatigue, headaches, rash and low-grade fever. All complaints spontaneously resolved within a few hours.

IVIG and disease activity as shown by MRI

Sørensen and colleagues[49] examined the effect of IVIG on disease activity using frequent gadolinium-enhanced MRI scans in a cross-over study of 26 patients with RRMS or secondary progressive MS with relapses. Inclusion criteria consisted of a disease duration of not longer than 10 years, an EDSS between 2.0 and 7.0, two or more acute exacerbations in the year before study entry and at least five cerebral lesions on T2-weighted images on a screening MRI. In a randomized fashion, one group of patients was first treated with IVIG for 6 months. After a 3-month washout period, patients were then treated with placebo for another 6 months. The second group was treated in reverse order. IVIG treatment consisted of infusions of 1 g/kg body weight per day for two consecutive days at monthly intervals. Human albumin (2%) administered with an identical regimen served as placebo. MRI was performed using a 1.5 Tesla scanner and a conventional double spin echo sequence with a slice thickness of 4 mm and no inter-slice gap. Post-contrast T1-weighted scans were obtained 10 minutes after injection of gadolinium in a dosage of 0.1 mmol/kg body weight. All scans were evaluated blindly by two independent radiologists for the presence of enhancing lesions. Lesion area measurements were obtained from proton-density images. In addition, all patients underwent careful neurological examination and neurophysiological studies with multimodal evoked potentials. Primary study end-points were the total number of gadolinium-enhancing lesions and the number of new enhancing lesions on serial MRI. Secondary end-points were the percentage of patients with active scans (scans with gadolinium-enhancing lesions), the total lesion load on T2-weighted MRI, changes in multimodal evoked potentials, number of exacerbations, number of exacerbation-free patients, number of severe exacerbations, changes in neurological function on the Scripps Neurological Rating Scale, and changes in EDSS ratings. Twenty-one patients were available for intention-to-treat analysis after completion of at least 1

month of follow-up and two MRIs in the second treatment period. Eighteen patients completed the entire cross-over study and constituted the per-protocol population.

Overall, IVIG treatment significantly reduced the mean number of new and total gadolinium-enhancing lesions by approximately 60% compared with placebo both in the per-protocol population (total number of lesions—baseline: 3.8 ± 8.3; IVIG: 1.2 ± 2.2; placebo 3.2 ± 5.9; $p = 0.03$) and according to intention-to-treat analysis (total number of lesions—baseline: 3.6 ± 7.7; IVIG: 1.3 ± 2.3; placebo 2.9 ± 5.4; $p = 0.003$). Disease activity on MRI decreased after 1 month of treatment with IVIG and then remained stable, whereas no changes in activity were observed during treatment with placebo. The average percentage of per-protocol patients with active scans on 6-monthly serial MRI scans was 37% during IVIG treatment and 68% when receiving placebo ($p < 0.01$). Four out of 18 patients did not have any gadolinium-enhancing lesions during the whole IVIG treatment period but none was free of new gadolinium-enhancing lesions while on placebo. Only four patients had a poor response to active treatment; a poor response was defined as more than 50% active scans during IVIG therapy and/or more active scans while on IVIG than on placebo. No significant between group differences were found in regard to the total T2 lesion load.

In IVIG treatment periods the number of relapses was 42% lower according to intention-to-treat analysis and 27% lower as per-protocol, but these differences did not reach statistical significance. However, a significantly greater number of patients were free of relapses when receiving IVIG (71%) than when receiving placebo medication (33%) ($p = 0.02$). Although a greater number of patients improved on IVIG than on placebo, no significant differences were found in regard to changes of the EDSS score between the two treatment periods. Multimodal evoked potentials also failed to demonstrate significant differences.

An unexpectedly high number of acute and chronic adverse events occurred in this study. More than 50% of patients experienced one or more adverse events from IVIG treatment. Acute adverse events consisted of headaches, nausea and urticarial rashes. Headache was usually mild, lasted for 1 or 2 days and was controlled by analgesics. A reduction in the IVIG infusion rate significantly decreased the occurrence of post-infusion headache and nausea. Urticarial rashes could be abolished or diminished by administration of an anti-histamine drug before the infusion. The most common major chronic side effect was severe eczema, which was observed in 11 patients during treatment with IVIG. The eczematous reaction developed 2–4 days after infusion and preferentially affected the palms of the hands. In six patients it also involved the soles of the feet and more proximal parts of the extremities and the eczema became generalized in two patients. In all patients, the eczema eventually resolved after discontinuation of IVIG therapy, but in some patients it persisted for several weeks after the last infusion. Differences in the concentration of cytokines between commercially available preparations of IVIG may have contributed to this unusual adverse effect profile because such observations have not been made as frequently in other indications for high-dose treatment. In addition, one patient developed hepatitis C and one experienced deep venous thrombosis and pulmonary emboli.

Comparison of IVIG with other immunomodulating drugs

Table 23.2 summarizes the results of the trials[47–49] discussed above as regards reduction of disease activity and progression of disability. As can be seen, observed treatment effects all went in the same direction and were uniformly in favour of IVIG. These results appear to demonstrate convincingly that IVIG treatment of patients with RRMS can reduce the frequency of relapses. To what extent this may be achieved is more difficult to determine. A comparison of the AIMS data with the results of studies assessing IFN-β[52–54] and glatiramer acetate[55] looks quite favourable for IVIG (*Fig. 23.1*). It is apparent that the placebo group of the AIMS trial experienced a more subtle decline in the annual relapse rate than noted in the other studies. Certainly this contributed to the observed magnitude of difference between placebo and active treatment groups and has been viewed as potential evidence for imperfect blinding (L Kappos; personal communication). However, this cannot question the absolute drop in relapses of IVIG-treated patients. It can also be argued that frequent and self-administration, on an 'as necessary' basis, of medications such as INF-β and glatiramer acetate are more likely to induce a true placebo effect as seen in the decline of relapse rates than are monthly intravenous infusions. In addition, Sørensen and colleagues confirmed a decrease in disease activity using the relatively objective method of serial contrast enhanced MRI scans.[49,56] The observed reduction in gadolinium-positive lesions of approximately 60% is close to that reported in trials of interferon-β 1a.[57]

Comparing the effects of different immunomodulatory treatments with regard to

Table 23.2 Clinical results of recent IVIG trials

	AIMS[47]		Achiron et al.[48]		Sørensen et al.[49]	
	IVIG	*Placebo*	*IVIG*	*Placebo*	*IVIG*	*Placebo*
Number of patients	75	73	20	20	21	21
Relapses						
Annual relapse rate						
baseline	1.3	1.41	1.85	1.55	—	—
on trial	0.52	1.26‡	0.59	1.61§	—	—
Number of relapses	62	116	—	—	11	19
Number of relapse-free patients	40	26†	6	0§	15	7†
Disability						
EDSS baseline	3.33	3.37	2.9	2.82	—	—
end of trial	3.09	3.49‡	2.6	2.97	—	—
Improved*	31	14	23	11	44	11
Stable	53	63	63	72	22	55
Worse*	16	23†	14	17†	34	34

* Percentage of patients with change of EDSS score by ≥ 1.
† $p < 0.05$.
‡ $p < 0.01$.
§ $p \leq 0.001$.

disease progression yields a similar picture (*Fig. 23.2*). Although the absolute rates of patient shifts in EDSS scores were somewhat different in patient groups on active or placebo medication between trials, the magnitude of treatment effects between trials appears similar.

Apart from these encouraging results for IVIG, the limitations of the currently available data certainly must be acknowledged. To date, the number of patients included in successful treatment trials of IVIG lags far behind that of patients involved in studies of INF-β. In addition, both the AIMS trial[47] and the study of Achiron and colleagues[48] had a duration of only 2 years, whereas observational periods of up to 5 years

for INF-β[58] and extended use of glatiramer acetate[59] have been reported. In view of the differences in the dosage of IVIG used in the various trials, data on dose efficacy relationship would be highly desirable. Finally, the lack of representative long-term MRI data for IVIG has to be noted, although presently such data can only serve to support certain morphology-related mechanisms of drug action and do not replace clinical measures of outcome. In the study by Achiron and colleagues[48] there was no significant difference in the change of a complex MRI lesion score between IVIG-treated and placebo patients, but limited sensitivity of the scoring method used and the small number of patients

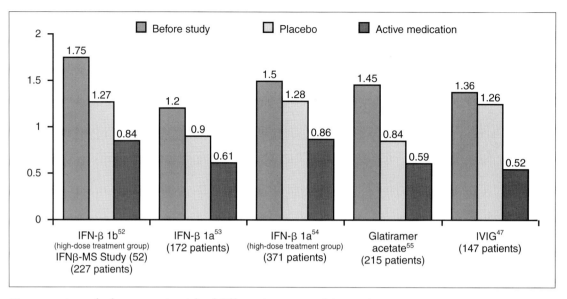

Fig. 23.1 Annual relapse rates in trials of different immunomodulatory drugs.

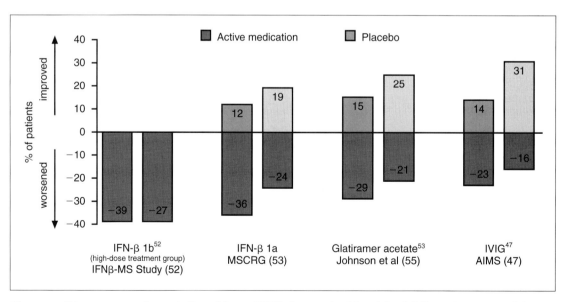

Fig. 23.2 Disease progression as indicated by an EDSS change of ≥ 1 in trials of different immunomodulatory drugs.

who underwent a final MRI exam have to be considered when interpreting these data.[60,61] Lack of a significant change of lesion area in the study by Sørensen and colleagues is readily explained by the short follow-up of only 6 months.[49] The possibility that the benefits of IVIG treatment might be reflected more readily by MRI variables other than the hyperintense lesion load also cannot be completely dismissed.

Current position of IVIG in the treatment of MS

At present, all available clinical evidence for a beneficial effect of IVIG treatment refers only to patients with RRMS. The magnitude of treatment effects of IVIG and the weight of evidence in comparison to approved immunomodulatory drugs have been considered above. This comparison is certainly in favour of IFN-β. The currently available body of evidence for the efficacy of glatiramer acetate is not very dissimilar to that for IVIG. It must also be considered that both frequency and routes of administration of IFN-β and glatiramer acetate are not easily acceptable for some patients, and local reactions at the injection site can become a problem, whereas monthly administration of IVIG (as in the AIMS trial[47]) or second-monthly administration (as in the trial by Achiron and colleagues[48]) is readily tolerated. At the dosages used in both these trials, side effects have been uniformly minor.[62] Several side effects, such as headache, myalgia, arthralgia, chills, fever, pruritus, rash, light headedness and malaise, may occur within the first hours of the infusion but they can be managed by temporarily stopping the infusion or by reducing the infusion rate. Treatment with analgesic drugs, antihistamines or corticosteroids may alleviate

these adverse reactions, but this is not generally required.[62] Treatment failures of IFN-β and glatiramer acetate may also warrant the consideration of IVIG as an alternative treatment option. However, it should be noted that there is at least anecdotal evidence against the use of IVIG in more severe forms of MS.[63] Finally, it should also be noted that IVIG has also been given successfully during pregnancy of MS patients in order to prevent a post-partum relapse.[64]

In the absence of clinical evidence for a more pronounced treatment effect, several factors presently argue against a high-dose regimen of IVIG in MS. Administration of large doses of IVIG can be associated with an increased risk of cardiovascular and renal complications and of thromboembolic events,[62] besides the frequent observation of chronic eczema by Sørensen and colleagues.[49] In contrast to a regimen as used in the AIMS trial, the costs of high dose IVIG treatment are significantly higher than those for IFN-β and glatiramer acetate.[65] Finally, concerns about the availability of IVIG have also been an argument against its use in MS, and this would become even more important if very large doses were required.[65]

DIRECTIONS OF FUTURE RESEARCH

Various questions will have to be resolved before the role of IVIG in the treatment of MS can be fully appreciated. Most importantly, the optimal dosage of IVIG for treating MS needs to be determined. The exact mechanism(s) of action will have to be clarified to appreciate the possible role of differences in the preparation of the product. This would also add valuable information in regard to the potential contribution of IVIG to combination therapies. Recently, almost complete cessation of relapses has been reported after the combined administration of IVIG and azathioprine.[66] The efficacy of IVIG in other than relapsing–remitting courses of the disease will have to be evaluated, for example in an ongoing study of 300 patients with secondary chronic progressive MS.

REFERENCES

1 Voltz R, Hohlfeld R. The use of intravenous immunoglobulins in the treatment of neuromuscular disorders. *Curr Opin Neurol* 1996; 9:360–366.

2 Stangel M, Hartung HP, Marx P et al. Intravenous immunoglobulin treatment of neurological autoimmune diseases. *J Neurol Sci* 1996; 153:203–214.

3 Dalakas MC. Use of intravenous immunoglobulin for neurologic diseases. *Neurology* 1998; 51 (suppl 5)S1–S45.

4 Van der Meché FGA, van Doorn PA. The current place of high-dose immunoglobulins in the treatment of neuromuscular disorders. *Muscle Nerve* 1997; 20:136–147.

5 Hartung HP, Toyka KV, Griffin JW. Guillain–Barré syndrome and chronic inflammatory demyelinating polyneuropathy. In: Antel J, Birnbaum G, Hartung HP, eds. *Clinical Neuroimmunology*. Oxford: Blackwell Science, 1998: 294–306.

6 Howard JF. Intravenous immunoglobulin for the treatment of acquired myasthenia gravis. *Neurology* 1998; 51 (Suppl 5):S30–S36.

7 Pestronk A. Multifocal motor neuropathy: diagnosis and treatment. *Neurology* 1998; 51 (Suppl 5): S22–S24.

8 Klein J, Horejsi V. *Immunology*. Oxford: Blackwell Science, 1997.

9 Deo YM, Graziano RF, Repp R et al. Clinical significance of Fc receptors and FcgammaR-directed immunotherapies. *Immunol Today* 1997; 18:127–134.

10 Jungi TW, Nydegger VE. Proposed mechanisms of action of intravenous IgG in autoimmune diseases. *Transfus Sci* 1992; 13:267–290.

11 Eibl MM, Wedgood RJ. Intravenous immunoglobulin: a review. *Immunodefic Rev* 1989; 1 (Suppl 1):1–42.

12 Yap PL, Williams PE. The safety of IVIG preparations. In: Yap PL, ed. *Clinical Applications of Intravenous Immunoglobulin Therapy*. Edinburgh: Churchill Livingstone, 1992, 43–62.

13 Cash J, Boyd K. Blood transfusion: Bayer's initiative. *Lancet* 1999; 353:691–692.

14 Sekul EA, Cupler EJ, Dalakas MC. Aseptic meningitis associated with high-dose intravenous immunoglobulin therapy: frequency and risk factors. *Ann Intern Med* 1994; 121:259–262.

15 Yu Z, Lennon VA. Mechanism of intravenous immune globulin therapy in antibody-mediated autoimmune diseases. *N Engl J Med* 1999; 340:227–228.

16 Lecky BRF. Gammaglobulin treatment in neurology: fundamentals and clinical applications. *J Neurol Neurosurg Psychiatry* 1994; 57 (Suppl 1): S1–S75.

17 Dalakas MC. Mechanism of action of intravenous immunoglobulin and therapeutic considerations in the treatment of autoimmune neurologic diseases. *Neurology* 1998; 51 (Suppl 5):S2–S8.

18 Roux KH, Tankersley DL. A view of the human idiotypic repertoire. Electron microscopic and immunologic analyses of spontaneous idiotype-anti-idiotype dimers in pooled human IgG. *J Immunol* 1990; 144:1387–1395.

19 Dietrich G, Kaveri SV, Kazatchkine MD. Modulation of autoimmunity by intravenous immune globulin through interaction with the function of the immune/idiotypic network. *Clin Immunol Immunopathol* 1992; 62:S73–S81.

20 Kazatchkine MD, Dietrich G, Hurez V et al. V region-mediated selection of autoreactive repertoires by intravenous immunoglobulin. *Immunol Rev* 1994; 139:79–107.

21 Diegel M, Rankin B, Bolen J et al. Cross linking of Fc receptor to surface immunoglobulin on B cells provides an inhibitory signal that closes the plasma membrane calcium channel. *J Biol Chem* 1994; 269:11409–11416.

22 Kurlander RJ, Hall J. Comparison of intravenous gamma globulin and a monoclonal anti-Fc receptor antibody as inhibitors of immune clearance in vivo in mice. *J Clin Invest* 1986; 77:2010–2018.

23 Miyagi F, Horiuchi H, Nagata I et al. Fc portion of intravenous immunoglobulin suppresses the induction of experimental allergic neuritis. *J Neuroimmunol* 1997; 78:127–131.

24 Ashman RF, Peckham DW, Stunz LL. Fc receptor off-signal in the B cell involves apoptosis. *J Immunol* 1996; 157:5–11.

25 Andersson J, Skansén-Saphir U, Sparrelid E et al.

Intravenous immune globulin affects cytokine production in T lymphocytes and monocytes macrophages. *Clin Exp Immunol* 1996; **104**:10–20.

26 Aukrust P, Müller F, Nordoy I et al. Modulation of lymphocyte and monocyte activity after intravenous immunoglobulin administration in vivo. *Clin Exp Immunol* 1997; **107**:50–56.

27 Svenson M, Hansen MB, Bendtzen K. Binding of cytokines to pharmaceutically prepared human immunoglobulin. *J Clin Invest* 1993; **92**:2533–2539.

28 Ross C, Svenson M, Hansen MB et al. High avidity IFN-neutralizing antibodies in pharmaceutically prepared human IgG. *J Clin Invest* 1995; **95**:1974–1978.

29 Dalakas MC, Illa I, Dambrosia JM et al. Efficacy of high-dose intravenous immunoglobulin in the treatment of dermatomyositis: a double-blind, placebo-controlled study. *N Engl J Med* 1993; **329**:1993–2000.

30 Lutz HU, Stammler P, Jelezarova E et al. High doses of immunoglobulin G attenuate immune aggregate-mediated complement activation by enhancing physiologic cleavage of C3b in C3bn–IgG complexes. *J Immunol* 1996; **88**:184–193.

31 Frank MM, Basta M, Fries LF. The effect of intravenous immune globulin on complement-dependent immune damage of cells and tissues. *Clin Immunol Immunpathol* 1992; **62**:(Part 2)S82–S86.

32 Leung DYM, Burns JC, Newburger JW et al. Reversal of lymphocyte activation in Kawasaki syndrome by intravenous immunoglobulin. *J Clin Invest* 1987; **79**:468–472.

33 Macey MG, Newland AC. CD4 and CD8 subpopulation changes during high dose intravenous immunoglobulin treatment. *Br J Haematol* 1990; **76**:513–520.

34 Marchalonis JJ, Kaymaz H, Dedeoglu F et al. Human autoantibodies reactive with synthetic autoantigens from T-cell receptor beta-chain, *Proc Natl Acad Sci U S A* 1992; **89**:3325–3329.

35 Kaveri S, Vassilev T, Hurez V et al. Antibodies to a conserved region of HLA class molecules, capable of modulating CD8 T cell-mediated function, are present in pooled normal immunoglobulin for therapeutic use. *J Clin Invest* 1996; **97**:865–869.

36 Takei S, Arora YK, Walker SM. Intravenous immunoglobulin contains specific antibodies inhibitory to activation of T cells by staphylococcal toxin superantigens. *J Clin Invest* 1993; **91**:602–607.

37 Blaszczyk R, Westhoff U, Grosse-Wilde H. Soluble CD4, CD8, and HLA molecules in commercial immunoglobulin preparations. *Lancet* 1993; **341**:789–790.

38 Prasad NK, Papoff G, Zeuner A et al. Therapeutic preparations of normal polyspecific IgG (IVIg) induce apoptosis in human lymphocytes and monocytes: a novel mechanism of action of IVIg involving the Fas apoptotic pathway. *J Immunol* 1998; **161**:3781–3790.

39 Zavazava N, Krönke M. Soluble HLA class I molecules induce apoptosis in alloreactive cytotoxic T lymphocytes. *Nature Med* 1996; **2**:1005–1010.

40 Rodriguez M, Lennon VA. Immunoglobulins promote remyelination in the central nervous system. *Ann Neurol* 1990; **27**:12–17.

41 Rodriguez M, Miller DJ, Lennon VA. Immunoglobulins reactive with myelin basic protein promote CNS remyelination. *Neurology* 1996; **46**:538–545.

42 Miller DJ, Sanborn KS, Katzmann JA et al. Monoclonal autoantibodies promote central nervous system repair in an animal model of multiple sclerosis. *J Neurosci* 1994; **14**:6230–6238.

43 Pavelko KD, van Engelen BGM, Rodriguez M. Acceleration in the rate of CNS remyelination in lysolecithin-induced demyelination. *J Neurosci* 1998; **18**:2498–2505.

44 Asakura K, Miller DJ, Murray K et al. Monoclonal autoantibody SCH94.03, which promotes central nervous system remyelination, recognizes an antigen on the surface of oligodendrocytes. *J Neurosci Res* 1996; **43**:273–281.

45 Sørensen PS. Treatment of multiple sclerosis with IVIg: potential effects and methodology of clinical trials. *J Neurol Neurosurg Psychiatry* 1994; **57** (**suppl**):62–64.

46 Achiron A, Barak Y, Sarova-Pinhas I. Use of intravenous immunoglobulin in multiple sclerosis. *BioDrugs* 1998; **9**:465–475.

47 Fazekas F, Deisenhammer F, Strasser-Fuchs S et al. for **the Austrian Immunoglobulin in Multiple Sclerosis Study Group.** Randomized placebo-controlled trial of monthly intravenous immunoglobulin therapy in relapsing–remitting multiple sclerosis. *Lancet* 1997; **349**:589–593.

48 Achiron A, Gabbay U, Gilad R et al. Intravenous immunoglobulin treatment in multiple sclerosis. Effect on relapses. *Neurology* 1998; **50**:398–402.

49 Sørensen PS, Wanscher B, Jensen CV et al. Intravenous immunoglobulin G reduces MRI activity in relapsing multiple sclerosis. *Neurology* 1998; **50**:1273–1281.

50 Fazekas F, Strasser-Fuchs S, Soelberg-Sørensen P. Intravenous immunoglobilin trials in multiple sclerosis. *Intern MS J* 1999; 6:14–21.

51 Fazekas F, Deisenhammer F, Strasser-Fuchs S et al. for the Austrian Immunoglobulin in Multiple Sclerosis Study Group. Treatment effects of monthly intravenous immunoglobulin on patients with relapsing–remitting multiple sclerosis: further analysis of the Austrian Immunoglobulin in MS Study. *Multiple Sclerosis* 1997; 3:137–142.

52 The IFNB Multiple Sclerosis Study Group. Interferon beta-1b is effective in relapsing–remitting multiple sclerosis: clinical results of a multicenter, randomized, double-blind, placebo-controlled trial. *Neurology* 1993; 43:655–661.

53 Jacobs DL, Cookfair DL, Rudick RA et al. Intramuscular interferon beta-1a for disease progression in relapsing multiple sclerosis. The Multiple Sclerosis Collaborative Research Group (MSCRG). *Ann Neurol* 1996; 39:6–16.

54 PRISMS (Prevention of Relapses and Disability by Interferon β-1a Subcutaneously in Multiple Sclerosis) Study Group. Randomised double-blind placebo-controlled study of interferon β-1a in relapsing/remitting multiple sclerosis. *Lancet* 1998; 352:1498–1504.

55 Johnson KP, Brooks BR, Cohen JA et al. Copolymer 1 reduces relapse rate and improves disability in relapsing–remitting multiple sclerosis: results of a phase III multicenter, double-blind, placebo-controlled trial. *Neurology* 1995; 45:1268–1276.

56 Miller DH, Albert PS, Barkhof F et al. Guidelines for using magnetic resonance techniques in monitoring the treatment of multiple sclerosis. *Ann Neurol* 1996; 39:6–16.

57 Pozzilli C, Bastianello S, Koudriavtseva T et al. Magnetic resonance imaging changes with recombinant human interferon-β-1a: a short term study in relapsing–remitting multiple sclerosis. *J Neurol Neurosurg Psychiatry* 1996; 61:251–258.

58 The IFNB Multiple Sclerosis Study Group, the University of British Columbia MS/MRI Analysis Group. Interferon beta-1b in the treatment of multiple sclerosis: final outcome of the randomized controlled trial. *Neurology* 1995; 45:1277–1285.

59 Johnson KP, Brooks BR, Cohen JA et al. Extended use of glatiramer acetate (Copaxone) is well tolerated and maintains its clinical effect on multiple sclerosis relapse rate and degree of disability. Copolymer 1 Multiple Sclerosis Study Group. *Neurology* 1998; 50:701–708.

60 Francis G. Intravenous immunoglobulin treatment in multiple sclerosis (letter). *Neurology* 1999; 52:214.

61 Achiron A, Barak Y. Intravenous immunoglobulin treatment in multiple sclerosis. *Neurology* 1999; 52:214.

62 Stangel M, Hartung HP, Marx P, Gold R. Side effects of high-dose intravenous immunoglobulins. *Clin Neuropharmacol* 1997; 20:385–393.

63 Francis GS, Freedman MS, Antel JP. Failure of intravenous immunoglobulin to arrest progression of multiple sclerosis: a clinical and MRI based study. *Multiple Sclerosis* 1997; 3:370–376.

64 Achiron A, Rotstein Z, Noy S et al. Intravenous immunoglobulin treatment in the prevention of childbirth-associated acute exacerbations in multiple sclerosis: a pilot study. *J Neurol* 1996; 243:25–28.

65 Lisak RP. Intravenous immunoglobulins in multiple sclerosis. *Neurology* 1998; 51 (Suppl 5):S25–S29.

66 Kalanie H, Tabatabai SS. Combined immunoglobulin and azathioprine in multiple sclerosis. *Eur Neurol* 1998; 39:178–181.

24
Therapeutic plasma exchange

Brian G Weinshenker

INTRODUCTION

Therapeutic plasma exchange (TPE), also known as plasmapheresis or apheresis, has been studied as a treatment for MS since 1980. Studies conducted over the past 18 years have not conclusively established whether TPE is effective for progressive multiple sclerosis (MS) or for acute attacks of MS. Noseworthy[1] has previously reviewed the benefits of TPE in progressive MS. Since that time, Vamvakas and colleagues[2] have published a review and meta-analysis of six prospective controlled studies published as of 1992 (the date of Noseworthy's previous review), but new studies have not been undertaken. Studies in progressive MS have been contradictory, although the meta-analysis suggests that TPE may have a weak beneficial effect in preventing deterioration at 12 months from initiation of treatment when combined with other immunosuppressive treatment.[2]

Perhaps more promising than the studies in patients with progressive MS are a series of uncontrolled observations suggesting that TPE can result in dramatic improvement in neurological function in patients with acute, severe attacks of demyelinating disease. In most instances, patients who appeared to benefit had severe neurological disability, apparently unresponsive to

corticosteroid therapy. A controlled study by Weiner and colleagues[3] failed to support the efficacy of TPE in acute attacks of MS when used as an adjunct to an intensive immunosuppressive treatment. However, a hint of benefit was observed in those who had relapsing–remitting MS (RRMS) with the most severe attacks. In order to address the putative benefit of TPE alone in patients with acute, severe attacks of demyelinating disease, investigators at the Mayo Clinic have conducted a 4-year, randomized, double-blind study of TPE in acute, severe attacks of inflammatory demyelinating disease.

This review briefly considers the results of the recent meta-analysis.[2] However, it concentrates on the status of treatment for acute severe attacks of demyelinating disease and on the rationale and methods utilized in the Mayo Clinic trial.

METHODS, ADVERSE EFFECTS, AND MECHANISMS OF ACTION

Plasma exchange consists of withdrawal of blood and separation of cellular elements from plasma by centrifugation, followed by reinfusion of the cellular elements in a replacement solution, usually consisting of albumin.[4] Plasma is rarely used as a replacement solution except in thrombotic, thrombocytopenic purpura; in this instance, plasma contains the active agent that is necessary to treat the disease. Recently, colloidal starch has been recommended as a suitable replacement solution.[5]

Plasma exchange is effective in the treatment of a number of non-neurological and neurological disorders. It is a life-saving treatment in Goodpasture's disease,[6] it is highly effective in managing acute exacerbations of myasthenia gravis,[7] and it is the treatment of choice for attacks of acute inflammatory demyelinating polyneuropathy with severe disability.[8] This is also an acute inflammatory demyelinating disease and may be particularly relevant to MS.

It is difficult to determine the critical plasma component responsible for improvement because all plasma proteins are removed by the TPE procedure. The immunopathogenic mechanisms of some diseases (e.g. myasthenia gravis) that are responsive to TPE are well established. In other diseases, the presence of circulating immune complexes appear to predict those patients who might respond.[9]

The role of antibodies is less well established for MS. However, myelin-reactive autoantibodies have been described in MS.[10] Circulating immune complexes are rarely present in patients with MS who have been reported to benefit from TPE,[9] although Stricker and colleagues[11] have reported circulating immune complexes in a patient with acute disseminated encephalomyelitis (ADEM) who appeared to respond to TPE. Other circulating factors that may be relevant to the therapeutic actions of TPE include pro-inflammatory cytokines (e.g., tumor necrosis factor-α, interferon-γ), and complement. Whether the action occurs at the level of the blood–brain barrier (e.g. by adhesion molecules), within the central nervous system or possibly in the periphery (e.g. by alteration of T-cell suppressor function), is unknown. As discussed below, the response described by many investigators in patients who receive TPE for acute attacks of MS is rapid, suggesting that the effect may be physiological rather than anti-inflammatory or associated with remyelination. Buchwald and colleagues[12] have recently found that IgG from patients with Guillain–Barré syndrome can interfere with neurotransmitter release and postsynaptic activation of muscle. Others have also described neuroelectric-blocking activity in the IgG fraction of MS sera that is capable of inhibiting the ventral root response in isolated, perfused spinal cords.[13] If patients who respond to treatment are prospectively identified, their pre-exchange blood may be helpful in distinguishing responders from non-responders by retrospective analysis of plasma or serum components.

TPE if often combined with other immunosuppressive therapy[3] to prevent rebound antibody production and to impair the function of the immune effector systems that perpetuate the disease process. However, as discussed below, many investigators have reported uncontrolled experience that suggests that the benefit of TPE can occur in the absence of any concomitant immunosuppression. In most instances, the benefit is sustained.

TPE is generally well tolerated. The most common adverse effects are hypotension and perioral paresthesias owing to the citrate in the citrate dextrose anti-coagulant. Other treatment-related complications include those of central line placement, which is required by a high proportion of patients who require frequent plasma exchange treatments. Serious complications are those related to central lines, including sepsis.[14] No such complications occurred in 22 patients who participated in the randomized study of TPE at the Mayo Clinic. However, multifactorial treatment-related anemia was observed frequently. Causes for the anemia include hemodilution caused by the replacement colloidal solution and loss of blood in the dead space of the tubing in the separator apparatus. Hemolysis does not occur. Anemia occurred to an equal extent in patients receiving active and sham treatment in the Mayo Clinic study, so it is not directly related to the removal of plasma and replacement with albumin.

TPE IN PROGRESSIVE MS

Noseworthy and colleagues[1] have reviewed seven non-randomized studies and four randomized studies up to until 1991 in 'chronic-progressive MS'. As of 1991, when the last of these studies was reported, it was not customary to differentiate between primary progressive MS (PPMS) and secondary progressive MS (SPMS). Most current studies enroll only patients with SPMS, since potentially important biological differences have been described between these two subtypes of MS.[15] Patients with PPMS have less inflammation, fewer MRI lesions, and possibly different immunogenetic factors, such as an excess of the MHC class II allele DR4.[16,17] Axonal degeneration may play a more dominant role in PPMS than in SPMS.[18] Accordingly, one might speculate that trials with a relative excess of patients with PPMS may be less likely to demonstrate benefit.

Vamvakas and colleagues[2] recently reported a meta-analysis of six prospective studies[19–24] that included patients with clinically definite, progressive MS and had a concurrent comparison group. The design and results of the individual studies were summarized in the paper. Of the six studies,

four were randomized[19–22] and two were double blinded with respect to the use of TPE.[19,22] One study was multicenter.[20] The treatment regimens were variable (between four and 20 treatments) as was the duration over which they were administered (2 weeks to 1 year), making comparison between the studies difficult. The homogeneity of the behavior of patients in these studies, assessed using the Q statistic,[25] although imperfect, allowed for meta-analysis. However, for analysis of mean change in disability status score (DSS), some patients in one study[19] were excluded because the conditions for homogeneity could not otherwise be met because these patients were 'outliers.'

The results of the meta-analysis are given in *Table 24.1*. There was significant, though modest, efficacy in reducing the odds of worsening at 12 months and in enhancing the odds of improving at 6 months and 12 months after undergoing TPE. Follow-up at 24–36 months revealed significant results only for the relative odds of worsening at 24 months.

The conclusions from this meta-analysis must remain tentative because:

(a) the 'control groups' were not strictly comparable (e.g. in the Canadian Cooperative Study, the 'control group' for the purposes of this analysis had received high-dose intravenous cyclophosphamide rather than oral cyclophosphamide, which the TPE group received);

(b) the effects of TPE and the other immunosuppressive treatments administered in these studies are difficult to disentangle; and

(c) the TPE regimes differed considerably in terms of the intensity of the exchanges and the durations over which they were applied.

Further investigation of TPE for progressive MS is of questionable benefit because:

Table 24.1 Meta-analysis of effect of plasma exchange in progressive MS

	Follow up			
	6 months		12 months	
	All	Controlled	All	Controlled
DSS	−0.171	−0.177 (−0.149)†	−0.212	−0.204 (−0.167)†
Relative odds of worsening	0.746	0.879	0.436*	0.441*
Relative odds of improvement	1.981*	2.321*	2.129*	2.258*

Based on review of six studies, four of which were controlled by Vamvakas et al.[2]
Values shown reflect difference in change in mean DSS or relative odds of worsening or improvement in treatment versus control group.
† After exclusion of 4 'outliers'. *$p < 0.05$.

(a) existing studies do not provide any indication of a subgroup that is likely to respond;
(b) other treatments for progressive MS exist; and
(c) TPE is an expensive, cumbersome treatment that is not well suited to chronic management of disease, particularly if other treatments are equally or more effective and if benefit is transient.

TPE IN ACUTE ATTACKS OF DEMYELINATING DISEASE

In contrast to the modest and equivocal results in patients with progressive MS, uncontrolled observations in patients treated with TPE for acute severe attacks suggest that patients may show dramatic recovery from devastating, apparently fixed, neurological deficits after treatment with a brief course of treatment. A controlled trial has recently been completed that should definitively answer this issue. The background of this study is reviewed here, concentrating on the

study by Rodriguez and colleagues[26] that led to this clinical trial. One previous randomized clinical trial of plasma exchange for acute attacks of MS[3] that left significant uncertainty about the role of TPE in this setting is considered.

The natural history of acute severe attacks of demyelinating disease has not been well studied. Ascertainment of cases in studies that address recovery from acute attacks is based on series of hospitalized patients, which are biased to patients with the most severe attacks.

The most complete data on this subject comes from Kurtzke's study of hospitalized US veterans.[27] The strengths of these data include the probable unbiased ascertainment (high likelihood that military recruits would have been hospitalized for these symptoms), the long duration of 'in-hospital' evaluation (mean 105 days), and the fact that most of the patients were experiencing a first attack. Pseudo-exacerbations caused by physiological perturbations such as fever were less likely to have an impact on this study because pseudo-exacerbations occur more frequently in patients with relatively more advanced disability. The outcome for 18 patients with the most severe attacks, whose admission DSS scores were 7–9 (i.e. not ambulatory), is shown in *Table 24.2.*

In this study, 56% of patients had either no or minimal recovery (DSS change ≤ 1) after a devastating acute attack that rendered them nonambulatory. Although Kurtzke concluded that severe attacks were as likely or more likely to be followed by improvement by 1 DSS point than mild attacks, it is important to point out that improvement by 1 DSS point is trivial for attacks that lead to an acute deterioration by 6 or more DSS points. Other studies conducted on patients with acute attacks support the conclusion that patients with relatively infrequent severe attacks may not recover, and indeed high-dose corticosteroid failure occurs in up to 40% of these patients.

The literature on the use of TPE in acute inflammatory demyelinating disease of the CNS is summarized in *Table 24.3.* Eleven series report favorable uncontrolled clinical experience with TPE in diverse idiopathic and symptomatic demyelinating disease syndromes in 28 patients. Fourteen of these patients had MS, nine had ADEM, two had acute transverse myelitis (ATM), and three had neuromyelitis optica (NMO). The patients had a variety of neurological deficits that led to treatment with TPE, most commonly coma in patients with ADEM and paraplegia or quadriplegia in patients with MS, ATM, and NMO. In some cases, there was an apparent underlying systemic autoimmune disease, such as Sjögren's disease[29] or mixed connective tissue disease.[30] In the vast majority of patients, TPE alone in the absence of concomitant corticosteroid or immunosuppressive treatment seemed to result in clinical benefit. The response was usually dramatic and evident in most cases within 1–4 days of initiation of TPE.

Table 24.2 Outcome of severe attacks of MS

DSS at dismissal*	
DSS	**Number of patients**
1	2
2	1
3	2
4	1
5	1
6	2
7	4
8	5
9	0

Improvement in DSS at dismissal*	
DSS	**Number of patients (%)**
0	7 (39)
1	3 (17)
2	0
3	8 (44)

Based on data from Kurtzke et al[28] on 18 US Second World War veterans admitted to hospital with acute exacerbations and a DSS of between 7 and 9.
*Mean hospital stay 105 days.

Many of these patients had failed to respond to high-dose corticosteroid therapy.

Rodriguez and colleagues[26] reported that dramatic benefit resulted from between six and nine courses of TPE administered without immunosuppressive treatment in six patients with acute attacks of MS. These patients had failed to

327

Table 24.3 Uncontrolled series of plasma exchange for acute attacks of inflammatory central nervous system demyelinating disease

Investigator	Year	Age and sex	Underlying illness	Dominant neurological deficit	Previous corticosteroid therapy (days)	Concomitant immunosuppression* during TPE	Number of days of TPE (total number of days)	Degree of improvement	Interval until improvement was first noted	Early relapse
Dau et al[31]	1980	28 male	MS	Paraplegia	Yes (14)	No	3 (14)	Marked	Immediate	Yes
		32 female	NMO	Paraparesis	Yes (7)	No	6 (25)	Marked	Immediate	No
		33 male	MS	Triparesis	Yes (14)	No	6 (42)	Marked	Immediate	No
Newton et al[32]	1981	12 female	ADEM	Quadriparesis	NS	No	3 (?)	Marked	2 weeks	No
		2 male	ATM		NS	No	2 (?)	Moderate	3 weeks	No
Valbonesi et al[33]	1981	26 male	MS	Paraparesis	No	No	2 (NS)	None		Yes
		60 male	MS	Hand inco-ordination	Yes (NS)	No	3 (6)+3(90)	Mild	Immediate	No
		26 female	MS	Spastic ataxic gait	No	Yes	3 (6)	Mild	Immediate	No
		50 male	MS	Quadriparesis	No	No	2 (2)	Moderate	Immediate	No
		27 female	MS	Spastic–ataxic hemiparesis	No	Yes	2 (NS) > 1	Marked	Immediate	Yes
		19 female	MS	Diplopia, mild weakness	Yes (5)	Yes	2 (3)	Mild	NS	No
Cotter et al[34]	1983	22 male	ADEM	Paraplegia, confusion	No	No	3 (4)	NS	2 days	Yes
Aguilera et al[35]	1985	26 female	NMO	Paraplegia	No	No	8 (14)+6(10†)	Marked	7 days	Yes
Konttinen et al[29]	1987	54 male	ATM, Sjögren's syndrome	Paraplegia	Yes (5)	Yes	3 (3)	Marked	7 days	No
Seales et al[36]	1991	50 female	ADEM	Coma; resp. failure	Yes (1)	Yes	5 (5)	Marked	9 days	No
Stricker et al[11]	1992	25 female	ADEM	Coma; resp. failure	No	NS	10 (NS)	Marked	NS	No
		31 female	ADEM	Coma; resp. failure; paraplegia	No	No	5 (NS)	Marked	Almost immediate	No
		5 male	ADEM	Confusion; weak arm	No	No	3 (3)	Marked	Immediate	No
		27 male	ADEM	Confusion, ataxia; ophthalmoparesis	No	Yes	8 (11)	Marked	Almost immediate	No
Rodriguez et al[26]	1993	22 male	MS	Paraplegia	Yes (14)	No	8 (18)	Marked	2 days	No
		27 female	MS	Quadriplegia	Yes (7)	No	9 (18)	Marked	4 days	No
		33 female	MS	Quadriplegia, respiratory failure	Yes (7)	Yes	6 (12)	Moderate	12 days	No
		22 female	MS	Hemiparesis, aphasia	Yes (5)	No	6 (13)	Marked	4 days	No
		40 female	MS	Hemiparesis, aphasia	Yes (NS)	No	9 (18)	Marked	4 days	No
		47 male	MS	Quadriplegia, respiratory failure	Yes (5)	No	9 (18)	Marked	3 days	No
Flechtner et al[30]	1994	19 female	NMO; MCTD	Quadriplegia, respiratory failure	Yes (NS)	No	6 (18)	Marked	Immediate	No
Kanter et al[37]	1995	20 male	ADEM	Coma	Yes (9)	No	5 (5)	Marked	2 days	No
		45 male	ADEM	Coma	Yes (6)	No	7 (7) + (NS)	Marked	Immediate	No

*Includes concomitant corticosteroid and/or cytotoxic drug treatment.

†Lymphocyte and plasma exchanges performed.

TPE, Therapeutic plasma exchange; NS, not started; NMO, neuromyelitis optica; ADEM, acute disseminated encephalomyelitis; ATM, acute transverse myelitis; MCTD, mixed connective tissue disease.

respond to standard treatment with intravenous corticosteroids. All were paraplegic, hemiplegic, or quadriplegic. In addition, two of these patients were aphasic and two were dependent on artificial ventilation. The mean improvement at the conclusion of TPE was 3.8 points on the expanded disability status score (EDSS) (range 0.5–6.0 points; median 4.5). Improvement was first evident at a median of 4.8 days (range 2–12 days) after starting TPE. Benefit was sustained over 6–35 months of follow-up.

The report of a randomized controlled study of TPE or immunoadsorption in 19 patients by Palm and colleagues provides few clinical details.[38] It is not possible to provide an adequate critique of the study on the basis of the report. However, the authors indicate that 'remarkable clinical improvements' were observed both in the patients treated with TPE and in those treated with immunoadsorption, whereas only modest or no improvement was observed in the patients who were treated with corticosteroids alone.

Weiner and colleagues[3] reported a randomized, controlled, parallel-design trial of 11 courses of true versus sham exchange over 8 weeks as a supplement to oral cyclophosphamide and adrenocorticotrophin hormone (ACTH) in 116 patients with RRMS or progressive MS with acute exacerbations. The primary end-point was improvement by 1 or 2 DSS points, depending on the baseline disability level (2 points constituted improvement below DSS 6, and 1 point constituted improvement above DSS 6). The overall difference between the patients and controls was not significant, but there was a trend in favor of treatment at 1 month, which was most evident in patients who had relapsing–remitting forms of MS with the most severe attacks.

The present author does not feel that the study by Weiner and colleagues[3] either proves or dis-

proves a beneficial effect, let alone a dramatic one, of TPE for acute attacks of MS. The limitations of this study included the facts that:

(a) patients with attacks of varying degrees of severity were included, including patients with mild attacks;

(b) patients with progressive MS were also included;

(c) all patients received ACTH and cyclophosphamide in addition to being randomized to receive true or sham plasma exchange; and

(d) the end-point was the DSS rather than the deficit targeted to the patient's specific attack-related neurological deficit, and the DSS can be quite insensitive to major improvements of cognitive dysfunction or upper-extremity dysfunction if these are the neurological deficits caused by the attack.

Mindful of the differences between the studies of Rodriguez[26] and Weiner,[3] a randomized, sham-controlled study focused on the patient subgroup of interest was developed at the Mayo Clinic in order to address these uncontrolled observations. Until these observations could be confirmed in a prospective, randomized, controlled, and blinded fashion, the findings of Rodriguez[26] would not achieve widespread acceptance and would not be incorporated into treatment strategies for MS.

The following principles were intrinsic to the design of the Mayo Clinic study:

(a) Patients for whom the diagnosis of demyelinating disease was virtually certain would be enrolled. In equivocal cases, biopsy material was obtained to confirm the diagnosis. The study included patients with atypical idiopathic inflammatory demyelinating diseases, such as ADEM, Devic's NMO, and focal demyelinating diseases of the brain with or without mass effect. By definition, patients qualifying for this protocol were atypical in that they had experienced a severe neurological deficit that was unresponsive to corticosteroids. Significant overlap between MS and 'atypical' inflammatory demyelinating diseases does exist, and exclusion of such patients would eliminate an important and not uncommon group of patients with severe demyelinating disease who might respond to TPE.

(b) Only patients with a high probability of having severe, permanent neurological deficits were included. All patients had a profound neurological deficit affecting one or more of the following: power in at least one extremity, language function, cognitive function, and consciousness. All patients enrolled had had a neurological deficit for 3 weeks and had experienced no or minimal improvement after 2 weeks of high-dose intravenous methylprednisolone therapy (minimum dose 7 mg/kg per day or the equivalent for 5 days). An exception was made for patients who had had an attack of inflammatory demyelinating disease for a minimum of 12 days and who had completed 5 days of intravenous methylprednisolone and experienced continued progression of their neurological deficit.

(c) The study was interested only in a functionally significant outcome and not in a 1-point change in the EDSS. Functionally important change was felt to be the standard required to justify this expensive and cumbersome treatment. Furthermore, the EDSS was not appropriate for some of the targeted neurological deficits, including global cognitive dysfunction and aphasia, which were included as targeted neurological deficits, since the EDSS is not sufficiently sensitive to these deficits. Accordingly, targeted neurological deficits were evaluated in a global

way by the two blinded evaluating neurologists. The study organizers avoided choosing demyelinating syndromes that are caused by more limited lesions such as optic neuritis or vertigo, for which the prognosis is generally felt to be less ominous. Objective and established scales were chosen to rate each of the outcomes, and consensus was reached about the degree of improvement that would be interpreted as mild, moderate, or marked improvement. However, the final decision about the degree of improvement was left up to the global opinion of the evaluating neurologist. This outcome measure was appropriate because it was expected that the masking would be very effective. Common adverse effects of TPE (e.g. hypotension, citrate toxicity) were independent of the active treatment, namely replacement of plasma by albumin. Moderate (functionally important) or marked improvements were required for treatment success in this study. However, perfect improvement (i.e. return to baseline function) was felt to be an excessive requirement.

(d) TPE was evaluated alone, without concomitant immunosuppression, since Rodriguez and colleagues[26] found that TPE alone seemed to provide the necessary clinical benefit.

A regimen that consisted of seven exchange treatments every other day was chosen, based on the study by Rodriguez.[26] A cross-over protocol was used. Although there could be some methodologic objections to cross-over, since the effect cannot be 'washed out,' recruitment to this sham-controlled study would not be feasible if exposure to the active treatment were not offered to half the patients in a parallel study design. Because the benefit was seen early in the course of treatment in the study of Rodriguez,[26] it was

Table 24.4 Outcome measures in the Mayo Clinic Plasma Exchange Study

First treatment	Cross-over	Second treatment	Z Score
1. Success	No	—	+1.0
2. Failure	Yes	Failure	0.0
3. Failure	Yes	Success	−1.0

felt that it would be unlikely that the benefit of TPE in the first treatment period would be detected first after cross-over.

If no carry-over effects occurred, cross-over would increase the power of the study. Patients would cross over only if they did not experience moderate or greater benefit from TPE. Three outcomes were possible for each patient (*Table 24.4*). Each outcome was assigned an arbitrary Z-score.

The difference in the distribution of the Z-scores between the two treatment groups was chosen as the primary outcome. The best outcome, from the point of view of TPE, would be a mean Z-score of +1.0 for the first active-treatment group and −1.0 for the first sham-treatment group. The magnitude and direction of the difference would be a measure of the effectiveness of TPE. The statistical test applied was a one-sided rank–sum test, since the hypothesis was that TPE was effective. On the basis of the outcome from the first (pre-cross-over) treatment phase, and setting $\alpha = 0.05$ and assuming 70% success with TPE and 20% success with sham, the power to detect treatment effect was 0.8 with the sample size of 22 patients.

Patients were followed for 6 months after treatment to determine if benefit was sustained and whether recurrent episodes of demyelinating disease occurred in the follow-up period.

Accrual was completed in October 1998, and the results of the study will be announced in mid-1999.

SUMMARY

The role of TPE in the treatment of MS remains undefined. There is equivocal evidence from a meta-analysis for a benefit from TPE as a supplement to immunosuppression, but TPE has not been evaluated as a stand-alone therapy. It is a cumbersome and expensive long-term treatment, and this is a significant limitation; further investigation will have to evaluate its role relative to other agents that may also provide benefit in progressive forms of MS, such as interferon-β 1b.[39]

TPE may cause rapid improvement in patients with acute, devastating attacks of demyelinating disease who fail to respond to high-dose corticosteroids. A study supported by the National Institutes of Health will shortly be reported that addresses this observation in a double-masked, randomized, sham-controlled, cross-over study.

ACKNOWLEDGMENTS

This work was supported by grant support from the National Institutes of Health (Grant NS32774 and Grant RR00585 to the Mayo Clinic General Clinical Research Center). Mrs Laura Irlbeck prepared the manuscript.

REFERENCES

1 **Noseworthy J.** Treatment of multiple sclerosis with plasma exchange. In: Rudick R, ed. *Treatment of Multiple Sclerosis*. London: Springer, 1992; 251–266.

2 Vamvakas EE, Pineda AA, Weinshenker BG. Meta-analysis of clinical studies of the efficacy of plasma exchange in the treatment of chronic progressive multiple sclerosis. *J Clin Apheresis* 1995; **10**:163–170.

3 Weiner HL, Dau PC, Khatri BO et al. Double-blind study of true vs. sham plasma exchange in patients treated with immunosuppression for acute attacks of multiple sclerosis. *Neurology* 1989; **39**:1143–1149.

4 Shumak KH, Rock GA. Therapeutic plasma exchange. *N Engl J Med* 1984; **310**:762–771.

5 Rock G, Sutton D, Freedman J et al. Pentastarch instead of albumin as replacement fluid for therapeutic plasma exchange. *J Clin Apheresis* 1997; **12**:165–169.

6 Rosenblatt S, Knight W, Bannayan G et al. Treatment of Goodpasture's syndrome with plasmapheresis. *Am J Med* 1979; **66**:689–696.

7 Klein H, Balow J, Dau P et al. Clinical applications of therapeutic apheresis. Report of the Clinical Applications Committee, American Society of Apheresism. *J Clin Apheresis* 1986; **3**:1–92.

8 Arnason B, Soliven B. Acute inflammatory demyelinating polyradiculoneuropathy, In: Dyck P, Thomas P, Griffin J et al., eds. *Peripheral Neuropathy.* Philadelphia: Saunders, 1993, 1476–1478.

9 Valbonesi M, Garelli S, Montani F et al. Plasma exchange and immune complex diseases: the predictability of immune complexes removal to clinical response. *Vox Sang* 1982; **42**:27–32.

10 Dau P. Plasmapheresis in acute multiple sclerosis: rationale and results. *J Clin Apheresis* 1991; **6**:200–204.

11 Stricker RB, Miller R, Kiprov DD. Role of plasmapheresis in acute disseminated (postinfectious) encephalomyelitis. *J Clin Apheresis* 1992; **7**:173–179.

12 Buchwald B, Toyka K, Zielasek J et al. Neuromuscular blockade by IgG antibodies from patients with Guillain–Barré syndrome: A macro-patch-clamp study. *Ann Neurol* 1998; **44**:913–922.

13 Schauf CL, Davis FA. Circulating toxic factors in multiple sclerosis: a perspective. *Adv Neurol* 1981; **31**:267–280.

14 Henze T, Prange H, Talartschik J, Rumpf K. Complications of plasma exchange in patients with neurological disease. *Klin Wochenschr* 1990; **68**:1183–1188.

15 Thompson A, Polman C, Miller D et al. Primary progressive multiple sclerosis. *Brain* 1997; **120**:1085–1096.

16 Olerup O, Hillert J, Fredrikson S et al. Primarily chronic progressive and relapsing/remitting multiple sclerosis: two immunogenetically distinct disease entities. *Proc Natl Acad Sci U S A* 1989; **86**:7113–7117.

17 Weinshenker B, Santrach P, Bissonett A et al. Major histocompatibility complex class II alleles and the course and outcome of multiple sclerosis: A population-based study, *Neurology* 1998; **51**:742–747.

18 Losseff N, Webb S, O'Riordan J et al. Spinal cord atrophy and disability in multiple sclerosis. A new reproducible and sensitive MRI method with potential to monitor disease progression. *Brain* 1996; **119**:701–708.

19 Khatri BO, McQuillen MP, Harrington GJ et al. Chronic progressive multiple sclerosis: double-blind controlled study of plasmapheresis in patients taking immunosuppressive drugs. *Neurology* 1985; **35**:312–319.

20 Noseworthy JH, Vandervoort MK, Penman M et al. Cyclophosphamide and plasma exchange in multiple sclerosis. *Lancet* 1991; **337**:1540–1541.

21 Hauser SL, Dawson DM, Lehrich JR et al. Intensive immunosuppression in progressive multiple sclerosis. A randomized, three-arm study of high-dose intravenous cyclophosphamide, plasma exchange, and ACTH. *N Engl J Med* 1983; **308**:173–180.

22 Gordon PA, Carroll DJ, Etches WS et al. A double-blind controlled pilot study of plasma exchange versus sham apheresis in chronic progressive multiple sclerosis. *Can J Neurol Sci* 1985; **12**:39–44.

23 Tindall RS, Walker JE, Ehle AL et al. Plasmapheresis in multiple sclerosis: prospective trial of pheresis and immunosuppression versus immunosuppression alone. *Neurology* 1982; **32**:739–743.

24 Trouillas P, Neuschwander P, Nighoghossian N et al. (Intensive immunosuppression in progressive multiple sclerosis. An open study comparing 3 groups: cyclophosphamide, cyclophosphamide–plasmapheresis and control subjects. Results after 3 years) Immunosuppression intensive dans la sclerose en plaques progressive. Etude ouverte comparant trois groupes: cyclophosphamide, cyclophosphamide–plasmaphereses et témoins. Résultats à trois ans. *Rev Neurol* 1989; **145**:369–377.

25 Yusuf S, Peto R, Lewis J et al. Beta blockade during and after myocardial infarction: an overview of the randomized trials. *Prog Cardiovasc Dis* 1985; **27**:335–371.

26 Rodriguez M, Karnes WE, Bartleson JD, Pineda AA. Plasmapheresis in acute episodes of fulminant CNS

inflammatory demyelination. *Neurology* 1993;
43:1100–1104.

27 **Kurtzke JF, Beebe GW, Nagler B et al.** Studies on the
natural history of multiple sclerosis. 7. Correlates of
clinical change in an early bout. *Acta Neurol Scand*
1973; **49**:379–395.

28 **Kurtzke JF, Beebe GW, Norman JE Jr.** Epidemiology
of multiple sclerosis in US veterans. 1. Race, sex, and
geographic distribution. *Neurology* 1979;
29:1228–1235.

29 **Konttinen YT, Kinnunen E, von Bonsdorff M et al.**
Acute transverse myelopathy successfully treated with
plasmapheresis and prednisone in a patient with
primary Sjögren's syndrome. *Arthritis Rheum* 1987;
30:339–344.

30 **Flechtner KM, Baum K.** Mixed connective tissue
disease: Recurrent episodes of optic neuropathy and
transverse myelopathy. Successful treatments with
plasmapheresis. *J Neurol Sci* 1994; **126**:146–148.

31 **Dau P, Johnson K, Panitch H, Bornstein M.**
Plasmapheresis in multiple sclerosis: preliminary
findings. *Neurology* 1980; **30**:1023–1028.

32 **Newton R.** Plasma exchange in acute post-infectious
demyelination, *Dev Med Child Neurol* 1981;
23:538–543.

33 **Valbonesi M, Garelli S, Mosconi L et al.** Plasma
exchange in the management of patients with multiple
sclerosis: preliminary observations. *Vox Sang* 1981;
41:68–73.

34 **Cotter F, Bainbridge D, Newland A.** Neurological
deficit associated with *Mycoplasma pneumoniae*
reversed by plasma exchange. *Br Med J* 1983; **286**:22.

35 **Aguilera AJ, Carlow TJ, Smith KJ, Simon TL.**
Lymphocytoplasmapheresis in Devic's syndrome.
Transfusion 1985; **25**:54–56.

36 **Seales D, Greer M.** Acute hemorrhagic
leukoencephalitis: a successful recovery. *Arch Neurol*
1991; **48**:1086–1088.

37 **Kanter DS, Horensky D, Sperling RA et al.**
Plasmapheresis in fulminant acute disseminated
encephalomyelitis. *Neurology* 1995; **45**:824–827.

38 **Palm M, Behm E, Schmitt E et al.** Immunoadsorption
and plasma exchange in multiple sclerosis:
Complement and plasma protein behaviour. *Biomater
Artif Cells Immobil Biotechnol* 1991; **19**:283–296.

39 **Kappos L, the European Study Group on Interferon
beta-1b in secondary-progressive MS.** Placebo-
controlled multicentre randomised trial of interferon
beta-1b in treatment of secondary progressive multiple
sclerosis. *Lancet* 1998; **352**:1491–1497.

25
Mitoxantrone

Hans-Peter Hartung, Richard Gonsette, Sean Morrissey, Hilmar Krapf and Franz Fazekas

INTRODUCTION

Mitoxantrone (1,4-dihydroxy-5,8-bis(((2-hydroxyethyl-amino)-ethyl)-amino)9,10-anthracenedione hydrochloride) is a synthetic anti-neoplastic agent with a molecular weight of 517 Da (*Fig. 25.1*). It was first discovered in 1978 and it has proven efficacy in the treatment of advanced breast cancer, non-Hodgkin's lymphoma, acute lymphoblastic leukaemia, chronic myeloid leukaemia and liver and ovarian carcinomas.[1–5] Soon after its introduction as a cytotoxic agent in cancer chemotherapy, it was found to be immunosuppressive. Wang and colleagues[6,7] showed that in vitro alloreactivity was almost completely abrogated by mitoxantrone, which appeared to affect the induction rather than the effector phase of the immune response. Furthermore, these investigators demonstrated that the drug interferes only with those lymphocytes that are capable of proliferating in response to newly presented antigens; it does not affect precursor populations. These effects were remarkably long-lasting. This prompted evaluation of the drug in experimental transplantation. It was found that mitoxantrone markedly prolonged the survival of heterotopic cardiac transplants.[8] This evidence stimulated several groups of neuroimmunologists to examine whether mitoxantrone could modulate the course of experimental autoimmune encephalomyelitis and indeed the drug was shown to suppress both actively induced experimental allergic encephalomyelitis (EAE) and T-cell transfer EAE in mice and guinea pigs.[9–12] At the same time, the crucial role of macrophages in causing myelin damage in EAE was proven, and in this context it was of great importance that Watson and colleagues,[13] in 1991, were able to demonstrate the blocking effect of mitoxantrone on in vitro myelin breakdown by macrophages retrieved from mice with EAE.

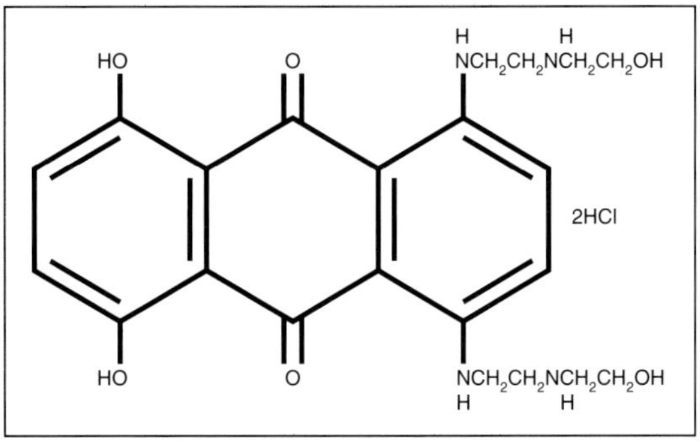

Fig. 25.1 Structure of mitoxantrone.

MECHANISMS OF ACTION

Cytotoxic actions

Mitoxantrone achieves its cytotoxicity by arresting the cell cycle at the G2–M and S interphase. It has been shown to induce DNA protein cross-links and protein-concealed single- and double-strand breaks in DNA as well as non-protein-associated strand breaks.[1,14] Further research has revealed that one molecular target of mitoxantrone is the enzyme DNA topoisomerase II, which is essential for efficient condensation–decondensation of chromatin and for the segregation of replicated daughter chromosomes at cell division. Topoisomerase II changes the topology of DNA strands by introducing transient, double-strand breaks through which an intact helix can pass. Topoisomerase II engages in a non-covalent protein–DNA complex that equilibrates with a so-called covalent-cleavable complex.[15,16] The cleavable complex formed between DNA and topoisomerase II is stabilized by mitoxantrone, which thereby prevents religation of transient double-stranded DNA.[15,17] In addition, mitoxantrone may induce aggregation and compaction of DNA by electrostatic cross-binding.[18]

Mitoxantrone has also been shown to evoke generation and release of highly reactive oxygen species to induce non-protein-associated DNA strand breaks.[3,19] There is evidence to suggest that metabolic oxidation of mitoxantrone to reactive 1,4-quinone and 5,8-di-iminequinone intermediates may be an important mechanism of activation of this agent and a prerequisite for its covalent binding to DNA.[18,20,21] This oxidation may take place in vivo through the action of nitrogen dioxide radicals.[20] Once cells are arrested in the G2 phase of the cell cycle, they may enter cell death pathways. As the under-standing of apoptosis (a physiological process to eliminate cells) grew, several investigators set out to study whether induction of apoptosis may be one of the mechanisms of the therapeutic action of mitoxantrone. Mitoxantrone was shown to induce programmed cell death of certain leukaemia cells.[22,23] This evidence was corroborated by the demonstration that natural resistance of acute myeloid leukaemia cells is associated with a lack of apoptosis.[24]

Immunosuppressive and immunomodulatory actions

In alloreactive mixed lymphocyte cultures, the proliferative response of lymphocytes to antigen is curtailed in the presence of mitoxantrone, and this drug also abolishes the generation of cytotoxic T cells.[6,7] T-helper cell activity was noted to be diminished, whereas T-suppressor cell function was enhanced.[25] Furthermore, mitoxantrone profoundly inhibits B lymphocyte function and antibody secretion.[26] Finally, as mentioned above, mitoxantrone inhibits macrophage-mediated myelin degradation ex vivo.[13] In an open trial of mitoxantrone in MS, Gonsette[27] followed patients' lymphocyte subsets for 3 years and noted a predilective immunosuppressive effect of mitoxantrone on CD4+ lymphocytes and a reduction of the number of B lymphocytes and HLA-DR2+ and IL-2R+ cells by approximately 60% on average. This reduction of the number of B cells and the decreased CD4+:CD8+ ratio was maintained for the whole duration of mitoxantrone therapy.[27] Similar effects have been observed by others.[28] Taken together, all pathogenetically relevant cell populations involved in the induction and effector phase of immune-mediated demyelination appear to be targets for the action of mitoxantrone (*Table 25.1*).

PHARMACOKINETICS

Pharmocokinetic studies have shown that mitoxantrone undergoes triphasic elimination with half-lives of 6–12 minutes, 1.1–3.1 hours and 23–215 hours.[2] Mitoxantrone can be identified in high concentration in autopsy tissues obtained more that 1 month after administration.[29] These pharmacokinetic data provide a rational basis for an intermittent dosing schedule. Seventy-eight percent of the drug is bound to plasma proteins, and the relationship between dose and area under the curve is linear. Clearance of mitoxantrone is reduced in patients with marked liver dysfunction.

CLINICAL TRIALS: SINGLE-ARM STUDIES

In 1987, Gonsette[27] designed a preliminary pilot trial in patients with relapsing–progressive multiple sclerosis (MS) in an active stage to evaluate safety and tolerability of mitoxantrone and determine its impact on circulating lymphocyte subsets. Mitoxantrone was administered by intravenous infusion at a concentration of $14\,mg/m^2$ every 3 weeks until lymphopenia of $\leq 10^3\,cells/ml$ was reached. Doses were adjusted according to the haematologic changes that were induced. In most of the patients, this occurred after three or four infusions. In a follow-up 18 patients over 1 year, it was observed that mitoxantrone was as active as cyclophosphamide in precipitating a marked and sustained lymphopenia and that it had a particularly profound effect on B cells and HLA-DR+ cells. Mitoxantrone therapy was better tolerated than cyclophosphamide. In a subsequent phase 2 trial, Gonsette[27] studied tolerability and the effects on disease activity of a regime that included an induction phase ($14\,mg/m^2$ administered at 3-week intervals) followed by maintained immunosuppression ($14\,mg/m^2$ every 3 months) for 2 years in 20 patients with relapsing–progressive active MS. In this patient population, only 20% progressed by at least 1.0 point on the expanded disability status scale (EDSS) and the mean annual relapse rate was reduced from 1.2 to 0.16. Side effects were acceptable. Importantly, there was no marked alopecia, but amenorrhoea was observed in 15% of the female patients.

Noseworthy and colleagues[30] treated 13 patients with progressive MS with mitoxantrone in an open trial. Patients received seven infusions of $8\,mg/m^2$ mitoxantrone every 3 weeks with dosage adjustments depending on their haematologic profile at the nadir. Treatment was generally well tolerated with the most common side effect being mild nausea. It was noted that four of seven women developed transient secondary amenorrhoea. Only three of 13 patients

Table 25.1 Immunosuppressive and immunomodulatory effects of mitoxantrone

Immunosuppressive effects on:
  CD4+ T cells
  B cells
  Macrophages
Immunomodulatory effects:
  Restores impaired suppressor cell function
Abrogates:
  Experimental autoimmune encephalomyelitis and experimental adjuvant arthritis
  Experimental cardiac transplant rejection

developed an increase in EDSS of more than 0.5 points. A comparison with two historical control groups from the Canadian Cooperative Trial of Cyclophosphamide and Plasma Exchange[31] did not suggest that mitoxantrone was efficacious. These results discouraged the investigators from proceeding with a randomized controlled trial, particularly since eight of 12 patients had evidence of activity on 13 of 29 follow-up magnetic resonance imaging (MRI) scans. An overview of single-arm trials is provided in *Table 25.2*.

CLINICAL TRIALS: RANDOMIZED CONTROLLED STUDIES

The first double-blind, placebo-controlled trial was conducted by the Italian mitoxantrone study group.[32] In this multicentre trial, 51 relapsing–remitting MS patients were enrolled to determine the clinical efficacy of mitoxantrone treatment over a period of 2 years. Patients were

allocated either to receive mitoxantrone (8 mg/m² monthly for 1 year (n = 27)) or placebo (n = 24) (*Tables 25.3, 25.4 and 25.5*).

EDSS was recorded by blinded examiners at baseline and at months 12 and 24. In addition, the number and the severity of relapses over the 24-month trial period were determined. The mean number of relapses was statistically significantly different between the mitoxantrone and placebo group during both the first year and the second year, with a reduction by approximately 70% in the mitoxantrone group. The proportion of patients with a 1.0 point increase on the EDSS was significantly reduced at month 24 in patients who had received mitoxantrone, although mean EDSS progression was no different between treatment arms (*Table 25.6*). The majority of side effects that were noted were considered to be mild (*Table 25.7*).

Forty-two of 51 patients (mitoxantrone n = 23; placebo n = 19) were examined by MRI at 0, 12 and 24 months using a 0.2T MR unit

Table 25.2 Single-arm studies in MS

Author	*Number of patients*	*Type of MS*	*Dose*
Gonsette and Demonty 1990[33]	16	relapsing–remitting	14 mg/m² every 3 weeks
	6	progressive	
Kappos et al 1990[34]	14	rapidly progressive	10 mg/m² every 3 weeks
Mauch et al 1992[35]	6	relapsing–remitting	12 mg/m² every 3 weeks
	4	progressive	
Noseworthy et al 1993[30]	13	progressive	8 mg/m² every 3 weeks
Ruggero 1993[36]	14	secondary progressive	6–10 mg/m² every 3 months
Reess et al 1998[37]	52	relapsing–remitting	12 mg/m² every 3–4 months
	23	secondary progressive	
Mesaroš et al 1998[38]	7	relapsing–remitting	20 mg monthly
	16	secondary progressive	
Total:	171		

Table 25.3 Study design of the Italian trial of mitoxantrone relapsing–remitting MS[32]

51 patients with relapsing–remitting MS and:

    disease history of 1–10 years

    EDSS of 2–5

    ≥ 2 exacerbations in previous 2 years

Stratification based on age, sex and EDSS

Mitoxantrone 8 mg/m² monthly for 12 months

    (27 patients)

Placebo monthly for 12 months (24 patients)

Evaluator blinded to study drug

with analysis of the MRI data performed by two masked neuroradiologists. There was a trend noticeable towards a reduction in the number of new lesions on T2-weighted images in the mitoxantrone group.

In a multicentre, open, randomized trial, the French and British Mitoxantrone Study Group assessed the efficacy of mitoxantrone on the development of inflammatory lesions by monthly MRI with gadolinium enhancement over a period of 6 months.[39] The target population were patients with very active severe disease (*Table 25.8*). During a 2-month baseline period, gadolinium-enhanced T1-weighted MRI scans were performed each month. After each scan, 1 g methylprednisolone was administered intravenously. Only patients who developed at least one gadolinium-enhancing MRI lesion during a 2-month baseline period were randomized to receive either 20 mg intravenous mitoxantrone each month plus 1 g intravenous methylprednisolone each month or only 1 g intravenous methylprednisolone each month. Clinical inclusion criteria were:

(a) age between 18 and 55 years;

(b) disease duration of less than 10 years;

(c) severe MS (i.e. immediate risk of having a major handicap such as loss of ambulation or loss of use of the upper limbs for writing, eating or dressing, or loss of vision);

(d) at least two relapses within the previous 12 months or progression by at least 2.0 points on the EDSS during this period, and

(e) EDSS ≥6.

The primary outcome criterion was the proportion of patients who developed new enhancing lesions on monthly gadolinium-enhanced

Table 25.4 Baseline characteristics of patients in the Italian mitoxantrone trial[32]

	Mitoxantrone	Placebo
Number of patients (male/female)	10/17	6/18
Mean age (years)	30.9	28.7
Mean age at onset (years)	23.7	24.3
Mean disease duration (years)	5.7	5.3
EDSS score		
mean	3.6	3.5
range	2–5	2–5
median	3.5	3.5
Mean number of exacerbations in the previous 2 years	2.8	2.8

Table 25.5 Efficacy assessment and safety monitoring in the Italian mitoxantrone trial[32]

Clinical parameters

    EDSS, exacerbation, medications

    Blinded neurologists

MRI parameters

    T2-weighted lesions at 0, 12 and 24 months

      (all patients)

    Gadolinium-enhanced lesions at 0, 2, 4, 6 and

      12 months (25 patients)

    Two reviewers blinded to study drug

Cardiac safety parameters

    ECG monthly

    Echocardiogram at 0, 6 and 12 months

Table 25.6 Summary of outcome measures in the Italian mitoxantrone trial[32]

Patients (%) with EDSS progression by $\geq$ 1 point

	Mitoxantrone	Placebo	p
Year 1	7	25	0.08
Year 2	0	25	0.01
Total	7	37	0.02

Patients (%) who were free of exacerbations over 2 years

Mitoxantrone	Placebo	p
63	21	0.006

Mean number of exacerbations over 2 years

Mitoxantrone	Placebo	p
0.89	2.62	0.0002

T1-weighted images. Secondary criteria included the mean number of new enhancing lesions per month and per patient and EDSS as determined at monthly visits. *Figure 25.2* depicts the study outline and *Fig. 25.3* depicts patient disposition in this trial. It is evident that a patient population with highly active disease was indeed enrolled (see *Table 25.8*). It is of note that the patients had had frequent exacerbations in the 12 months before entry.

Table 25.7 Adverse events recorded in the Italian mitoxantrone trial[32]

	Number of patients (%) with adverse events			
Adverse event	*Total*	*Mild*	*Moderate*	*Severe*
Nausea and/or vomiting	9 (18)	7 (14)	2 (4)	0 (0)
Upper respiratory tract infection	2 (4)	1 (2)	1 (2)	0 (0)
Urinary tract infection	3 (6)	1 (2)	2 (4)	0 (0)
Headache	3 (6)	3 (6)	0 (0)	0 (0)
Diarrhoea	1 (2)	0 (0)	1 (2)	0 (0)
Cardiac events	0 (0)	0 (0)	0 (0)	0 (0)
Alopecia	0 (0)	0 (0)	0 (0)	0 (0)
Haematological events	0 (0	0 (0)	0 (0)	0 (0)
Amenorrhoea	5/35*			
Total number of patients:	51(100%)			

* 5 of 35 female patients (14%)

Table 25.8 Baseline characteristics of patients in the French–British mitoxantrone trial[39]

	Mitoxantrone + methylprednisolone	*Methylprednisolone only*
Number of patients (male/female)	6/15	10/11
Mean age (years)	31.4	32.2
Mean duration disease (years)	6.9	5.7
Mean EDSS at month 2	4.4	4.7
Number of exacerbations in the previous 12 months	3.1	2.4

At baseline, the percentage of patients without new enhancing lesions was 10% in the mitoxantrone and 4.8% in the methylprednisolone group. Between months 2 and 6 of the treatment in the mitoxantrone group, this percentage progressively increased to 9.5% (*Tables 25.9 and 25.10*). The difference was highly significant after 6 months. *Figure 25.4* depicts the mean number of new gadolinium-enhancing lesions per scan over the 6-month period. Differences at months 2, 3 and 5 were also significant and in favour of mitoxantrone. Regarding secondary clinical end-

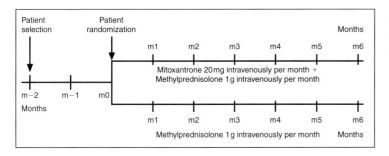

Fig. 25.2 *Trial design of the French–British mitoxantrone trial* [39].

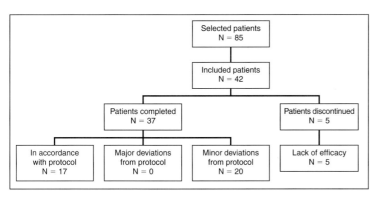

Fig. 25.3 *Patient disposition in the French–British mitoxantrone trial* [39].

Table 25.9 Primary outcome measure (enhancing lesions on MRI) in the French–British mitoxantrone trial[39]

	Mitoxantrone + methylprednisolone (n = 21)	*Methylprednisolone only (n = 21)*	p
Patients (%) without new enhancing lesions at 6 months	90.5	30.3	< 0.001
Mean number of new enhancing lesions at 6 months	0.1	2.9	< 0.001
Mean total number of enhancing lesions at 6 months	1.4	3.1	< 0.001

Table 25.10 MRI efficacy parameters in the French–British mitoxantrone trial[39]

	Mitoxantrone + methylprednisolone	*Methylprednisolone only*	p
Total period (2 yrs)			
Number of new lesions			
mean	3.5	7.3	0.05
median	2	5	
Number of enlarging lesions			
mean	4.3	4.3	NS
median	3	3	

NS, not significant

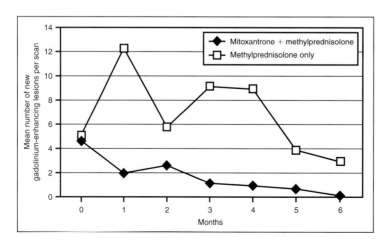

Fig. 25.4 Primary outcome measure (number of new gadolinium-enhancing lesions on MRI scan). Modified from Edan et al, 1998.[39]

points, there was a marked and statistically significant effect in terms of disease progression (*Table 25.11*), and the majority of mitoxantrone-treated patients scored at least 1.0 point better on the EDSS at the conclusion of the trial. The change in the EDSS score in the two treatment groups over the 6-month trial period is shown in *Fig. 25.5*.

Twice as many patients on mitoxantrone experienced no relapses during the 6-month trial period as patients receiving methylprednisolone alone. This difference was statistically significant. *Figure 25.6* shows the number of new relapses recorded each month in the two groups studied.

Table 25.12 summarizes adverse events noted in the two treatment groups. Again, secondary amenorrhoea occurred frequently in female patients. Adverse effects were more frequent in the mitoxantrone group than in the methylprednisolone-only group, and most of these adverse effects were expected. None of the enrolled patients developed signs of cardiotoxicity.

Table 25.11 Clinical efficacy parameters in the French–British mitoxantrone trial[39]

	Mitoxantrone + methylprednisolone (n = 21)	Methylprednisolone only (n = 21)	p
Number of patients with Δ ≥ 1.0 point on EDSS by study end			
improved	12	3	
stable	8	12	< 0.01
worse	1	6	
Number of patients who were free of relapse at 6 months	14	7	< 0.05

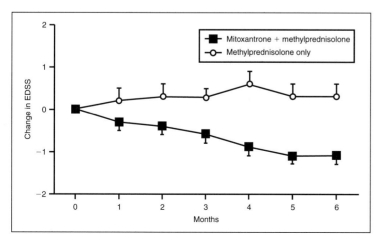

Fig. 25.5 Change in EDSS from baseline in patients in the French–British mitoxantrone trial.[39]

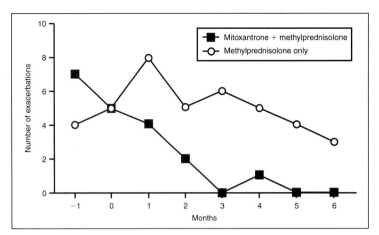

Fig. 25.6 Number of exacerbations in patients in the French–British mitoxantrone trial.[39]

Laboratory abnormalities included raised liver enzymes and creatinine levels. As expected, mitoxantrone induced drops in the white blood cell count. The leukopenia was always a neutropenia. A mild decrease in the platelet count was also noted in some patients, although platelets never fell below 10^5 cells/mm³. Four patients in the mitoxantrone group had a continuous decrease of the erythrocyte count that persisted throughout the study but this was also true for five patients in the methylprednisolone only group.

The authors concluded that their study was specifically targeted to severely affected patients with highly active disease. The trial provided evidence that in this selected group, mitoxantrone was effective in improving both clinical and MRI parameters of disease activity over a 6-month period and that methylprednisolone alone was not. There was no event to generate

Table 25.12 Adverse events recorded in the French–British mitoxantrone trial[39]

	Number of patients with adverse events	
Adverse event	**Mitoxantrone + methylprednisolone**	**Methylprednisolone only**
Amenorrhoea	8	0
Alopecia	7	0
Nausea and/or vomiting	1	0
Other gastrointestinal event	6	1
Asthenia	5	0
Upper respiratory tract infection	5	2
Urinary tract infection	5	1
Neurological event unrelated to MS	3	0
Anaemia	4	1
Cardiac event	0	0

major safety concerns. The authors surmised that the rapid action of mitoxantrone may render this drug suitable as rescue therapy or for initiation of immunosuppression when an abrupt containment of the inflammatory process of MS is desirable.

THE EUROPEAN MITOXANTRONE IN MULTIPLE SCLEROSIS (MIMS) TRIAL

In 1992, a group of neurologists from Germany, Belgium, Hungary and Poland rallied to initiate a large double-blind, randomized, placebo-controlled, phase 3 trial[40] in patients in an active stage of MS using a three-group parallel design of $12\,mg/m^2$ or $5\,mg/m^2$ of mitoxantrone or placebo every 3 months for a period of 2 years. Inclusion criteria were:

(a) patients with clinically or laboratory-supported definite MS of the relapsing–progressive or secondary progressive form in an active stage of the disease with evidence of deterioration (e.g. deterioration of at least 1.0 point on the EDSS in the 18 months before entry);

(b) EDSS between 3 and 6; and

(c) age between 18 and 55 years.

Patients who had been treated with immunosuppressant agents in the preceding 9 months, patients with cardiac risk factors (history of congestive heart failure or myocardial infarction or with reduced left ventricular ejection fraction), patients who had received corticosteroids in the preceding 8 weeks, and patients with an attack in the 8 weeks before entry were excluded.

Patients who were blinded to the treatment received the study drug every 3 months from month 0 to month 21. Methylene blue was used as placebo to match the blue color of the mitox-

antrone infusion. The EDSS rater was blinded, whereas a treating physician who was in charge of overall medical care was not blinded. Sixty-three patients were randomized to receive mitoxantrone $12\,mg/m^2$, 66 to receive mitoxantrone $5\,mg/m^2$ and 65 to receive placebo. For intention-to-treat analysis 60, 64 and 64 patients respectively were available at the conclusion of the trial. Primary outcome criteria were clinical; they included an assessment of the change in EDSS from baseline, the change in ambulation index from baseline, the number of relapses requiring corticosteroid therapy and the time to first relapse requiring corticosteroid therapy. Secondary outcome criteria were the percentage of patients that experienced confirmed EDSS deterioration by at least 1.0 point at 3 months, the percentage of patients without relapses that required treatment, the mean number of relapses and the time to first relapse. In a subgroup of 110 patients, annual MRI examinations were carried out at months 0, 12 and 24. MRI scans were done on 0.5 Tesla or 1.0 Tesla units. Conventional double-spin echoes and T1-weighted scans after administration of 0.1 mmol/kg gadolinium were applied. Lesions were determined by two experienced neuroradiologists who were masked as to the allocation of the patients to the treatment groups. Assessment was done independently during one session.[41]

Randomization was successful in that there were no significant differences in baseline characteristics between the three treatment arms. Mean duration of the disease was close to 10 years, mean EDSS between 4.4 and 4.7, and patients had deteriorated on EDSS by 1.5–1.6 points and had experienced between 1.2 and 1.42 relapses in the 12 months before entry.

At this time, the full data have not been published. Overall, all primary outcome criteria and most of the secondary criteria were met. Mitoxantrone 12 mg/m^2 was significantly more efficacious than placebo. By and large, medication was well tolerated. As expected, nausea and alopecia occurred more frequently in the mitoxantrone group. Amenorrhoea was observed in close to 20% of mitoxantrone-treated female patients and leukopenia was recorded in 9–19% of mitoxantrone-treated patients. Particular attention was paid to adverse cardiac events because of the known cardiotoxicity of the drug.[42] All patients had ECG and echocardiography before and during the trial. In 19 patients on mitoxantrone and nine on placebo, left ventricular ejection fraction decreased by ≥10%, but none of the patients had clinical evidence of a cardiomyopathy.

therapy in rapidly progressing patients with highly active disease, with the aim of stabilizing them and then switching to other established immunomodulatory therapy. Alternatively, patients who deteriorate on established immunomodulatory therapy may receive benefit from mitoxantrone, and it is conceivable that after a defined treatment interval they may be responsive again to other forms of immunotherapy. The exact place of mitoxantrone in the management of MS needs to be determined. Currently, plans are being made to examine mitoxantrone in combination or in sequence with interferon-β.

Mitoxantrone has certainly enlarged our armamentarium for the treatment of this crippling disease.

CONCLUSIONS

This chapter has reviewed evidence that has emerged over the past decade to indicate that mitoxantrone is effective in the treatment of active relapsing–progressive and secondary progressive MS. Mitoxantrone is the second drug that has been shown to be efficacious in secondary progressive MS. It is well tolerated but one has to keep in mind that the duration of treatment is limited by cumulative cardiotoxicity. Due to limited experience, the risk of cardiac toxicity in patients with multiple sclerosis is difficult to estimate accurately. In cancer patients, the probability of developing congestive heart failure is about 3% for mitoxantrone cumulative doses up to 100 mg/m^2 and about 5% for doses between 140 and 160 mg/m^2 in the absence of prior cardiac risk factors.[5,42,43] Asymptomatic decrease in the left ventricular ejection fraction may occur at lower dose. Hence, cardiac monitoring is recommended.

Mitoxantrone may be considered as rescue

REFERENCES

1 **Alberts DS, Peng YM, Bowden GT et al.** Pharmacology of mitoxantrone: mode of action and pharmacokinetics. *Invest New Drugs* 1985; 3:101–107.

2 **Faulds D, Balfour JA, Chrisp P, Langtry HD.** Mitoxantrone: a review of its pharmacodynamic and pharmacokinetic properties, and therapeutic potential in the chemotherapy of cancer. *Drugs* 1991; 41:400–499.

3 **Lenk H, Müller U, Tanneberger S.** Mitoxantrone: mechanisms of action, antitumor activity, pharmacokinetics, efficacy in the treatment of solid tumors and lymphomas, and toxicity. *Anticancer Res* 1987; 7:1257–1264.

4 **Koeller J, Eble M.** Mitoxantrone: a novel anthracycline derivative. *Clin Pharm* 1998; 7:574–581.

5 **Shenkenberg TD, Von Hoff D.** Mitoxantrone: a new anticancer drug with significant clinical activity. *Ann Intern Med* 1986; 105:67–81.

6 **Wang BS, Murdock KC, Lumanglas AL et al.** Relationship of chemical structures of anthraquinones with their effects on the suppression of immune responses. *Int J Immunopharmacol* 1987; 9:733–739.

7 **Wang BS, Lumanglas AL, Ruszala-Mallon VM et al.** Induction of alloreactive immunosuppression by 1,4-bis [(2-aminoethyl)amino]-5,8-dihydroxy-9,10-

anthracenedione dihydrochloride (CL 232,468). *Int J Immunopharmacol* 1984; **6**:475–482.

8 Schneider T, Kupiec-Weglinski JW, Towpik E et al. Mitoxantrone: an immunosuppressive agent potentially useful in the organ transplantation (abstract). *Fedn Proc Am Socs Exp Biol* 1985; **44**:1681.

9 Bisteau M, Devos G, Brucher JM, Gonsette RE. Prevention of subacute experimental allergic encephalomyelitis in Guinea-pigs with desferrioxamine, isoprinosine and mitoxantrone. In: Gonsette RE, Delmotte P, eds. *Recent Advances in Multiple Sclerosis Therapy*. International Congress Series 863. Elsevier Science Publishers, 1989, 299–300.

10 Levine S, Saltzman A. Regional suppression therapy after onset and prevention of relspses in experimental allergic encephalomyelitis by mitoxantrone. *J Neuroimmunol* 1986; **13**:175–181.

11 Lublin FD, Lavasa M, Viti C, Knobler RL. Suppression of acute and relapsing experimental allergic encephalomyelitis with mitoxantrone. *Clin Immunol Immunopathol* 1987; **45**:122–128.

12 Ridge SC, Sloboda AE, McReynolds RA et al. Suppression of experimental allergic encephalomyelitis by mitoxantrone. *Clin Immunol Immunopathol* 1985; **35**:35–42.

13 Watson CM, Davison AN, Baker D et al. Suppression of demyelination by mitoxantrone. *Int J Immunopharmacol* 1991; **13**:923–930.

14 Bowden GT, Roberts R, Alberts DS et al. Comparative molecular pharmacology in leukemic L 1210 cells of the anthracene anticancer drugs mitoxantrone and bisantrene. *Cancer Res* 1985; **45**:4915–4920.

15 Holden JA. Human deoxyribonucleic acid topoisomerases: molecular targets of anticancer drugs. *Ann Clin Lab Sci* 1997; **27**:402–412.

16 Smith PJ, Blunt NJ, Desnoyers R et al. DNA topoisomerase II-dependent cytoxicity of alkylaminoanthraquinones and their N-oxides. *Cancer Chemother Pharmacol* 1997; **39**:455–461.

17 Fox ME, Smith PJ. Long-term inhibition of DNA synthesis and persistence of trapped topoisomerase II complexes in determining the toxicity of the antitumor DNAN intercalators mAMSA and mitoxantrone. *Cancer* 1990; **50**:5813–5818.

18 Fisher GR, Patterson LH. DNA strand breakage by peroxidase-activated mitoxantrone. *J Pharm Pharmacol* 1990; **43**:65–68.

19 Basra J, Wolf CR, Brown JR, Patterson LH. Evidence

for human liver mediated free-radical formation by doxorubicin and mitoxantrone. *Anticancer Drug Des* 1985; **1**:45–52.

20 Reszka KJ, Matuszak Z, Chignell CF. Lactoperoxidase-catalyzed oxidation of the anticancer agent mitoxantrone by nitrogen dioxide ($NO_2^{\bullet}$) radicals. *Chem Res Toxicol* 1997; **10**:1325–1330.

21 Panousis C, Kettle AJ, Phillips DR. Neutrophil-mediated activation of mitoxantrone to metabolites which form adducts with DNA. *Cancer Lett* 1997; **113**:173–178.

22 Bhalla K, Ibrado AM, Tourkina E et al. High-dose mitoxantrone induces programmed cell death or apoptosis in human myeloid leukemia cells. *Blood* 1993; **82**:3133–3140.

23 Bellosillo B, Colomer D, Pons G, Gil J. Mitoxantrone, a topoisomerase II inhibitor, induces apoptosis of B-chronic lymphocytic leukaemia cells. *Br J Haematol* 1998; **100**:142–146.

24 Bailly JD, Skladanowski A, Bettaieb A et al. Natural resistance of acute myeloid leukemia cell lines to mitoxantrone is associated with lack of apoptosis. *Leukemia* 1997; **11**:1523–1532.

25 Fidler JM, Quinn DeJoy S, Gibbons JJ Jr. Selective immunomodulation by the antineoplastic agent mitoxantrone. I. Suppression of B lymphocate function. *J Immunol* 1986; **137**:727–732.

26 Fidler JM, Quinn DeJoy S, Smith FR, Gibbons JJ Jr. Selective immunomodulation by the antineoplastic agent mitoxantrone. II. Nonspecific adherent suppressor cells derived from mitoxantrone-treated mice. *J Immunol* 1986; **136**:2747–2754.

27 Gonsette RE. Mitoxantrone immunotherapy in multiple sclerosis. *Multiple Sclerosis* 1996; **1**: 329–332.

28 Zaffaroni M, Ghezzi A, Baldini SM, Zibetti A. Effetti immunosuppressori del mitoxantrone nella sclerosi multipla cronica-progressiva. In: Ghezzi A, Zaffaroni M, Zibetti A et al, eds. *La ricerca sulla sclerosi multipla in Italia: confronto di esperienze*. Salerno: Momento Medico, 1995: 112–114.

29 Stewart DJ, Green RM, Mikhael NZ et al. Human autopsy tissue concentrations of mitoxantrone. *Cancer Treat Rep* 1986; **70**:1255–1261.

30 Noseworthy JH, Hopkins MB, Vandervoort MK et al. An open-trial evaluation of mitoxantrone in the treatment of progressive MS. *Neurology* 1993; **43**:1401–1406.

31 Noseworthy JH, Ebers GC, Gent M et al. The Canadian Cooperative trial of cyclophosphamide and

plasma exchange in progressive multiple sclerosis. *Lancet* 1991; 337:441–446.

32 Millefiorini E, Gasperini C, Pozzilli C et al. Randomised placebo-controlled trial of mitoxantrone in relapsing-remitting multiple sclerosis: a 24–month clinical and MRI outcome. *J Neurol* 1997; 244:153–159.

33 Gonsette RE, Demonty L. Immunosuppression with mitoxantrone in multiple sclerosis: a pilot study for 2 years in 22 patients. *Neurology* 1990; 40(suppl 1): 262.

34 Kappos L, Gold R, Künstler E et al. Mitoxantrone in the treatment of rapidly progressive MS: a pilot study with serial gadolinium-enhanced MRI. *Neurology* 1990; 40(suppl 1):261.

35 Mauch E, Kornhuber HH, Krapf H et al. Treatment of multiple sclerosis with mitoxantrone. *Eur Arch Psych Clin Neurosci* 1992; 242:96–102.

36 Ruggero C, Marciano N. Mitoxantrone therapy of secondary progressive multiple sclerosis: pilot study. *Neurology* 1993; 43(Suppl 2):A281.

37 Reess J, Eisenmann S, Mauch E. Results of an open study with 75 MS-patients treated with mitoxantrone. *Multiple Sclerosis* 1998; 4:382.

38 Mesaroš Š, Lević Z, Drulović J et al. Treatment of multiple sclerosis with mitoxantrone. *Multiple Sclerosis* 1998; 4:387.

39 Edan G, Miller D, Clanet M et al. Therapeutic effect of mitoxantrone conbined with methylprednisolone in multiple sclerosis: a randomised multicentre study of active disease using MRI and clinical criteria. *J Neurol Neurosurg Psychiatry* 1997; 62:112–118.

40 Hartung HP, Gonsette R, and the MIMS Study Group. Mitoxantrone in progressive multiple sclerosis: a plcebo-controlled, randomised, observer-blind phase III trial: clinical results and three-year follow-up. *Neurology* 1999; 52(suppl 2):A290.

41 Krapf H, Morrissey SP, Zenker O et al. the MIMS Study Group. Mitoxantrone in progressive multiple sclerosis: MRI results of the European phase III trial. *Neurology* 1999; 52(suppl 2):A495.

42 De Castro S, Cartoni D, Millefiorini E et al. Noninvasive assessment of mitoxantrone cardiotoxicity in relapsing remitting multiple sclerosis. *J Clin Pharmacol* 1995; 35:627–632.

43 Dukart G, Barone JS. An overview of cardiac episodes following mitoxantrone administration. *Cancer Treat Symp* 1984; 3:35–41.

26
Methylprednisolone

R Philip Kinkel

INTRODUCTION

Treatment of multiple sclerosis (MS) with pulses of high dose methylprednisolone (HDMP) has gained increased acceptance over the past two decades and has supplanted adrenocorticotrophic hormone (ACTH) as the treatment of choice for MS relapses. More recent evidence suggests that HDMP not only hastens recovery from MS relapses but may modify the course of relapsing–remitting MS (RRMS) as well as secondary progressive MS (SPMS). This chapter reviews the evidence supporting the use of HDMP for these indications. For a comprehensive review of clinical trials pertaining to the use of ACTH or other preparations of glucocorticosteroids (GSC) in MS, the reader is referred to Dr LW Myers' review.[1]

BACKGROUND

Pharmacology

Methylprednisolone (MP) is a synthetic GCS that differs from hydrocortisone (cortisol) by the addition of a double bond at the 1,2 position and a methyl group at the 6 position.[2] These structural differences increase the relative glucocorti-coid effect, decrease the mineralocorticoid effect, and increase the duration of action (*Table 26.1*). The biologically active sterol is highly insoluble in aqueous solutions and must be administered intravenously as a sodium hemisuccinate ester. Following intravenous administration, 10% of the ester is excreted unchanged in the urine before it can be converted to the biologically active sterol compound. At normal or low concentrations, 80–90% of GCS are bound to corticosteroid-binding globulin (CBG), a protein with high affinity but low capacity for binding GCS. A smaller percentage of GCS binds to albumin, which displays a higher binding capacity but lower affinity. At the high concentrations achieved with HDMP, the protein-binding capacity in serum is exceeded and a greater proportion of serum GCS exists in a free state. This is of relevance for two reasons. First, only the unbound fraction of GCS is able to enter cells and interact with specific receptors. Secondly, rapid penetration of the central nervous system (CNS) requires high doses of GCS, since the blood–brain barrier (BBB) is relatively impermeable to bound GCS.[3] Presumably for this reason, peak levels in the cerebrospinal fluid (CSF) are delayed for over 6 hours after a 1500 mg bolus of HDMP, whereas peak levels in the plasma occur within 2 hours.[4] Since the mean plasma residence time is less than

Table 26.1 Relative potency and biological activity of glucocorticosteroids

Preparation	Glucocorticoid activity	Mineralocorticoid activity	Duration of action	Equivalent strength (mg)
Cortisone	0.8	0.8	Short	25
Cortisol	1	1	Short	20
Prednisone	4	0.8	Intermediate	5
Prednisolone	4	0.8	Intermediate	5
Methylprednisolone	5	0.5	Intermediate	4
Dexamethasone	25	0	Long	0.75

4 hours after a 1000 mg intravenous bolus of MP, high CSF concentrations persist at a time when serum concentrations are negligible.[5,6]

In addition to intravenous formulations, oral preparations of MP as the parent sterol compound are available up to a maximum strength of 32 mg. Although they are well absorbed, the relatively small size of the tablet formulation renders oral administration of high doses (500–2000 mg/day) impractical. As an alternative to oral megadose administration, recent studies suggest that the intravenous solution may be taken orally, since oral doses up to 1000 mg per day are well absorbed and well tolerated.[5] Concerns about a potential increase in gastrointestinal side effects with oral HDMP appear to be unfounded, since oral administration does not increase gastrointestinal permeability or the incidence of endoscopically identified lesions in the gastric mucosa compared to intravenous administration.[7,8] Further studies of the tolerability, efficacy, and pharmacokinetics of HDMP pulses administered orally are required before this route is established as an alternative to intravenous administration.

Molecular biology

Unbound MP freely diffuses across plasma membranes and exerts its effects through interaction with widely distributed intracellular glucocorticoid receptors. The glucocorticoid receptor consists of a DNA-binding domain, a steroid-binding domain, and an immunogenic domain.[9] In the steroid-free state, the receptor exists as an oligomer complexed to heat-shock protein (HSP)-90, which facilitates its interaction with glucocorticoids and immunophilin (IP).[10] Binding of the sterol to the receptor complex causes dissociation from HSP and IP and allows the steroid-receptor complex to translocate into the nucleus, where it binds to glucocorticoid responsive elements (GRE) on the 5'-flanking region of certain genes.[11] This may lead to an enhancement of transcription in certain instances (e.g. during glucose metabolism) or to inhibition of transcription in the case of many anti-inflammatory effects.[12] GCS also regulate RNA processing, RNA transport, RNA translation, and protein secretion.[11]

An important inhibitory effect on inflammation is mediated through direct interaction of the steroid-receptor complex with the activator protein (AP)-1 complex.[13] The AP-1 complex is activated by pro-inflammatory stimuli, and it enhances the transcription of many genes involved in the inflammatory response. Inter-action with the steroid-receptor complex results in inactivation of AP-1, and this in turn inhibits transcription of pro-inflammatory growth factors and cytokines.

Mechanisms of action

GCS have many biologic effects of potential ther-apeutic benefit in MS. The effects on the immune system result in restoration of the BBB, reduction in tissue edema, suppression of inflammation, and immunomodulation (*Table 26.2*). In very high doses, MP suppresses lipid peroxidation associated with progressive neuronal degenera-tion following spinal cord injury.[40] All of these effects are complex, inter-related, and dose-dependent in ways that are only partly under-stood. No particular biological activity of GCS has been causally linked to the clinical benefits observed in MS patients, in part because of the pleotropic effects of GCS on cell function and survival.

Although GCS, even at low doses, produce significant immunomodulatory and anti-inflammatory effects, short-term or chronic administration of low-dose GCS has not been demonstrated to alter the course of MS signifi-cantly.[1] In contrast, there is accumulating evid-ence to suggest that HDMP administered in 'pulses' may have more profound biologic effects that are favorable to the course of MS with fewer adverse reactions. The next section focuses on neuroimaging studies that suggest that HDMP may have biologic effects that are capable of altering the course of MS and of hastening recov-ery from relapses.

EFFECTS OF HDMP ON DISEASE ACTIVITY MEASURED BY COMPUTED TOMOGRAPHY AND MAGNETIC RESONANCE IMAGING

Shortly after development of computed tomogra-phy (CT) imaging, it became clear that GCS produce a rapid, dose-dependent reduction in contrast enhancement.[41–43] This effect is evident within 8 hours, presumably represents an effect on the BBB, and is associated with rapid clinical improvement. Resolution of contrast enhance-ment raised the possibility that the rapid benefits of GCS therapy were attributable to abrupt reso-lution of edema, followed later by reduction of inflammation. Consistent with this interpretation, intravenous mannitol was found to reduce edema rapidly, although it produced only a transient improvement in MS symptoms. In contrast, GCS reduced CT contrast enhancement and clinical symptoms for up to 4 months.[43,44] Later resumption of clinical symptoms and CT disease activity suggested that GCS therapy had little effect on the long-term course of the disease.[1]

After the application of quantitative magnetic resonance imaging (MRI) techniques in MS patients, increased T1 and T2 relaxation times were noted in normal appearing white matter (NAWM) of MS brains (see Chapter 7). This finding is consistent with the diffuse, microscopic pathological changes described in MS tissue.[45,46] It was subsequently noted that HDMP (0.5 g for 5 days) resulted in a significant reduction in T1 relaxation times in NAWM, despite development of discrete new T2 lesions in nine out of 50 cases

Table 26.2 Potential mechanisms of action of glucocorticosteroids in MS

Effects on cellular immune system function and inflammation

Redistribution of T cells with transient reduction in T cell counts (CD4$^+$ T-cell count > CD8$^+$ T-cell count)[14,15]

Decreased T-cell responses to antigen and mitogen[16]

Decreased synthesis and/or release of pro-inflammatory cytokines and growth factors (IL-1, IL-2, IL-6, IFN-γ, IL-8, TNF-α)[17,18]

Up-regulation of TGF-β and IL-10 expression[17,19–21]

Inhibition of IFN-γ up-regulation of MHC class II expression by macrophages and microglia[22]

Decreased eicosanoid production by monocytes[23]

Decreased Fc receptor expression by macrophages[24]

Decreased immunoglobulin levels 2–4 weeks after treatment[25]

Increased synthesis of lipocortin-1 and reduced transcription of the cyclo-oxygenase-2 gene[26,27]

Effects on endothelial cell function and permeability

Down-regulation of endothelial cell adhesion molecule expression[28]

Reduced activity of matrix metalloproteinase (gelatinase B) and increased activity of tissue inhibitors of metalloproteinases[29]

Effects on cerebrospinal fluid immune compartment

Transient, dose-dependent decrease in T-cell count (CD3$^+$ T cells, CD4$^+$ T cells, and CD8$^+$ T cells)[30,31]

Transient, dose-dependent decrease in IgG and IgM synthesis[16,30,32–36]

Decreased sICAM[37,38]

Decreased TNF-α[39]

Decreased antibodies to myelin basic protein[35]

IL, interleukin; IFN, interferon; TNF, tumor necrosis factor; TGF, transforming growth factor; SICAM, soluble intercellular adhesion molecule.

as early as 10 days after treatment.[47] The investigators hypothesized that symptomatic improvement following HDMP is primarily the result of a reduction in white matter edema and that there is no effect on the underlying disease-specific pathology. Since this study was done without gadolinium administration, another possible explanation is that the new lesions may have been new enhancing lesions at baseline that did not develop a 'T2 footprint' until the follow-up imaging study 10 days after the administration of

HDMP.[48,49] Indeed, it is now recognized that the first visible manifestation of acute perivascular inflammation on MRI is the gadolinium enhancing lesion [50,51] (see Chapter 5).

Studies over the past decade confirm that HDMP produces a rapid reduction in gadolinium enhancement. In early studies that were focused on immediate pre- and post-HDMP treatment,[52–55] there was an 84–96% reduction in gadolinium enhancement within 1–4 days of treatment.[27,28] Other studies found that this effect correlated with clinical improvement.[52,55] Serial gadolinium-enhanced MRI scans done for 1 month after HDMP treatment for acute relapses demonstrated that many lesions re-enhanced within days and new lesions frequently appeared within 1 month despite continued clinical improvement.[54] In an uncontrolled study, the effect of HDMP on gadolinium enhancement persisted for an average of 9.7 weeks.[56]

These studies suggested that HDMP had only transient effects on gadolinium enhancement and inflammation. However, this interpretation may be incorrect. First, the studies did not include sufficient serial observation of MRI lesion activity before treatment with HDMP to determine the effect of treatment on subsequent MRI activity. Secondly, the studies did not include randomized, placebo or dose–response control groups for comparison. Two recent studies that address these methodological concerns suggest that HDMP may have dose-dependent effects on subsequent MRI disease activity. A study by Smith and colleagues[57] included nine patients with RRMS studied with monthly gadolinium-enhanced MRI scans in a natural history study. The investigators noted an increase in the total number of enhancing lesions, new enhancing lesions, and an increase in the total area of enhancement in the month that preceded clinical worsening. Interestingly, HDMP treatment for clinical worsening resulted in a 33% reduction in new lesions over the subsequent 6 months, despite no significant change in the average total number of enhancing lesions per month during the entire study. A second study, by Oliveri and colleagues,[58] was a double-blind, randomized comparison of two doses of intravenous MP (0.5 g for 5 days versus 2.0 g for 5 days) using gadolinium-enhanced MRI obtained at baseline and at 7, 15, 30, and 60 days after the beginning

of treatment as the main outcome measure. Both doses of intravenous MP resulted in early dramatic reduction in the number of enhancing lesions followed by a rebound of enhancing lesions on day 15.[53,54] However, there was a significant dose-dependent reduction in the total number of enhancing lesions and the number of new enhancing lesions beginning 30 days after the start of treatment and persisting for the duration of the study.

These studies suggest that HDMP may have prolonged dose-dependent benefits involving early events in lesion formation or lesion propagation, in addition to more transient beneficial effects on established areas of inflammation and demyelination. These results are particularly interesting in the light of recent studies of NAWM that have revealed that new enhancing lesions arise in areas with decreased magnetization transfer ratios (MTR) in the 3–6 months before the occurrence of a detectable enhancing lesion.[59,60] An effect of HDMP on MTR in NAWM would suggest that HDMP affects events early in lesion formation. Regardless, currently available MRI studies suggest a role of HDMP for relapse management as well as disease modification.

CLINICAL TRIALS OF HDMP FOR MS RELAPSES

The use of GCS as an MS treatment was first reported in 1951.[61] Seven subsequent clinical trials between 1954 and 1979 failed to show a convincing benefit of low to intermediate doses of daily or alternate-day oral GCS, as reviewed by Myers.[1] Although the design of these studies would be considered suboptimal in comparison to current standards, there developed a consensus

Table 26.3 Clinical trials of HDMP versus ACTH for MS relapses

Study	Treatment regimens	Number of subjects	Study design	Comments
Abbruzzese et al, 1983[73]	Intravenous MP 20 mg/kg per day for 3 days, 10 mg/kg per day for 4 days, 5 mg/kg per day for 3 days, 1 mg/kg per day for 5 days	30	Open, randomized	No difference at any time between treatments
	Intravenous ACTH 0.5 mg bd for 15 days	30		
Barnes et al, 1985[74]	Intravenous MP 1 g qd for 7 days	14	Single blind, randomized	MP better at 3, 7, and 28 days but not 3 months after treatment
	Intramuscular ACTH 60 U for 7 days, 40 U for 7 days, 20 U for 7 days	11		
Thompson et al, 1989[75]	Intravenous MP 1 g qd for 3 days	29	Double blind, randomized	No difference at 3, 7, 14, 28 or 90 days after treatment; MP better tolerated
	Intramuscular ACTH 40 U bd for 7 days, 20 U bd for 4 days, 20 U qid for 3 days	32		

that chronic GCS administration in low doses does not prevent disease progression. If not for positive results of the ACTH Cooperative Study,[62] subsequent studies of GCS would probably have been curtailed.

During the 1970s, HDMP pulses were reported to be beneficial in acute allograph rejection,[63] and shortly after this therapeutic benefits of pulse HDMP were reported in lupus nephritis,[64] Goodpasture's syndrome,[65] crescentric glomerulonephritis, [66] polyarteritis nodosa,[67] and rheumatoid arthritis.[68] These reports were followed by several uncontrolled, short, open trials of intravenous HDMP for MS relapses. Rapid improvement was reported in the majority of patients with few adverse effects.[16,69–72]

Because ACTH was considered the standard of treatment for MS relapses until the 1980s, there followed a series of three randomized trials (*Table 26.3*) to assess the relative benefit of intravenous HDMP versus ACTH.[73–75] In these trials, a small number of patients were treated with a single course of HDMP or ACTH and then followed for a brief period of time. Therefore, the studies lack statistical power to detect small but significant differences between treatments, and the trial durations were too short to assess the benefits on the disease course. The most influential of these trials was randomized, placebo-controlled, double-blind comparison of intravenous HDMP for 3 days versus intramuscular ACTH for 14 days.[75] Both treatment groups improved significantly but there were no significant differences between the groups at 3, 7,

Table 26.4 Placebo-controlled trials of HDMP for MS relapses

Study	Treatment regimens	Number of subjects	Study design	Comments
Durelli, 1986[32]	Intravenous MP 15 mg/kg per day for 3 days, 10 mg/kg per day for 3 days, 5 mg/kg per day for 3 days, 2.5 mg/kg per day for 3 days, 1 mg/kg per day for 3 days	12	Double blind, randomized	MP better than placebo at the end of treatment. No further follow-up comparison
	Placebo	8		
Milligan, 1987[76]	Intravenous MP 500 mg per day for 5 days	13	Double blind, randomized	MP better than placebo at 1 and 4 weeks after treatment
	Placebo	9		
Sellebjerg, 1998[77]	Oral MP 500 mg per day for 5 days	26	Double blind, randomized	More MP treated patients improved ≥1.0 EDSS point at 1, 3 and 8 weeks after treatment
	Placebo	25		

14, 28, and 90 days after treatment. The investigators concluded that intravenous HDMP was an effective alternative to ACTH, required a shorter treatment duration, and was better tolerated. This led many clinicians to abandon the use of ACTH for clinical relapses in favor of intravenous HDMP. This practice was supported by three randomized, double-blind placebo-controlled trials of intravenous or oral HDMP for relapses in MS (*Table 26.4*).[32,76,77] Although these studies followed only a small number of patients for only 2–8 weeks, all three studies found a significant benefit of HDMP compared to placebo. A single injection of 1.0 g MP was not found to be beneficial compared to a 5-day regimen in a small randomized trial,[78] leading to

the conclusion that a course of HDMP for 3–5 days is necessary to treat MS relapses effectively.

More recent randomized studies of GCS have focused on the relative benefit of different preparations, doses, and routes of administration (*Table 26.5*). Some of these studies were driven by a desire to reduce the cost of medical therapy. The first of these studies was a randomized, placebo-controlled comparison of oral versus intravenous HDMP.[79] Mean change in Disability Status Scores (DSS) between the two groups were compared 28 days after the start of treatment. There were no significant differences, nor were there increased gastrointestinal side effects in the patients who received oral MP.

The second study of this type was a random-

Table 26.5 Clinical trials of different types and doses of glucocorticosteroids for MS relapses

Study	Treatment regimens	Number of subjects	Study design	Comments
Alam et al, 1993[79]	Intravenous MP 500 mg/day for 5 days	20	Double blind, randomized	No difference at 5 or 28 days after treatment; side effects minor and equally distributed between treatments
	Oral MP 500 mg/day for 5 days	15		
La Mantia et al, 1994[80]	Intravenous MP 1 g/day for 3 days, 500 mg/day for 3 days, 250 mg/day for 3 days, 125 mg/day for 3 days, 62.5 mg/day for 2 days	10	Double blind, randomized	High rate of worsening in low-dose MP group during month after treatment (Note: groups of unequal disease duration)
	Intravenous MP 40 mg/day for 7 days, 20 mg/day for 4 days, 10 mg/day for 3 days	10		
	Intravenous dexamethasone 8 mg/day for 7 days, 4 mg/day for 4 days, 2 mg/day for 3 days	11		
Barnes et al, 1997[81]	Intravenous MP 1 g/day for 3 days	38	Double blind, randomized	No significant difference in median change in EDSS at 1, 4, 12, or 24 weeks after treatment
	Oral MP 48 mg/day for 7 days, 24 mg/day for 7 days, 12 mg/day for 7 days	42		

ized, double-blind comparison of intravenous dexamethasone and intravenous MP in equivalent low dose versus intravenous HDMP.[80] Intravenous administration was used to simplify the blinding procedure, but the lower dose preparations could have been administered orally. Mean change in Expanded Disability Status Scale (EDSS) and the percentage of patients improved ≥1.0 point on EDSS were compared on days 2, 4, 7, and 14 and then 1, 2, 4, 6 and 12 months after the end of treatment. The authors of the study reported a high rate of symptomatic wors-

ening in the low-dose MP group during the first month after treatment with fewer low-dose MP patients achieving ≥1.0 point improvement in EDSS. They also reported a lower relapse rate in the HDMP group than in the low dose MP group during the year after treatment, but the significance of this finding is unclear given the small number of patients studied and differing duration of disease in the three treatment groups. No significant differences in mean EDSS change was noted at any time after treatment.

The third study to compare different doses of

MP was reported by Barnes and colleagues in 1997.[81] This was a double-blind, placebo-controlled, randomized trial comparing intravenous HDMP for 3 days with low-dose oral MP for 3 weeks. Treatment was started within 4 weeks of an MS relapse. The authors reported no significant difference in median EDSS change 1, 4, 12, and 24 weeks after treatment. They concluded that there was no more benefit from 3 days of intravenous HDMP than from 3 weeks of low-dose oral therapy. It is unclear whether this conclusion is justified given the limitations of the trial: specifically, the trial was designed solely to determine if the rate and extent of recovery following an MS relapse differed between the treatment groups, as determined by EDSS change. However, it is unlikely that statistical power existed to detect differences between the treatment groups.[82] Additionally, the study by Barnes[81] assessed only the effect of therapy on relapse and did not assess the impact of GCS on subsequent disease activity.

CLINICAL TRIALS OF HDMP ON MS DISEASE COURSE

Optic Neuritis Treatment Trial

The benefits of GCS treatment on subsequent disease activity has only recently been addressed by rigorous clinical trials. The first and most influential of these trials was the Optic Neuritis Treatment Trial (ONTT).[83] In this trial, 457 patients with acute monocular optic neuritis of less than 8 days' duration (mean 5 days) were randomized into three groups to receive treatment with oral prednisone (1 mg/kg per day for 14 days), intravenous HDMP (250 mg qid for 3 days followed by oral prednisone 1 mg/kg per day for 11 days), or oral placebo. The two groups receiving oral treatment alone were masked to treatment, but the patients receiving HDMP were not. Baseline characteristics, including the severity of baseline MRI abnormalities, were well matched in all these groups. In a series of publications based on pre-planned analyses, the investigators systematically reported the effects of treatment on the speed of recovery, the extent of recovery, and the subsequent disease course. Compared with placebo, intravenous HDMP resulted in more rapid recovery of vision, which was most evident during the first 2 weeks. The extent of recovery from visual field deficits, contrast sensitivity, and color vision were significantly better in the HDMP group at 6 months but not at 12 months, indicating little difference in final visual outcome.[84] The group receiving intravenous HDMP had a rate of recurrent optic neuritis in either eye over the subsequent 2 years of 14%; this compared to 16% in the placebo group and 30% in the oral prednisone group. This surprising result indicated that oral prednisone, in addition to being ineffective at improving vision, was also associated with an increased recurrence rate of optic neuritis.

In subsequent reports from the ONTT, the rate of conversion to clinically definite MS, was evaluated in a cohort of 389 patients without definite or probable MS at study onset.[84–86] Unexpectedly, the group receiving intravenous HDMP had a significantly lower rate of conversion to clinically definite MS (7.5%) during the subsequent 2 years than the placebo group (16.7%) or the oral prednisone group (14.7%). Most of this benefit occurred in patients with abnormal MRI scans at study entry, because this group of patients was at highest risk of a recurrence involving a different past of the CNS. Among those patients with Beck grade 3 or 4

MRI scans (i.e. two or more typical white matter lesions), clinically definite MS developed in 35.9%, 32.4% and 16.2% of the placebo, prednisone, and intravenous HDMP groups, respectively. Possibly because the patients received only a single course of treatment, the benefit on conversion to clinically definite MS was no longer evident 3–5 years after treatment.[85,87]

These results from the ONTT generated considerable controversy in the neurological community. Beck and colleagues[88] have clearly addressed the various concerns, and the ONTT results appear to be valid. One major question is whether the results of the ONTT also apply to patients with established RRMS.[89] Although the ONTT did not perform on-study MRI scans to study the effect of a single treatment on subsequent MRI activity, recent studies by Smith and colleagues[57] and Oliveri and colleagues[58] suggest that HDMP has a dose-dependent benefit that lasts for up to 6 months. Furthermore, a recent study by the author's group suggests that patients with isolated monosymptomatic demyelinating syndromes and abnormal MRI scans (grade 3 or 4 by the Beck criteria) experience a frequency of new enhancing lesions over the course of the subsequent year similar to that of RRMS patients.[90] These studies provide a strong rationale for further studies of pulsed HDMP as a treatment for RRMS.

Bimonthly HDMP pulses for SPMS

The majority of patients with RRMS eventually experience gradual progression of disability occurring between attacks or in the absence of attacks—the secondary progressive stage of MS[91] (see Chapters 1 and 32). Despite the lack of definitive controlled trials, it was widely held

that chronic GCS administration does not alter the disease course in SPMS. In the first study to assess the role of pulses of HDMP for SPMS, Goodkin and colleagues[92] conducted a double-blind, dose-comparison study of second-monthly MP 'pulses' in patients with early SPMS. Between 1991 and 1995, 109 patients with SPMS were randomized to pulses of intravenous HDMP (500 mg/day for 3 days followed by oral MP 64 mg/day for 2 days, 48 mg/day for 2 days, 32 mg/day for 2 days, 24 mg/day for 2 days, 8 mg/day for 3 days) or low-dose intravenous MP (10 mg/day for 3 days followed by oral MP 10 mg/day for 2 days, 8 mg/day for 2 days, 6 mg/day for 2 days, 4 mg/day for 2 days, 2 mg/day for 3 days) every 8 weeks for 2 years. The low-dose regimen was used to improve the success of blinding, since it was anticipated that HDMP pulses would produce side effects that would unmask patients.

The primary outcome measure was the proportion of sustained treatment failures in each treatment arm during the 2-year study. The sample size requirement, 92 patients, was derived from two assumptions: the rate of treatment failure in the low-dose MP group would be 62%, and there would be a 50% reduction in the proportion of patients experiencing sustained treatment failure over 2 years in the HDMP group.

Confirmed treatment failure was defined using criteria from a composite outcome measure (*Table 26.6*). A patient was considered at risk for treatment failure upon worsening for the first time by the requisite amount on any individual component of the composite measure. In the case of the relapse criterion, a patient was considered at risk to fail upon the occurrence of two relapses in the previous 11 months requiring early treatment with HDMP. To satisfy criteria for sustained treatment failure, worsening on any

Table 26.6 Composite outcome measure in second-monthly HDMP study[92]

Component	Composite outcome	
	Entry score	Required worsening for treatment failure
EDSS	4.0–5.0	1.0 (sustained for ≥ 5 months)
EDSS	5.5–6.5	0.5 (sustained for ≥ 5 months)
Ambulation Index	2.0–6.0	1.0 (sustained for ≥ 5 months)
9-Hole Peg Test	Best of two trials	20% or more, either hand (sustained for ≥ 5 months)
Box/Block Test	Best of two trials	20% or more, either hand (sustained for ≥ 5 months)
Exacerbations	≥ 1 in 2 years	≥ 3 in 12 consecutive months

component of the composite outcome measure had to be sustained for at least 5 months, or a patient needed to experience a third relapse in any consecutive 12 months of the study. Survival analysis using Kaplan–Meier curves to estimate treatment failure rates over the course of the study was a pre-planned secondary analysis.

Participation was offered to all patients with SPMS who satisfied all of the following criteria:

(a) one or more documented relapses with or without recovery in the previous 2 years;
(b) worsening of ≥0.5 points on the EDSS sustained for 5 or more months over the previous 2 years;
(c) an EDSS score of 4.0–6.5;
(d) Ambulation Index of 2.0–6.0;
(e) age 21–60 years; and
(f) disease duration of longer than 1 year.

Baseline characteristics of study participants is shown in *Table 26.7*. Unexpectedly, there were more males in the HDMP group. With this exception, baseline characteristics were similar between groups.

An accounting of study patients is given in *Table 26.8*. Forty-five patients completed treatment according to protocol in each treatment group. Primary results from the study are shown in *Table 26.9*. Of the 108 patients who initiated therapy, 29 of 54 (53.7%) low-dose MP and 21 of 54 (38.9%) HDMP recipients met criteria for sustained treatment failure (between-group difference 14.8%; 95% CI −3.8% to 33.4%; $p = 0.18$). The pre-planned secondary analysis, a log rank comparison of survival curves by treatment group, showed significant differences between groups in estimates of overall sustained treatment failure ($p = 0.04$) (*Fig. 26.1*).

Methodologic differences probably account for the slight differences in statistical significance using the primary and secondary outcome results. The primary outcome analysis (the proportion of treatment failures in either arm) utilizes only the entry and 2 years examination data, whereas the secondary outcome analysis (using survival analysis) takes into account both the distribution

Table 26.7 Baseline characteristics of study groups in second-monthly HDMP study[92]

| Variable | Baseline characteristics by dose (N = 54) | | |
	HDMP	Low-dose MP	Significance (p)*
Age (years; mean, SD)	39.8 (7.38)	39.4 (6.7)	0.73
Duration (years; mean, SD)	10.0 (5.87)	8.7 (6.9)	0.29
Female (%)	48	72	0.01
EDSS (mean, SD)	5.3 (1.1)	5.3 (1.1)	0.49
9-Hole Peg Test (right)	34.8 (15.6)	32.8 (13.6)	0.49
9-Hole Peg Test (left)	34.8 (17.2)	41.6 (53.85)	0.38
Box and Block Test (right)	43.6 (10.8)	44.6 (11.9)	0.65
Box and Block Test (left)	43.7 (10.0)	42.4 (10.6)	0.52
Exacerbations	1.52 (0.82)	1.65 (0.81)	0.41

*T test, except sex distribution, which is chi-square test.
SD, standard deviation.

Table 26.8 Accounting of patients in second-bimonthly HDMP study[92]

Patient status	HDMP	Low-dose MP	Total
Randomized to treatment	54	55	109
Started treatment	54	54	108
Stopped drug	3	0	3
Lost to follow-up	6	9	15
Completed protocol	45	45	90

of treatment failure and the time when treatment failures occurred. Although the difference in the proportion of treatment failures at 24 months was not statistically significant, the distribution of sustained treatment failures throughout the 24-month course of the study significantly favored the HDMP group. It is also relevant to recall that the study was designed to detect a 50% reduction in sustained treatment failure using the primary outcome measure, whereas the observed difference was 15%.

Additionally, the requirement that failure be

Table 26.9 Sustained treatment failure analysis in second-bimonthly HDMP study[92]

Failure parameter	Treatment		Chi-square test
	HDMP	Low-dose MP	p-value
Composite outcome	21	29	0.18
EDSS	3	2	1.00*
Ambulation Index	2	2	1.00*
9-Hole Peg Test	4	4	1.00*
Box and Block Test	2	1	1.00*
Relapses	2	6	0.27*
EDSS, Ambulation Index	6	7	0.77
EDSS, 9-Hole Peg Test	0	2	0.49
9-Hole Peg Test, Box and Block Test	0	2	0.49
EDSS, Ambulation Index, 9-Hole Peg Test	2	1	1.00
EDSS, Ambulation Index, 9-Hole Peg Test, Box and Block Test	0	2	0.49

*Exact chi-square test.
Composite outcome is sustained failure on EDSS, Ambulation Index, 9-Hole Peg Test, Box and Block Test, or three or more relapses treated with unscheduled doses of MP during any 12-month period.

sustained for 5 months had an impact on the sensitivity of the study by effectively shortening the study period from 24 months to 19 months. Any subject who worsened by the requisite amount after the 19-month time point could not, by the definitions used in the study, achieve the primary disability outcome. To determine the possibility that this influenced the study results, a post hoc analysis was performed assuming that patients at risk of failure when lost to follow-up or after 19 months on study would have become sustained treatment failures (*Table 26.10*). Using that approach, a significant treatment effect was evident using a comparison of treatment failures in either arm. Although post hoc analyses are exploratory and based on assumptions that cannot be verified, the results of the secondary analyses were interpreted as being sufficiently encouraging to warrant a phase 3 trial of HDMP in patients with SPMS.

A concern during the analysis was the disparity in the number of males in the two groups (52%

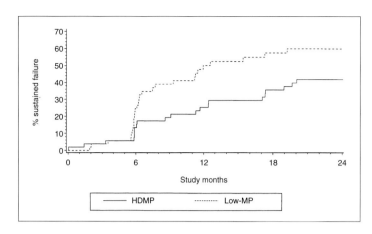

Fig. 26.1 *Kaplan–Meier analysis of treatment failure rates in bimonthly HDMP study (*p = 0.04*). Reprinted with permission from Goodkin et al.[9]*

Table 26.10 Post hoc analysis from second-bimonthly HDMP study[92] assuming sustained treatment failure for patients at risk of failing when lost to follow-up or after the 19th month on study

Failure parameter	High Dose (n = 54) Number of patients failing (%)	Low Dose (n = 54) Number of patients failing (%)
Composite (*p* = 0.02)	28 (51.9)	40 (74.1)
Individual parameters:		
EDSS (*p* = 0.04)	16 (29.6)	26 (49.1)
Ambulation Index (*p* = 0.05)	15 (27.8)	24 (46.2)
9-Hole Peg Test (*p* = 0.15)	12 (23.1)	17 (36.2)
Box and Block Test (*p* = 0.10)	6 (11.8)	11 (24.4)
Exacerbations (*p* = 0.38)	5 (9.3)	8 (14.8)

of the HDMP group was male; 28% of the low-dose MP group was male). A Cox regression model was applied to examine potential interactions between sex and treatment arm. The Cox model, which included the sex, the dose group and their interactive effect, revealed that only the treatment arm was significantly related to the time to sustained failure.

TOXICITY OF HDMP PULSES

Side effects of intravenous HDMP are listed in *Table 26.11*. GCS toxicity is theoretically related to the daily dose, the cumulative dose, and the frequency of administration. In general GCS toxicity is reduced with short-term 'pulse' administration of HDPM (1 g/day for 3–5 days).[93–96] Osteoporosis, aseptic osteonecrosis, cushingoid

Table 26.11 Side effects associated with HDMP treatment

Side effects that occur during therapy

Insomnia and mild euphoria

Anxiety

Mania, psychosis, or both*

Metallic taste during infusion

Increased appetite and weight gain

Nausea or vomiting*

Gastrointestinal upset or pain†

Flushing and increased sweating

Headache

Myalgias

Easy bruising

Intractable hiccups*

Pancreatitis*

Cardiac arrhythmias*

Glaucoma*

Side effects that occur early in patients with underlying risk factors

Peptic ulcer disease

Diabetes mellitus

Hypertension

Acne

Depression

Side effects that occur with repetitive use‡

Osteoporosis

Osteonecrosis

Posterior subcapsular cataracts

Fatty liver

Cushingoid features

Infection diathesis

Impaired healing

*Rare.
†More common with oral administration.
‡Rare compared to chronic daily or alternate day therapy.

features, infections, and hypothalamic–pituitary axis suppression are rare with pulses of HDMP at this dose for 3–5 days (even with a brief oral GCS tapering regimen).

Most of the common side effects are treatable or can be avoided with proper education. One of the commonest side effects is a feeling of well-being or mild euphoria. Moderate to severe anxiety, especially in patients who are newly diagnosed, is common and should be treated with reassurance and short-acting anxiolytic medication. Manic episodes and psychosis are rare and should be avoided in future treatment courses by pre-medication with anti-psychotic agents or lithium carbonate, as appropriate. Depression is uncommon, but it occurs more frequently than psychosis. It can be avoided with judicial co-administration of anti-depressants in high-risk patients or those with a history of depression during GCS therapy. Insomnia is so frequent that most patients require a short-acting sedative or hypnotic to be used as needed. Most other acute side effects require only education, symptomatic treatment if they occur and dietary modifications. Anaphylactoid reactions are very rare, but patients should receive their first dose under medical supervision.[97,98] Subsequent doses can be safely administered in the patient's home unless there is a medical contraindication (e.g. a cardiac condition or diabetes mellitus).

Side effects associated with repeated pulses of HDMP have been assessed only in the study by Goodkin and colleagues.[92] Adverse effects occurred significantly more frequently in the HDMP group than in the low-dose MP group (chi-square: $p = 0.009$). Nevertheless, cessation of study drug because of side effects occurred in only one patient. Side effects attributable to HDMP included weight gain (31.5% in the HDMP group; 13% in the low-dose MP group),

Table 26.12 Serious adverse events in second-bimonthly HDMP study[92]

Adverse event	Number of patients affected	Relationship to treatment	Treatment arm
Relationship between treatment and serious adverse events			
Relapses	3	Unrelated	Low (2 patients), High (1 patient)
Death: aspiration pneumonia*	1	Unrelated	Low
Death: hepatic necrosis second to intravenous drug abuse	1	Unrelated	High
Cervical cancer	1	Unrelated	High
Prostate cancer	1	Unrelated	High
Psychosis	1	Drug related	High
Compression fracture†	1	Drug related	High
Aseptic meningitis	1	Unlikely	High

*Patient and family elected not to treat this adverse event.
†No neurological sequelae.

insomnia (32.5% in the HDMP group; 5.6% in the low-dose MP group), depression (26% in the HDMP group; 5.6% in the low-dose MP group), infections (38.9% in the HDMP group; 20.4% in the low-dose MP group), and headache (26% in the HDMP group; 13% in the low-dose MP group). Most of the infections were of the lower urinary tract. Serious adverse effects were rare (*Table 26.12*). One HDMP recipient who was known to have dysphagia before initiating treatment died of aspiration pneumonia. This death would have been treatable, but the patient and family elected not to treat the infection. One patient required cessation of HDMP after development of psychosis.

The relative risk of osteoporosis in MS patients treated with repeated pulses of HDMP compared with chronic daily or alternate-day GCS is unknown. This is relevant since bone mineral density is decreased and the incidence of fractures is increased in MS patients.[99] Although only one patient experienced a fracture in the study by Goodkin and colleagues,[92] patients were not monitored for osteoporosis. One recent study[100] found no relationship between single or repeated pulses of HDMP and bone mineral density of the lumbar spine or femoral head in MS patients. In fact, bone mineral density of the lumbar spine increased for 6 months after a pulse of HDMP, presumably because of improved mobility with treatment. This finding is consistent with a reported association between low bone mineral density and decreased mobility, as well as low 25-hydroxy-vitamin D levels.[99] It is possible that improved mobility with pulses of HDMP, especially in pre-menopausal women with MS, may offset declines in bone mineral density related to GCS.

Although additional studies are needed, recommendations to prevent GCS-induced osteoporosis can be made at this time based on guidelines developed by the American College of Rheumatology.[101] Patients starting 'pulse' therapy with HDMP should have bone mineral density measurements in the lumbar spine and femoral heads and should begin vitamin D replacement (50 000 units three times weekly or calcitriol 0.5–1.0 µg/day) and calcium supplementation to achieve a total daily intake of 1500 mg of calcium per day. Serum and urine calcium levels should be monitored if calcitriol is prescribed in excess of 0.25 µg per day. Patients should be advised to stop smoking and to limit alcohol intake. Regular stretching, strengthening and aerobic exercise should be instituted to optimize mobility. Additional treatments should be determined by the degree of bone mineral density loss. Options include thiazide diuretics in patients with high urinary calcium levels, hormonal replacement in post-menopausal women, oral contraceptives in pre-menopausal women, testosterone in men with low testosterone levels, calcitonin, and biphosphonates.

IMPLICATIONS FOR PRACTICE

The evidence reviewed above suggests that HDMP hastens recovery from MS relapses and may have a beneficial impact on subsequent clinical and MRI disease activity. The latter effects have been demonstrated in patients with optic neuritis, who are at high risk for MS, and in SPMS patients. However, the available data is limited, since there are only three clinical trials that have assessed the effects of HDMP on the disease course.

The appropriate dose, route, and frequency of administration for HDMP pulses are unknown. Doses of HDMP ranging from 500 mg to 1000 mg/day (intravenous or oral) for 3–5 days have been found to hasten recovery from MS relapses. However, a recent study reported that HDMP at a dose of 2000 mg/day for 5 days significantly reduced new and total enhancing MRI lesion counts for 2 months.[58] This raised the possibility that doses in excess of 500 mg/day may be required to alter subsequent disease activity significantly. Further studies are required to clarify this issue. In the interim, doses of 500–1000 mg/day (intravenous or oral) for 3–5 days are appropriate for the treatment of MS relapses that are associated with significant functional decline. Conventional doses of oral GCS, such as the regimen studied by Barnes and colleagues,[56] cannot be currently recommended.

It is currently unclear whether results from the ONTT can be generalized to other isolated monosymptomatic demyelinating syndromes (IMDS). There is little reason to believe that patients with MRI scans typical for MS who present with partial transverse myelitis or brainstem syndromes carry a risk of subsequent relapse different from patients presenting with optic neuritis and similar MRI abnormalities.[102,103] Furthermore, a recent study suggests that all IMDS groups with abnormal MRI scans at onset experience a frequency of enhancing lesion activity over the course of the subsequent year similar to that of RRMS patients.[90] Therefore, such patients are likely to experience the same temporary, disease-modifying benefit from HDMP as optic neuritis patients. More importantly, IMDS patients are not likely to receive significant benefit from conventional doses of oral GCS, which should be avoided in the absence of future controlled clinical trials.

The role of pulse HDMP treatment in RRMS is unknown. Similarly, the role of pulse HDMP as additive therapy for patients who fail conventional treatment with interferon-β or glatiramer acetate is unclear. Both areas are ripe for controlled clinical trials.

Lastly, the relative role of pulse HDMP therapy in SPMS remains uncertain. The study by Goodkin and colleagues[92] suggests that second-monthly pulses of HDMP at a dose of 500 mg for 3 days delays the development of disability progression and has few significant side effects in a population of patients with few treatment options. However, the optimal dose of pulse HDMP therapy is unknown, as are the effects on MRI, and the efficacy relative to interferon-β needs to be determined. As with RRMS, it is likely that future studies will focus on HDMP treatment as additive therapy for patients who fail conventional treatment with interferon-β.

ACKNOWLEDGEMENTS

Supported in part by a grant from the National Multiple Sclerosis Society (DEG: RG 2350-A-3) and Bracco diagnostics (RPK).

REFERENCES

1 Myers LW. Treatment of multiple sclerosis with ACTH and corticosteroids. In: Rudick RA, Goodkin DE, eds. *Treatment of Multiple Sclerosis: Trial Design, Results, and Future Perspectives* (London: Springer, 1992); 6:135–156.

2 Schimmer BP, Parker KL. Adrenocorticotropic hormone; adrenocortical steroids and their synthetic analogs; inhibitors of the synthesis and actions of adrenocortical hormones. In: Hardman JG, Limbird LE, eds. *Goodman and Gilman's Pharmacological Basis of Therapeutics* 9th edn. (St Louis Missouri: McGraw-Hill, 1996); 1459–1485.

3 Pardridge WM, Mietus LJ. Transport of steroid hormones through the rat blood–brain barrier: primary role of albumin bound hormone. *J Clin Invest* 1979; 64:145–154.

4 Defer GL, Barre J, Ledudal P et al. Methylprednisolone infusion during acute exacerbation of MS: plasma and CSF concentrations. *Eur Neurol* 1995; 35:143–148.

5 Hayball PJ, Cosh DG, Ahern MJ et al. High dose oral methylprednisolone in patients with rheumatoid arthritis: pharmacokinetics and clinical response. *Eur J Clin Pharmacol* 1992; 42:85–88.

6 Narang PK, Wilder R, Chatterji DC et al. Systemic bioavailability and pharmacokinetics of methylprednisolone in patients with rheumatoid arthritis following 'high-dose' pulse administration. *Biopharm Drug Dispos* 1983; 4:233–248.

7 Metz LM, Sabuda D, Enns R et al. Safety and tolerability of high-dose oral prednisone in the treatment of multiple sclerosis (Abstract). *Neurology* 1998; 50:A63.

8 Chassard D, Banzet O, Lamy F et al. Tolerance gastro-duodenale de la methylprednisolone: étude de la voie orale versus voie veineuse chez le volontaire sain. *Presse Med* 1994; 23:515–517.

9 Hollenberg SM, Weinberger C, Ong ES et al. Primary structure and expression of a functional human glucocorticoid receptor cDNA. *Nature* 1985; 318:635–641.

10 Smith DF, Toft DO. Steroid receptors and their associated proteins. *Mol Endocrinol* 1993; 7:4–11.

11 Boumpas DT, Chrousos GP, Wilder RL et al. Glucocorticoid therapy for immune-mediated diseases: basic and clinical correlates (Review). *Ann Intern Med* 1993; 119:1198–1208.

12 Diamond MI, Miner JN, Yoshinaga SK, Yamamoto KR. Transcription factor interactions: selectors of positive or negative regulation from a single DNA element. *Science* 1990; 249:1266–1272.

13 Jonat C, Rahmsdorf HJ, Par KK et al. Antitumor promotion and antiinflammation: down-modulation of AP-1 (Fos/Jun) activity by glucocorticoid hormone. *Cell* 1990; 62:1189–1204.

14 Crockard AD, Treacy MT, Droogan AG et al. Transient immunomodulation by intravenous methylprednisolone treatment of multiple sclerosis. *Multiple Sclerosis* 1995; 1:20–24.

15 Fauci AS, Dale DC, Balow JE. Glucocorticosteroid therapy: mechanisms of action and clinical considerations. *Ann Intern Med* 1976; 84:304–315.

16 Trotter JL, Garvey WF. Prolonged effects of large-dose methylprednisolone infusion in multiple sclerosis. *Neurology* 1980; **30**:702–708.

17 Almawi WY, Beyhum HN, Rahme AA, Rieder MJ. Regulation of cytokine and cytokine receptor expression by glucocorticoids (review). *J Leukoc Biol* 1996; **60**:563–572.

18 Joyce DA, Steer JH, Abraham LJ. Glucocorticoid modulation of human monocyte/macrophage function: control of TNF-alpha secretion (review). *Inflamm Res* 1997; **46**:447:451.

19 Ossege LM, Sindern E, Voss B, Malin JP. Corticosteroids induce expression of transforming-growth-factor-beta1 mRNA in peripheral blood mononuclear cells of patients with multiple sclerosis. *J Neuroimmunol* 1998; **84**:1–6.

20 Gayo A, Mozo L, Suarez A et al. Glucocorticoids increase IL-10 expression in multiple sclerosis patients with acute relapse. *J Neuroimmunol* 1998; **85**:122–130.

21 Gelati M, Lamperti E, Dufour A et al. IL-10 production in multiple sclerosis patients, SLE patients and healthy controls: preliminary findings. *Ital J Neurol Sci* 1997; **18**:191–194.

22 Loughlin AJ, Woodroofe MN, Cuzner ML. Modulation of interferon-gamma-induced major histocompatibility complex class II and Fc receptor expression on isolated microglia by transforming growth factor-beta 1, interleukin-4, noradrenaline and glucocorticoids. *Immunology* 1993; **79**:125–130.

23 Kirk PF, Williams JD, Petersen MM, Compston DA. The effect of methylprednisolone on monocyte eicosanoid production in patients with multiple sclerosis. *J Neurol* 1994; **241**:427–431.

24 Ruiz P, Gomez F, King M et al. In vivo glucocorticoid modulation of guinea pig splenic macrophage Fc gamma receptors. *J Clin Invest* 1991; **88**:149–157.

25 Cupps TR, Gerrard TL, Falkoff RJ et al. Effects of in vitro corticosteroids on B cell activation, proliferation, and differentiation. *J Clin Invest* 1985; **75**:754–761.

26 Gold R, Pepinsky RB, Zettl UK et al. Lipocortin-1 (annexin-1) suppresses activation of autoimmune T cell lines in the Lewis rat. *J Neuroimmunol* 1996; **69**:157–164.

27 Crofford LJ, Wilder RL, Ristimaki AP et al. Cyclooxygenase-1 and -2 expression in rheumatoid synovial tissues. Effects of interleukin-1 beta, phorbol, ester, and corticosteroids. *J Clin Invest* 1994; **93**:1095–1101.

28 Cronstein BN, Kimmel SC, Levin RI et al. A mechanism for the anti-inflammatory effects of corticosteroids: the glucocorticoid receptor regulates leukocyte adhesion to endothelial cells and expression of endothelial-leukocyte adhesion molecule 1 and intercellular adhesion molecule 1. *Proceedings of the National Academy of Sciences of the United States of America* 1992; **89**:9991–9995.

29 Rosenberg GA, Dencoff JE, Correa NJ et al. Effect of steroids on CSF matrix metalloproteinases in multiple sclerosis: relation to blood–brain barrier injury. *Neurology* 1996; **46**:1626–1632.

30 Compston DA, Milligan NM, Hughes PJ et al. A double-blind controlled trial of high dose methylprednisolone in patients with multiple sclerosis: 2. Laboratory results. *J Neurol Neurosurg Psychiatry* 1987; **50**:517–522.

31 Durelli L, Poccardi G, Cavallo R. CD8+ high CD11b+ low T cells (T suppressor-effectors) in multiple sclerosis cerebrospinal fluid are increased during high dose corticosteroid treatment. *J Neuroimmunol* 1991; **31**:221–228.

32 Durelli L, Cocito D, Riccio A et al. High-dose intravenous methylprednisolone in the treatment of multiple sclerosis: clinical–immunologic correlations. *Neurology* 1986; **36**:238–243.

33 Anderson TJ, Donaldson IM, Sheat JM, George PM. Methylprednisolone in multiple sclerosis exacerbation: changes in CSF parameters. *Aust N Z J Med* 1990; **20**:794–797.

34 Staugatis SM, Shapshak P, Myers LW et al. Azathioprine and steroids are not more effective in decreasing multiple sclerosis intra-blood–brain-barrier IgG synthesis than steroids alone. *Ann Neurol* 1985; **18**:356–357.

35 Warren KG, Catz I, Jeffrey VM, Carroll DJ. Effect of methylprednisolone on CSF IgG parameters, myelin basic protein and anti-myelin basic protein in multiple sclerosis exacerbations. *Can J Neurol Sci* 1986; **13**:25–30.

36 Frequin ST, Barkhof F, Lamers KJ et al. CSF myelin basic protein, IgG and IgM levels in 101 MS patients before and after treatment with high-dose intravenous methylprednisolone. *Acta Neurol Scand* 1992; **86**:291–297.

37 Franciotta D, Piccolo G, Zardini E et al. Soluble CD8 and ICAM-1 in serum and CSF of MS patients treated with 6-methylprednisolone. *Acta Neurol Scand* 1997; **95**:275–279.

38 Trojano M, Avolio C, Simone IL et al. Soluble

intercellular adhesion molecule-1 in serum and cerebrospinal fluid of clinically active relapsing–remitting multiple sclerosis: correlation with Gd–DTPA magnetic resonance imaging-enhancement and cerebrospinal fluid findings. *Neurology* 1996; **47**:1535–1541.

39   **Spuler S, Yousry T, Scheller A et al.** Multiple sclerosis: prospective analysis of TNF-alpha and 55 kDa TNF receptor in CSF and serum in correlation with clinical and MRI activity. *J Neuroimmunol* 1996; **66**:57–64.

40   **Hall ED.** Neuroprotective actions of glucocorticoid and nonglucocorticoid steroids in acute neuronal injury (Review). *Cell Mol Neurobiol* 1993; **13**:415–32.

41   **Sears ES, Tindall RS, Zarnow H.** Active multiple sclerosis. Enhanced computerized tomographic imaging of lesions and the effect of corticosteroids. *Arch Neurol* 1978; **35**:426–434.

42   **Troiano R, Hafstein M, Ruderman M et al.** Effect of high-dose intravenous steroid administration on contrast-enhancing computed tomographic scan lesions in multiple sclerosis. *Ann Neurol* 1984; **15**:257–263.

43   **Troiano R, Hafstein MP, Zito G et al.** The effect of oral corticosteroid dosage on CT enhancing multiple sclerosis plaques. *J Neurol Sci* 1985; **70**:67–72.

44   **Stefoski D, Davis FA, Schauf CL.** Acute improvement in exacerbating multiple sclerosis produced by intravenous administration of mannitol. *Ann Neurol* 1985; **18**:443–450.

45   **Miller DH, Johnson G, Tofts PS.** Precise relaxation time measurements of normal-appearing white matter in inflammatory central nervous system disease. *Magn Reson Med* 1989; **11**:331–336.

46   **Allen IV, McKeown SR.** A histological, histochemical and biochemical study of the macroscopically normal white matter in multiple sclerosis. *J Neurol Sci* 1979; **41**:81–91.

47   **Kesselring J, Miller DH, MacManus DG et al.** Quantitative magnetic resonance imaging in multiple sclerosis: the effect of high dose intravenous methylprednisolone. *J Neurol Neurosurg Psychiatry* 1989; **52**:14–17.

48   **Grossman RI, Braffman BH, Brorson JR et al.** Multiple sclerosis: serial study of gadolinium-enhanced MR imaging. *Radiology* 1988; **169**:117–122.

49   **Miller DH, Barkhoff F, Nauta JJ.** Gadolium enhancement increases the sensitivity of MRI in detecting disease activity in multiple sclerosis. *Brain* 1993; **116**:1077–1094.

50   **Kermode AG, Thompson AJ, Tofts PS et al.** Breakdown of the blood–brain barrier precedes symptoms and other MRI signs of new lesions in multiple sclerosis. *Brain* 1990; **113**:1477–1489.

51   **Katz J, Taubenberger J, Raine C et al.** Gadolinium enhancing lesion on magnetic resonance imaging: neuropathological findings. *Ann Neurol* 1990; **28**:243.

52   **Burnham JA, Wright RR, Dreisbach J, Murray RS.** The effect of high-dose steroids on MRI gadolinium enhancement in acute demyelinating lesions. *Neurology* 1991; **41**:1349–1354.

53   **Barkhof F, Hommes OR, Scheltens P, Valk J.** Quantitative MRI changes in gadolinium-DTPA enhancement after high-dose intravenous methylprednisolone in multiple sclerosis. *Neurology* 1991; **41**:1219–1222.

54   **Miller DH, Thompson AJ, Morrissey SP et al.** High dose steroids in acute relapses of multiple sclerosis: MRI evidence for a possible mechanism of therapeutic effect. *J Neurol Neurosurg Psychiatry* 1992; **55**:450–453.

55   **Barkhof F, Frequin ST, Hommes OR et al.** A correlative triad of gadolinium-DTPA MRI, EDSS, and CSF-MBP in relapsing multiple sclerosis patients treated with high-dose intravenous methylprednisolone. *Neurology* 1992; **42**:63–67.

56   **Barkhof F, Tas MW, Frequin ST et al.** Limited duration of the effect of methylprednisolone on changes on MRI in multiple sclerosis. *Neuroradiology* 1994; **36**:382–387.

57   **Smith ME, Stone LA, Albert PS et al.** Clinical worsening in multiple sclerosis is associated with increased frequency and area of gadopentetate dimeglumine-enhancing magnetic resonance imaging lesions. *Ann Neurol* 1993; **33**:480–489.

58   **Oliveri RL, Valentino P, Russo C et al.** Randomized trial comparing two different high doses of methylprednisolone in MS: a clinical and MRI study. *Neurology* 1998; **50**:1833–1836.

59   **Goodkin DE, Rooney WD, Sloan R et al.** A serial study of new MS lesions and the white matter from which they arise. *Neurology* 1998; **51**:1689–1697.

60   **Filippi M, Rocca MA, Martino G et al.** Magnetization transfer changes in the normal appearing white matter precede the appearance of enhancing lesions in patients with multiple sclerosis. *Ann Neurol* 1998; **43**:809–814.

61   **Jonsson B, von Reis G, Sahlgren E.** Experience of ACTH and cortisone treatment in some organic

neurological cases. *Acta Psychiatr Neurol Scand* 1951(Suppl 74):60–63.

62 Rose AS, Kuzme JW, Kurtzke JF et al. Cooperative study in the evaluation of therapy in multiple sclerosis: ACTH vs placebo. Final report. *Neurology* 1970; **20**:1–59.

63 Bell PR, Briggs JD, Calman KC et al. Reversal of acute clinical and experimental organ rejection using large doses of intravenous prednisolone. *Lancet* 1971; **1**:876–880.

64 Cathcart ES, Idelson BA, Scheinberg MA, Couser WG. Beneficial effects of methylprednisolone 'pulse' therapy in diffuse proliferative lupus nephritis. *Lancet* 1976; **1**:163–166.

65 de Torrente A, Popovtzer MM, Guggenheim SJ, Schrier RW. Serious pulmonary hemorrhage, glomerulonephritis, and massive steroid therapy. *Ann Intern Med* 1975; **83**:218–219.

66 Bolton WK, Couser WG. Intravenous pulse methylprednisolone therapy of acute crescentic rapidly progressive glomerulonephritis. *Am J Med* 1979; **66**:495–502.

67 Neild GH, Lee HA. Methylprednisolone pulse therapy in the treatment of polyarteritis nodosa. *Postgrad Med J* 1977; **53**:382–387.

68 Fan PT, Yu DT, Clements PJ et al. Effect of corticosteroids on the human immune response: comparison of one and three daily 1 gm intravenous pulses of methylprednisolone. *J Lab Clin Med* 1978; **91**:625–634.

69 Dowling PC, Bosch VV, Cook SD. Possible beneficial effect of high-dose intravenous steroid therapy in acute demyelinating disease and transverse myelitis. *Neurology* 1980; **30**:33–36.

70 Buckley C, Kennard C, Swash M. Treatment of acute exacerbations of multiple sclerosis with intravenous methyl-prednisolone. *J Neurol Neurosurg Psychiatry* 1982; **45**:179–180.

71 Newman PK, Saunders M, Tilley PJ. Methylprednisolone therapy in multiple sclerosis (letter). *J Neurol Neurosurg Psychiatry* 1982; **45**:941–922.

72 Goas JY, Marion JL, Missoum A. High dose intravenous methyl prednisolone in acute exacerbations of multiple sclerosis (letter). *J Neurol Neurosurg Psychiatry* 1983; **46**:99.

73 Abbruzzese G, Gandolfo C, Loeb C. 'Bolus' methylprednisolone versus ACTH in the treatment of multiple sclerosis. *Ital J Neurol Sci* 1983; **4**:169–172.

74 Barnes MP, Bateman DE, Cleland PG et al.

Intravenous methylprednisolone for multiple sclerosis in relapse. *J Neurol Neurosurg Psychiatry* 1985; **48**:157–159.

75 Thompson AJ, Kennard C, Swash M et al. Relative efficacy of intravenous methylprednisolone and ACTH in the treatment of acute relapse in MS. *Neurology* 1989; **39**:969–971.

76 Milligan NM, Newcombe R, Compston DA. A double-blind controlled trial of high dose methylprednisolone in patients with multiple sclerosis: 1. Clinical effects. *J Neurol Neurosurg Psychiatry* 1987; **50**:511–516.

77 Sellebjerg F, Frederiksen JL, Nielsen PM, Olesen J. Double-blind, randomized, placebo-controlled study of oral, high-dose methylprednisolone in attacks of MS. *Neurology* 1998; **51**:529–534.

78 Bindoff L, Lyons PR, Newman PK, Saunders M. Methylprednisolone in multiple sclerosis: a comparative dose study (letter). *J Neurol Neurosurg Psychiatry* 1988; **51**:1108–1109.

79 Alam SM, Kyriakides T, Lawden M, Newman PK. Methylprednisolone in multiple sclerosis: a comparison of oral with intravenous therapy at equivalent high dose. *J Neurol Neurosurg Psychiatry* 1993; **56**:1219–1220.

80 La Mantia L, Eoli M, Milanese C et al. Double-blind trial of dexamethasone versus methylprednisolone in multiple sclerosis acute relapses. *Eur Neurol* 1994; **34**:199–203.

81 Barnes D, Hughes RA, Morris RW et al. Randomised trial of oral and intravenous methylprednisolone in acute relapses of multiple sclerosis. *Lancet* 1997; **349**:902–906.

82 Barkhof F, Polman C. Oral or intravenous methylprednisolone for acute relapses of MS? (comment) (published erratum appears in *Lancet* 1997 7; **349**:1704). *Lancet* 1997; **349**:893–894.

83 Beck RW, Cleary PA, Anderson MMJ et al. A randomized, controlled trial of corticosteroids in the treatment of acute optic neuritis. The Optic Neuritis Study Group. *N Engl J Med* 1992; **326**:581–588.

84 Beck RW, Cleary PA, Optic Neuritis Study Group. Optic Neuritis Treatment Trial: one-year follow-up results. *Arch Ophthalmol* 1993; **111**:773–775.

85 Beck RW. The Optic Neuritis Treatment Trial: three-year follow-up results. *Arch Ophthalmol* 1995; **113**:136–137.

86 Cleary PA, Beck RW, Bourque LB et al. Visual symptoms after optic neuritis. Results from the Optic

Neuritis Treatment Trial. *J Neuroophthalmol* 1997; 17:18–23.

87 **Optic Neuritis Study Group.** The 5-year risk of MS after optic neuritis. Experience of the optic neuritis treatment trial. Optic Neuritis Study Group. *Neurology* 1997;49:1404–1413.

88 **Beck RW, Trobe JD.** The Optic Neuritis Treatment Trial. Putting the results in perspective. The Optic Neuritis Study Group. *J Neuroophthalmol* 1995; 15:131–135.

89 **Kupersmith MJ, Kaufman D, Paty DW et al.** Megadose corticosteroids in multiple sclerosis (editorial). *Neurology* 1994; 44:1–4.

90 **Kinkel RP, Simon JH, Baron B.** Bi-monthly cranial MRI activity following an isolated monosymptomatic demyelinating syndrome: potential outcome measures for future multiple sclerosis 'prevention' trials. *Multiple Sclerosis* 1999; in press.

91 **Lublin FD, Reingold SC.** Defining the clinical course of multiple sclerosis: results of an international survey. *Neurology* 1996; 46:907–911.

92 **Goodkin DE, Kinkel RP, Weinstock-Guttman B et al.** A phase II study of i.v. methylprednisolone in secondary–progressive multiple sclerosis. *Neurology* 1999; 52:896–897.

93 **Lyons PR, Newman PK, Saunders M.** Methylprednisolone therapy in multiple sclerosis: a profile of adverse effects. *J Neurol Neurosurg Psychiatry* 1988; 51:285–287.

94 **Smith MD, Ahern MJ, Roberts-Thomson PJ.** Pulse methylprednisolone therapy in rheumatoid arthritis: unproved therapy, unjustified therapy, or effective adjunctive treatment. *Ann Rheum Dis* 1990; 49:265.

95 **Levic Z, Micic D, Nikolic J et al.** Short-term high dose steroid therapy does not affect the hypothalamic–pituitary–adrenal axis in relapsing multiple sclerosis patients. Clinical assessment by the insulin tolerance test. *J Endocrinol Invest* 1996; 19:30–34.

96 **Miro J, Amado JA, Pesquera C et al.** Assessment of the hypothalamic–pituitary–adrenal axis function after corticosteroid therapy for MS relapses. *Acta Neurol Scand* 1990; 81:524–528.

97 **Pryse-Phillips WE, Chandra RK, Rose B.** Anaphylactoid reaction to methylprednisolone pulsed therapy for multiple sclerosis. *Neurology* 1984; 34:1119–1121.

98 **van der Berg JS, van Eikema H, Wuis EW et al.** Anaphylactoid reaction to intravenous methylprednisolone in a patient with multiple sclerosis (letter). *J Neurol Neurosurg Psychiatry* 1997; 63:813–814.

99 **Cosman F, Nieves J, Komar L et al.** Fracture history and bone loss in patients with MS. *Neurology* 1998; 51:1161–1165.

100 **Schwid SR, Goodman AD, Puzas JE et al.** Sporadic corticosteroid pulses and osteoporosis in multiple sclerosis. *Arch Neurol* 1996; 53:753–757.

101 **Anonymous.** Recommendations for the prevention and treatment of glucocorticoid-induced osteoporosis. *Arthritis Rheum* 1996; 39:1–22.

102 **Morrissey SP, Miller DH, Kendall BE et al.** The significance of brain magnetic resonance imaging abnormalities at presentation with clinically isolated syndromes suggestive of multiple sclerosis. A 5-year follow-up study. *Brain* 1993; 116:135–146.

103 **Filippi M, Horsfield MA, Morrissey SP et al.** Quantitative brain MRI lesion load predicts the course of clinically isolated syndromes suggestive of multiple sclerosis. *Neurology* 1994; 44:635–641.

27
Hematopoietic stem cell transplantation

William H Burns and Richard K Burt

BACKGROUND

Clearly there is a need for more effective treatments for progressive multiple sclerosis (MS). Although the pathogenesis of MS has not been fully defined, T-cell-mediated immune destruction of myelin-producing cells is thought to be an important element. This view of MS as an autoimmune disease is supported by the fact that immunosuppression and immunomodulation are currently the most effective therapies for MS. Since bone marrow transplant procedures (BMT; here referred to as hematopoietic stem cell transplantation (HSCT)), often ablate the immune system along with the hematopoietic system, HSCT represents the ultimate clinical extension of immunosuppression. Indeed, patients undergoing HSCT must be reimmunized with the usual vaccines because they lose immunological memory, especially if the donor graft is depleted of T cells to prevent graft-versus-host disease (GVHD). Since immunosuppression is an effective but often temporary treatment of MS, the authors and others have hypothesized that HSCT might be useful in MS.[1–8] Furthermore, improvement or cure of other autoimmune diseases (e.g. rheumatoid arthritis, ulcerative colitis, psoriasis) coincident in patients receiving HSCT for other diseases has been reported.[9–12]

Animal studies that the authors and others have performed provide an experimental basis for the therapeutic use of HSCT in MS. Studies in SJL/J mice and Buffalo and Lewis rats suggest that after adoptive transfer of encephalitogenic lymphocytes or after active immunization with myelin basic protein (MBP) or proteolipid protein (PLP), immune ablation and syngeneic marrow rescue can prevent or ameliorate clinical symptoms.[13–16] In Lewis rats, after immunization with a unique peptide fragment of MBP, the effector cells that initiate experimental allergic encephalomyelitis (EAE) are skewed towards over-utilization of the $V_\beta 8.2$ T-cell receptor.[17,18] Since in this model the T lymphocyte subset (CD4, $V_\beta 8.2$) that initiates EAE is well defined, the authors used it as a molecular marker of residual disease. When analysed by reverse transcriptase polymerase chain reaction and in situ hybridization, $V_\beta 8.2$ T cells are absent from the central nervous system (CNS) after syngeneic HSCT.[15] Therefore, BMT was able to eliminate the effector lymphocytes responsible for autoimmune disease from the CNS and the new immune system established after transplant did not recapitulate the disease process.

With the above human observations and animal studies as a basis, the authors formulated a therapeutic approach using HSCT as extreme immunoablation to treat MS. It was hoped that any original (unknown) inciting factors of MS in these patients might be absent at the time of transplant. Furthermore, since vaccine immunization of HSCT patients is usually unsuccessful for many months after transplant, it was also hoped that the blood–brain barrier would be repaired at the site of CNS lesions before the patient's immune system was reconstituted, thus lessening the presentation of MS-specific antigens to the new immune system. On the basis of the authors' transplant data in EAE animals, it was hoped that the new immune system would not recapitulate the disease. Moreover, in the autologous transplant setting it seemed desirable to deplete T cells from the stem cell source in order to avoid continuation of the disease. The authors recently reported Phase 1 study results for patients with severe, rapidly progressive MS and are now completing this study.[19,20] The results of a concomitant European study[21] published before these results is reviewed first.

CLINICAL STUDIES

European study

The first report of HSCT for MS was from the Greek transplant group headed by Dr Fassas.[21] Fifteen patients with primary and secondary progressive MS, all having an increase of 1.0 on the Kurtzke expanded disability status scale (EDSS) during the previous year and with a median EDSS score of 6 (5–7.5) and a median Scripps Neurological Rating Scale (NRS) score of 42 (33–62) at the beginning of the procedure, received autologous transplants. Stem cells were from unselected peripheral blood stem cells (PBSC) collected by apheresis following mobilization with cyclophos-

phamide and growth factors (granulocyte colony stimulating factor (G-CSF) and granulocyte–macrophage colony stimulating factor (GM-CSF)). Patients were treated in preparation for the transplant with BEAM (Bis-chloroethyl nitrosourea (BCNU), Etoposide, Cytosine arabinoside, and Melphalan), a regimen often used in transplants for lymphoma. BCNU and melphalan are the most immunosuppressive drugs in this regimen. Because the stem cells were not separated from lymphocytes in the apheresis product, anti-thymocyte globulin (ATG) was given for 2 days after the infusion of the PBSC as an in vivo 'purge' of lymphocytes. In this study, mobilization of stem cells was better achieved with G-CSF than with GM-CSF because of allergic reactions experienced with the latter. Allergic reactions were also a problem with administration of ATG.

At the time of the report, the median follow-up time was only 6 months. Patients tolerated their transplants well. All patients improved over the first 6 months after transplant as judged by increases in NRS scores (10–41 points), but two patients have subsequently experienced decreased NRS scores. On the EDSS scale, seven patients showed improvement, four of them by at least 1.5 points. The EDSS scores of the other eight patients became stable.

Although this study suffers from a short follow-up, it is important because it is the first demonstration of the safety and initial efficacy of transplantation for MS using a familiar transplant regimen. The dependence on an in vivo lymphocyte purge rather than an efficient in vitro stem-cell separation from lymphocytes before infusion of the graft may be an important deficiency for long-term treatment benefits. The preparative regimen also may not be the most immunoablative regimen achievable. Even so, stabilization and improvement observed in these patients is encouraging.

USA study

The rationale that determined the protocol is recounted and the results are reviewed.

Type of transplant

To justify any new therapy such as HSCT, the risk of dying from the disease must be higher than that expected from its treatment, or the morbidities associated with the disease must justify the treatment risks. Survival in MS correlates inversely with the level of disability. Less than 6% of patients with an unrestricted activity level are dead within 10 years, and there is increased mortality for patients with increasing disability. Autologous transplant has a mortality of 1–3% in breast cancer patients and up to 10–15% in patients with lymphomas and other malignancies. The latter patients usually have been heavily treated before transplant and the accumulation of treatment toxicities is thought to play a role in their increased transplant-related mortality. Since allogeneic transplantation carries a much higher mortality, mainly because of GVHD, it was reasoned that it should be tried only if clinical benefits achieved with autologous transplants were not realized or were of short duration. Furthermore, it was reasoned that the collected stem cells could be depleted of T cells, thus achieving a very high level of immunoablation with less risk using autologous stem cell transplants. It was thought that increased mortality in MS patients with increasing disability and functional impairments along with increasing morbidities justified the relatively low expected risk of mortality of autologous HSCT. The transplant mortality rate was expected to be closer to that of breast cancer patients than lymphoma patients since the MS patients would not previously have received intensive chemotherapy.

Pre-transplant regimen

Most pre-transplant regimens are designed for their anti-tumor effects. The most immunosuppressive regimen and the one with the best chance of affecting the CNS lesions would be one incorporating total body irradiation (TBI). The authors were concerned about possible toxicities that might occur following irradiation of MS CNS lesions, since this had been reported in the rat EAE model.[14] It was encouraging that no untoward toxicities were noted when total lymphoid irradiation (TLI), which includes irradiation of the spinal cord, was used for the treatment of MS. In fact, patients receiving TLI doses that produced the most profound lymphopenia had the most improvement, although it was transient, in their MS symptoms.[22–26] Furthermore, craniospinal irradiation to high doses is used to treat CNS leukemia and there is little evidence that there is hemorrhage or other acute toxicities at lesion sites as a result of the irradiation. For these reasons it was felt that a regimen containing TBI could be used, thereby achieving the maximum possible immunosuppression in the CNS. Other groups in the USA have proposed using busulfan and cyclophosphamide. However, busulfan has relatively little immunosuppressive effects compared to TBI.[27–29] As described earlier, European groups have agreed on BEAM, although in the authors' opinion the BEAM regimen would not be expected to penetrate the CNS as reliably as TBI.

Procurement of stem cells

Initially, it was planned to harvest bone marrow by multiple bone marrow aspirations with the patient under anesthesia. This was modified after inadequate harvests were achieved in the first three patients, for reasons that are unclear. The protocol was modified to mobilize stem cells by administering G-CSF to the patients and collecting stem cells by apheresis; subsequent bone marrow harvest was performed only if needed to supplement the PBSC.

In vitro T-cell purge

In the phase 1 study, the CellPro Ceprate® column that selects for cells bearing the CD34 antigen was used. With this procedure, the authors routinely achieved > 2-log depletion of T cells with good recovery of the CD34+ cells.

Patient selection

It was anticipated that the best results from immunoablation and HSCT would occur in younger patients with a short duration of progressive disease and a low burden of neurologic deficits. Since gadolinium enhancement on magnetic resonance imaging (MRI) indicates blood–brain barrier breakdown at areas of acute inflammation, it was also anticipated that patients with gadolinium-enhancing lesions on MRI would be more likely to respond than patients with non-enhancing plaques, which represent areas of axonal degeneration and glial scarring. T2-weighted hyperintensities are histologically nonspecific, with underlying pathology ranging from non-destructive edema to significant myelin or axonal loss and gliosis. To prevent inherent bias in outcome due to spontaneous fluctuation of disease, patients with relapsing–remitting disease were not considered to be candidates for HSCT in this study. Since variable relapse and progression rates with spontaneous remissions could limit the determination of treatment efficacy (a secondary end-point in this phase 1 study), patients with progressive disease, severe impairments, and marked deterioration in their baseline neurologic function during the 12 months before enrollment were chosen. All

immunosuppressive and immunomodulatory medications were stopped before transplantation.

The neurological criteria for entry into the study were:
(a) an established clinical diagnosis of MS;
(b) a Kurtzke EDSS score of 5.0–8.0 at the time of pre-transplant evaluation and an increase in score by 1.5 points over the previous 12 months in patients with an EDSS score ≤5.5 at the start of the evaluation period, or an increase of 1.0 points in patients with an EDSS score ≥6 at the start of the evaluation period;
(c) failure to stabilize active clinical progression with intravenous methylprednisolone given for a minimum of 3 days at 1 g/day.

Although not mandatory, selecting patients with evidence of active disease as reflected by blood–brain barrier disruption on MRI (gadolinium enhancement) in either the spinal cord or the brain was stressed.

Results

Nine patients have been transplanted and are now 7–28 months post-transplant. Eight patients had secondary progressive MS and one had primary progressive disease. Seven of the nine had enhancing lesions present just before transplantation was performed. All had rapid, cumulative impairment or disability during the year before transplant and all had failed corticosteroid therapy and other immunomodulatory therapies. The EDSS scores just before transplant ranged from 6.0 to 8.5 (five patients had EDSS scores ≥ 8.0).

Harvest of bone marrow from the first three patients was performed with the patients receiving general anesthesia and was without incident. However, insufficient CD34+ cells were obtained (< 2 × 10^6 per kg) after selection on the Ceprate®

columns. These patients and subsequent ones were mobilized with G-CSF and generally one apheresis collection was sufficient 5 days later to obtain the required number of cells. No increase in MS symptoms related to G-CSF during the mobilization phase was noted.

All patients received cyclophosphamide (60 mg/kg) daily for 2 days, followed by TBI administered 150 cGy twice per day for 4 days (a total of 1200 cGy). Methylprednisolone (1 g) was given on the same days as the TBI. This pre-transplant regimen was well tolerated and there were no MS-specific toxicities. Stem cells were infused the day after TBI ended. G-CSF was chosen over GM-CSF as a post-transplant growth factor because of the known maturing and activating influence of GM-CSF on dendritic cells involved in antigen presentation. The authors wanted to minimize the potential of immunizing the new immune system with CNS antigens. The

median time to reach absolute neutrophil counts > 500 cells/μl and platelet counts > 20,000 cells/μl was 10 days and 14 days, respectively. Peri-transplant infections were not unusual in type or numbers for autologous BMT.

Since transplant, no patients have received immunosuppressive or immunomodulatory medications. MRI scans with gadolinium are performed on a schedule at 3, 6, 12, 18, and 24 months post-transplant and to date none have shown new lesions or gadolinium-enhancing lesions. All patients have had stabilization of their disease and in some cases slight improvement in motor function (*Table 27.1*).

Preliminary conclusions from the phase 1 study

The authors' preliminary conclusions are:

(a) the use of PBSC is preferable to bone marrow as a source of stem cells for these transplants;

Table 27.1 Phase 1 study results (February 1999)

Patient	Months post-HSCT	Number of relapses	Pre-HSCT EDSS and most recent EDSS	Pre-HSCT NRS and most recent NRS	MRI findings
1	28	0	8.5/8.5	15/16	No new lesions
2	28	0	8.0/8.0	30/29	No new lesions
3	24	0	8.0/8.0	34/37	No new lesions
4	18	0	6.5/6.0	49/63	No new lesions
5	15	0	7.0/6.5	29/38	No new lesions
6	15	0	6.0/6.0	51/61	No new lesions
7	9	0	7.0/*	67/*	No new lesions
8	7	0	8.0/*	33/*	*
9	7	0	8.5/8.5	17/24	No new lesions

* Pending current evaluation.

(b) mobilization of stem cells with G-CSF has been well tolerated by these patients;

(c) TBI can be safely employed in the immunoablative regimen without observable CNS toxicities specific for MS;

(d) despite a median 2.3-log depletion of T cells using the Ceprate® CD34+ selection system as a method of T-cell depletion, engraftment has occurred rapidly in these patients and no unexpected infections have been encountered;

(e) the use of this treatment regimen has resulted in no MS-specific toxicities and appears at this point to be a well-tolerated regimen.

Although the main purpose of the phase 1 study was to determine toxicities and feasibility, it is also notable as a secondary observation that the disease has stabilized in all nine patients treated to date, although the follow-up is short (median 1 year). Furthermore, no patients have received immunosuppressive or immunomodulatory drugs since their transplant. Gadolinium-enhancing MRI lesions that were present at the time of transplant have not been present after transplant, and no new lesions have been observed.

Future studies

On the basis of the two published reports reviewed here, phase 2 clinical trials are indicated. Neither of these trials revealed MS-specific toxicities associated with the transplant procedures. The transplant-related toxicities and risks were acceptable to patients and investigators, given the poor prognoses of progressive MS and the limited therapeutic options. Future trials should be done under carefully considered protocols that further establish the toxicities and benefits for well-defined patient populations. These trials should incorporate correlative laboratory studies that examine the degree of immunosuppression and the characteristics of immune reconstitution after transplantation so that the reasons for success or failure can be determined and further improvements in the procedure can be made. These studies should also enable comparison of different preparative regimens and of different methodologies of lymphocyte purging. It is important for future studies to incorporate the vast amount of information that has been gained in recent therapeutic trials of MS that relate to study design (often specific to MS), and to include disease measurement and outcome definitions. This will require close collaboration between the bone marrow transplant and neurology communities.

IMPLICATIONS FOR CLINICAL PRACTICE

Immunoablative therapy followed by stem cell reconstitution represents a new approach to the treatment of MS. The therapy is based on experience with immunoreconstitution following autologous and allogeneic HSCT and the understanding that reconstitution of the hematopoietic system may not follow the same course of development as had led to the onset of the disease. As described above, the preliminary results appear promising. A deeper understanding of the therapy is needed to determine the extent to which it can be a viable alternative to other treatment modalities. Therefore these transplants should only be performed in carefully conceived clinical trials.

It is important that the patient selection criteria and availability of these trials be widely distributed to neurologists. Where appropriate, neurologists should be encouraged to enter patients into these trials so that the role of this procedure can be determined as quickly as possible. Definitive clinical trials to define the role of stem cell transplants for breast cancer have been difficult because the availability of the procedure was established before the efficacy studies could be performed. Only now, years later, are these studies maturing to the point of definitive interpretations. There is the danger that this scenario will be repeated for MS. Hence, participation in rigorous clinical trials is considered essential to progress in this field.

ACKNOWLEDGEMENTS

We wish to thank the following for their collaboration in our study: Lorri Lobeck, Bruce Cohen, Cass Terry, Karin Karlin, Henry McFarland, and Jerry Wolinsky.

REFERENCES

1 van Bekkum DW. BMT in experimental autoimmune diseases. *Bone Marrow Transplant* 1993; **11**:183–187.

2 Slavin S, Karussis D, Weiss L et al. Immunohematopoietic reconstitution by allogeneic and autologous bone marrow grafts as a means for induction of specific unresponsiveness to donor-specific allografts and modified self in autoimmune disorders. *Transplant Proc* 1993; **25**:1274–1275.

3 Marmont AM. Immune ablation followed by allogeneic or autologous bone marrow transplantation: a new treatment for severe autoimmune diseases? *Stem Cells* 1994; **12**:125–135.

4 Ikehara S. Intractable diseases and bone marrow transplantation. *Pathol Int* 1994; **44**:817–826.

5 Burt RK, Burns W, Hess A. Bone marrow transplantation for multiple sclerosis. *Bone Marrow Transplant* 1995; **16**:1–6.

6 Marmont AM, van Bekkum DW. Stem cell

transplantation for severe autoimmune diseases: new proposals but still unanswered questions. *Bone Marrow Transplant* 1995; **16**:497–498.

7 Tyndall A, Gratwohl A. Haematopoietic stem cell and progenitor cells in the treatment of severe autoimmune diseases. *Ann Rheum Dis* 1996; **55**:149–151.

8 Burt RK, Burns WH, Miller SD. Bone marrow transplantation for multiple sclerosis: returning to Pandora's box. *Immunol Today* 1997; **18**:559–561.

9 Baldwin JL, Storb R, Thomas ED, Mannik M. Bone marrow transplantation in patients with gold-induced marrow aplasia. *Arthritis Rheum* 1977; **20**:1043–1048.

10 Jacobs P, Vincent MD, Martell RW. Prolonged remission of severe refractory rheumatoid arthritis following allogeneic bone marrow transplantation for drug induced aplastic anemia. *Bone Marrow Transplant* 1986; **1**:237–239.

11 Lui Yin JA, Jowitt SN. Resolution of immune-mediated diseases following bone marrow transplantation for leukemia. *Bone Marrow Transplant* 1992; **9**:31–33.

12 Lowenthal RM, Cohen ML, Atkinson K, Biggs JC. Apparent cure of rheumatoid arthritis by bone marrow transplantation. *J Rheumatol* 1993; **20**:137–140.

13 Karussis DM, Vourka-Karussis U, Lehmann D et al. Prevention and reversal of adoptively transferred, chronic relapsing experimental autoimmune encehalomyelitis with a single high dose cytoreductive treatment followed by syngeneic bone marrow transplantation. *J Clin Invest* 1993; **92**:765–772.

14 van Gelder M, Kinwel-Bohre EP, van Bekkum DW. Treatment of experimental allergic encephalomyelitis in rats with total body irradiation and syngeneic BMT. *Bone Marrow Transplant* 1993; **11**:233–241.

15 Burt RK, Burns W, Ruvolo P et al. Syngeneic bone marrow transplantation eliminates V beta 8.2 T lymphocytes from the spinal cord of Lewis rats with experimental allergic encephalomyelitis. *J Neurosci Res* 1995; **41**:526–531.

16 van Gelder M, van Bekkum DW. Effective treatment of relapsing experimental autoimmune encephalomyelitis with pseudoautologous bone marrow transplantation. *Bone Marrow Transplant* 1996; **18**:1029–1034.

17 Acha-Orbea H, Mitchell DJ, Timmermann L et al. Limited heterogeneity of T cell receptors from lymphocytes mediating autoimmune encehphalomyelitis allows specific immune intervention. *Cell* 1988; **54**:263–273.

18 Burns FR, Li XB, Shen N et al. Both rat and mouse T cell receptors specific for the encephalitogenic determinant of myelin basic protein use similar V alpha and V beta chain genes even though the major histocompatibility complex and encephalitogenic determinants being recognized are different. *J Exp Med* 1989; **169**:27–39.

19 Burt RK, Traynor AE, Cohen B et al. T cell-depleted autologous hematopoietic stem cell transplantation for multiple sclerosis: report on the first three patients. *Bone Marrow Transplant* 1998; **21**:537–541.

20 Burt RK, Traynor AE, Pope R et al. Treatment of autoimmune disease by intense immunosuppressive conditioning and autologous hematopoietic stem cell transplantation. *Blood* 1998; **92**:3505–3514.

21 Fassas A, Anagnostopoulos A, Kazis A et al. Peripheral blood stem cell transplantation in the treatment of progressive multiple sclerosis: first results of a pilot study. *Bone Marrow Transplant* 1997; **20**:631–638.

22 Devereux CK, Vidaver R, Hafstein MP et al. Total lymphoid irradiation for multiple sclerosis. *Intl J Rad Oncol Biol Phys* 1988; **14**:197–203.

23 Devereux C, Troiano R, Zito G et al. Effect of total lymphoid irradiation on functional status in chronic multiple sclerosis: importance of lymphopenia early after treatment – the pros. *Neurology* 1988; **38** (**suppl 2**):32–37.

24 Cook SD, Devereux C, Troiano R et al. Effect of lymphoid irradiation on clinical course, lymphocyte count, and T-cell subsets in chronic progressive multiple sclerosis. *Ann N Y Acad Sci* 1988; **540**:533–534.

25 Cook SD, Devereux C, Troiano R et al. Total lymphoid irradiation in multiple sclerosis: blood lymphocytes and clinical course. *Ann Neurol* 1987; **22**:634–638.

26 Cook SD, Devereux C, Troiano R et al. Effect of total lymphoid irradiation in chronic progressive multiple sclerosis. *Lancet* 1986; **1**:1405–1409.

27 Santos GW, Tutschka PJ. Effect of busulfan on antibody production and skin allograft survival in the rat. *J Natl Cancer Inst* 1974; **53**:1775–1780.

28 Tutschka PJ, Santos GW. Bone marrow transplantation in the busulfan-treated rat. I. Effect of cyclophosphamide and rabbit anti-rat thymocyte serum as immunosuppression. *Transplantation* 1975; **20**:101–106.

29 Tutschka PJ, Santos GW. Bone marrow transplantation in the busulfan-treated rat. II. Effect of cyclophosphamide and antithymic serum on the presensitized state. *Transplantation* 1975; **20**:116–122.

28
Emerging disease-modifying therapies

Emmanuelle Waubant and Donald E Goodkin

This chapter reviews published results of phase 1 and 2 trials of selected promising disease-modifying therapies for multiple sclerosis (MS) (*Table 28.1*). Treatments that target the cytokine environment are reviewed first, followed by treatments that may stabilize the blood–brain barrier. Finally, treatments directed against inflammatory cells (either by targeting autoreactive T cells or the tri-molecular complex are reviewed). A list of on-going studies for which there are no published data in patients with MS is also provided (*Table 28.2*).

THERAPIES THAT TARGET CYTOKINES

Transforming growth factor-β2

Rationale and mode of action
Transforming growth factor (TGF)-β is a pleiotropic cytokine that down-regulates interferon (IFN)-γ-induced class II major histocompatibility complex (MHC) expression, inhibits generation of cytotoxic lymphocytes, and possibly inhibits tumor necrosis factor (TNF)-α. TGF-β 1 and TGF-β 2 suppress experimental allergic encephalomyelitis (EAE), and anti-TGF antibodies exacerbate the disease.[23,24] TGF-β expression has been associated with clinical remission of MS.[25,26]

Study design
Twelve patients with clinically definite MS have been treated with recombinant TGF-β 2 (Celtrix Pharmaceuticals, Santa Clara, California, USA) administered intravenously at doses of 0.2 µg/kg, 0.6 µg/kg, and 2.0 µg/kg three times weekly for up to 4 weeks.[27] Primary outcome was tolerability and secondary outcomes included Expanded Disability Status Score (EDSS) and MRI activity.

Results
Eleven patients completed this study. Only two patients receiving 2.0 µg/kg completed therapy because of toxicity, and three patients were added to the 0.6 µg/kg cohort. A transient anemia was reported in 10 patients during the dosing period. Five patients had a more than three-fold increase in their transaminase levels, which lasted up to 8 weeks after discontinuing the drug. Serum creatinine levels were increased in four patients. Three patients (two in the 0.6 µg/kg group and one in the 2.0 µg/kg group) discontinued injections because of a decline in glomerular filtration; this returned to normal 4 weeks after discontinuing therapy. Two patients developed transient hypertension. One patient

Table 28.1 Available and emerging disease-modifying therapies

Therapeutic strategy	Treatment options	Putative mechanisms of action
Global immunosuppression		
	Cyclophosphamide*	Globally reduces T-cell population
	Azathioprine*	
	Methotrexate*	
	Total lymphoid irradiation*	
	2-Chlorodeoxyadenosine*	
	Mitoxantrone*	
	Glucocorticosteroids*	
	Paclitaxel[†]	
Immunomodulation		
Inhibit interaction between T-cell receptor, peptide, and MHC class II molecules	Copolymer[‡] Altered peptide ligands[†]	Blocks or competes with the binding of encephalitogenic peptides to the MHC class II molecule
	TCR vaccination and TCR peptide vaccination[†]	Generates antibodies against peptides within the T-cell receptor
	IL-10,[†] TGF-β,[†] IFN-β[‡]	Immunomodulation; reduces MHC class II molecule expression
Induce T-cell anergy	Antibodies to B7 or CD28 molecules[§]	T-cells are anergized when interaction between the T-cell receptor, the peptide and the MHC class II molecule occurs in the absence of co-signaling
	Soluble MHC-II/peptide complexes[†]	
Delete autoreactive T cells	Anti-CD4, anti-CD52[†]	Depletes T cells targeted by the antibodies
Reduce T-cell trafficking across blood–brain barrier	Glucocorticosteroids TGF-β,[†] IFN-β[‡]	Decreases the expression of adhesion molecules on T cells and vascular endothelial cells
	Antibodies to adhesion molecules (Antegren, anti-CD11/CD18)[¶]	Decreases the attachment of T cells to vascular endothelial cells
	Matrix metalloprotease inhibitors,[†] IFN-β[‡]	Inhibits proteases that facilitate T-cell trafficking across the blood–brain barrier

Alter the balance of pro-inflammatory (T-helper 1) and immunomodulatory (T-helper 2) cytokines	Antibodies to TNF-α,[†] IL-1,[†] Soluble IL-2 or TNF-α receptors Antagonists to IL-1 receptor[§]	Reduces pro-inflammatory (T-helper 1) cytokine activity
	Oral myelin[¶]	Increases immunomodulatory (T-helper 2) cytokine production
	IFN-β,[‡] IFN-α[†]	Antagonize production of pro-inflammatory cytokines induced by IFN-γ
	Glucocorticosteroids[*]	Reduces T-helper 1 cytokine secretion and macrophage function
	Matrix metalloprotease inhibitors[†]	Blocks cleavage of pro-TNF to TNF
	Methotrexate[*]	Reduces level of soluble IL-2 receptor
	Intravenous immunoglobulin[*]	Reduces pro-inflammatory cytokines
	Anti-CD40 ligand[§]	Blocks T-helper 1 differentiation and effector function, inhibits IFN-γ production
	Roquinimex (Linomide)[¶]	Inhibits TNF production
Neuroprotection	Riluzole,[†] IGF-1,[†] Eliprodil[†]	Prevents neuronal death
Reduce gliosis	Pirfenidone[†]	Prevents gliosis; blocks TNF synthesis
Promote remyelination	Insulin-like growth factor[†]	Promotes oligodendrocyte survival and maturation of precursors in vitro
	Intravenous immunoglobulin[*¶] Oligodendrocyte grafts[§] Eliprodil[§]	Promotes remyelination

[*] Unlabeled use in the USA and Europe.
[†] Phase I-II clinical trials.
[‡] Approved for use in relapsing forms of MS in the USA and Europe.
[§] Preclinical testing.
[¶] Phase III clinical trials.

Adapted from Waubant et al 1997.[1]

Table 28.2 On-going studies for which there are no published data in patients with MS

Drug	Mode of action	Design of trial	Form of MS	Primary outcome(s)	Secondary outcome(s)	Sponsor
Antegren™	Prevents leukocyte migration to central nervous system	Placebo-controlled	Treatment of relapse	Time to recovery	New gadolinium-enhancing MRI lesions	Athena
BB-3644 [2–6]	Matrix metallo protease inhibitor; prevents leukocyte migration to central nervous system	Double-blind, dose comparison	(Healthy volunteers)	Tolerance; safety	Pharmakokinetic parameters	British Biotech
Insulin growth factor-1	Prevents inflammation, promotes remyelination and neuroprotection	Open-label, single cross-over	RRMS SPMS	MRI activity	MRI lesion load; magnetization transfer ratio; magnetic resonance spectroscopy; EDSS; immunologic function	Cephalon
IL-10 [13–16]	Immunomodulation	Placebo-controlled	Relapsing MS	Tolerance; safety	new gadolinium-enhancing MRI lesions	Schering–Plough
Paclitaxel [17,18]	Suppresses T cells, Inhibits MMP	Open-label Dose comparison	SPMS	Tolerance; safety	Disability; MRI parameters	Angiotech
Pirfenidone [19]	Antigliotic Anti-TNF	Open-label	SPMS	EDSS; Scripps	New MRI lesions; Quality of Life	Marnac
Riluzole [20–22]	Neuroprotection	Open-label, single cross-over	PPMS	Tolerance; safety	MRI atrophy; EDSS	Rhone–Poulenc–Rorer

developed bilateral maculopathy that resolved 1 month after treatment. EDSS scores and MRI activity did not change significantly over 25 weeks.

Comments
TGF-β 2 as administered in this pilot study was associated with significant drug-related adverse events and there was no suggestion of efficacy.

Tumor necrosis factor-α antagonists

Rationale and mode of action
Tumor necrosis factor (TNF) is a pro-inflammatory cytokine produced by macrophages, T cells, and astrocytes. In vitro, TNF α causes selective damage to myelin and oligodendrocytes,[28] induces gliotic proliferation,[29] and up-regulates expression of MHC class II molecules and adhesion molecules on vascular endothelial cells and macrophages. Blood mononuclear TNF-α production appears to increase before the onset of an acute exacerbation[30] but not before new MRI activity.[31] Administration of soluble TNF-α receptors[32] or TNF-α antibodies[29,33] prevents EAE.

Study design
TNF-α antagonists have been evaluated in patients with MS in phase 1 and phase 2 studies. In the phase 1 study, two patients with rapidly progressive MS were treated with two alternate weekly intravenous infusions of humanized chimeric mouse monoclonal antibody cA2 (Centocor Inc, Malvern, Pennsylvania, USA).[34] The primary outcome was tolerability. Secondary outcome measures included the number of new T2-weighted and gadolinium-enhancing MRI lesions, the EDSS score, and the number of cells and IgG index in the cerebrospinal fluid (CSF).

In the phase 2 trial,[35] 167 patients with relapsing–remitting MS (RRMS) and secondary progressive MS (SPMS) received placebo or Lenercept (sTNFR–IgG p55; Roche, Basel, Switzerland) administered intravenously at doses of 10 mg, 50 mg, and 100 mg each month as part of a 48-week study. The primary outcome was tolerability. Secondary outcome measures included MRI and neurological evaluations.

Results
In the phase 1 study, infusions were clinically well tolerated. One patient developed transient hypotension during infusions. Neurological examination findings were unchanged. The number of gadolinium-enhancing lesions appeared to increase in both the patients after the first infusion compared to a baseline MRI. CSF lymphocytes counts and IgG index were higher after treatment than before treatment.[34]

In the phase 2 study,[35] transient episodes of flushing and dyspnea occurred after the injection of Lenercept at doses of 50 mg and 100 mg. An increase in the occurrence of headaches was noted at all doses. The number of patients with exacerbations and the total number of exacerbations were greater in the active treatment groups (respectively, $p = 0.007$, chi-square; $p = 0.009$, Kruskal–Wallis test). Additionally, when compared to placebo recipients, the time to first relapse was shorter in Lenercept recipients. The changes in EDSS scores after 24 weeks and 48 weeks of treatment did not differ across treatment groups. Although analysis of the MRI activity (new active lesions, percentage of active scans and burden of disease) was similar across treatment groups, high-dose recipients may have experienced more MRI activity than low-dose recipients.

Comments

Despite suggestion that TNF-α production is increased before clinical exacerbations, Lenercept as administered in this study appeared to increase disease activity.

THERAPIES THAT TARGET THE BLOOD–BRAIN BARRIER

Antegren™

Rationale and mode of action

Increased expression of adhesion molecules facilitates attachment of inflammatory cells to vascular endothelial cells and transmigration through blood vessel walls into the central nervous system (CNS). Antegren™ (Elan Pharmaceuticals; South San Francisco, CA, USA) is a humanized monoclonal antibody to α4β1 integrin that blocks the interaction of very late antigen 4 (VLA-4), an adhesion molecule found on activated leukocytes, with vascular cell adhesion molecule 1 (VCAM-1), an adhesion molecule expressed on endothelial cells, thereby preventing development of EAE in Lewis rats.[36]

Study design

Antegren™ has been evaluated in patients with MS in phase 1 and phase 2 studies. In the phase 1 study,[37] 28 patients with stable RRMS or SPMS were randomized to groups of four treated incrementally with a single dose of Antegren™, 0.03 mg/kg, 0.1 mg/kg, 0.3 mg/kg, or with placebo, and groups of eight treated with Antegren™, 1.0 mg/kg or 3.0 mg/kg drug, or with placebo. In each group, 75% of the patients received the active drug and 25% the placebo. The primary outcome was tolerability. Secondary outcomes were EDSS for all patients, brain MRI scans in the groups receiving the 1.0 mg/kg and 3.0 mg/kg of the active drug, Antegren™ pharmacokinetics, and total and neutralizing anti-Antegren™ antibody levels.

In the phase 2 trial,[38] 72 patients with RRMS or SPMS were randomly assigned to treatment with Antegren™ 3 mg/kg or placebo, administered intravenously at weeks 0 and 4. The primary outcome was MRI activity, which was measured at weeks −4, 0, 1, 2, 4, 6, 8, 12, 16, 20, and 24.

Results

In the phase 1 study,[37] mild headache, pain, nausea, sore throat, upper respiratory infections, and fatigue were reported with similar frequency in both treatment groups. Three patients reporting five events were considered drug related: headache, nausea (in two patients), shakiness, and urticaria. All these events were mild and transient. No treatment effect was detected by EDSS or brain MRI outcomes. Three patients who received 3.0 mg/kg Antegren™ had detectable immune response against the drug at week 8, and this reponse persisted in two patients at week 12.

In the phase 2 trial,[38] formation of new gadolinium-enhancing lesions was significantly reduced ($p < 0.017$) in Antegren™ recipients for up to 12 weeks. Antegren™ levels were undetectable beyond week 8. Total numbers of adverse events were comparable in the Antegren™ and placebo groups. No evidence of efficacy was detected by EDSS or Guy's Neurological Disability Ratings.

Comments

Antegren™ as administered in these studies was generally well tolerated. Although a treatment effect was evident by MRI, there was no evidence of clinical efficacy. Results of a second study are awaited with interest (see *Table 28.2*).

Anti-CD11–CD18 antibodies

Rationale and mode of action

The CD11–CD18 integrin mediates leukocyte adhesion and migration. Treatment of rodent and primate EAE with monoclonal antibodies to CD11–CD18, Hu23F2G (LeukArrest™) (ICOS, Bothel, Washington, USA) suggests clinical efficacy and a reduction in brain MRI lesion area.

Study design

LeukArrest™ has been tested in phase 1 and phase 2 studies. Twenty-four patients with primary progressive MS (PPMS) and or SPMS were enrolled in an uncontrolled phase 1 single dose escalation study of intravenous drug at doses 0.01–4.0 mg/kg.[39] The primary outcome was safety. Secondary outcome measures included pharmacology, immunogenicity of the drug, brain MRI, and clinical evaluation.

In the phase 2 study,[40] 169 patients were randomly assigned to intravenous treatment with placebo (43 patients), methylprednisolone 1 g daily for 3 days (41 patients), LeukArrest™ 1 mg/kg (44 patients), or LeukArrest™ 2 mg/kg (41 patients) within 7 days of onset of acute exacerbation. Efficacy end-points included change in Neurologic Rating Scale and EDSS from day 0 to day 90, and change in brain MRI activity from day 0 to day 5.

Results

In the phase 1 trial,[39] adverse events included two cases of urinary tract infection and two cases of gingivitis. Six of 12 patients receiving the three highest doses had transient leukocytosis. A marked decrease in leukocyte migration in response to cutaneous inflammation was found in eight of nine patients after treatment with Hu23F2G 1.0 mg/kg, 2.0 mg/kg or 4.0 mg/kg.

No antibodies against Hu23F2G were detected. No significant disease activity was detected clinically or by brain MRI.

In the phase 2 study,[40] no treatment effect was evident by clinical or MRI measures. However, the proportion of patients rescued with methylprednisolone was significantly lower in the methylprednisolone recipients than in the placebo and LeukArrest™ groups: 35% in the placebo group, 15% in the methylprednisolone group, 43% in the group that received LeukArrest™ 1 mg/kg, and 29% in the group that received LeukArrest™ 2 mg/kg.

Comments

Treatment with LeukArrest™ was tolerated at doses that achieved high degrees of leukocyte CD11/CD18 saturation.[39] LeukArrest™ as administered in the phase 2 study did not hasten recovery of exacerbations.[40] However, patients treated with methylprednisolone were less likely to require corticosteroid rescue for exacerbations of MS. Another phase 2 study with various doses is on-going.

THERAPIES THAT ACT BY DELETION OF AUTOREACTIVE T CELLS

Anti-CD4 antibodies

Rationale and mode of action

The CD4 molecule is a co-receptor that is involved in presentation of antigens to T cells. Activated CD4+ T cells are believed to play a major role in the development of EAE and MS. Deletion of CD4+ T cells by treatment with antibodies to CD4 prevents onset of EAE and delays relapses in established EAE.[41,42]

Study design

Anti-CD4 antibodies have been tested in patients with MS in phase 1 and phase 2 studies. In the phase 1 study,[43] 29 patients with MS were enrolled in an open-label, dose-escalating trial of cM-T412, a chimeric murine–human monoclonal anti-CD4 antibody. The first 25 patients received a single intravenous infusion of cM-T412, five each receiving 10 mg, 50 mg, 100 mg, 150 mg, and 200 mg. The last four patients each received three doses of 50 mg every other day. The primary outcome was tolerability. Secondary outcomes included EDSS, number of T2-weighted and gadolinium-enhancing MRI lesions, lymphocyte count, cM-T412 pharmacokinetics, and immune response against cM-T412.

In the first phase 2 study,[44] 21 patients with MS (both RRMS and SPMS) were enrolled to receive 100 mg of cM-T412 each month for three months. The primary outcome was the number of new lesions on serial brain MRIs. In the second phase 2 study,[23] 71 patients with RRMS or SPMS were randomly assigned to intravenous treatment with placebo or cM-T412 50 mg monthly for 6 months.[45] The primary outcome was the number of new gadolinium-enhancing lesions and new or enlarging T2-weighted lesions during 9-monthly MRI scans.

Results

In the phase 1 study,[43] the treatment was well tolerated but the majority of patients noted mild flu-like symptoms following the infusion. The most common side effects were headache, nausea, myalgia, fever, and tachycardia occurring in the first few hours of treatment. CD4+ lymphopenia lasted for 6 or more months. EDSS scores remained stable 6 months after therapy. No statistical difference could be demonstrated in the number of gadolinium-enhancing lesions on serial MRI scans during the period of low CD4+ T-cell counts. Twenty-three percent of the patients had a transient low titer of antibodies to cM-T412.

In the first phase 2 study,[44] because cM-T412 depleted CD4+ T-cell counts more effectively than expected, most patients received only one or two of the planned treatments. The 21 patients received 36 treatments, with only two patients receiving all three planned doses. Seventeen patients experienced a prolonged decrease in CD4+ T-cell counts for longer than 4 months. MRI measures were not significantly affected by treatment. Most patients were clinically stable 1 year after treatment.

In the second phase 2 study,[45] there was no significant effect of therapy on MRI activity. However, patients with lower CD4+ T-cell counts developed significantly fewer active lesions over 18 months ($p = 0.04$) than patients with higher CD4+ T-cell counts. There was also a decrease in the number of clinical relapses in anti-CD4 antibody recipients ($p = 0.02$), but the study was not effectively blinded. EDSS score and the number of intravenous methylprednisolone treatments were not affected by treatment. Some patients experienced a transient increase in the severity of pre-existing neurologic symptoms after infusions.

Comments

CD4 antibody therapy as administered in these studies was safe and may decrease clinical activity of the disease.

Anti-CDw52 antibodies

Rationale and mode of action

CD52 is a pan-lymphocyte glycoprotein, the function of which is unknown. It is also found on some monocytic populations. Anti-CDw52 antibody (CAMPATH-1H (Leuko Sites, UK)) is a humanized antibody to CD52. It causes a rapid induction of intense lymphopenia.[46]

Study design

Seven patients with SPMS or PPMS were enrolled in an open-label trial[46,47] of 10 days (interrupted by a weekend) of a daily intravenous infusion of 12 mg CAMPATH-1H. The primary outcome was tolerability. Secondary outcomes were neurologic examination, number and size of new gadolinium-enhancing lesions and new or enlarging T2-weighted lesions on MRI.

In the open-label phase 2 trial,[48] 27 patients received a single pulse of intravenous CAMPATH-1H. The primary outcome was change in MRI activity.

Results

In the phase 1 study,[46,47] lymphopenia was rapid and profound within hours of the first infusion in all patients, and it lasted at least 6 months. There was a decrease in MRI activity after treatment compared to before treatment.[46] Seven more patients were later added to the initial study,[47] and 12 of the 14 patients exhibited worsening of pre-existing symptoms lasting several hours after the first infusion. This correlated with increased levels of TNF-α, INF-γ, and IL-6 in serum. The two patients who did not experience this clinical worsening or the increased serum levels of pro-inflammatory cytokines had been pre-medicated with intravenous methylprednisolone (500 mg).

The phase 2 study[48] demonstrated a 50% reduction in MRI activity, but patients continued to worsen clinically. One third of the patients developed autoimmune thyroid (Grave's) disease.

Comments

CAMPATH-1H showed preliminary evidence of efficacy as measured by decreased MRI activity.

IMMUNOTHERAPIES THAT TARGET THE 'TRIMOLECULAR COMPLEX'

Antigen presentation modifiers

Rationale and mode of action

Myelin basic protein (MBP[84–102]) is an immunodominant peptide epitope of MBP. An in vitro study[49] has indicated that peripheral blood T cells cloned from MS patients who are responsive to MBP[84–102] are rendered non-reactive or undergo apoptosis following incubation with HLA-DR2:MBP[84–102] complexes. Administration of soluble MHC class II–peptide complexes to mice with chronic relapsing EAE ameliorates disease in a dose-dependent manner. Soluble MHC molecules loaded with MBP[84–102] (AG284; Anergen Inc, Redwood City, California, USA) may render T cells in MS unresponsive to MBP[84–102] and prevent new MS lesions.

Study design

Thirty-three patients with SPMS heterozygous for HLA-DR2(B1*1501) were grouped into cohorts of four (one to receive placebo, three to receive AG284) and randomly assigned to three alternate-day identical doses of intravenous placebo or AG284. The patients were observed for 12 weeks after the first infusion.[50] Cohorts were treated sequentially, and the dose of AG284 increased in stages (0.6 μg/kg, 2.0 μg/kg, 6.0 μg/kg, 20.0 μg/kg, 60.0 μg/kg, 105 μg/kg, 150 μg/kg). The primary outcome was tolerability. Secondary outcomes included the number and area of new focal gadolinium-enhancing lesions and T2-weighted lesions on MRI (MRIs were done on days −25, −4, 7, and 28), EDSS, 9-Hole Peg Test, and T-cell reactivity (on ELISPOT assay) to whole MBP and MBP[84–102].

Results

There was no dose-limiting toxicity. The number and severity of exacerbations and the number of treatments with intravenous methylprednisolone were similar across treatment groups. None of the other adverse events, which included headache, pain at the injection site, cardiac flow murmurs, hypertonia, urinary tract infections, and low absolute lymphocyte counts, was clinically significant, and the proportion of subjects experiencing adverse events was similar across treatment groups.

There were no differences between groups in change in clinical or MRI measures and there was no trend suggesting change in clinical or MRI measures related to the dose of AG284.

After controlling for the occurrence of exacerbations, a significant treatment effect was observed as measured by the number of T2-weighted lesions on MRI. This result should be interpreted cautiously since the number of subjects experiencing new T2-weighted lesions was small. Further, this apparent treatment effect was not evident when measured by the number or area of new gadolinium-enhancing lesions.

No serum antibody to HLA-DR developed after treatment with AG284. The result of T-cell reactivity is not yet available.

Comments

AG284 as administered in this study is safe and well tolerated. Exploratory analyses suggest a possible treatment effect measured by the number of new T2-weighted lesions. Further studies of AG284 as a promising treatment for MS are warranted.

Altered peptide ligands

Rationale and mode of action

Altered peptide ligands (APLs), which may differ by as few as one or two amino acids from the peptide generating the full immune response, can bind to the T-cell receptor without triggering complete T-cell activation. Some APLs can modulate the cytokine pattern of T cells and reverse EAE.[51] Some can induce a form of 'anergy' in T cells.[52]

CGP 77116 (Novartis, Basel, Switzerland, Neurocrine Biosciences, San Diego, CA, USA) is an APL based on the immunodominant epitope of human MBP. Immune responses directed against this epitope may be involved in the pathogenesis of MS. In vitro, CGP 77116 fails to induce T-cell proliferation and selectively reduces the production of inflammatory cytokines by pathogenic T cells. In the EAE model, CGP 77116 markedly reduces the severity of disease and induces a specific T-cell response that downregulates the inflammatory process.

Study design

Thirty patients with RRMS or SPMS were treated in a phase 1, double-blind, placebo-controlled, dose-escalation study.[53] Seven patients received placebo and 23 patients received CGP 77116 (at doses of 1 mg, 3 mg, 10 mg, 20 mg, or 50 mg) subcutaneously once a week for 4 consecutive weeks; they were followed for 12 weeks after the first injection. The primary outcome was tolerability. Secondary outcome measures included EDSS and gadolinium-enhanced brain MRI scans.

Results

CGP 77116 (now called MSP771) was in general well tolerated, with the most common side effect being local, transient injection site reactions. There were no significant changes on the MRI measures or on the EDSS scores during the period of the study.

Comments

CGP 77116 in doses up to 50 mg appears to be well tolerated. Studies to evaluate safety and efficacy further are on-going.

VACCINATION WITH T CELLS OR T-CELL RECEPTOR PEPTIDE

Rationale and mode of action

There is a restricted use of T-cell receptor genes for autoantigen presentation in EAE[54] and possibly in MS.[55] Consequently, attempts have been made to delete or render non-responsive those cells that react to self-antigens.[56]

T-cell vaccination relies on the injection of autologous autoantigen-specific T-cell clones that have been attenuated or inactivated in vitro. Similar strategies make use of vaccinated peptides of the T-cell receptor complementarity determining region of auto-aggressive T cells. It is believed that vaccination with such peptides stimulates counter-regulatory T cells, which recognize (through their T-cell receptor) the immunizing T-cell receptor peptides (anti-idiotypic regulation).[52] Vaccination with attenuated encephalitogenic T cells induces cell- mediated protection against EAE.[57]

T cell vaccination

Study design

In the first pilot trial of T-cell vaccination, eight MS patients (five with RRMS and three with progressive MS) were vaccinated subcutaneously on three occasions with irradiated autologous immunodominant MBP peptide-specific T-cell clones.[58,59] Before the study, these patients were paired to control patients with MS.

In the second phase 1 study,[60] four patients with CPMS were vaccinated with autologous bovine myelin-reactive irradiated T-cell lines. The cells were injected subcutaneously at baseline, and again after 6–12 weeks at a dose of 40×10^6 cells. After each vaccination, the patients were monitored for routine blood parameters, immunological responses towards the vaccine, proportion of T cells reactive to bovine myelin, proteolipid protein (PLP), MBP and myelin oligo-dendrocyte glycoprotein (MOG) peptides, and clinical characteristics.

Results

In the first phase 1 trial,[58,59] treatment was well tolerated and induced a progressive decline in circulating MBP-reactive T cells. In the majority of the recipients, MBP-reactive T cells remained undetectable in the circulation over a period of 1–3 years after vaccination. In three of eight patients, MBP-reactive T cells reappeared during clinical exacerbation.[61] In the 2 years before and after vaccination, the total number of exacerbations decreased from 16 to three in five vaccinated patients with RRMS, and from 12 to 10 in the matched control patients.[59] MRI lesion load increased by 8.0% in the vaccinated patients, compared to a 39.5% increase in the controls. In the patients with CPMS, vaccination did not appear to alter the clinical course. This may reflect the possibility that the encephalitogenic immune response might involve other myelin proteins, such as PLP, myelin associated glyco-protein (MAG) or MOG.

In the second phase 1 trial,[60] no significant side effects were associated with the injection of the inoculates. Three patients showed stable EDSS over time. After the second inoculation, there was a progressive decline (75–80%) in levels of circulating bovine myelin-reactive

T cells, and a complete depletion of circulating T cells reactive to human MBP 143-168, PLP 104-117, and MOG 43-55 peptide. In contrast, the frequency of tetanus toxoid-reactive T cells remained unchanged. T-cell vaccination was also associated with a decline in bovine myelin-specific IL-2 and IFN-γ-secreting T cells. Twelve T-cell lines that could specifically recognize the inoculates were selected from two patients. These regulatory T-cell lines lysed the inoculates by MHC class I-restricted cytolytic activity and preferentially secreted IFN-γ, TNF, and TGF-β.

Comments

T-cell vaccination using MBP-reactive or bovine myelin-reactive T cell lines is well tolerated and promotes effective depletion of circulating myelin-reactive T cells.

Vaccination with T-cell receptor peptide

Study design

Twenty-three HLA-DRB1*1501-positive patients with CPMS were enrolled in the first controlled double-blind phase 1 study of native Vβ5.2-38-58 peptide, a 1:1 mixture of the native peptide and Y49T-substituted Vβ5.2-38-58 peptide.[62] Drug was administered weekly for 4 weeks and then monthly for an additional 10 months, giving a total of 14 injections. The primary outcome was safety and tolerability. Secondary outcomes included neurological status and T-cell response to Vβ5.2 peptides and MBP. A second open-label, single-center, phase 1 trial[63] was conducted in 10 patients with MS. Patients were pre-screened for over-representation of Vβ6 in activated CSF T cells expanded in culture. A peptide of 20 amino acids from the CDR2 region of Vβ6 was administered intramuscularly in incomplete Freund's adjuvant in two 1.0 ml doses of either 100 μg or 300 μg to 10 patients (five patients for each dose). Patients were monitored for safety, immune parameters, and changes in the number and profile of the CSF T cells for 24 weeks.

Results

In the first phase 1 study,[62] the T-cell receptor peptide vaccine from the Vβ5.2 sequence boosted peptide-reactive T cells. Vaccine responders had a reduced MBP response and remained clinically stable without side effects during 1 year of therapy, whereas non-responders had an increased MBP response and progressed clinically. Peptide-specific T-helper 2 cells directly inhibited MBP-specific T-helper 1 cells in vitro, possibly through the release of IL-10. These findings suggest that bystander suppression may be used to advantage to treat MS and other auto-immune diseases.

In the second phase 1 study,[63] the immunization appeared safe, with no adverse event attributable to the drug. The disease course in these patients remained stable (as assessed by EDSS, activities of daily living (ADL), MRI). Cell-mediated immunity to the peptide was noted in all 10 patients, and four of 10 patients (two in each dosage group) developed delayed type hypersensitivity as measured by skin test. At the higher vaccine dose, there was a marked reduction in the ability to grow CSF T cells, and the frequency of Vβ6 T cells was significantly reduced in these five patients.[63] No antibody to the peptide was detected.

Comments

Vaccination with T-cell receptor peptide was well tolerated and further studies are warranted to determine the clinical and MRI treatment effect.

REFERENCES

1 **Waubant E, Oksenberg J, Goodkin D.** Pathophysiology of MS lesions. *Sci Med* 1997; 4:32–41

2 **Gijbels K, Galardy R, Steinman L.** Reversal of experimental autoimmune encephalomyelitis with a hydroxamate inhibitor of matrix metalloproteases. *J Clinical Invest* 1994; 94:2177–2182.

3 **Leppert D, Waubant E, Galardy R et al.** T cell gelatinases mediate basement membrane transmigration *in vitro*. *J Immunol* 1995; 154:4379–4389.

4 **Liedtke W, Cannella B, Mazzaccaro RJ et al.** Effective treatment of models of multiple sclerosis by matrix metalloproteinase inhibitors. *Ann Neurol* 1998; 44:35–46.

5 **Lee MA, Palace J, Stabler G et al.** Serum gelatinase B, TIMP-1 and TIMP-2 levels in multiple sclerosis: a longitudinal clinical and MRI study. *Brain* 1999; 122:191–197.

6 **Waubant E, Gee L, Sloan R et al.** Serum levels of matrix metalloprotease-9 (MMP-9) and natural tissue inhibitor of matrix metalloprotease-type 1 (TIMP-1) predict MRI activity in relapsing–remitting patients (abstract). *Neurology* 1999; 52(suppl 2):A567.

7 **Lewis ME, Neff NT, Contreras PC et al.** Insulin-like growth factor-1: potential for treatment of motor neuronal disorders. *Exp Neurol* 1993; 124:73–88.

8 **Liu X, Yao DL, Webster H.** Insulin-like growth factor 1 treatment reduces clinical deficits and lesion severity in acute demyelinating experimental autoimmune encephalomyelitis. *Multiple Sclerosis* 1995; 1:2–9.

9 **Yao DL, Xia L, Hudson LD, Webster HV.** Insulin-like growth factor-1 given subcutaneously reduces clinical deficits, decreases lesion severity and upregulates synthesis of myelin proteins in experimental autoimmune encephalomyelitis. *Life Sci* 1996; 16:1301–1306.

10 **Lai EC, Felice KJ, Festoff BW et al.** Effect of recombinant human insulin-like growth factor-I on progression of ALS. A placebo controlled study. *Neurology* 1997; 49:1621–1630.

11 **Li W, Quigley L, Yao DL et al.** Chronic relapsing experimental autoimmune encephalomyelitis: effects of insulin-like growth factor-I treatment on clinical deficits, lesion severity, glial responses, and blood brain barrier defects. *J Neuropathol Exp Neurol* 1998; 57:426–438.

12 **Borasio GD, Robberecht W, Leigh PN et al.** A placebo-controlled trial of insulin growth factor-I in amyotrophic lateral sclerosis. European ALS/IGF-I Study Group. *Neurology* 1998; 51:583–586.

13 **Kennedy M, Torrance D, Picha K, Mohler K.** Analysis of cytokine mRNA expression in the central nervous system of mice with experimental autoimmune encephalomyelitis reveals that IL-10 mRNA expression correlates with recovery. *J Immunol* 1992; 149:2496–2505.

14 **Chernoff AE, Granowitz EV, Shapiro L et al.** A randomized controlled trial of IL-10 in humans. Inhibition of inflammatory cytokine production and immune responses. *J Immunol* 1995; 154:5492–5499.

15 **Salmaggi A, Dufour A, Eoli M et al.** Low serum interleukine-10 levels in multiple sclerosis: further evidence for decreased systemic immunosuppression? *J Neurol* 1996; 243:13–17.

16 **Samoilova EB, Horton JL, Chen Y.** Acceleration of experimental autoimmune encephalomyelitis in IL-10 deficient mice: roles of IL-10 in disease progression. *Cell Immunol* 1998; 188:118–124.

17 **Munkarah A, Chuang L, Lotzova E et al.** Comparative studies of taxol and taxotere on tumor growth and lymphocyte functions. *Gynecol Oncol* 1994; 55:211–216.

18 **White CM, Martin BK, Lee LF et al.** Effects of paclitaxel on cytokine synthesis by unprimed human monocytes, T lymphocytes, and breast cancer cells. *Cancer Immunol Immunother* 1998; 46:104–112.

19 **Cain WC, Stuart RW, Lefkowitz DL et al.** Inhibition of tumor necrosis factor and subsequent endotoxin shock by pirfenidone. *Int J Immunopharmacol* 1998; 20:685–695.

20 **Bensimon G, Lacomblez L, Meininger V, for the ALS/Riluzole Study Group.** A controlled trial of riluzole in amyotrophic lateral sclerosis. *N Eng J Med* 1994; 330:585–591.

21 **Peluffo H, Estevez A, Barbeito L, Stutzman JM.** Riluzole promotes survival of rat motoneurons in vitro by stimulating trophic activity produced by spinal astrocyte monolayers. *Neurosci Lett* 1997; 228:207–211.

22 **Bezard E, Stutzmann JM, Imbert C et al.** Riluzole delayed appearance of parkinsonian motor abnormalities in a chronic MPTP monkey model. *Eur J Pharmacol* 1998; 356:101–104.

23 **Racke MK, Dhib-Jalbut S, Cannella B et al.** Prevention and treatment of chronic relapsing experimental allergic encephalomyelitis by transforming growth factor-β1. *J Immunol* 1991; 146:3012–3017.

24 Racke MK, Sriram S, Carlino J et al. Long term treatment of chronic relapsing experimental allergic encephalomyelitis by transforming growth factor-β2. *J Neuroimmunol* 1993; **46**:175–183.

25 Beck J, Rondot P, Jullien P et al. TGF-beta-like activity produced during regression of exacerbations in multiple sclerosis. *Acta Neurol Scand* 1991; **84**:452–455.

26 Rieckmann P, Albrecht M, Kitze B et al. Tumor necrosis factor-α messenger RNA expression in patients with relapsing–remitting multiple sclerosis is associated with disease activity. *Ann Neurol* 1995; **37**:82–88.

27 Calabresi PA, Fields NS, Maloni HW et al. Phase 1 trial of transforming growth factor beta 2 in chronic progressive MS. *Neurology* 1998; **51**:289–292.

28 Selmaj K, Raine CS. Tumour necrosis factor mediates myelin and oligodendrocyte damage in vitro. *Ann Neurol* 1988; **23**:339–346.

29 Selmaj K, Raines CS, Cross AH. Anti-TNF alpha therapy abrogates autoimmune demyelination. *Ann Neurol* 1991; **30**:694–700.

30 Beck J, Rondot P, Catinot L et al. Increased production of interferon-gamma and tumor necrosis factor precedes clinical manifestation in multiple sclerosis: do cytokines trigger off exacerbations? *Acta Neurol Scand* 1988; **78**:318–323.

31 Van Oosten BW, Barkhof F, Scholten PET et al. Increased production of tumor necrosis factor α, and not interferon γ, preceding disease activity in patients with multiple sclerosis. *Arch Neurol* 1998; **55**:793–798.

32 Selmaj K, Papierz W, Glabinski A, Kohno T. Prevention of chronic relapsing experimental autoimmune encephalomyelitis by soluble tumor necrosis factor receptor I. *J Neuroimmunol* 1995; **56**:135–141.

33 Ruddle NH, Bergman CM, McGrath ML et al. An antibody to lymphotoxin and tumor necrosis factor prevents transfer of experimental allergic encephalomyelitis. *J Exp Med* 1990; **172**:1193–1200.

34 Van Oosten BW, Barkhof F, Truyen L et al. Increased MRI activity and immune activation in two multiple sclerosis patients treated with monoclonal anti-tumor necrosis factor antibody cA2. *Neurology* 1996; **47**:1531–1534.

35 The Lenercept Multiple Sclerosis Study Group, the UBC MS/MRI Analysis Group. TNF neutralization induces an increase in relapses in patients with multiple sclerosis (abstract). *Canadian J Neurol Sci* 1998; **25** (suppl 2):S31–S32.

36 Yednock TA, Cannon C, Fritz LC et al. Prevention of experimental autoimmune encephalomyelitis by antibodies against α4β1 integrin. *Nature* 1992; **356**:63–66.

37 Sheramata W, Vollmer T, Stone L et al. A placebo-controlled, safety, tolerability, dose escalation, PK study of various doses of intravenous Antegren in patients with MS (abstract). *Neurology* 1998; **50** (suppl):A63.

38 Tubridy N, Miller DH, Moseley IF, Donoghue S. UK Antegren MS trial group. A preliminary study of humanised monoclonal antibody to alpha-4 beta-1 integrin on brain lesion activity detected by MRI in multiple sclerosis (abstract). *J Neurol* 1998; **245**:386.

39 Bowen JD, Petersdorf SH, Richards TL et al. Phase I study of a humanized anti-CD11/CD18 monoclonal antibody in multiple sclerosis. *Clin Pharmacol Ther* 1998; **64**:339–346.

40 Lublin F, Hu23F2G MS Study Group. A phase 2 trial of anti-CD11/CD18 monoclonal antibody in acute exacerbations of multiple sclerosis (abstract). *Neurology* 1999; **52**(suppl 2):A290.

41 Brostoff SW, Mason DW. Experimental allergic encephalomyelitis: successful treatment in vivo with a monoclonal antibody that recognizes T helper cells. *J Immunol* 1984; **133**:1938–1942.

42 Waldor M, Sriram S, Hardy R et al. Reversal of experimental allergic encephalomyelitis with monoclonal antibody to a T-cell subset marker. *Science* 1985; **227**:415–417.

43 Lindsey JW, Hodgkinson S, Mehta R et al. Phase I clinical trial of chimeric monoclonal anti-CD4 antibody in multiple sclerosis. *Neurology* 1994; **44**:413–419.

44 Lindsey JW, Hodgkinson S, Mehta R et al. Repeated treatment with chimeric anti-CD4 antibody in multiple sclerosis. *Ann Neurol* 1994; **36**:183–189.

45 Van Oosten BW, Lai M, Hodkinson S et al. Treatment of multiple sclerosis with the monoclonal anti-CD4 antibody cM-T412: results of a randomized, double-blind, placebo-controlled, MR-monitored phase 2 trial. *Neurology* 1997; **49**:351–357.

46 Moreau T, Thorpe J, Miller D et al. Preliminary evidence from magnetic resonance imaging for reduction in disease activity after lymphocyte depletion in multiple sclerosis. *Lancet* 1994; **344**:298–301.

47 Moreau T, Coles A, Wing M et al. Transient increase in symptoms associated with cytokine release in patients with multiple sclerosis. *Brain* 1996; **119**:225–237.

48 Coles AJ, Paolillo A, Molyneux P et al. Monoclonal antibody treatment exposes three mechanisms underlying the clinical course of multiple sclerosis (abstract). *Ann Neurol* 1998; **44**:464.

49 Nag B, Kendrick T, Arimilli S et al. Soluble MHC II-peptide complexes induce antigen-specific apoptosis in T cells. *Cell Immunol* 1996; **170**:25–33.

50 Goodkin DE, Andersson PB, Waubant E et al. A double blind, dose escalation study of safety and tolerability of IV AG 284 in patients with secondary progressive multiple sclerosis (abstract). *Multiple Sclerosis* 1998; **4**:508.

51 Brocke S, Gijbels K, Allegretta M et al. Treatment of experimental encephalomyelitis with a peptide analogue of myelin basic protein. *Nature* 1996; **379**:343–346.

52 Holfeld R. Biotechnical agents for the immunotherapy of multiple sclerosis. Principles, problems and perspectives. *Brain* 1997; **120**:865–916.

53 Lindsey JW, Lublin F, Stark S et al. Double-blind, randomized, placebo-controlled evaluation of safety, tolerability, and pharmacokinetics of CGP 77116 in patients with multiple sclerosis (abstract). *Neurology* 1998; **50 (suppl)**:A149.

54 Acha-Orbea H, Mitchell DJ, Timmerman L et al. Limited heterogeneity of T cell receptors from lymphocytes mediating autoimmune encephalomyelitits allows specific immune intervention. *Cell* 1988; **54**:263–273.

55 Oksenberg J, Stuart S, Begovitch AB et al. Limited heterogeneity of rearranged T-cell receptor V alpha transcripts in brains of multiple sclerosis patients. *Nature* 1990; **345**:344–346.

56 Ben-Nun A, Wekerle H, Cohen IR. Vaccination against autoimmune encephalomyelitis with T-lymphocytes cell lines reactive against myelin basic protein. *Nature* 1981; **292**:60–61.

57 Lider O, Reshef T, Beraud E et al. Anti-idiotypic network induced by T cell vaccination against experimental autoimmune encephalomyelitis. *Science* 1988; **239**:181–183.

58 Zhang J, Medaer R, Stinissen P et al. MHC-restricted depletion of human myelin basic protein-reactive T cells by T cell vaccination. *Science* 1993; **261**:1451–1454.

59 Medaer R, Stinissen P, Truyen L et al. Depletion of myelin-basic-protein-autoreactive T cells by T-cell vaccination: pilot trial in multiple sclerosis. *Lancet* 1995; **346**:807–808.

60 Correale J, McMillan M, McCarthy K, Weiner L. T cell vaccination in multiple sclersosis. Results of a phase 1 clinical trial (abstract). *Neurology* 1998; **50 (suppl)**:A63.

61 Zhang J, Vandevyver C, Stinissen P, Raus J. In vivo clonotypic regulation of human myelin basic protein-reactive T cells by T cell vaccination. *J Immunol* 1995; **155**:5868–5875.

62 Vandenbark AA, Chou YK, Witham R et al. Treatment of multiple sclerosis with T-cell receptor peptides: results of a double-blind pilot trial. *Nature Med* 1996; **2**:1109–1115.

63 Wilson DB, Smith RA, Richieri SP et al. Results of a phase 1 clinical trial of a T-cell receptor vaccine in patients with multiple sclerosis (abstract). *Neurology* 1996; **46**:A406.

29
Combination therapies

Christian Confavreux

BACKGROUND

Since 1993, the field of multiple sclerosis (MS) therapeutics has changed dramatically. Positive results of well-designed and well-conducted, prospective, multicentre, randomized double-blind, placebo-controlled phase 3 trials have been published. This led to approval by US and European regulatory agencies of interferon (IFN)-β 1b (Betaseron®),[1–3] IFN-β 1a (Avonex® and Rebif®),[4,5] and glatiramer acetate (Copaxone®)[6] for patients with relapsing–remitting MS (RRMS). The same process is likely to lead to approval of IFN-β 1b for patients with secondary progressive MS (SPMS).[7]

To date, thousands of patients have used one or more of these disease-modifying agents. The experience has not always been positive. The number of MS patients treated with IFN-β has stabilized in the USA over the past few years at around 60 000. This implies that as many new patients are discontinuing treatment as are starting it. This may not be surprising when considering the evidence regarding efficacy of the presently approved disease-modifying agents. Although the study results are consistent, the magnitude of clinical efficacy is limited to a one third reduction in relapse rate and an approximate 10% absolute reduction of the proportion

of patients with sustained worsening by at least 1.0 point on the Kurtzke expanded disability status scale (EDSS).[1,3–8] In daily practice it appears that some patients respond well to current therapies while other patients are much less responsive. Current therapies are also limited by the need for parenteral administration and by local and systemic adverse effects. Consequently, there is a clear and urgent need for more effective therapies.

There are several possible approaches to future experimental therapeutics in the MS field. First, we can proceed with studies of immunoactive drugs used as monotherapy in the hope that a new agent will be superior to presently available agents in terms of efficacy, acceptability, tolerance, immediate and long-term safety, and cost. There are large numbers of promising new drugs to be tested in MS,[9,10] some of which are already in phase 1 studies (see Chapter 28). There are no clear approaches to prioritizing these promising agents, since our understanding of the pathogenesis of MS (see Chapter 19) or the mechanisms of the drugs are not adequate to predict the results of clinical trials. This is problematic, given the limited number of patients suitable for clinical trials and the finite resources available for MS studies.

Secondly, we can base new trials on new

disease concepts. A promising instance could be lessons recently gathered from the study of pregnancy and MS. The effect of pregnancy on MS measured by clinical[11] and MRI activity[12] is more marked than is the effect of current disease-modifying agents.[1–7] Better understanding of the biological mechanisms by which the fetal allograft is tolerated during pregnancy could lead to new and effective therapeutic strategies in MS.

Thirdly, we could focus studies on optimizing use of available agents. For example, the use of current drugs beginning at the first episode of MS may result in improved long-term benefits (see Chapter 31). Two prospective therapeutic trials using IFN-β beginning with the first symptom are eagerly awaited.

Fourthly, we can develop an approach to testing drugs in combination with currently available disease-modifying agents. This approach is the subject of this chapter.

RATIONALE FOR COMBINATION THERAPIES IN MS

Combination therapy has been used successfully for years in neoplastic and infectious diseases. For instance, combinations of various antibiotics was necessary to prevent emergence of drug-resistant strains of *Mycobacterium tuberculosis* and to effect cure in active tuberculosis. More recently, the introduction of triple-drug combinations for human immunodeficiency virus (HIV) infection reduced the viral load to undetectable serum levels and dramatically changed the clinical course and the prognosis in patients with acquired immune deficiency syndrome. Similar progress is observed in patients with chronic hepatitis C.[13] The addition of ribavirin, a synthetic guanosin analogue with in vitro activity against several viruses, to IFN-α 2b resulted in a sustained virological response and the disappearance of hepatitis C viraemia in 31–43% of patients when used as initial therapy[14,15] and 49% of patients when used for the treatment of a relapse after initial treatment with IFN.[16] Comparative rates achieved in these trials with IFN monotherapy range from 5 to 19%.

Combination therapy has also been explored in autoimmune diseases, notably rheumatoid arthritis.[17,18] Results show that all combinations are not equivalent in terms of efficacy and toxicity. For instance, addition of gold[19] or azathioprine[20] to methotrexate was not more effective than monotherapy. Addition of hydroxychloroquine to gold was marginally more effective, but also more toxic than gold alone.[21] In contrast, addition of cyclosporine to methotrexate,[22] of sulphasalazine and hydroxychloroquine to methotrexate,[23] of step-down prednisolone and methotrexate to sulphasalazine,[24] or of infliximab (a chimeric anti-tumour necrosis factor (TNF)-α monoclonal antibody, to methotrexate[25] were significantly more beneficial than monotherapy, without significant additional toxicity.

Combination therapy can provide dramatically better outcomes than monotherapy. For instance, when recombinant tumor necrosis factor receptor–Fc fusion protein was added to methotrexate,[26] the proportion of patients with a 20% improvement in clinical disease activity at 24 weeks increased from 27% for monotherapy to 71% with the combination; the proportion of patients with a 50% improvement increased from 3% with monotherapy to 27% for the combination.

Combination therapy in MS will probably be required, since multiple environmental and genetic factors appear to play a role in the disease.[27] Viruses may trigger the disease, although no persistent viral infection has been clearly demonstrated during the clinically overt stage of MS. Chronic immune dysregulation ultimately targeting central nervous system (CNS) myelin is postulated to result in CNS injury. The mechanism is postulated to be cell-mediated autoimmunity, possibly resulting from defective T-cell suppressor function and from an altered immunological balance with a shift away from anti-inflammatory T-helper 2 (Th$_2$) responses towards pro-inflammatory T-helper 1 (Th$_1$) responses. Owing in part to epitope spreading, there is not a single myelin antigen involved in MS pathogenesis. For these and other reasons, there are presumably different subtypes of MS. This may explain why patients respond in variable degree to each effective monotherapy.[27] Lastly, to cover the full scope of MS pathology, strategies for brain repair through protection and regeneration of axons and myelin will need to be implemented.[28]

GUIDELINES FOR COMBINATION THERAPIES IN MS

The first and most important question is what therapy to include in the combination. To improve the chances of additive or synergistic beneficial effects, a candidate drug for combination therapy should have a beneficial effect on the outcome criteria and should have a mechanism of action that is different from the standard monotherapy. In the case of MS, drugs could be targeted at different therapeutic domains, such as tissue destruction and tissue repair. But the concept also holds within a given therapeutic domain. For example, presently available therapies presumably act by modulating the immune system, but none of them fully controls the disease process. Theoretically, in vitro or animal data could direct the choice among several candidate therapies. Unfortunately, results from such experiments do not necessarily predict results in MS patients. For example, oral myelin ingestion is a potent method of inducing myelin tolerance. This therapeutic strategy is highly effective in experimental allergic encephalomyelitis (EAE).[29] Despite the encouraging results of a small pilot trial,[30] a large scale North American phase 3 trial failed to demonstrate significant benefits, either clinical or as measured by magnetic resonance imaging (MRI), over placebo (Weiner HL, personal communication). Importantly, safety and tolerability must also be taken into account. Each therapy in the combination must have an acceptable profile in this respect. Ideally, toxicity might be lessened by the combination through, for instance, decreasing the dosage of each individual agent. This has been one of the rationales for combining azathioprine and corticosteroids in the treatment of myasthenia gravis.[31] In practice, in a disease such as MS, which afflicts rather young subjects and does not reduce life expectancy significantly, drugs with a low level of side effects and a good safety profile in the long run should be selected preferentially.

The second question is how to test combination therapy in MS patients. A preliminary evaluation of safety and tolerability of the combination is clearly needed. This serves three aims:

(a) checking, by monitoring clinical and biological parameters at regular intervals, that the combination is acceptably safe and well tolerated with respect to vital functions;

(b) assessing, through appropriate pharmacological follow-up, the impact of the combination on the pharmacokinetics of each individual drug in the combination; and

(c) searching for hints of efficacy or, conversely, adverse interaction by using relatively sensitive clinical criteria, such as relapses, or surrogate markers, such as brain MRI activity on serial T2–weighted or gadolinium-enhanced T1 sequences.

The design of such phase 2 studies is simple when the combination consists of two drugs, A and B (*Fig. 29.1*). It obviously becomes more complex when the combination consists of more agents. (A tentative solution to this problem is illustrated in the lower panel of *Fig. 29.1*.) The study begins with a run-in period of each single therapy, then with the addition of a second agent to each monotherapy, and eventually with a third drug to each double combination of agents, and so on. Appropriate clinical and paraclinical monitoring must be done throughout the study.

Such phase 2 studies should take place before a large phase 3 efficacy study, but this strategy may prove time consuming and may delay a phase 3 study. This is a major problem in MS, where definitive phase 3 trials require years with presently available outcome criteria. In order to save time and money, an alternative could be to combine phase 2 and phase 3 studies with rigorous monitoring of safety and tolerability of the drug combination during the initial stages of the trial. Completion of the trial could be contingent on analysis of the initial part of the trial.

The third question is how to design the phase 3 efficacy trial. Ideally, a full factorial 2 × 2 design is recommended, with the use of a placebo for each single agent. Combining two single agents, A and B, results in four cells, one with patients taking placebo A + placebo B (*Table 29.1*). In practice, such a design becomes unrealistic when three or more agents are combined. Even the combination of two drugs is arguably inappropriate on ethical grounds and may not be feasible when one of the drugs is licenced and approved for use as standard therapy. The study design, therefore, will be influenced by currently available treatments. At the present time, combination therapy in RRMS will be compared with monotherapy with IFN-β 1a, IFN-β 1b or glati-

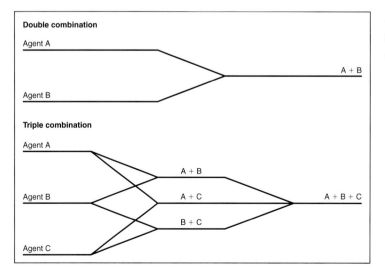

Fig. 29.1 Suggested design for phase 2 studies of combination therapies.

Table 29.1 Principle of the full 2 × 2 factorial design of a placebo-controlled trial of two agents (A and B) to be tested as a single therapy or as a combination

	B	*Placebo B*
A	A + B	A + Placebo B
Placebo A	Placebo A + B	Placebo A + Placebo B

ramer acetate. For SPMS, combination therapy will be compared (currently) with IFN-β 1b. In these clinical situations, a placebo arm is not acceptable. By contrast a placebo arm is acceptable and appropriate for studies in primary progressive MS (PPMS).

These considerations concern combination therapies in which agents are used in parallel. For combination strategies of the sequential type (e.g. an induction phase followed by a maintenance phase) a conventional parallel design is appropriate.

PRESENTLY AVAILABLE DATA ON COMBINATION THERAPIES IN MS

Published data are scarce. From experimental models of MS, there are some indications that the therapeutic response is greater with drugs in combination than with either single drug. This has been shown with antagonists of the pro-inflammatory cytokines TNF-α and interleukin (IL)-1 in EAE in Lewis rats,[32] and with the anti-inflammatory cytokines IL-4 and IL-10 in Theiler's virus-induced encephalomyelitis.[33] There are also in vitro studies that demonstrate additive effects of glatiramir acetate and IFN-β

1b on inhibition of cellular immune reactivity to myelin basic protein.[34] However, addition of glatiramer acetate to IFN-β proved to be of no benefit in acute murine EAE.[35] Lastly, all-trans-retinoic acid was shown to potentiate the ability of IFN-β 1b to augment suppressor cell function in MS.[36]

Results of relatively prolonged combination therapy in MS were first published for progressive MS. In a randomized, placebo-controlled, single-masked trial,[37] 57 patients received low-dose oral cyclophosphamide and prednisone and weekly plasma exchanges for 22 weeks. They were followed for a mean of 30 months. Comparison with 56 patients receiving placebo medication and sham plasma exchanges did not show any significant difference in terms of the proportion of patients with a confirmed worsening of at least 1.0 point on the EDSS. More recently, in a pilot trial involving 11 patients with a randomized, single-masked, cross-over design, brain MRI activity was assessed during a 24-week period of plasma exchange in combination with azathioprine and a control period of similar duration.[38] No significant difference was found between the two periods.

In RRMS, initiation of IFN-β therapy is associated with a flu-like syndrome and transient induction of TNF-α and IFN-γ. As recently shown in a pilot trial,[39] clinical symptoms and cytokine changes can be significantly reduced by the phosphodiesterase inhibitor pentoxifylline. Furthermore, this combination enhances induction of the anti-inflammatory cytokine IL-10 obtained with IFN-β 1b alone. The net result is normalization of the disturbed cytokine balance characteristic of MS with a shift from a Th_1 to a Th_2 profile. However, long-term effects of this combination therapy on the course of MS have not yet been assessed. By contrast, monthly infusions of intravenous immunoglobulins were added to daily azathioprine for 3 years in an open pilot trial involving 38 MS patients.[40] According to the authors, this combination resulted in reduced relapses, and a slight decrease in the EDSS score.

PRESENT AND FUTURE

At present, there is a trial planned in North America that combines glatiramer acetate and IFN-β (Lublin F, personal communication). This small trial is focused on safety. A total of 32 patients with relapsing–remitting MS will be studied over 9–10 months to determine if combined therapy causes increased MRI-detected lesions in the brain, increased side effects or increased MS relapses. If results from this study are reassuring, a larger study of possible efficacy will be considered.

An open pilot trial combining IFN-β 1a (6×10^6 IU/week), prednisone (7.5–15 mg/day) and azathioprine (100–150 mg/day) is progressing in 18 MS patients who showed persisting relapses despite IFN-β and prednisone (OJ Kolar, personal communication). The median duration of treatment is 1 year. No serious side effects have been reported. With respect to neurological findings, three patients have improved, nine have stabilized and six have worsened.

A French and Italian prospective randomized, controlled trial with blinded assessment at endpoint has been launched to assess the efficacy on clinical progression of an induction therapy with monthly infusions of mitoxantrone for a 6-month period followed by a maintenance therapy with INF-β 1b (G Edan, personal communication). Comparison will be made with a control group treated with IFN-β 1b alone. Treatment will be

for 36 months. Eligible patients have clinically active RRMS and a total of 220 patients will be enrolled.

A phase 3 trial aiming at assessing the efficacy of the combination of IFN-β 1a and azathioprine is soon to be launched in RRMS in the ERAZIMUS project (EaRly AZathioprine and Interferon-β in MUltiple Sclerosis).[9] These drugs in combination may have additive or synergistic efficacy, per-haps because of their immunosuppressive, immunomodulatory and anti-inflammatory effects, with different mechanisms of action. One potential mechanism of synergy could be prevention of anti-IFN antibody production by azathioprine treatment, since neutralizing antibodies may cause waning therapeutic efficacy in IFN-treated patients.[41,42] A phase 2 study aimed at assessing the clinical and biological safety and tolerability of the combination is under way. Thirty RRMS patients already receiving azathioprine treatment for at least 6 months have been enrolled. Three different dose groups of 10 subjects each have been studied consecutively: 50 mg, 100 mg or 150 mg daily (*Fig. 29.2*). After enrolment, the patients received the first intramuscular injection of IFN-β 1a (6×10^6 IU) followed by a weekly injection for 4 months. The safety profile of the combination was evaluated through haematology and biochemistry parameters, and clinical assessments were done at specific times throughout the study. Possible metabolic interaction of the two drugs was evaluated through measurements of serum neopterin and erythrocyte 6-thioguanine nucleotides. This phase 2 trial is just being completed. Preliminary results concerning the first 20 patients confirm biological and clinical safety and tolerability of IFN-β 1a combined with low doses (50 mg and 100 mg) of azathioprine.[43] If the results of the third and last group of 10 patients receiving

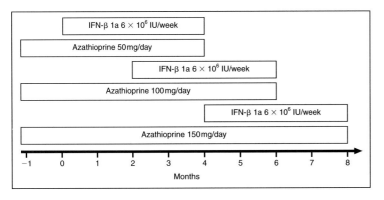

Fig. 29.2 Design of the ERAZIMUS phase 2 trial. Three subgroups of 10 patients each with increasing daily doses of azathioprine.

150 mg of azathioprine daily for at least 6 months are confirmative, the project will enter a phase 3 trial.

CONCLUSION

Combination therapy is an exciting, emerging field in MS.[44] There are a number of drugs that deserve to be tested in combination therapies. Realistically, combination therapy will include at least one drug already known to be beneficial. Protocols will incorporate the add-on type of design. This is the case for all forms of MS excepted PPMS. Assessment of efficacy should be done in comparison to the known therapeutic effects of the reference treatment. The sensitivity of conventional outcome measures, however, is low in untreated MS patients, and it is even lower in the face of the reference treatment. Another problem is that some conventional therapies (i.e. the IFNs), so dramatically reduce new MRI lesions that it may not be possible to measure additive effects on that parameter. In practice, this leads to an increased sample size and longer trial durations. One solution to this might be found by defining new outcome criteria with higher sensitivity, reliability and predictive value. Great efforts are being made to that end, but their validity has not yet been demonstrated. Alternatively, efficacy of combined therapies could be assessed more quickly and convincingly by focusing on particular clinical situations such as very active disease or individual cases for which the reference treatments have proved to be unsuccessful in monotherapy. Escalating doses of the add-on therapy, depending on the clinical response, could also be an appropriate strategy within pilot trials. Another difficulty is collaboration of different drug companies that may be required for implementation of such trials. Despite the difficulties, drug combinations represent a new and promising era in MS therapy. Results with this approach in HIV and hepatitis C virus infections are strongly encouraging.

REFERENCES

1 The IFNβ Multiple Sclerosis Study Group. Interferon beta-1b is effective in relapsing–remitting multiple sclerosis. I. Clinical results of a multicenter, randomized, double-blind, placebo-controlled trial. *Neurology* 1993; 43:655–661.

2 Paty DW, Li DKB, the UBC MS/MRI Study Group, the IFNB Multiple Sclerosis Study Group. Interferon beta-1b is effective in relapsing–remitting multiple sclerosis. II. MRI analysis results of a multicenter, randomized, double-blind, placebo-controlled trial. *Neurology* 1993; 43:662–667.

3 The IFNB Multiple Sclerosis Study Group, the University of British Columbia MS/MRI Analysis Group. Interferon beta-1b in the treatment of multiple sclerosis: final outcome of the randomized controlled trial. *Neurology* 1995; 45:1277–1285.

4 Jacobs LD, Cookfair DL, Rudick RA et al. Intramuscular interferon beta-1a for disease progression in relapsing multiple sclerosis. *Ann Neurol* 1996; 39:285–294.

5 PRISMS (Prevention of Relapses and Disability by Interferon b-1a Subcutaneously in Multiple Sclerosis) Study Group. Randomised double-blind placebo-controlled study of interferon b-1a in relapsing/remitting multiple sclerosis. *Lancet* 1998; 352:1498–1504.

6 Johnson KP, Brooks BR, Cohen JA et al. Copolymer 1 reduces relapse rate and improves disability in relapsing–remitting multiple sclerosis: results of a phase III multicenter, double-blind, placebo-controlled trial. *Neurology* 1995; 45:1268–1276.

7 European Study Group on Interferon β-1b in Secondary Progressive MS. Placebo-controlled multicentre randomised trial of interferon β-1b in treatment of secondary progressive mutliple sclerosis. *Lancet* 1998; 352:1491–1497.

8 Kurtzke JF. Rating neurological impairment in multiple sclerosis: an expanded disability status scale (EDSS). *Neurology* 1983; 33:1444–1452.

9 Confavreux C, Moreau T. Emerging treatments in multiple sclerosis: azathioprine and mofetil. *Multiple Sclerosis* 1996; 1:379–384.

10 Noseworthy J, Miller DH. Measurement of treatment efficacy and new trial results in multiple sclerosis. *Curr Opin Neurol* 1997; 10:201–210.

11 Confavreux C, Hutchinson M, Hours MM et al. Rate of pregnancy-related relapse in multiple sclerosis. *N Engl J Med* 1998; 339:285–291.

12 Van Walderveen MAA, Tas MW, Barkhof F et al. Magnetic resonance evaluation of disease activity during pregnancy in multiple sclerosis. *Neurology* 1994; 44:327–332.

13 Liang TJ. Combination therapy for hepatitis C infection. *N Engl J Med* 1998; 339:1549–1550.

14 McHutchinson JG, Gordon SC, Schiff ER et al. Interferon alfa-2b alone or in combination with ribavirin as initial treatment for chronic hepatitis C. *N Engl J Med* 1998; 339:1485–1492.

15 Poynard T, Marcellin P, Lee SL et al. Randomised trial of interferon α2b plus ribavirin for 48 weeks or for 24 weeks versus interferon α2b plus placebo for 48 weeks for treatment of chronic infection with hepatitis C virus. *Lancet* 1998; 352:1426–1432.

16 Davis Gl, Esteban-Mur R, Rustgi V et al. Interferon alfa-2b alone or in combination with ribavirin for the treatment of relapse of chronic hepatitis C. *N Engl J Med* 1998; 339:1493–1499.

17 Madhok R, Capell HA. Outstanding issues in use of disease-modifying agents in rheumatoid arthritis. *Lancet* 1999; 353:257–258.

18 O'Dell JR. Anticytokine therapy. A new era in the treatment of rheumatoid arthritis? *N Engl J Med* 1999; 340:310–312.

19 Williams HJ, Ward JR, Reading JC et al. Comparison of auranofin, methotrexate and the combination of both in the treatment of rheumatoid arthritis. A controlled clinical trial. *Arthritis Rheum* 1992; 35:259–269.

20 Willkens RF, Sharp JT, Stablein D et al. Comparison of azathioprine, methotrexate, and the combination of the two in the treatment of rheumatoid arthritis. *Arthritis Rheum* 1995; 38:1799–1806.

21 Scott DL, Dawes PT, Tunn E et al. Combination therapy with gold and hydroxychloroquine in rheumatoid arthritis: a randomized, placebo-controlled study. *Br J Rheumatol* 1989; 28:128–133.

22 Tugwell P, Pincus T, Yocum D et al. Combination therapy with cyclosporine and methotrexate in severe rheumatoid arthritis. *N Engl J Med* 1995; 333:137–141.

23 O'Dell JR, Haire CE, Erikson N et al. Treatment of rheumatoid arthritis with methotrexate alone, sulfasalazine and hydroxychloroquine, or a combination of all three medications. *N Engl J Med* 1996; 334:1287–1291.

24 Boers M, Verhoeven AC, Markusse HM et al. Randomised comparison of combined step-down prednisolone, methotrexate and sulphasalazine with

sulphasalazine alone in early rheumatoid arthritis. *Lancet* 1997; **350**:309–318.

25 Maini RN, Breedveld FC, Kalden JR et al. Therapeutic efficacy of multiple intravenous infusions of anti-tumor necrosis factor α monoclonal antibody combined with low-dose weekly methotrexate in rheumatoid arthritis. *Arthritis Rheum* 1998; **41**:1552–1563.

26 Weinblatt ME, Kremer JM, Bankhurst AD et al. A trial of etanercept, a recombinant tumor necrosis factor receptor: Fc Fusion protein, in patients with rheumatoid arthritis receiving methotrexate. *N Engl J Med* 1999; **340**:253–259.

27 Weiner HL. A 21 point unifying hypothesis on the etiology and treatment of multiple sclerosis. *Can J Neurol Sci* 1998; **25**:93–101.

28 Compston A. Brain repair. *J Intern Med* 1995; **237**:127–134.

29 Weiner HL. Oral tolerance: immune mechanisms and treatment of autoimmune diseases. *Immunol Today* 1997; **18**:335–343.

30 Weiner HL, Mackin GA, Matsui M et al. Double-blind pilot trial of oral tolerization with myelin antigens in multiple sclerosis. *Science* 1993; **259**:1321–1324.

31 Palace J, Newsom-Davis J, Lecky B, the Myasthenia Gravis Study Group. A randomized double-blind trial of prednisolone alone or with azathioprine in myasthenia gravis. *Neurology* 1998; **50**:1778–1783.

32 Wieman B, Van GY, Danilenko DM et al. Combined treatment of acute EAE in Lewis rats with TNF-binding protein and interleukin-1 receptor antagonist. *Exp Neurol* 1998; **149**:455–463.

33 Hill KE, Pigmans M, Fujinami RS, Rose JW. Gender variations in early Theiler's virus induced demyelinating disease: differential susceptibility and effects of IL-4, IL-10 and combined IL-4 with IL-10. *J Neuroimmunol* 1998; **85**:44–51.

34 Milo R, Panitch H. Additive effects of copolymer-1 and interferon β-1b on the immune response to myelin basic protein. *J Neuroimmunol* 1995; **61**:185–193.

35 Mizrachi-Koll R, Karussis D, Abramsky O. Synergistic in vivo effects of COP-1 and interferon-β on hyperacute experimental autoimmune encephalomyelitis (EAE). *Neurology* 1997; **48**:A422.

36 Qu ZX, Dayal A, Jensen MA, Arnason BG. All-trans retinoic acid potentiates the ability of interferon beta-1b to augment suppressor cell function in multiple sclerosis. *Arch Neurol* 1998; **55**:315–321.

37 Canadian Cooperative Multiple Sclerosis Study Group. The Canadian cooperative trial of cyclophosphamide and plasma exchange in progressive multiple sclerosis. *Lancet* 1991; **337**:441–446.

38 Sorensen PS, Wansher B, Szpirt W et al. Plasma exchange combined with azathioprine in multiple sclerosis using serial gadolinium-enhanced MRI to monitor disease activity: a randomized single-masked cross-over pilot study. *Neurology* 1996; **46**:1620–1625.

39 Weber F, Polak T, Günther A et al. Synergistic immunomodulatory effects of interferon-β1b and the phosphodiesterase inhibitor pentoxifylline in patients with relapsing–remitting multiple sclerosis. *Ann Neurol* 1998; **44**:27–34.

40 Kalanie H, Tabatabai SS. Combined immunoglobulin and azathioprine in multiple sclerosis. *Eur Neurol* 1998; **39**:178–181.

41 The IFNB Multiple Sclerosis Study Group, the University of British Columbia MS/MRI Analysis Group. Neutralizing antibodies during treatment of multiple sclerosis with interferon beta-1b: experience during the first three years. *Neurology* 1996; **47**:889–894.

42 Pachner AR. Anticytokine antibodies in beta interferon-treated MS patients and the need for testing: plight of the practicing neurologist. *Neurology* 1997; **49**:647–750.

43 Moreau T, Blanc S, Riche G, Confavreux C. ERAZIMUS: EaRly AZathioprine versus beta-Interferon treatment in MUltiple Sclerosis. Results of a pilot safety study. *Multiple Sclerosis* 1998; **4**:325.

44 Lublin FD, Reingold SC. Combination therapy for treatment of multiple sclerosis. *Ann Neurol* 1998; **44**:7–9.

PART IV

Disease modifying drug therapy in clinical practice

30
To treat or not to treat?

Giancarlo Comi and Gianvito Martino

INTRODUCTION

Although the aetiology of multiple sclerosis (MS) is still unknown, convincing pathological and experimental evidence indicates that the pathogenic process underlying MS is T-cell-mediated inflammation that leads to patchy central nervous system (CNS) demyelination. Epidemiologic evidence suggests that the disease is triggered by some still unknown environmental factors in genetically susceptible subjects.[1–3] Based on current concepts on pathogenesis, various non-specific immunosupressive agents have been tested over the past 25 years, with marginal benefits on the natural evolution of the disease and frequent short- and long-term adverse effects.[4] Owing to their unfavourable toxicity profiles, these therapies have usually been limited to patients with progressive courses or high clinical activity. The effects of these therapies in the early phases of the disease have never been investigated. The purpose of this chapter is to discuss approaches to determining which MS patients should be treated with currently available disease-modifying drugs.

APPROVED TREATMENTS FOR MS

In more recent years, three large controlled clinical trials involving about 1000 patients with relapsing–remitting MS (RRMS) have demonstrated that interferon (IFN)-β 1a and IFN-β 1b reduce significantly the frequency of clinical attacks and the accumulation of new brain lesions measured by magnetic resonance imaging (MRI).[5–7] In addition to IFN-β, glatiramir acetate has also been found effective in reducing disease activity in RRMS patients.[8] The mechanisms of action of these two drugs are, however, still not completely clarified. IFN-β has a broad spectrum of immunomodulatory activity that ranges from down-regulation of pro-inflammatory cytokines such as IFN-γ and tumor necrosis factor (TNF)-α to up-regulation of anti-inflammatory molecules such as interleukin (IL)-1 receptor antagonist and IL-10.[9] Glatiramer acetate seems to have a more restricted immuno-suppressive profile, since it has been shown that it down-regulates T-cell reactivity against myelin antigens such as myelin basic protein (MBP).[10] Both IFN-β and glatiramer acetate have favourable short-term and long-term safety profiles and, although they have only partial therapeutic effects (relapses and disability progression are reduced but not eliminated), they have substantially changed the philosophy of MS treatment.

The use of IFN-β 1a, (Avonex®; Biogen Inc Cambridge MA, USA) IFN-β 1b, (Betaseron®; Schering Berlin, Germany) and glatiramer acetate

(Copaxone®; TEVA Kfar-Saba, Israel) in selected RRMS patients has been approved in the USA by the Food and Drug Administration (FDA). The European Agency for the Evaluation of Medicinal Products (EMEA) licensed Avonex®, Betaseron® and another IFN-β 1a agent (Rebif®; Serono Geneva, Switzerland) for RRMS and Betaseron® for secondary progressive MS (SPMS). Policies by insurance companies or public health systems for reimbursing patients for these drugs generally follow the inclusion and exclusion criteria utilized in clinical trials that demonstrated their efficacy. For instance, in many countries, IFN-β 1a can be prescribed to RRMS patients with an EDSS score below 4.0, while Betaseron® (IFN-β 1b) can be prescribed to RRMS patients with an EDSS score between 1.0 and 5.5. The purpose of this chapter is not to comment on comparison of therapeutic effects of different types of IFN-β. However, it should be pointed out that a neurologist may wish to take into account the dosage, route of administration, side effect profile, and published results in making a treatment decision for a particular agent in a given patient.

CANDIDATES FOR TREATMENT

All patients with a diagnosis of definite MS who are in an active phase of the disease are candidates for treatment that may favourably modify the disease course. However, the decision to treat should be individualized according to a careful evaluation of clinical and paraclinical variables and a meaningful discussion with the patient and her or his family. Patients with RRMS, progressive relapsing MS (PRMS), and SPMS may benefit from IFN-β, and patients with RRMS patients may also benefit from glatiramer acetate.

In the authors' opinion, patients with RRMS who have already accumulated some degree of disability and who have clinical evidence of disease activity require immediate treatment. Patients with an evident benign course or with long-standing quiescent disease should also be treated if they experience recurrent clinical relapses. The decision is somewhat more difficult in RRMS patients who do not have clinical disability but who present with a clinical relapse after a long period of clinical inactivity. It is reasonable in these cases to obtain a cranial MRI scan to determine whether treatment is required. With incomplete recovery from the relapse, or with multiple new lesions, treatment is warranted. In some patients, an additional follow-up MRI scan may be helpful to help to determine if there is an active disease process, as evidenced by new lesions, to indicate the need for treatment.

Cranial MRI scanning is emerging as very important in evaluating the need for treatment for individual MS patients. It is at least 10 times more sensitive in revealing disease activity than clinical evaluation is.[11] The number of active lesions on MRI is predictive of short-term clinical and MRI disease activity,[12–14] although the predictive value of a single MRI scan decreases over time and is lost after 2 years.[13] Importantly, the T2-weighted lesion load is predictive of future disability.[15] From the practical point of view, patients with a high brain MRI lesion load or multiple active lesions should be considered to be at high risk of subsequent disease activity and disability progression, and should be considered as candidates for treatment.

The European Study on IFN-β 1b in SPMS[16] showed that treatment is effective in patients with disability progression without relapses as well as in patients with progression and superimposed relapses. Because observation is required to enable disability progression to be detected prospectively, treatment seems warranted in patients with SPMS with or without relapses.

To date there is no convincing evidence that treatment may be beneficial in patients with primary progressive MS (PPMS). These patients have disease onset at an older age, disability that is mostly related to spinal cord involvement, infrequent cognitive dysfunction and a low brain MRI lesion load. These aspects suggest that pathogenetic mechanisms may be at least partially different in RRMS and PPMS and that, consequently, the therapeutic approach may also be different.

In patients with clinically isolated syndromes suggestive of MS, the presence of typical cranial MRI findings and intrathecal IgG synthesis is predictive of conversion to clinically definite MS. The rate of conversion is about 50% in 5 years.[17–19] Moreover, the number of cranial MRI lesions at the time of clinical presentation is predictive of disability both 5 and 10 years later.[20] Ideally, patients with clinically isolated syndromes suggestive of MS who have typical cranial MRI and CSF oligoclonal bands should be treated because they have MS and are in an active phase of the disease. However, about 20% of these patients will not develop significant disability in the next 15 years, and an additional 5% will never develop a clinical relapse. At the present, patients with clinically isolated syndromes should probably not be treated until they convert to clinically definite MS. This opinion could change in the near future, depending on results of two ongoing clinical trials testing the efficacy of IFN-β 1a in such patients. In fact, there is a strong scientific rationale for early treatment in MS patients, and some clinical evidence supports this strategy.

RATIONALE FOR EARLY TREATMENT IN MS

The Northeast Cooperative MS Trial on intermittent cyclophosphamide pulse therapy in chronic progressive MS documented that the drug is effective only in patients younger than 40 years of age who have an EDSS score > 4.0 at entry.[21] The multicentre North American trial of glatiramer acetate in RRMS showed a higher reduction in relapse rate in patients with lower disability at entry into the trial.[8] In the PRISMS study,[7] both low doses (22 µg three times weekly) and high doses (44 µg three times weekly) of IFN-β 1a (Rebif®, Serono) significantly reduced clinical and MRI disease activity in RRMS patients with an EDSS score > 4.0 at entry. A post hoc analysis showed that only the higher dose was effective in more disabled patients (EDSS > 3.5). This result suggests that a ceiling effect occurs in the earlier phases of the disease, while in the more advanced phases higher doses of the drug may be more effective. The Optic Neuritis Treatment Trial[22] showed that a short course of high-dose intravenous methylprednisolone (MP) reduced conversion to clinically definite MS from 35.9% in the placebo group to 16.2% in the intravenous MP group. This favourable effect of intravenous MP was evident after 2 years of follow-up, but it had disappeared by 5 years, indicating that the treatment was effective in delaying but not in preventing the conversion to clinically definite MS.

How can the rationale for the early use of immunomodulatory drugs in RRMS patients be explained on a pathophysiological basis? The pathogenic mechanisms in MS are orchestrated by two different populations of immune cells. The first population determines the organ specificity of the process by specifically recognizing the target organ. The second population consists of effector cells that circulate systemically[2,3] and enter the brain secondarily. Activated T cells recognizing several myelin components such as MBP, myelin oligodendrocyte glycoprotein (MOG) and proteolipid protein (PLP)[1] constitute the first cell population, while effector cells consist of B cells as well as antigen-non-specific T cells and macrophages. In MS, and in autoimmunity more generally, autoreactive T cells tend to recognize more epitopes within the same antigen and more antigens within the same organ over time as the disease progresses, a process termed 'epitope spreading'.[23] Early immunomodulatory treatment may lead to down-regulation of antigen-specific T cells and may inhibit epitope spreading at an early stage of immune pathogenesis. Additional pathological findings comparing the inflammatory response in new and old plaques suggests that the inflammatory process may have different characteristics as the disease progresses, and specifically that the pathological process may persist locally in CNS lesions.[24] Since peripherally administered immunomodulatory drugs may not cross the blood–brain barrier and accumulate within the CNS,[25,26] it may be most effective to treat at a disease stage when pathogenic cells are present systemically. Moreover, increasing localization of the pathogenic response in the CNS over time could diminish the efficiency of reparative mechanisms.[27,28]

Recent MRI studies have demonstrated that axonal damage in normal-appearing white matter plays an important role in chronic disability in MS patients.[29,30] Because axonal damage appears to occur early during the course of MS,[31] the nervous system is able to protect against clinical manifestations until a large proportion of nervous axons is involved. Any further loss of axons reduces the 'safety factor' of the nervous system, however, providing an important additional rationale for early treatment with drugs that reduce inflammation, demyelination, and axonal injury.

CLINICAL TRIALS IN PATIENTS WITH CLINICALLY ISOLATED SYNDROMES SUGGESTIVE OF MS

In July 1994, the Working Group for Treatment Trials of the European Charcot Foundation planned the Early Treatment of MS (ETOMS) study for patients with a first clinical episode suggestive of MS and with cranial MRI strongly suggestive of MS (Paty's criteria, modified).[32] For inclusion in the study, patients had to have symptom onset suggestive of MS no more than 3 months before study entry. Patients were randomized to receive IFN-β 1a (Rebif®, Serono) 6×10^6 IU by subcutaneous injection once a week or placebo. The primary objective of the study is to investigate the efficacy of IFN-β 1a in reducing conversion to clinically definite MS during 2 years of treatment. Secondary outcomes from the study are the time to conversion to clinically definite MS, cranial MRI disease activity and cranial MRI disease burden. Fifty-four European centres are involved in the study. Patient recruitment started in August 1995 and was completed in June 1997 with the enrolment of 311 patients. The study will be completed in June 1999.

A similar study is ongoing in North America. Patients within 2 weeks of onset of a monosymptomatic attack suggestive of MS having two or more lesions on cranial MRI are randomized to receive IFN-β 1a 30 μg by intramuscular injection once a week or placebo. The primary endpoint of the study is time to conversion to clinically definite MS. Accrual into the study was complete in spring 1998.

Results from the European and the North American studies will clarify whether or not IFN-β delays conversion to clinically definite MS. These studies have a relatively short duration, however, and will not define the extent to which early treatment per se can halt the disease. It would follow that treatment that delayed the occurrence of the second relapse would have a favourable effect on the long-term evolution of the disease. Indeed, epidemiological studies suggest that a short interval between the initial relapse and the second relapse is associated with a poor outcome.[33–35]

CONCLUSIONS

For the first time two types of treatments, IFN-β and glatiramer acetate, have been approved as therapies able to modify the disease course in MS. Patients with RRMS and SPMS may benefit from treatment, and in a short time ongoing clinical trials will clarify if such therapies are effective for patients with PPMS. Available immunological, clinical and pathological data suggest that early treatment of RRMS with immunomodulatory drugs could be advantageous compared to late treatment. Ideally, treatment should be started at clinical presentation, but ongoing clinical trials in patients with clinically isolated syndromes suggestive of MS should provide empirical evidence as to whether this has significant advantages compared to delayed treatment.

Restricting treatment to patients with at least two relapses in the previous 2 years, a restriction applied by insurance companies in some countries, is not a rational basis for the decision, but rather merely reflects inclusion criteria utilized in clinical trials performed to date. There is no evidence that the level of therapeutic response is related to relapse frequency during the pretreatment period. The brain and spinal cord MRI reflects the pathological process in MS more clearly than clinical variables during the RRMS stage, making this technique a powerful complement to the clinician in selecting appropriate candidates for treatment. Future studies will help clarify whether genetic or immunological markers could play a role in treatment decisions.

In deciding whether to start treatment to modify the MS disease course, even in the presence of clear clinical indications, the neurologist should consider physical, psychological and social implications. Many patients feel worse for a time after starting therapy, and side effects from medication may have a significant impact on the patient's quality of life. Only through adequate patient education about the goals of therapy can long-term compliance be optimized.

REFERENCES

1 **Martina R, McFarland HF, McFarlin DE.** Immunological aspects of demyelinating diseases. *Annu Rev Immunol* 1992; 10:153–187.

2 **Steinman L.** Multiple sclerosis: a coordinated immunological attack against myelin in the central nervous system. *Cell* 1996; 85:299–302.

3 **Steinman L.** A few autoreactive cells in an autoimmune infiltrate control a vast population of nonspecific cells: a tale of smart bombs and the infantry. *Proc Natl Acad Sci U S A* 1996; 93:2253–2256.

4 **Polman CH, Hartung HP.** The treatment of multiple sclerosis: current and future. *Curr Opin Neurol* 1995; 8:200–209.

5 **The IFNB Multiple Sclerosis Group.** Interferon beta-1b is effective in relapsing–remitting multiple sclerosis. Clinical results of a multicenter, randomized, double-blind, placebo-controlled trial. *Neurology* 1993; 43:655–661.

6   Jacobs LD, Cookfair DL, Rudick RA et al. Intramuscular interferon beta-1a for disease progression in relapsing multiple sclerosis. The Multiple Sclerosis Collaborative Research Group (MSCRG). *Ann Neurol* 1996; **39**:285–294.

7   PRISMS (Prevention of Relapses and Disability by Interferon beta-1a Subcutaneously in Multiple Sclerosis) Study Group. Randomised double-blind placebo-controlled study of interferon beta-1a in relapsing/remitting multiple sclerosis. *Lancet* 1998; **352**:1498–1504.

8   Johnson KP, Brooks BR, Cohen JA et al. Extended use of glatiramer acetate (Copaxone) is well tolerated and maintains its clinical effect on multiple sclerosis relapse rate and degree of disability. Copolymer 1 Multiple Sclerosis Study Group. *Neurology* 1998; **50**:701–708.

9   Weinstock-Guttman B, Ransohoff RM, Kinkel RP, Rudick RA. The inteferons: biological effects, mechanisms of action, and use in multiple sclerosis. *Ann Neurol* 1995; **37**:7–15.

10 Fridkis-Hareli M, Teitelbaum D, Gurevich E et al. Direct binding of myelin basic protein and synthetic copolymer 1 to class II major histocompatibility complex molecules on living antigen-presenting cells — specificity and promiscuity. *Proc Natl Acad Sci U S A* 1994; **91**:4872–4876.

11 Miller DH, Barkhof F, Nauta JJ. Gadolinium enhancement increases the sensitivity of MRI in detecting disease activity in multiple sclerosis. *Brain* 1993; **116**:1077–1094.

12 Molyneux PD, Filippi M, Barkhof F et al. Correlation between monthly enhanced MRI lesion rate and changes in T2 lesion volume in multiple sclerosis. *Ann Neurol* 1998; **43**:332–339.

13 Kappos L, Moeri D, Radue EW et al. Predictive value of gadolinium-enhanced MRI for relapse rate and changes in disability/impairment in multiple sclerosis: a metaanalysis. *Lancet* 1999; **353**:964–969.

14 Koudriavtseva T, Thompson AJ, Fiorelli M et al. Gadolinium enhanced MRI predicts clinical and MRI disease activity in relapsing-remitting multiple sclerosis. *J Neurol Neurosurg Psychiatry* 1997; **62**:285–287.

15 Filippi M, Horsfield MA, Morissey SP et al. Quantitative brain MRI lesion load predicts the course of clinically isolated syndromes suggestive of MS. *Neurology* 1994; **44**:635–641.

16 European Study Group on Interferon β-1b in Secondary Progressive MS. Placebo-controlled multicentre randomised trial of interferon β-1b in treatment of secondary progressive multiple sclerosis. *Lancet* 1998; **352**:1491–1497.

17 Jacobs LD, Kaba SE, Miller CM et al. Correlation of clinical, magnetic resonance imaging, and cerebrospinal fluid findings in optic neuritis. *Ann Neurol* 1997; **41**:392–398.

18 Beck RW, Cleary PA, Trobe JD et al. The effect of corticosteroids for acute optic neuritis on the subsequent development of multiple sclerosis. The Optic Neuritis Study Group. *New Engl J Med* 1993; **329**:1764–1769.

19 Paolino E, Fainardi E, Ruppi P et al. A prospective study on the predictive value of CSF oligoclonal bands and MRI in acute isolated neurological syndromes for subsequent progression to multiple sclerosis. *J Neurol Neurosurg Psychiatry* 1996; **60**:572–575.

20 O'Riordan JI, Thompson AJ, Kingsley DP et al. The prognostic value of brain MRI in clinically isolated syndromes of the CNS. A 10-year follow-up. *Brain* 1998; **121**:495–503.

21 Weiner HL, Mackin GA, Orav EJ et al. Intermittent cyclophosphamide pulse therapy in progressive multiple sclerosis: final report of the Northeast Cooperative Multiple Sclerosis Treatment Group. *Neurology* 1993; **43**:910–918.

22 Optic Neuritis Study Group. The 5-year risk of MS after optic neuritis. Experience of the optic neuritis treatment trial. Optic Neuritis Study Group. *Neurology* 1997; **49**:1404–1413.

23 Tuohy VK, Yu M, Weinstock-Guttman B, Kinkel RP. Diversity and plasticity of self recognition during the development of multiple sclerosis. *J Clin Invest* 1997; **99**:1682–1690.

24 Lucchinetti CF, Bruck W, Rodriguez M, Lassmann H. Distinct patterns of multiple sclerosis pathology indicates heterogeneity on pathogenesis. *Brain Pathol* 1996; **6**:259–274.

25 Khan OA, Dhib-Jalbut SS. Serum interferon beta-1a (Avonex) levels following intramuscular injection in relapsing–remitting MS patients. *Neurology* 1998; **51**:738–742.

26 Khan OA, Xia Q, Bever CT Jr et al. Interferon beta-1b serum levels in multiple sclerosis patients following subcutaneous administration. *Neurology* 1996; **46**:1639–1643.

27 Storch M, Lassmann H. Pathology and pathogenesis of demyelinating diseases. *Curr Opin Neurol* 1997; **10**:186–192.

28 Bruck W, Bitsch A, Kolenda H et al. Inflammatory

central nervous system demyelination: correlation of magnetic resonance imaging findings with lesion pathology. *Ann Neurol* 1997; **42**:783–793.

29 **Filippi M, Iannucci G, Tortorella C et al.** Comparison of MS clinical phenotypes using conventional and magnetization transfer MRI. *Neurology* 1999; 52:588–594.

30 **Fu L, Matthews PM, De Stefano N et al.** Imaging axonal damage of normal appearing white matter in multiple sclerosis. *Brain* 1998; **121**:103–113.

31 **Trapp BD, Peterson J, Ransohoff RM et al.** Axonal transection in the lesions of multiple sclerosis. *N Engl J Med* 1998; **338**:278–285.

32 **Comi G, Barkhoff F, Durelli L et al.** Early treatment of multiple sclerosis with Rebif (recombinant human interferon beta): design of the study. *Multiple Sclerosis* 1995; **1(suppl 1)**:S24–S27.

33 **Confavreux C, Aimard G, Devic M.** Course and prognosis of multiple sclerosis assessed by the computerized data processing of 349 patients. *Brain* 1980; **103**:281–300.

34 **Wienshenker BG, Bass B, Rice GP et al.** The natural history of multiple sclerosis: a geographically based study. 2. Predictive value of the early clinical course. *Brain* 1989; **112**:1419–1428.

35 **Weinshenker BG, Rice GP, Noseworthy JH et al.** The natural history of multiple sclerosis: a geographically based study. 3. Multivariate analysis of predictive factors and models of outcome. *Brain* 1991; **114**:1045–1056.

31

Treatment for patients with relapsing–remitting multiple sclerosis

Elliot M Frohman

INTRODUCTION

Multiple sclerosis (MS) patients most commonly present when the anatomic and clinical burden of disease is limited. We therefore have a unique opportunity to substantially influence the natural history of this disabling disease if effective disease-modifying strategies can be implemented early. Upon achieving success in limiting disease progression, the entire landscape of what constitutes MS will be dramatically altered over the next few decades. MS has traditionally been viewed as an enigmatic, untreatable, and almost uniformly disabling neurological disease. However, remarkable progress has been achieved over the past few years in identifying disease modifying therapies that can favorably influence the disease process in MS. Furthermore, new insights into the underlying disease mechanisms that culminate in inflammatory demyelination has yielded a number of novel therapeutic strategies. Powerfully persuasive evidence is now available to confirm the premise that the disease process in MS is constitutive, even in early-stage patients who appear to be well. Neuropathological and brain imaging data, coupled with our inability to predict the clinical course in individual patients, supports the notion of early treatment for all patients.

In this chapter an approach is outlined for treating relapsing–remitting MS (RRMS) with abortive strategies during relapses as well as disease-modifying therapies to stabilize the disease and slow the progression of disability. RRMS is defined and selection criteria for treatment, treatment options, duration of therapy, and treatment approaches to patients with isolated syndromes are discussed. A major challenge in the management of MS is how to monitor disease activity effectively, which is necessary to determine whether therapies are effective and adequate. Because the disease may be active without clinical symptoms, it follows that methods are needed to determine when patients are truly in remission. We need to understand better what measures can be taken to control ongoing disease activity when patients are already on treatment with disease-modifying agents (DMAs). A practical treatment algorithm for converting patients to alternative therapies is needed. The role of neutralizing antibodies in therapeutic decisions needs to be clarified. There is a broad diversity of potential adjunctive agents that could be used in combination with standard therapy to treat MS; their potential benefits and side effects are discussed here. Other important considerations include management of DMA-related side effects, treatment of MS in childhood, and pregnancy and family planning issues as they relate to treatment recommendations.

The therapeutic approach described in this chapter represents the opinion of one dedicated MS physician. In some instances, there is little literature-based evidence to support opinions. Therefore, some of these positions are controversial. Nevertheless, as consensus about treatment paradigms evolves, individual neurologists must take a position regarding optimal disease management for current patients. As such, the present author adheres to the premise that the disease produces progressive disability in most patients and that it is likely that early treatment intervention with the currently available DMAs provides the best opportunity of limiting such disability.

Despite the availability of effective treatments, there is still widespread reluctance to implement therapy aggressively as soon as the diagnosis of MS is confirmed. It is hoped that this chapter will serve to challenge nihilism about our ability to treat MS effectively. To observe patients in the early stages of MS without DMAs is, in the author's estimation, analogous to observing a patient with known hypertension and waiting for stroke or myocardial infarction. New guidelines endorsing early therapy for patients with MS must be widely disseminated.

RELAPSING–REMITTING MS

Laboratory-supported diagnostic criteria evolved initially to satisfy entry criteria into MS clinical drug trials.[1] However, these criteria take on additional importance given the availability of drugs that reduce clinical relapses, decrease new brain lesions, and slow disability progression. During the relapsing–remitting phase of MS,

patients typically experience partial or complete recovery form each relapse and there is usually no clinical evidence of progressive deterioration between attacks. Unfortunately, many patients do not fully recover from relapses and are left with residual neurological deficits. Hence, disability progression in MS can occur by incomplete recovery from relapse or by more gradually progressive deterioration. In fact, the majority of patients with an initial relapsing–remitting phase of the disease pass to a secondary progressive form of MS (SPMS). The course of SPMS can also be punctuated by relapses, adding further to more severe long-term disability. It is during SPMS that patients accrue most of the disability associated with MS.

Manifestations and relevance of relapses

Given partial or complete recovery from individual relapses, some physicians and patients assume incorrectly that RRMS is a non-progressive stage of the disease. However it is unequivocal that patients do accrue significant elements of fixed functional disability during RRMS. The broad diversity of clinical manifestations that can occur during RRMS predisposes patients to a constellation of chronic neurological deficits.[2] As such, the ability to improve the frequency, severity, and recovery from disease-related relapses represents a fundamental therapeutic objective. Effectively reducing relapses may also delay the transition from RRMS to SPMS.

On outward appearance and by the expanded disability status scale (EDSS), many RRMS patients appear to have benign disease, yet many suffer from some 'invisible' aspects of MS. These include severe fatigue, sensory disturbances, bowel, bladder, and sexual abnormalities, and cognitive decline. Compared with other clinical measures, cognitive abnormalities appear to be more strongly correlated with disease burden as measured by magnetic resonance imaging (MRI).[3–11] In addition to intellectual deterioration, deconditioning, depression, demoralization, and helplessness also can contribute to severe disability.

Patients with MS will, on occasion, exhibit episodes of reversible neurological dysfunction that are not linked to new inflammatory demyelinating events. In these circumstances neurological symptoms that have been previously experienced during a bona fide exacerbation reemerge to produce symptoms that are familiar to the patient. For example, after recovery from optic neuritis, visual dysfunction can reoccur after exercise, on exposure to high temperatures such as a hot bath or shower, or with infection. Originally described by Uhthoff[12] in patients with optic neuritis after exercise, this phenomenon can produce reversible dysfunction in a multitude of neuroanatomical pathways and lead to highly distinctive clinical manifestations. The mechanisms that underlie these pseudorelapses probably relate to worsening conduction or conduction block within demyelinated pathways. This is most commonly precipitated by exposure to high temperature, infection, or during metabolic derangement. Recognition of pseudorelapses is important to avoid excessive treatment with corticosteroids. Symptoms that persist despite treatment of infection, metabolic derangement, or elevated body temperature should raise suspicion of a bone fide MS relapse.

Treatment objectives in relapsing forms of MS

Table 31.1 lists the treatment objectives that together promote clinical stabilization and limit

Table 31.1 Objectives of treatment in RRMS

Accelerate recovery from relapses

Promote more complete recovery from relapses

Reduce the risk of exacerbation

Slow or halt progression of disability

Optimize restoration of function

Aggressively treat symptomatic complaints

long-term disability. In patients with an acute relapse the objective of treatment is to accelerate recovery and maximize restoration of neurological function. Therapies are also needed to reduce the risk of future relapses and to slow or halt disease progression. For patients with static neurological deficits, novel therapies are needed to promote restoration of function. Symptomatic therapies are needed to mitigate common complaints and interdisciplinary rehabilitation approaches are needed to reintegrate patients into their home, work, and social environments.

Treatment of acute relapses

Most acute relapses are associated with new gadolinium-enhancing lesions on brain or spinal cord MRI, and indicate new inflammation.[13] As such, corticosteroids remain the agents of choice for acute relapses. The therapeutic effects probably relate to the multiple mechanisms by which they attenuate inflammation (see Chapter 26).[14–25] The therapeutic effects of steroids may also improve neuronal conduction, leading to enhanced fidelity of neuronal transmission mechanisms. In MRI studies, corticosteroids diminish the duration and degree of gadolinium enhancement, which appears to correspond to clinical stabilization.[21,26–29] This may be significant in that a high MRI activity rate may correlate with less favorable clinical outcome.[30]

Use of high dose corticosteroids appears to accelerate resolution of gadolinium enhancement.[26,27,31,32] However, following steroid treatment, a second burst of inflammatory activity can occur in association with new gadolinium enhancement.[33] It appears that this phenomenon may relate to the rate of corticosteroid discontinuation. The dose of corticosteroids may also be crucial. In one study, Oliveri and colleagues[34] compared two doses of intravenous methylprednisolone (IVMP) in RRMS; one group received 0.5 g/day for 5 days; the other group received 2 g/day for 5 days. The higher dose was associated with a reduction in the number of gadolinium-enhancing lesions on MRI and a reduction of new gadolinium-enhancing lesions seen at 30 and 60 days after onset of therapy. Clinical worsening following cessation of corticosteroids was correlated with a burst of new gadolinium-enhancing lesions, signifying recrudescence of disease activity.[28,35] It has also been shown in a small cohort of RRMS patients that a short course of IVMP can decrease the rate of new lesion development at 6 months.[35]

Corticosteroid withdrawal is well known for precipitating re-emergence of disease activity in other immune-mediated disorders in humans, such as systemic lupus erythematosus and acute disseminated encephalomyelitis.[36,37] Reder and colleagues[38] suggested that abrupt withdrawal of corticosteroids may simulate a temporary adrenalectomy-like hypoglucocorticoid state until adrenal function and glucocorticoid receptor levels rebound. In experimental allergic encephalomyelitis (EAE), abrupt withdrawal of dexamethasone was found to lead to severe clinical and histological relapses, whereas a slow taper of corticosteroids was associated with a prevention of relapses.[38]

The Optic Neuritis Treatment Trial (ONTT)[39] found that IVMP followed by a prednisone taper was favorable compared to placebo and oral prednisone in terms of faster recovery, decreased episodes of recurrent optic neuritis, and longer time to confirmed MS. Patients treated with low-dose oral prednisone experienced twice the number of recurrent episodes of optic neuritis compared to the patients treated with IVMP and a prednisone taper. Conspicuously, Herishanus and colleagues[40] showed that 66% of patients with optic neuritis who were treated with IVMP for 3 days at 1 g/day without a taper experienced recurrent episodes. In this study, MS was confirmed in 83% of treated patients within 18 months.

On the basis of the ONTT findings, it has been suggested that oral corticosteroids should not be used for clinical relapses. However, the available data suggest that the route of administration may be less important than the total dose of corticosteroids and the use of a taper. The present author has been impressed with the response that patients exhibit to high-dose oral corticosteroids and has found it difficult to appreciate differences in effectiveness based on route of administration (*Table 31.2*). This may be at least partially related to the excellent gastrointestinal absorption of corticosteroids.[41,42] However, some patients some seem to respond more favorably to one preparation or route of administration than another. For mild to moderate relapses that do not require hospitalization, outpatient oral corticosteroid regimens, usually with prednisone or dexamethasone, can be used (see *Table 31.2*).

For more severe relapses requiring hospitalization for hydration, rehabilitation or observation, or because of severe deficits, high-dose IVMP at 1–2 g/day for 3–7 days can be used, depending upon the circumstances. After intravenous corticosteroids one of a number of oral tapering regi-

Table 31.2 Corticosteroid regimens

Agent	Exacerbations	Adjunctive
Intravenous methylprednisolone	1–2 g/day intravenously for 3–7 days, followed by an oral corticosteroid taper (see below)	1–2 g monthly or second-monthly intravenously for 1–2 days
Prednisone	*Taper* 200 mg for 4 days, then 100 mg for 4 days, then decreasing by 10 mg daily until off *Primary treatment* 400 mg for 4 days, then 200 mg for 4 days, then 100 mg for 2 days, then decreasing by 10 mg increments daily until off	*Monthly* 400 mg for 2–4 days *Every other month* 400 mg for 2 days, then 200 mg for 2 days, then 100 mg for 2 days, then can add 10 mg progressive taper
Dexamethasone	*Taper* 12 mg for 4 days, then 8 mg for 4 days, then 4 mg for 4 days *Primary treatment* 16–40 mg for 4 days then reduce by half: 8–20 mg for 4 days, then 4–12 mg for 4 days, then decreasing by 4 mg increments every 4 days	*Monthly* 12–24 mg for 2–4 days *Every other month* 16–24 mg for 2 days then reduce by half: 8–12 mg for 2 days, then 4–8 mg for 2 days

mens generally lasting 2–4 weeks can be used (see *Table 31.2*). If a patient presents with a second phase of disease activity after completion of the treatment regimen, the oral regimen can be started again from the beginning. If we can demonstrate unequivocally that high-dose oral and intravenous corticosteroid regimens are equally effective, this would have important ramifications related to cost and convenience.

RATIONALE FOR EARLY TREATMENT WITH DISEASE MODIFYING THERAPY

The disease eventually results in progressive neurologic disability in the majority of patients

Natural history studies have shown that 50% of patients reach an EDSS score of 6.0 within 15 years of disease onset, at which time 10% are restricted to a wheelchair.[2] It also appears that the frequency of early relapses influences the rate of disability progression. In patients with five or more relapses in the first year, the median time to an EDSS score of 6.0 is less than 7 years, compared with 13 years for patients with between two and four relapses in the first year and 18 years for patients with only one or two relapses.[43,44] Short intervals between relapses and failure to recover completely also carry a less favorable prognosis. Currently available DMAs all significantly decrease the number of new relapses.[45–47] Recognition that a high frequency of relapses in the first 2 years after onset of MS is associated with a less favorable long-term outcome should prompt early treatment intervention with agents known to reduce the relapse rate.

About half of RRMS patients will pass to SPMS within 10 years.[2,48,49] However, longitudinal analysis of a large MS population demonstrates that the mean time for this transition may occur as early as 6 years.[2] Patients who present at a more advanced age typically exhibit a more fulminant disease course, with earlier conversion to SPMS. Ultimately, 25 years after disease onset, approximately 90% of MS patients have developed progressive disease. In addition, some 45–65% of patients experience intellectual decline that serves to disable them further.[3]

Despite these studies, there is great individual variability in disease severity, and prognostic markers are not strong enough to use reliably in the individual patient. Therefore, the benign MS designation can only be used in retrospect, after it is clear that a patient has long-standing MS with minimal disease progression.

Recurrent waves of inflammatory demyelination occur much more commonly than clinical symptoms do. Therefore most clinically quiescent patients continue to experience constitutive disease activity that can culminate in chronic inflammation that leads to demyelination, axonal dysfunction, axonal loss and wallerian degeneration, and ultimately neurodegeneration. During this process, sequestered antigens within the immunologically privileged central nervous system can be released and recognized by activated immune cells. This process leads to 'epitope spreading,' with diversified immune responses against brain antigens.[50] Each new phase of disease activity may augment these immune responses and in essence constitutes a booster immunization against the CNS.

MRI activity supports early and indefinite treatment intervention

Early in the disease course, 80% of MS patients exhibit new gadolinium-enhancing lesions within a three month period.[51] Ongoing MRI activity in early RRMS predisposes patients to an increased frequency of relapses, making progression to higher levels of disability more likely. Typically there are between five and 10 times as many new MRI lesions as there are clinical relapses. In addition to new gadolinium-enhancing lesions, some T2-weighted lesions progress without new gadolinium enhancement. One particular study[52] demonstrated that lipid mobilization, as evidenced by lipid signals on magnetic resonance spectroscopy (MRS), can occur in the absence of enhancement.

The enhancement phase of lesion development signifies the early inflammatory component of the MS plaque. Agents that stabilize blood–brain barrier integrity, such as corticosteroids, probably have a prominent effect on this aspect of plaque development. However, the evidence that some plaques emerge without enhancement suggests the possibility that demyelination and axonal loss can occur in the absence of perivenular inflammatory processes. This implies that the number of gadolinium-enhancing lesions should not be the exclusive measure of the MS disease process. In fact, therapeutic agents that markedly reduce the number of new gadolinium-enhancing lesions may not necessarily influence the overall disease process. This point underscores the necessity of formulating composite imaging algorithms that use different techniques for measuring the various distinctive components of the disease process. Such measurements, when taken together, will probably provide a more accurate estimation of disease activity by which therapeutic agents can be judged.

In general, there appears to be only a weak correlation between the anatomic burden of disease, as measured by brain MRI, and clinical disability.[53,54] This may relate to frequent involvement of non-eloquent neuroanatomic pathways by the disease process. In contrast, disability appears to correlate better with brain and spinal cord atrophy, which is probably a consequence of demyelination and axonal loss.[55–57]

Stevenson and colleagues[58] have demonstrated that spinal cord imaging with analysis of spinal cord cross-sectional area (at the second cervical level) is strongly correlated with disability and disease duration. In a longitudinal study, baseline spinal cord cross-sectional area measurements were significantly different between controls and MS patients with primary progressive and secondary progressive disease, but not between control subjects and RRMS or benign MS groups. However, over a 12-month period there was a significant increase in spinal cord atrophy in the RRMS and primary progressive patients, suggest-

ing that even early in the disease process, RRMS patients are at risk of spinal cord atrophy.

The development of advanced magnetic resonance techniques should yield novel information about the disease process in MS. MRS analysis of MS lesions characteristically shows decreased N-acetyl aspartate (NAA), a chemical component that appears to be restricted to neurons and their processes, including axons.[59,60] There appears to be a strong correlation between MS histopathology, disability and diminished levels of NAA.[52,61–63] Other imaging measures that correlate pathology with EDSS include black holes as seen on T1-weighted MRI.[64,65] Magnetization transfer ratios (MTR) appear to strongly correlate with disability.[66,67] What has also become clear is that normal-appearing white matter may in fact harbor microscopic evidence of demyelination and axonal damage.[68]

MRI is increasingly used as a surrogate marker of disease activity. Compared to conventional MRI, MTR and MRS may demonstrate abnormalities that are a better reflection of the principal pathological hallmarks of MS, namely demyelination and axonal loss. It should, however, be recognized that such abnormalities are dynamic and potentially reversible.[52,69,70] Normalization of MTR and MRS abnormalities may be the natural consequence of repair mechanisms within the CNS or they may represent reversible metabolic derangements that occur during episodes of inflammatory demyelination. The presence of such a repair apparatus suggests that the recovery process may be subject to therapeutic influences, the activity of which might be able to be monitored by changes in MTR and MRS.

In patients with monosymptomatic syndromes consistent with the first MS relapse, MRI provides important predictive information about the risk of developing clinically definite MS. The ONTT clearly demonstrated that the number of lesions present in patients with monosymptomatic optic neuritis is a strong predictor of the likelihood of developing MS.[71,72] In the ONTT, patients with no evidence of brain MRI lesions had a less than 5% chance of having confirmed definite MS at 2 years. In patients with three or more lesions, the risk was 30%. Filippi and colleagues[73] found that 86% of patients with clinically isolated syndromes suggestive of MS with a T2-weighted lesion load of more than 1.23 cm^3 developed definite MS at 5 years compared to only 3% in those with a normal MRI.[73]

These findings indicate that the MS disease process is active and ongoing in MS patients even before the first relapse. Furthermore, it seems likely that the burden of disease as measured by MRI represents the 'tip of the iceberg' with respect to the underlying disease process. MS immunopathogenesis (see Chapter 19) involves a process of chronic inflammation working with terminal injury effector mechanisms and leading to the development of the plaque lesion. The ontogeny of an MS plaque probably involves the migration of activated T and B lymphocytes from the blood compartment into the CNS. During the initial process, cells become adherent to the vascular endothelium through interaction of specific adhesion molecules and associated receptors.[74,75] Cells then use matrix metalloproteinases to digest basement membrane collagen and fibronectin in order to pass into the brain.[76] On entry, activated lymphocytes can interact with resident antigen-presenting cells, such as microglia, and undergo a second round of stimulation. Pro-inflammatory cytokines and injury molecules can then be elaborated by activated lymphocytes and macrophages, with consequent damage to the oligodendrocyte–myelin– axonal

unit.[77] Axonal integrity may be at risk not so much because of a direct immunological attack, but rather as a secondary effect of a loss of trophic support from the myelin–oligodendrocyte complex.

The evidence is now unequivocal that axonal loss is an inevitable pathological feature in MS.[68] Axonal injury probably culminates in wallerian degeneration and neurodegeneration. However, it appears that such injury may be minimal during the earliest stages of the disease. This provides an early therapeutic window of opportunity to promote axonal preservation and functional integrity of CNS white matter pathways.[68,78] Suppression of inflammatory mechanisms may facilitate CNS repair processes that may allow for the recruitment of progenitor oligodendrocytes with an ability to promote plaque remyelination.[79,80]

Pathological studies have shown that lesions derived from an individual patient exhibit a stereotypic pattern of inflammation, demyelination, axonal loss, gliosis, and remyelination. There appears to be a consistent pattern of histopathology across different lesions within the same patient, whereas recent studies have shown that there is substantial heterogeneity in lesion pathology between different patients.[81] Luccinetti and colleagues[82] have codified five discrete lesional characterizations that appear to be uniform within an individual patient. This suggests that individual differences in the pathology may account for the clinical variability seen within the MS population. In a similar fashion, subtypes of immune-mediated inflammatory neuropathies with demyelinating and axonal components have been delineated.[83] If subtypes of MS are confirmed, this would have significant ramifications for the design of future clinical trials. For example, the response to individual or multicomponent therapeutic regimens may vary between patients with distinctly different underlying pathological substrates. In contrast, responses may be more robust in clinically and pathologically uniform MS populations.

A REVOLUTION IN MS: THE EMERGENCE OF DISEASE-MODIFYING THERAPIES

On the subject of treatment for MS, Charcot in 1877 stated that '... the time has not yet come when such a subject can be seriously considered.'[84] Until very recently the situation was still much the same. Perhaps the most significant advance in MS therapeutics has been the approval of three DMAs: interferon (IFN)-β 1b (Betaseron®, Berlex Laboratories, Richmond CA, USA) in 1993, IFN-β 1a (Avonex®, Biogen, Cambridge MA, USA) in 1996, and glatiramer acetate (Copaxone®, TEVA Marion Partners, Kansas City MO, USA) in 1996.[45–47]

IFN-β

IFN-β has been shown to decrease clinical relapses, reduce brain MRI activity, and slow progression of disability.[45,46] The IFN-β 1b trial confirmed a dose response on clinical and imaging outcome measurements.[45,85] Whereas the IFN-β 1b trial used subcutaneous dosing every second day, the IFN-β 1a trial used a once-weekly 30 μg intramuscular dosing. The IFN-β 1a trial showed similar effects on relapses; additionally, patients treated with IFN-β 1a exhibited a (statistically significant) 37% reduction in the relative risk of disability progression, defined by a ≥ 1.0 point EDSS worsening sustained for at

least 6 months.[46] Furthermore, significantly fewer patients treated with IFN-β 1a progressed to sustained higher levels of disability compared to placebo-treated patients.[86] Failure to demonstrate a statistically significant effect on disability progression in the initial IFN-β 1b trial may have been related to trial design and placebo dropouts. More recently, IFN-β 1b has been shown to slow disability progression significantly in patients with SPMS (EDSS 3.0–6.5).[87]

Results from a trial of another form of IFN-β 1a (Rebif®, Ares Serono International, Geneva, Switzerland) were recently published, confirming therapeutic effects of IFN-β 1a on relapses and disability progression.[88] The study did not provide compelling evidence in favor of the high-dose versus low-dose groups in terms of the number of relapses, severity of relapses, odds ratio for hospital admission, change in EDSS, or the first quartile time to sustained disability progression.[89] The study found that patients treated with the higher dose developed fewer active MRI lesions. For a subset of patients with EDSS scores over 3.5, higher dose recipients had longer times to disability progression. This last, post hoc observation will need to be confirmed prospectively.

IFN neutralizing antibodies

Essentially, all patients treated with IFN-β develop antibodies to the IFN molecule.[90] Most of these antibodies bind to the molecule but do not interfere with the receptor-binding portion of the molecule. Consequently, most binding antibodies do not neutralize the effect of IFN-β. Only neutralizing antibodies (Nab) are clearly associated with loss of biological activity. Khan and colleagues[91] found that the presence of Nab was associated with undetectable serum levels of IFN.

Pachner[92] reviewed techniques used to detect

IFN antibodies. Enzyme-linked immunosorbent assay (ELISA) techniques measure binding antibodies to all epitopes. Immunoblotting methods detect denatured IFN separated electrophoretically. The myxovirus associated antigen (MXA) assay quantifies an IFN-inducible protein that is diminished in the presence of Nab. Cytopathic effect assays (CPE) detect Nab by demonstrating neutralization of IFN inhibition of virally mediated cell lysis. Most laboratories currently use the CPE assay.

In the phase III IFN-β 1b trial, approximately 38% of patients developed Nab. Efficacy of IFN-β 1b appeared to be lost in Nab-positive patients.[90] It was suggested that increased disease activity in Nab-positive patients reflected inherently greater disease severity at baseline, but there were no significant differences with respect to pre-study EDSS score or relapse rate between patients that were eventually Nab-positive compared to the other patients.[90] In the phase III IFN-β 1a trial, 22% of patients became Nab-positive. Rudick and colleagues[93] subsequently showed, using a two-step assay, that 39% of patients treated with IFN-β 1b and 6% of patients treated with IFN-β 1a developed Nab. In this method, patient sera were screened by ELISA for IFN-β-binding antibodies, and positive sera were then tested in a CPE assay. In the Rebif® trial, the low-dose and high-dose groups developed Nab in 24% and 13% of the cases, respectively.[87] It was speculated that 'high zone tolerance' explained the lower rate of Nab in the high-dose group. However, a similar effect was not seen in the IFN-β 1b trial when comparing low-dose and high-dose groups.[90] The explanation for the lower Nab rates in the higher dose group is not currently known.

Lower immunogenicity with IFN-β 1a may relate to a number of factors. IFN-β has an amino acid sequence that is identical to naturally occurring IFN-β, and it is glycosylated. Glycosylation is important for the molecular configuration of IFN-β. It was shown that non-glycosylated IFN-β exhibits a reduction in anti-inflammatory, antiviral, and anti-proliferative effects.[94] Lack of glycosylation may account for the formation of IFN-β 1b aggregates.[95,96] Aggregate forms of IFN-β have decreased biological activity, diminished ability to interact with the IFN receptor, and potentially increased immunogenicity. Another factor that may account for the increased immunogenicity seen with IFN-β 1b is the subcutaneous route of administration. The skin is an active immune organ with immunocompetent antigen-presenting cells that mediate humoral and cellular immune responses. In contrast, muscle is immunologically quiescent.

The intramuscular route of administration for IFN-β 1a may also be associated with greater overall bioavailability than that derived from the subcutaneous route. While this difference appears to have been demonstrated for the Avonex® form of IFN-β 1a, the Rebif® product apparently produces no significant differences in serum levels irrespective of whether the drug is administered by the subcutaneous or intramuscular route.[97] It is not yet clear what accounts for these disparate observations.

Mechanisms of action of IFN

Much has been learned about potential mechanisms of action of IFN-β in MS. IFN-β inhibits T cell proliferation and reduces the production of T-helper 1 pro-inflammatory cytokines such as interleukin (IL)-2, tumor necrosis factor (TNF)-α, and IFN-γ, while at the same time increasing T-helper 2 cytokines such as IL-4 and IL-10.[98,99] IFN-β inhibits antigen presentation, decreases cellular adhesion and cell trafficking, and regulates co-stimulatory molecules.[100] The activity of matrix metalloproteinases are reduced by IFN-β, which may relate to the significant reduction in new brain MRI lesions in patients treated with these agents.[101–104] Matrix metalloproteinases also are known to promote the conversion of pro-TNF-α to mature TNF-α. TNF can contribute to the death of oligodendrocytes by apoptotic mechanisms.[105] Nitric oxide (NO) can damage oligodendrocytes and is a potent vasodilator that has potential effects on the integrity of the blood–brain barrier.[106] NO synthesis results from inducible nitric oxide synthetase (iNOS). In MS lesions, microglial cells, macrophages, and astrocytes express iNOS.[107,108] IFN-β has been shown to selectively decrease IL-1β and IFN-γ induced iNOS expression in astrocytes.[109] Co-cultures of microglial cells and T lymphocytes pre-treated with IFN-β show increased production of IL-10 and a decreased production of TNF-α.[99] Finally, IFN-β increases elaboration of nerve growth factor from astrocytes, which may have implications for axonal integrity. These anti-inflammatory properties may augment the effects of corticosteroids. In that regard, IFN-β 1a was found to decrease the risk of recurrent gadolinium enhancement on MRI after corticosteroid treatment.[110]

Glatiramer acetate

Glatiramer acetate has a composition similar to myelin basic protein (MBP) and consists of a mixture of four principal amino acids (L-glutamic acid, L-lysine, L-alanine, and L-tyrosine). In a large prospective trial in RRMS, glatiramer acetate significantly reduced the relapse rate, although the effect on disability progression and MRI lesion activity is less certain (see Chapter 21).[47,111] Glatiramer acetate is administered daily as a subcutaneous injection. Unlike IFN-β, it is not associated with flu-like symptoms and is the best tolerated of the three DMAs. It is, however, associated with a number of characteristic symptomatic side effects. Most commonly, patients experience injection site reactions characterized by mild erythema and induration. Occasional patients describe short periods of chest tightness or pressure, and some experience flushing, dyspnea, palpitations, or anxiety. One distinct advantage of this agent is the lack of evidence for Nab.

Glatiramer acetate was originally designed to simulate MBP with an intent of blocking MBP antigen presentation. Glatiramer acetate produces immunological effects that probably confer benefit on the MS disease process. Glatiramer acetate is able to cross-react with monoclonal antibodies and T cells generated to MBP.[112,113] It induces antigen-specific suppressor T cells,[114] and can bind to major histocompatibility (MHC) class II molecules, thereby inhibiting antigen presentation and potentially displacing MBP or other relevant peptides that are involved in lymphocyte activation.[115,116]

PRACTICAL MANAGEMENT STRATEGIES

When should disease-modifying therapy be started and for which MS patients?

Evidence from controlled clinical trials supports the use of IFN-β and glatiramer acetate in RRMS and the use of IFN-β in SPMS. Given the evidence, reviewed above, that MS becomes progressive in most patients over time, the present author believes that all patients with a confirmed diagnosis of RRMS or SPMS should be offered treatment. Some may reasonably suggest that patients with a long quiescent course should be excluded from therapy on the basis of actuarial evidence for benign disease. However, it is not uncommon to observe patients with recrudescent disease activity after a long period of apparent stabilization. Furthermore, patients who fail to exhibit outward evidence of disease activity may in fact have subclinical ongoing pathological changes that remain occult until critical thresholds are exceeded, at which point symptoms and disability emerge.

Patients who are newly diagnosed with MS often have limited limited clinical symptoms and little anatomic disease burden. As such, some neurologists have surmised that such patients are 'too mild to treat.' However, the author believes that this is a fundamental error that reflects inadequate awareness of the chronicity and magnitude of disease activity that is constitutive over time. In addition, a high frequency of attacks during the first 2 years of MS onset is associated with a less favorable long-term outcome.[43] It is plausible to suggest that reducing the relapse frequency in the early years will promote stabilization of the disease process and limit later disability.

The author sees many patients in practice who indicate they would have started therapy if their physician had recommended it. MS becomes progressive in most patients; the disease process is constitutively active; and we now have treatment that, although not curative, can favorably influence the disease process and the clinical course. Ultimately, we have a responsibility to advocate strongly for the implementation of treatment in patients with a confirmed diagnosis of MS.

Should monosymptomatic patients receive disease-modifying therapy

One patient population that generates considerable debate is the monosymptomatic group, where a diagnosis of clinically definite MS cannot be rendered. Currently two important studies are in progress to answer the question of whether treatment of monosymptomatic disease confers long-term benefit (the European Treatment Trial of Monosymptomatic MS (ETOMS) study of Rebif®; and the Controlled trial of high risk subjects in an MS Prevention Study (CHAMPS) of Avonex®). Until results of these trials are available, we are confronted with the difficult decision of whether to treat such patients or to follow them until there is an expression of new disease activity. In the author's opinion, delay in diagnosis until a second clinical relapse, when alternative etiologies have been reasonably excluded, may represent excess reliance on diagnostic criteria that is not in the interest of the patient. The MRI scan can be helpful in deciding on treatment. If the monosymptomatic patient has no evidence of multicentric lesions in the brain or spinal cord, it is reasonable to observe the patient with repeat MRI studies, commonly every 6 months. New clinical relapses, emergent abnormalities on the neurological exam, or the evolution of new MRI lesions all prompt the recommendation of treatment.

Characteristic lesions on MRI at the time of presentation in a monosymptomatic patient indicate that the patient is at high risk of subsequent MRI lesions and clinical relapses. There is a strong correlation between the presence and number of brain MRI lesions and progression to clinically definite MS in those with clinically isolated syndromes.[72,117,118] For these patients, the author typically recommends treatment. While this approach may be aggressive, the vast majority of monosymptomatic patients with characteristic MRI lesions have clinically definite MS within a couple of years. Therefore, until the results from the monosymptomatic trials are available, it is reasonable to elect to treat such patients in most cases.

Which drug should be recommended for individual patients?

Efficacy on relapse frequency appears to be similar for IFN-β preparations and glatiramer acetate. However, there are differences with significant practical consequences. Moreover, there may be differences on the MRI effects of the drugs (*Table 31.3*). When counseling a patient on currently available DMAs, the author generally does not recommend IFN-β 1b (Betaseron®) as a first-line agent, primarily because of skin lesions with a small risk of abscess formation and necrosis, and also because IFN-β 1b is less well tolerated than weekly IFN-β 1a (Avonex®) injections. IFN-β 1b is also associated with a substantially higher frequency of Nab that may abrogate biological activity of the drug. Since IFN-β 1a and IFN-β 1b antibodies are cross-reactive,[119] patients developing Nab to IFN-β 1b may not respond to IFN-β 1a. Because IFN-β 1b has demonstrated efficacy, changing drugs in patients who are doing well on IFN-β 1b is not recommended. For patients contemplating therapy with an IFN-β, the author favors IFN-β 1a because of convenience, the low risk of Nab formation, tolerability, and documented efficacy.

Glatiramer acetate is well tolerated by patients. Despite the need for daily injections, patients remain highly compliant with glatiramer acetate. The author has been impressed with its stabilizing effects in patients with limited disability. The effect on relapse rate is similar to the IFNs, although the effect on disability progression is less clear. Similarly, we await the results of recent investigations concerning the effect on MRI disease activity.

For patients with the lowest levels of disability who are early in the course of the illness, the author generally favors treatment with either IFN-β 1a or glatiramer acetate. For patients with more advanced disability or with a component of secondary progression, the author favors the use of IFN-β.

What role do patients play in the choice of DMA?

Comprehensive information about MS and the available treatments will have a beneficial impact on long-term compliance. Patients must play an active role in this process since they must take responsibility for using these agents properly and accept the potential risk of adverse reactions. Most patients in the author's practice self-administer their injections, although some have this performed by family members or friends. Therefore, it is important that family members and caregivers are also educated about the treatments and receive information about expectations and potential side effects.

How long should treatment be continued?

Treatment with a DMA should be continued indefinitely. Justifiable reasons for terminating therapy include intolerable side effects, lack of efficacy, or substitution with a superior agent. It is helpful to explain to patients that MS is analo-

Table 31.3 Disease-modifying agents for RRMS

Trade name	*Avonex®*	*Rebif®*	*Betaseron®*	*Copaxone®*
Generic name	IFN-β 1a	IFN-β 1a	IFN-β 1b	Glatiramer acetate (amino acid polymer)
Route of administration	Intramuscular	Subcutaneous	Subcutaneous	Subcutaneous
Frequency of administration	Weekly	3 times weekly	Every other day	Daily
Reduction in exacerbations	+ + +	+ + +	+ + +	+ + +
Reduction in progression in disability	+ + +	+ + +	+	+
Neutralizing antibodies	+	+ +	+ + +	–
Reduction in MRI lesions	+ +	+ + +	+ + +	?
Most common side effects	Flu-like symptoms, fatigue, spasiticity, weakness	Flu-like symptoms, skin lesions, fatigue, spasticity, weakness	Flu-like symptoms, skin lesions, spasticity, weakness	Skin reaction, flushing, shortness of breath, chest pressure, anxiety

gous to other chronic illnesses that require long-term intervention. Using examples like hypertension or diabetes mellitus helps them understand this concept. In the future, it is likely that greater control over the disease process will be achieved through the use of combination drug regimens. The author generally tells patients about future prospects for new and more effective treatments, and indicates that they can discuss potential changes in their medication at future visits.

How should efficacy and disease activity be monitored?

Given the sensitivity of MRI over clinical examination, MRI is expected to play an increasing role in monitoring DMA therapy. While the clinical effects of DMAs are of paramount importance, evidence for ongoing MRI changes probably signifies that the disease process is not adequately controlled. Consequently, patients on DMAs should be monitored by serial neurological examinations, with documentation of relapses and disability, and periodic MRI analyses.

Despite the economic implications of MRI studies, high levels of lesion activity may signal loss of drug efficacy before the clincal changes become evident. This provides an opportunity to consider addition of adjunctive therapy, dosage adjustments of DMAs, or alternative monotherapy. The high cost of DMAs justifies the use of yearly MRI scans as part of an efficacy assessment strategy.

Should Nab titers be used to influence treatment decisions?

As detailed above, the evidence suggests that persistently high titers of Nab abrogate biological activity, ultimately diminishing the therapeutic response to IFN-β. While there are no validated practice guidelines related to use of Nab titers in patients treated with IFN-β the author generally checks titers after 12–18 months of therapy. If titers are < 1:20, repeating the assay is not necessary unless there is a major worsening in the patient's clinical course. For a patient who appears to be under control but has increased titers, the test can be repeated after 3 months, along with a cranial MRI scan. In the absence of evidence for new disease activity, therapy should be continued and the patient followed closely despite the Nab results. If the patient has relapses or new MRI lesions in the face of Nab titers > 1:20, they can be switched to glatiramer acetate.

When should patients be converted to an alternative agent?

The DMAs are not curative, in that they do not completely arrest relapses or disability progres-

sion in many patients. Nevertheless, continued relapses or disability progression while on treatment should prompt reassessment of the treatment plan. Drug intolerability is another indication for considering an alternative DMA. An occasional patient will request a change to an alternative agent on the basis of practical considerations. For example, a patient who travels frequently for business may find daily injections prohibitive. Alternately, an occasional patient may find it difficult to overcome persistent IFN-related side effects or may have difficulty with the longer needle used for intramuscular injections. Glatiramer acetate is appropriate for these patients. With continued disease activity despite treatment with IFN-β, the author often elects to switch to glatiramer acetate. Similarly, patients with relapses despite treatment with glatiramer acetate should be offered treatment with IFN-β.

What adjunctive therapy is appropriate and when should it be added?

Adjunctive therapy involves the use of a second DMA in combination with IFN-β or glatiramer acetate. Currently there is little evidence to support combination therapies for the treatment of MS, and in most instances the safety of combination therapy has not been rigorously evaluated. The rationale for using the agents described below derives principally from studies testing the drugs as monotherapy. For the majority of these drugs, there have been a limited number of well-designed, randomized, placebo-controlled studies. Therefore, in many circumstances these agents are used on empirical grounds in patients who are not adequately responsive to first-line therapeutic approaches.

For acute relapses, corticosteroid therapy is the standard of care and a variety of regimens can be used as previously outlined (see *Table 31.2*). For patients on IFN-β who have repeated relapses (with negative Nab titer), the author frequently adds intermittent pulses of corticosteroids (see *Table 31.2*). In general, chronic corticosteroid therapy in MS patients is best avoided, so in this situation the addition of a steroid-sparing agent such as azathioprine should be considered.

A variety of other adjunctive agents can be used in combination with DMAs. It is important to emphasize that many neurologists have limited experience with the use of some of these agents in the treatment of MS patients with highly active disease. Referral of these patients to centers that routinely use more aggressive treatment protocols should be encouraged.

Intravenous immune globulin

Intravenous immune globulin (IVIg) improves suppressor cell function, blocks Fc receptors on macrophages, reduces T-helper 1 pro-inflammatory cytokines, and appears to promote remyelination in an animal model of inflammatory demyelination.[120] Clinically, IVIg may reduce MS relapses, although the effect on MRI activity and progression of disability is less certain. Fazekas and colleagues[121] studied monthly IVIg in a well-designed, 2-year, randomized, double-blind, placebo-controlled trial in 148 RRMS patients. There was a 59% reduction in relapses in addition to a small beneficial effect on EDSS. In another 2-year study, Achiron and colleagues[122] randomized 40 RRMS patients to placebo or IVIg treatment with 0.4 g/kg per day for 5 days followed by second-monthly boosters of 0.4 g/kg. A significant 38.6% reduction in relapse rate was observed in the IVIg group. Six of the IVIg-treated patients but none of the placebo patients remained relapse free for the entire 2 years. The median time to first relapse was 233 days in the treated group and 82 days in the placebo group. No significant effects on EDSS or MRI were seen, although the study was not powered to demonstrate this effect.

In an attempt to determine whether IVIg promotes myelin repair in MS, a recent study found no evidence of functional restoration in MS patients with fixed motor deficits.[123,124] Another study is under way to determine whether IVIg can promote improvement in visual function in those with chronic optic neuropathy. Restoration of visual function in patients with stable visual deficits caused by optic neuritis has already been documented.[125]

IVIg is generally well tolerated, but it can be associated with a number of adverse reactions (*Table 31.4*). When patients experience relapses and a switch to an alternative DMA is not indicated, the author often begins monthly IVIg treatment with 1 g/kg per day for 2 days initially followed by monthly or second-monthly boosters of 1 g/kg. This therapy is highly effective in individual patients. This approach is limited by drug availability and financial constraints.

Azathioprine

Azathioprine is a nucleoside analogue pro-drug of 6-mercaptopurine that impairs DNA and RNA synthesis. Studies of this agent in the treatment of MS have yielded mixed results, perhaps because of differences in trial design, study duration, and the number of patients studied. A retrospective meta-analysis of all randomized, blinded controlled trials involving 793 patients in 75 studies demonstrated a reduction in relapses.[126] In a different meta-analysis, the probability of remaining free of relapses at the conclusion of 2 years of therapy was analysed for azathioprine

Table 31.4 Adjunctive immunotherapy

Agent	Regimen	Laboratory studies	Adverse events
Intravenous immune globulin	*Induction* 1 g/kg per day for 2 days *Maintenance* 1 g/kg per month	Quantitative IgA, plasma viscosity, blood urea nitrogen, creatinine, liver function tests	Aseptic meningitis, anaphylaxis, rash, acute renal insufficiency, viral hepatitis, cerebral ischemia, hypercoagulable state
Azathioprine	*Induction* 50 mg/day for 1 week *Titration* 50 mg/week until 2–3 mg/kg	White blood cell count < 3000 cells/microliter Lymphocyte count 800–1000 Mean corpuscular volume > 100 femtoliters	Allergic reaction in 15%, lymphopenia, anemia, transaminitis, alopecia, pancreatitis, latent viral infections, slight risk of lymphoma
Methotrexate	*Induction* 2.5 mg/week *Titration* 2.5 mg/week until at 7.5–20 mg/week Folic acid 1 mg/day	Liver function tests, chest X-ray	Liver dysfunction including cirrhosis, interstitial pneumonitis, gastrointestinal upsets, mucositis
Cyclophosphamide (CYP)	*Preparation* 1. Place Foley catheter (unless patient performs clean intermittent self-catheterization) 2. Antibiotic suppression 3. Hydration *Maintenance* 1. Intravenous Mesna at 20% of cyclophosphamide dose 30 minutes before and 4 and 8 hours after cyclophosphamide infusion 2. Anti-emetics along with each Mesna dose 3. Intravenous cyclophosphamide, 1 g/m^2 4. Hydration	Before and 2 weeks after treatment Full blood count with differential, liver function tests, blood urea nitrogen, creatinine, electrolytes, urinalysis with microscopy	Nausea, vomiting, alopecia, hepatorenal toxicity, hemorrhagic cystitis, myelosuppression, amenorrhea, risk of sterility, long-term risk of cancer

and the newly available DMAs and the results compared to those from corresponding placebo groups.[127] The odds ratio for being free of relapses at 2 years were 1.37 for glatiramer acetate, 1.68 for IFN-β 1a, 2.38 for IFN-β 1b, 2.07 for IVIg, and 2.04 for azathioprine. Currently, little is known about the effect of azathioprine on disability progression or MRI activity. However, the author has found azathioprine particularly effective in stablizing MS patients who exhibit strong corticosteroid responsiveness.

The author uses azathioprine as a first-line agent in patients with Devic's disease (neuromyelitis optica) and as a second-line agent (after DMAs) in those patients with recurrent transverse myelitis. The author also uses azathioprine in patients who, for one reason or another, are not able to use first-line DMAs. For MS patients with ongoing disease activity who have not responded to DMAs alone or in combination with pulse corticosteroids or IVIg, azathioprine can be added (see *Table 31.4*). One of the well-recognized limitations of azathioprine is that many months may be required before clinical benefits become evident. Likewise, the expected laboratory changes that correspond to drug activity, such as mild leukopenia and elevated mean corpuscular volume (MCV) may not be achieved for 3–6 months.[128]

The author generally begins therapy with 50 mg daily for 1 week and subsequently increases it by 50 mg weekly until a dose of 2–3 mg/kg per day is achieved (see *Table 31.4*). The full blood count with differential should be followed and the MCV should be kept above 100 femtoliters, the WBC at approximately 3000, and the absolute lymphocyte count at about 800–1000 cells per microliter. Haematology is done weekly for the first month and monthly thereafter. Liver enzymes should also be checked for evolving transaminitis.

Azathioprine is well tolerated and easy to use in most patients. There are, however, well-recognized adverse effects (see *Table 31.4*). While there has been concern about the long-term risk of malignancy (particularly lymphoma) in those treated with this agent, there has been no substantiated increased risk of malignancy in MS patients.[129]

Methotrexate

Methotrexate is an inhibitor of dihydrofolate reductase and has a number of properties that are at least theoretically beneficial in MS. Methotrexate has anti-inflammatory activity, is able to decrease the levels of pro-inflammatory cytokines and augment suppressor cell function, and has been shown to benefit upper extremity function in secondary progressive MS patients.[130] In addition, Fischer and colleagues[131] have reported beneficial effects of methotrexate on neurocognitive function, including improved information processing speed. A standard regimen is 7.5 mg orally, given weekly. This dose is well tolerated by most patients. Potential side effects include liver dysfunction, including cirrhosis, interstitial pneumonitis, and gastrointestinal upset. The risk of potential side effects can, however, be reduced by the use of folate supplementation without apparent loss of drug efficacy.[132,133]

The author has used more aggressive methotrexate protocols, which have been well tolerated by patients without evident toxicity (see *Table 31.4*). The weekly dose of methotrexate can be increased from 7.5 mg to 15–20 mg by 2.5 mg increments each week. Folic acid supplements (1 mg/day) are given.

Cyclophosphamide

Cyclophosphamide is an alkylating agent that has a diversity of immunological actions. It can induce immune suppression and produce myelosuppression, is lympholytic, decreases IFN-γ production, and increases the levels of IL-4 and IL-10. Many studies of cyclophosphamide have been completed with the majority showing only modest benefit or no benefit.[134] However, the number of randomized, double-blind, placebo-controlled studies is small and most have studied patients with progressive MS. There is, therefore, a lack of sufficiently well designed studies examining the role of cyclophosphamide in RRMS or in early stage patients with progressive MS. A small cross-sectional study[135] has demonstrated that monthly infusions of cyclophosphamide and methylprednisolone increases IL-4 and IL-10 levels to an extent greater than either agent alone and to a greater extent than with IFN-β 1b. Long-term therapy is associated with an eventual decrease in IFN-γ production as well. The authors of this study suggest that the cyclophosphamide–methylprednisolone regimen induces a favorable immune deviation toward a T-helper 2 state. Monthly boosters of the two agents may avoid many of the side effects associated with prolonged oral administration protocols such as those used in systemic lupus.[136,137]

In the author's experience, monthly combination therapy is very well tolerated. This form of treatment can be reserved for patients who continue to experience relapses or disability progression despite first- and second-line therapeutic intervention. Therapy is begun with the placement of a Foley catheter and hydration with 1–2 liters of fluids. Patients are treated concomitantly with oral antibiotics such as nitrofurantoin in order to prevent a urinary tract infection. The placement of the Foley catheter is especially important in MS patients with high post-void residual volumes since this can prolong the exposure of the bladder wall to cyclophosphamide and its metabolites. Foley catheters are not placed in those patients who already perform clean intermittent self-catherization.

Methylprednisolone, 1–2 g, is infused over 2 hours, followed by intravenous cyclophosphamide, 1 g/m^2, over 2–3 hours. Mesna at 20% of the cyclophosphamide dose is given along with anti-emetics at 30 minutes before and 4 and 8 hours after the cyclophosphamide infusion. Mesna decreases the conversion of cyclophosphamide to its toxic metabolites and thereby decreases the risk of adverse events, including hemorrhagic cystitis. Post-therapy hydration is administered with 1–2 liters of intravenous fluids. Laboratory studies, including full blood count, liver function tests, and urinalysis with microscopic analysis at baseline and at 2 weeks after treatment, should be performed. Patients are referred for intensive physical therapy and rehabilitation and they return monthly for repeat infusions. After 6 months of treatment, patients are re-evaluated and it is determined whether to continue, reduce, or discontinue therapy.

Impressive responses have been seen in some patients with aggressive disease progression or frequent relapses. A number of severely disabled patients have regained ambulation without assistance. However, not many favorable responses have been seen in more advanced progressive patients with static neurological deficits. Therefore cyclophosphamide should probably be restricted to patients who are refractory to standard first-line agents and who exhibit unrelenting disease progression.

How should DMA-related adverse events be managed?

The author suggests a fractionated dosing scheme when initiating DMA for both IFN-β and glatiramer acetate. In the case of IFN-β, the author generally begins therapy at one quarter of the recommended dose and increases it by one quarter increments weekly. The vast majority of patients find this approach psychologically and physically more tolerable than starting at the full dose. Although some patients experience only mild adverse reactions with the full dose, the 'go slow' approach allows patients the opportunity to execute the injection technique with a minimal degree of potential side effects. This quickly builds confidence and reinforces expectation of long-term tolerability.

Most post-injection side effects can be mitigated with over-the-counter agents such as naproxen, acetaminophen, ibuprofen, or aspirin. Patients who experience increased body temperature following IFN-β treatment despite these agents can be encouraged to use ice-cold liquids, lower the ambient temperature, and avoid hot food or liquids. Patients with persistent side effects from IFN-β can be started on pentoxifylline, amantidine, or low-dose corticosteroids on the day of injection and the following day for weekly IFN-β 1a, and daily for every second-day subcutaneous IFN-β 1b. This is continued for 4–6 weeks.

Pentoxifylline (PTX) is a methylxanthine phosphodiesterase inhibitor that can reduce T-helper 1 cytokine secretion.[138] Rieckmann and colleagues[139] have demonstrated that PTX, 800 mg bid can decrease levels of IFN-γ, TNF-α, IL-12, IL-2 receptor, and ICAM-1 and increase levels of IL-4 and IL-10 in vivo. It has also been demonstrated that PTX reduces TNF-α, and IFN-γ production by microglial cells.[140] These immunologic effects may underlie beneficial effects of PTX on IFN-β side effects.[141] PTX is well tolerated by most patients, although some have difficulty with headache, nausea, and gastrointestinal distress.

When starting therapy with glatiramer acetate,

patients can start with one half of the recommended dose for the first 2–3 days. Many patients have no adverse events following injections, but some experience flushing, chest pressure, dyspnea, and anxiety. For patients with this reaction, the dose can be reduced by 50%. These same patients describe similar side effects of significantly less severity with a transient reduction in dose. In almost all cases they go on to tolerate escalation to full dose with long-term tolerability.

How should we approach treatment of children with MS?

Unfortunately there is currently no available literature that provides any specific treatment recommendations about the treatment of MS in childhood. Consequently, the author's approach to treatment of MS in children is virtually indistinguishable from that in adults. As with the adult population, a fractionated dosing scheme can be used when starting patients on DMAs. The dose of DMAs, especially IFN-β, may need to be adjusted in young children with smaller body weights to avoid intolerable side effects.

How should pregnancy and family planning issues influence treatment?

The use of DMAs in women with MS who are of child-bearing age is an area that requires active patient participation in the decision-making process. Unfortunately, there are few studies to guide decisions. There is currently little evidence to suggest that any of the DMAs are teratogenic in humans. Spontaneous abortion has been observed in patients treated with IFN-β, although the relationship to drug treatment has not been confirmed. When counseling patients who are considering pregnancy and who would otherwise be starting therapy with a DMA, the author recommends withholding therapy until the pregnancy and breast-feeding periods are completed. However, if patients are clearly having difficulty achieving pregnancy, the author recommends starting therapy until they become pregnant. Many women with MS will forego therapy in order to become pregnant, a process that may require considerable time, thereby exposing patients to long periods without treatment. For patients already on treatment with a DMA and who are interested in having a child, the author does not recommend withdrawing therapy until they have become pregnant. Such patients must be observed closely and must be reliable. If there are concerns about patient reliability then the author suggests terminating therapy until the post partum period is completed. Of course patients must be informed of potential risks of using DMAs while attempting to become pregnant.

In one study,[142] IVIg was administered to a small cohort of MS patients with a documented history of post partum relapses. Treatment was implemented during the first week after childbirth and at 6 and 12 weeks thereafter. None of the patients relapsed during the 6-month period after delivery, although two had a relapse at 8 months and one at 10 months after childbirth. Further investigations are needed to determine whether early post partum therapy is effective in reducing disease activity following childbirth. In the meantime, the author recommends initiating DMAs immediately after delivery or breast-feeding, because of the documented increase in relapses in the 3–6 months following pregnancy.[143]

ADDITIONAL COMMENTS ON MS THERAPY

The understanding of the immunopathological mechanisms that underlie MS is undergoing rapid expansion, as are the available therapeutic options. An idiopathic inflammatory demyelinating syndrome, MS is probably a spectrum of disorders, all of which culminate in a final common pathway of injury processes. Although we have yet to identify triggering mechanisms that initiate the disease process in individual patients, greater insights have been achieved in decoding the sequence of pathogenetic steps that occur following established disease. These insights have catalysed the accelerated pace of new clinical trial initiatives that focus on influencing these specific steps in the disease process. Biological agents that can influence antigen presentation, cytokine profiles, cell adhesion, trafficking mechanisms, and terminal injury effector molecules are already under investigation in human MS clinical drug trials. Furthermore, the advent of rational combination immunotherapy protocols is already under investigation. The enormous list of potential therapeutic strategies underscores the limitations and partial effectiveness of the currently available agents (*Table 31.5*). Ultimately though, the time has now arrived when the subject of treatment for MS can be 'seriously considered'.

The heterogeneity of clinical phenotypes in MS may relate to distinct histopathological differences between patients and may account for the differences in disease course, duration, and extent of disability. The author suspects that our ability to control the disease process effectively in individual patients will be contingent upon the recognition of distinctive populations of MS patients. Characterization of these patient subgroups will be crucial in developing new strategic therapeutic

Table 31.5 Emerging therapeutic strategies

IFN/glatiramer acetate combination

IFN + X (steroids, IVIg, Imuran, MTX, PTX)

Oral IFNs and glatiramer acetate

Antiviral agents (HHV-6)

Antibacterial regimens (*Chlamydia pneumoniae*)

Anti-adhesion molecules

Matrix metalloproteinase inhibitors

Co-stimulatory modulators

Antioxidants

NOS inhibitors

Excitatory amino acid receptor antagonists

Macrophage/microglial cell inhibitors

T-cell receptor peptide vaccines

T-cell receptor blocking peptides

Chemotherapy

Lymphocyte depletion

Bone marrow transplantation

Oligodendroglial cell activation (remyelination)

Retinoic acid

Mitoxantrone

Plasmapheresis

Thalidomide

Vitamin D

interventions that can uncouple specific mechanisms of the disease that lead to inflammatory demyelination, sclerosis, axonal injury, and ultimately to neurodegeneration.

Other sections of this text address a multitude of issues relating to the treatment of symptomatic side effects in MS. It cannot, however, be overemphasized that optimal care for our patients is rendered when interdisciplinary strategies are in place to facilitate the process of treating the 'whole patient'. The comprehensive management of MS is highly labor-intensive and

requires great commitment and endurance. The implementation of disease-modifying strategies constitutes the initial treatment framework to which other therapeutic and rehabilitation measures should be added. Improved quality of life for MS patients will result with the identification of anti-fatigue measures, improved training techniques, proper sleep management, prevention strategies to optimize bone and mineral metabolism, proper management of bowel and bladder function, and with the open discussion of problems relating to sexuality and sexual dysfunction. Furthermore, agents that can optimize the physiological function of demyelinated pathways, such as aminopyridines, may prove to be beneficial for improving function and for enhancing rehabilitation strategies aimed at promoting restoration of neurological function in disabled MS patients.

REFERENCES

1 Poser CM, Paty DW, Scheinberg L et al. New diagnostic criteria for multiple sclerosis: guidelines for research protocols. *Ann Neurol* 1983; 13:227–231.
2 Weinshenker BG, Bass B, Rice GPA et al. The natural history of multiple sclerosis: a geographically based study. I. Clinical course and disability. *Brain* 1989; 112:133–146.
3 Rap SM, Leo GJ, Bernardin L, Unverzagt F. Cognitive dysfunction in multiple sclerosis. I. Frequency, patterns, and prediction. *Neurology* 1991; 41:685–691.
4 Pozzilli C, Fieschi C, Perani D et al. Relationship between corpus collosum atrophy and cerebral metabolic asymmetries in multiple sclerosis. *J Neurol Sci* 1992; 112:51–57.
5 Baumhefner RW, Syndulko K, Ke D et al. Relationship between total MRI lesion area above the spinal cord and clinical and neuroperformance outcome assessments in chronic progressive multiple sclerosis. *Neurology* 1994; 44 (suppl 2):A39.

6   Franklin GM, Heaton RK, Nelson LM et al.
    Correlation of neuropsychological and MRI findings
    in chronic/progressive multiple sclerosis. *Neurology*
    1988; **38**:1826–1829.

7   Izquierdo G, Campoy F Jr, Mir J. Memory and
    learning disturbances in multiple sclerosis. MRI
    lesions and neuropsychological correlation. *Eur J
    Radiol* 1991; **13**:220–224.

8   Medaer R, Eeckhout C, Gautama K, Vermijlen C.
    Lymphocytapheresis therapy in multiple sclerosis: a
    preliminary study. *Acta Neurol Scand* 1984;
    69:111–115.

9   Pozzilli C, Passafiume D, Bernardi S et al. SPECT,
    MRI, and cognitive functions in multiple sclerosis. *J
    Neurol Neurosurg Psychiatry* 1991; **54**:110–115.

10 Reischies FM, Baum K, Brau H et al. Cerebral
    magnetic resonance imaging findings in multiple
    sclerosis. *Arch Neurol* 1988; **45**:1114–1116.

11 Clark CM, James G, Li DKB et al. Ventricular size,
    cognitive function and depression in patients with
    multiple sclerosis. *Can J Neurol Sci* 1992;
    19:352–356.

12 Uhthoff W. Untersuchungen über bei multiplen
    Herdsklerose vorkommenden Augenstorungen. *Arch
    Psychiatr Nervenkrankh* 1890; **21**:55–116, 303–410.

13 Katz D, Taubenberger JK, Cannella B et al.
    Correlation between magnetic resonance imaging
    findings and lesion development in chronic, active
    multiple sclerosis. *Ann Neurol* 1993; **34**:661–669.

14 Drews J. Glucocorticoids. In: Drews J, ed.
    Immunopharmacology. New York: Springer, 1990.

15 McCombe PA, Nickson I, Tabi Z, Pender MP.
    Corticosteroid treatment of experimental
    autoimmune encephalomyelitis in the Lewis rat
    results in loss of Vβ8.2 and myelin basic protein-
    reactive cells from spinal cord, with increased total
    T-cell apoptosis but reduced apoptosis of Vβ8.2
    cells. *J Neuroimmunol* 1996; **70**:93–101.

16 Nieto MA, Lopez-Rivas A. IL-2 protects T-
    lymphocytes from glucocorticoid-induced DNA
    fragmentation and cell death. *J Immunol* 1989;
    143:4166–4170.

17 Zubiaga AM, Munoz E, Huber BT. IL-4 and IL-2
    selectively rescue Th cell subsets from glucocorticoid-
    induced apoptosis. *J Immunol* 1992; **149**:107–112.

18 Tuosto L, Cundari E, Montani MS, Piccoletta E.
    Analysis of susceptibility of mature human T-
    lymphocytes to dexamethasone-induced apoptosis.
    Eur J Immunol 1994; **24**:1061–1065.

19 Kupersmith MJ, Kaufman D, Paty DW et al.

20 Elovaara I, Lalla M, Spare E et al.
    Methylprednisolone reduces adhesion molecules in
    blood and cerebrospinal fluid in patients with MS
    Neurology 1998; **51**:1703–1708.

21 Durelli L, Cocito D, Riccio A et al. High-dose
    intravenous methylprednisolone in the treatment of
    multiple sclerosis: clinical–immunological
    correlations. *Neurology* 1986; **36**:238–243.

22 Ohno R, Katsunhiko H, Sowa K et al. High-dose
    intravenous corticosteroids in the treatment of
    multiple sclerosis. *Jpn J Med* 1987; **26**:212–216.

23 Milligan NM, Newcomb R, Compston DAS. A
    double-blind controlled trial of high dose
    methylprednisolone in patients with multiple
    sclerosis: 1. Clinical effects. *J Neurol Neurosurg
    Psychiatry* 1987; **50**:511–516.

24 Milanese C, La Manita L, Salmaggi A et al. Double-
    blind randomized trial of ACTH versus
    dexamethasone versus methylprednisolone bouts in
    multiple sclerosis. *Eur Neurol* 1989; **29**:10–16.

25 Rosenberg GA, Dencoff JE, Correa N et al. Effects of
    steroids on CSF matrix-metalloproteinases in
    multiple sclerosis: relation to blood–brain barrier
    injury. *Neurology* 1996; **46**:1626–1632.

26 Barkhof F, Hommes OR, Scheltens P, Valk J.
    Quantitative MRI changes in gadolinium-DPTA
    enhancement after high-dose intravenous
    methylprednisolone in multiple sclerosis. *Neurology*
    1991; **41**:1219–1222.

27 Burnham JA, Wright RR, Driesbach J, Murray RS.
    The effect of high-dose steroids on MRI gadolinium
    enhancement in acute demyelinating lesions.
    Neurology 1991; **41**:1349–1354.

28 Miller DH, Thompson AJ, Morrissey SP et al. High
    dose steroids in acute relapses of multiple sclerosis:
    MRI evidence for a possible mechanism of
    therapeutic effect. *J Neurol Neurosurg Psychiatry*
    1992; **55**:450–453.

29 Thompson AJ, Kennard C, Swash M et al. Relative
    efficacy of intravenous methylprednisolone and
    ACTH in the treatment of acute relapses in MS.
    Neurology 1989; **39**:969–971.

30 Paty DW, Koopmans RA, Li DKB, Oger JJF.
    Magnetic resonance imaging (MRI) as an outcome
    measure in multiple sclerosis. *J Neurol Rehabil* 1993;
    7:117.

31 Kappos L, Staedt D, Rohrbach E et al. Time course
    of gadolinium enhancement in MRI of patients with

Megadose corticosteroids in multiple sclerosis.
    Neurology 1994; **44**:1–4.

multiple sclerosis: effects of corticosteroid treatment. *J Neurol* 1988; **235**:10.

32 Barkhof F, Scheltens P, Frequin ST et al. Relapsing–remitting multiple sclerosis: sequential enhanced MR imaging vs clinical findings in determining disease activity. *AJR Am J Roentgenol* 1992; **159**:1041–1047.

33 Barkhof F, Tas MW, Frequin STFM et al. Limited duration of the effect of methylprednisolone on changes on MRI in multiple sclerosis. *Neuroradiology* 1994; **36**:382–387.

34 Oliveri RL, Valentino P, Russo C et al. Randomized trial comparing two different high doses of methylprednisolone in MS. *Neurology* 1998; **50**:1833–1836.

35 Smith ME, Stone LA, Albert PS et al. Clinical worsening in multiple sclerosis is associated with increased frequency and area of gadopentate dimeglumine-enhancing magnetic resonance imaging lesions. *Ann Neurol* 1993; **33**:480–489.

36 Buchanan WW, Stephen LJ, Buchanan HM. Are 'homeopathic' doses of oral corticosteroids effective in rheumatoid arthritis? *Clin Exp Rheumatol* 1988; **6**:281–284.

37 Ziegler DK. Acute disseminated encephalitis:some therapeutic and diagnostic considerations. *Arch Neurol* 1966; **14**:476–488.

38 Reder AT, Thapar M, Jensen MA. A reduction in serum glucocorticoids provokes experimental allergic encephalomyelitis: implications for treatment of inflammatory brain disease. *Neurology* 1994; **44**:2289–2294.

39 Beck RW, Clearly PA, Anderson MM et al. A randomized, controlled trial of corticosteroids in the treatment of acute optic neuritis. *N Engl J Med* 1992; **326**:581–588.

40 Herishanu YO, Badarna S, Sarov B et al. A possible harmful late effect of methylprednisolone therapy on a time cluster of optic neuritis. *Acta Neurol Scand* 1989; **80**:569–574.

41 Gambertoglio JG, Amend WJC Jr, Benet LZ. Pharmacokinetics and bioavailability of prednisone and prednisolone in healthy volunteers and patients: a review. *J Pharmacokinet Biopharm* 1980; **8**:1–52.

42 Gucuyener K, Hasanoglu A, Tunaoglu S, Ozturk G. Oral megadose methylprednisolone in a patient with chronic progressive multiple sclerosis. *Neurology* 1993; **43**:230.

43 Weinshenker BG, Bass B, Rice GPA et al. The natural history of multiple sclerosis: a geographically

based study. II. Predictive value of the early clinical course. *Brain* 1989; **112**:1419–1428.

44 Kurtzke JF. Rating neurological impairment in multiple sclerosis: an expanded disability status scale (EDSS). *Neurology* 1983; **33**:1444–1452.

45 The IFNB Multiple Sclerosis Study Group. Interferon beta-1b is effective in relapsing–remitting multiple sclerosis. I. Clinical results of a multicenter, randomized, double-blind, placebo-controlled trial. *Neurology* 1993; **43**:655–661.

46 Jacobs LD, Cookfair DL, Rudick RA et al. Intramuscular interferon beta-1a for disease progression in relapsing multiple sclerosis. *Ann Neurol* 1996; **39**:285–294.

47 Johnson KP, Brooks MD, Cohen JA et al. Copolymer 1 reduces relapse rate and improves disability in relapsing–remitting multiple sclerosis: results of a phase III multicenter, double-blind, placebo-controlled trial. *Neurology* 1995; **45**:1268–1276.

48 Minderhoud JM, van der Hoeven JH, Prange AJ. Course and prognosis of chronic progressive multiple sclerosis. Results of an epidemiological study. *Acta Neurol Scand* 1988; **78**:10–15.

49 Runmarker B, Andersen O. Prognostic factors in a multiple sclerosis incidence cohort with twenty-five years of follow-up. *Brain* 1993; **116**:117–134.

50 Hohlfeld R. Biotechnological agents for the immunotherapy of multiple sclerosis. Principals, problems and perspectives. *Brain* 1997; **120**:865–916.

51 McFarland HF, Stone LA, Calabresi PA et al. MRI studies of multiple sclerosis: implications for the natural history of the disease and for monitoring effectiveness of experimental therapies. *Multiple Sclerosis* 1996; **2**:198–205.

52 Narayana PA, Doyle TJ, Lai D, Wolinsky JS. Serial proton magnetic resonance spectroscopic imaging, contrast enhanced magnetic resonance imaging, and quantitative lesion volumetry in multiple sclerosis. *Ann Neurol* 1998; **43**:56–71.

53 IFNB Study Group, University of British Columbia MS/MRI Analysis Group. Interferon β-1b in the treatment of MS: final outcome of the randomized controlled trial. *Neurology* 1995; **45**:1277–1285.

54 Thompson AJ, Kermode AG, MacManus DG et al. Patterns of disease activity in multiple sclerosis: clinical and magnetic resonance imaging study. *Br Med J* 1990; **300**:631–634.

55 Davie CA, Barker GJ, Webb S et al. Persistent functional deficit in multiple sclerosis and autosomal

dominant cerebellar ataxia is associated with axonal loss. *Brain* 1995; **118**:1583–1592.

56 Losseff NA, Webb SL, O'Riordan JI et al. Spinal cord atrophy and disability in multiple sclerosis. A new reproducible and sensitive MRI method with potential to monitor disease progression. *Brain* 1996; **119**:701–708.

57 Losseff NA, Wang L, Lai HM et al. Progressive cerebral atrophy in multiple sclerosis: a serial study. *Brain* 1997; **119**:2009–2019.

58 Stevenson VL, Leary SM, Losseff NA et al. Spinal cord atrophy and disability in MS. A longitudinal study. *Neurology* 1998; **51**:234–238.

59 Simmons ML, Frondoza CG, Coyle JT. Immunocytochemical localization of *N*-acetyl-aspartate with monoclonal antibodies. *Neuroscience* 1991; **45**:37–45.

60 Moffett JR, Namboodiri MAA, Cangro CB, Neale JH. Immunohistochemical localization of *N*-acetylaspartate in rat brain. *NeuroReport* 1991; **2**:131–134.

61 De Stefano N, Mathews PM, Antel JP et al. Chemical pathology of acute demyelinating lesions and its correlation with disability. *Ann Neurol* 1995; **38**:901–909.

62 Narayana S, Fu L, Pioro E et al. Imaging of axonal damage in multiple sclerosis: spatial distribution of magnetic resonance imaging lesions. *Ann Neurol* 1997; **41**:385–391.

63 Hirohiko K, Grossman RI, Lenkinski RE, Gonzalez-Scarano F. Proton MR spectroscopy and magnetization transfer ratio in multiple sclerosis: correlative findings of active versus irreversible plaque disease. *AJNR* 1996; **17**:1539–1547.

64 Truyen L, van Waesberghe JHTM, van Walderveen MAA et al. Accumulation of hypointense lesions ('black holes') on T1 spin-echo MRI correlates with disease progression in multiple sclerosis. *Neurology* 1996; **47**:1469–1476.

65 van Walderveen MAA, Kamphorst W, Scheltens P et al. Histopathological correlate of hypointense lesions on T1-weighted spin-echo MRI in multiple sclerosis. *Neurology* 1998; **50**:1282–1288.

66 Gass A, Barker GJ, Kidd D et al. Correlation of magnetization transfer ratio with clinical disability in multiple sclerosis. *Ann Neurol* 1994; **36**:62–67.

67 Van Buchem MA, Grossman RI, Miki Y et al. Correlation of quantitative volumetric magnetization transfer ratio measurements with clinical and neuropsychological data in multiple sclerosis.

Radiology 1996; **201P** (suppl):174–175.

68 Trapp B, Peterson J, Ransohoff RM et al. Axonal transection in the lesions of multiple sclerosis. *N Engl J Med* 1998; **338**:278–285.

69 Davie CA, Hawkins CP, Barker GJ et al. Serial proton magnetic resonance spectroscopy in acute multiple sclerosis lesions. *Brain* 1994; **117**:49–58.

70 Lai HM, Davie CA, Gass A et al. Serial magnetization transfer ratios in gadolinium enhancing lesions in multiple sclerosis. *J Neurol* 1997; **224**:308–311.

71 Beck RW, Arrington J, Murtagh FR. Brain magnetic imaging in acute optic neuritis: experience of the Optic Neuritis Study Group. *Arch Neurol* 1993; **50**:841–846.

72 Beck RW, Cleary PA, Trobe JD et al. The effect of corticosteroids for acute optic neuritis on the subsequent development of multiple sclerosis: the Optic Neuritis Study Group. *N Engl J Med* 1993; **329**:1764–1769.

73 Filippi M, Horsfield MA, Morrissey SP et al. Quantitative brain MRI lesion load predicts the course of clinically isolated syndromes suggestive of multiple sclerosis. *Neurology* 1994; **44**:635–641.

74 Cannella B, Raine CS. The adhesion molecule and cytokine profile of multiple sclerosis lesions. *Ann Neurol* 1995; **37**:424–435.

75 Tsukada N, Matsuda M, Miyagi K, Yanagisawa N. Adhesion of cerebral endothelial cells to lymphocytes from patients with multiple sclerosis. *Autoimmunity* 1993; **14**:329–333.

76 Rosenberg GA, Kornfeld M, Estrada E et al. TIMP-2 reduces proteolytic opening of the blood–brain barrier by type IV collagenase. *Brain Res* 1992; **576**:203–207.

77 Sriram S, Rodriquez M. Indictment of the microglia as the villain in multiple sclerosis. *Neurology* 1997; **48**:464–470.

78 Ferguson B, Matyszak MK, Esiri MM, Perry VH. Axonal damage in acute multiple sclerosis lesions. *Brain* 1997; **120** (Pt 3):393–399.

79 Raine CS, Scheinberg L, Waltz JM. Multiple sclerosis: oligodendrocyte survival and proliferation in an active established lesion. *Lab Invest* 1981; **45**:534–546.

80 Selmaj K, Brosnan CF, Raine CS. Expression of heat shock protein-65 by oligodendrocytes in vivo and in vitro: implications for multiple sclerosis. *Neurology* 1992; **42**:795–800.

81 Lucchinetti CF, Brueck W, Rodriquez M, Lassman

H. Distinct patterns of multiple sclerosis pathology indicates heterogeneity in pathogenesis. *Brain Pathol* 1996; **6**:259–274.

82 Lucchinetti CF, Brueck W, Rodruquez M, Lassman H. Multiple sclerosis: lessons from neuropathology. *Semin Neurol* 1998; **18**:337–349.

83 Saperstein DS, Amato AA, Katz JS, Barohn RJ. Immune mediated polyneuropathies. In: Pourmand R, ed. *Neuromuscular Diseases: Expert Clinical Views*. Newton: Butterworth Heinemann, in press.

84 Charcot JM (translated by Sigerson G. *Lectures on Diseases of the Nervous System*. London: The New Sydenham Society, 1877: 222.

85 Paty DW, Li DKB, the UBC MS/MRI Study Group, the IFNB Multiple Sclerosis Study Group. Interferon beta-1b is effective in relapsing–remitting multiple sclerosis. II. MRI analysis results of a multicenter, randomized, double-blind trial. *Neurology* 1993; **43**:662–667.

86 Rudick RA, Goodkin DE, Jacobs LD et al. Impact of interferon beta-1a on neurologic disability in relapsing multiple sclerosis. *Neurology* 1997; **49**:358–363.

87 European Study Group on Interferon β1b in Secondary Progressive MS. Placebo-controlled multicentre randomised trial of interferon β1b in treatment of secondary progressive multiple sclerosis. *Lancet* 1998; **352**:1491–1497.

88 PRISMS Study Group. Randomised double-blind placebo-controlled study of interferon β1a in relapsing/remitting multiple sclerosis. *Lancet* 1998; **352**:1498–1504.

89 Goodkin DE. Interferon β therapy for multiple sclerosis. *Lancet* 1998; **352**:1486–1487.

90 The IFNB Multiple Sclerosis Study Group. Neutralizing antibodies during treatment of multiple sclerosis with interferon beta-1b. *Neurology* 1996; **47**:889–894.

91 Khan QA, Xia Q, Bever CT, Johnson KP et al. Interferon beta-1b serum levels in multiple sclerosis patients following subcutaneous administration. *Neurology* 1996; **46**:1639–1643.

92 Pachner AR. Anticytokine antibodies in beta interferon-treated MS patients and the need for testing: plight of the practicing neurologist. *Neurology* 1997; **49**:647–650.

93 Rudick RA, Simonian NA, Alam JA et al. Incidence and significance of neutralizing antibodies to interferon beta-1a in multiple sclerosis. *Neurology* 1998; **50**:1266–1272.

94 Runkel L, Werner M, Blake R et al. Structural and functional differences between glycosylated and non-glycosylated forms of human interferon-β (IFN-β). *Pharm Res* 1998; **15**:641–649.

95 Hochuli E. Interferon immunogenicity: technical evaluation of interferon-alpha 2a. *J Interferon Cytokine Res* 1997; **17**(suppl):S15–S21.

96 Wang C, Eufemi M, Turano C, Giartosio A. Influences of the carbohydrate moiety on the stability of glycoproteins. *Biochemistry* 1996; **35**:7299–7307.

97 Munafo A, Trinchard-Lugan I, Nguyen TXQ, Buraglio M. Bioavailability of recombinant human interferon-β-1a after intramuscular and subcutaneous administration. *Eur J Neurol* 1998; **5**:187–193.

98 Noronha A, Toscas A, Jensen MA. Interferon β decreases T cell activation and interferon γ production in multiple sclerosis. *J Neuroimmunol* 1993; **46**:145–154.

99 Yong VW, Chabot S, Stuve O, Williams G. Interferon beta in the treatment of multiple sclerosis. Mechanisms of action. *Neurology* 1998; **51**:682–689.

100 Genc K, Dona DL, Reder AT. Increased CD80(+) B cells in active multiple sclerosis and reversal by interferon beta-1b. *J Clin Invest* 1997; **99**:2664–2671.

101 Stuve O, Dooley NP, Uhm JH et al. Interferon β-1b decreases the migration of T lymphocytes in vitro: effects on matrix metalloproteinase-9. *Ann Neurol* 1996; **40**:853–863.

102 Leppert D, Waubant E, Burk MR et al. Interferon beta-1b inhibits gelatinase secretion and in vivo migration of human T cells: a possible mechanism for treatment efficacy in multiple sclerosis. *Ann Neurol* 1996; **40**:846–853.

103 Stuve O, Chabot S, Jung SS et al. Chemokine-enhanced migration of T lymphocytes is antagonized by interferon beta 1b through an effect on matrix metalloproteinase-9. *J Neuroimmunol* 1997; **80**:38–46.

104 Pollard JD, Westland KW, Harvey GK et al. Activated T cells of nonneuronal specificity open the blood–nerve barrier to circulating antibody. *Ann Neurol* 1994; **37**:467–475.

105 Louis JC, Magal E, Takayama S, Varon S. CNTF protection of oligodendrocytes against natural and tumor necrosis factor α-induced death. *Science* 1993; **259**:689–692.

106 Merrill JE, Ignarro LJ, Sherman MP et al. Microglial

cell cytotoxicity of oligodendrocytes is mediated through nitric oxide. *J Immunol* 1993; **151**:2132–2141.

107 Bo L, Dawson TM, Wesselingh S et al. Induction of nitric oxide synthase in demyelinating regions of multiple sclerosis brains. *Ann Neurol* 1994; **36**:778–786.

108 Bagastra O, Michaels FH, Zheng YM et al. Activation of the inducible form of nitric oxide synthase in the brains of patients with multiple sclerosis. *Proc Natl Acad Sci U S A* 1995; **92**:12041–12045.

109 Hua LL, Liu JSH, Brosnan CF, Lee SC. Selective inhibition of human glial inducible nitric oxide synthetase by interferon-β Implications for multiple sclerosis. *Ann Neurol* 1998; **43**:384–387.

110 Gasperini C, Pozzilli C, Bastianello S et al. Effect of steroids on Gd-enhancing lesions before and during recombinant beta interferon 1a treatment in relapsing–remitting multiple sclerosis. *Neurology* 1998; **50**:403–406.

111 Johnson KP, Brooks BR, Cohen JA et al. Extended use of glatiramer acetate (Copaxone) is well tolerated and maintains its clinical effect on multiple sclerosis relapse rate and degree of disability. *Neurology* 1998; **50**:701–708.

112 Teitelbaum D, Aharoni R, Sela M, Arnon R. Cross-reactions and specificities of monoclonal antibodies against myelin basic protein and against the synthetic copolymer-1. *Proc Natl Acad Sci U S A* 1991; **88**:9528–9532.

113 Teitelbaum D, Milo R, Arnon R, Sela, M. Synthetic copolymer-1 inhibits human T-cell lines specific for myelin basic protein. *Proc Natl Acad Sci U S A* 1992; **89**:137–141.

114 Lando Z, Teitelbau, D, Aron R. Effect of cyclophosphamide on suppressor cell activity in mice unresponsive to EAE. *J Immunol* 1979; **123**:2156–2160.

115 Racke MK, Martin R, McFarland H, Fritz RB. Copolymer-1-induced inhibition of antigen-specific T cell activation: interference with antigen presentation. *J Neuroimmunol* 1992; **37**:75–84.

116 Fridkis-Hareli M, Teitelbaum D, Gurevich E et al. Direct binding of myelin basic protein and synthetic copolymer 1 to class II major histocompatibility complex molecules on living antigen-presenting cells: specificity and promiscuity. *Proc Natl Acad Sci U S A* 1994; **91**:4872–4876.

117 Morrissey SP, Miller DH, Kendall BE et al. The significance of brain magnetic resonance imaging abnormalities at presentation with clinically isolated syndromes suggestive of multiple sclerosis. *Brain* 1993; **116**:135–146.

118 Barkhof F, Filippi M, Miller DH et al. Comparison of MRI criteria at first presentation to predict conversion to clinically definite multiple sclerosis. *Brain* 1997; **120**:2059–2069.

119 Khan OA, Dhib-Jalbut SS. Neutralizing antibodies to interferon β-1a and interferon β-1b in MS patients are cross-reactive. *Neurology* 1998; **51**:1698–1702.

120 Van Engelen BGM, Miller DJ, Pavelko KD et al. Promotion of remyelination by polyclonal immunoglobulin and IVIg in Theiler's virus induced demyelination and in MS. *J Neurol Neurosurg Psychiatry* 1994; **57** (suppl 1):65–68.

121 Fazekjas F, Deisenhammer F, Strasser-Fuchs S et al. Randomised placebo-controlled trial of monthly intravenous immunoglobulin therapy in relapsing–remitting multiple sclerosis. *Lancet* 1997; **349**:589–593.

122 Achiron A, Gabbay U, Gilad R et al. Intravenous immunoglobulin treatment in multiple sclerosis. *Neurology* 1998; **50**:398–402.

123 Noseworthy J, O'Brien P, van Engelen B, Rodriquez M. Intravenous immunoglobulin therapy in multiple sclerosis: progress from the Theiler's virus model to a randomized, double-blinded, placebo-controlled clinical trial. *J Neurol Neurosurg Psychiatry* 1994; **57** (suppl):11–14.

124 Noseworthy J, Weinshenker B, O'Brien P. Intravenous immunoglobulin (IVIg) does not reverse recently acquired, apparently permanent weakness in multiple sclerosis (MS) (abstract). *Ann Neurol* 1997; **42**:421.

125 Van Engelen BGM, Hommes OR, Pinckers A et al. Improved vision after intravenous immunoglobulin in stable demyelinating optic neuritis. *Ann Neurol* 1992; **32**:834–835.

126 Yudkin PL, Ellison GW, Ghezzi A et al. Overview of azathioprine treatment in multiple sclerosis. *Lancet* 1991; **338**:1051–1055.

127 Palace J, Rothwell P. New treatments and azathioprine in multiple sclerosis. *Lancet* 1997; **350**:261.

128 Witte AS, Cornblath DR, Schatz NJ, Lisak RP. Monitoring azathioprine therapy in myasthenia gravis. *Neurology* 1986; **36**:1533–1534.

129 Kappos L, Stolle U, Wilhelm U. Occurrence of cancer after long-term treatment with azathioprine in

multiple sclerosis and myasthenia gravis. *Annu Rep Max Planck Soc Clin Res Unit Multiple Sclerosis* 1985; 3:3–17.

130 Goodkin DE, Rudick RA, vanderBrug-Medendorp S et al. Low-dose (7.5 mg) oral methotrexate reduces the rate of progression in chronic progressive multiple sclerosis. *Ann Neurol* 1995; 37:30–40.

131 Fischer JS, Goodkin DE, Rudick RA et al. Low-dose (7.5 mg) oral methotrexate improves neuropsychological function in patients with chronic progressive multiple sclerosis. 119th Annual Meeting of the American Neurological Association. *Ann Neurol* 1994; 36:54.

132 Shiroky JB, Neville C, Esdaile JM. Low-dose methotrexate with leucovorin (folinic acid) in the management of rheumatoid arthritis:results of a multicenter, double-blind, placebo-controlled trial. *Arthritis Rheum* 1993; 36:795–803.

133 Morgan SL, Baggott JE, Vaughn WH. Supplementation with folic acid during methotrexate therapy for rheumatoid arthritis: a double-blind, placebo-controlled trial. *Ann Intern Med* 1994; 121:833–841.

134 Paty DW, Hashimoto SA, Ebers GC. Management of multiple sclerosis and interpretation of clinical trials. In: Paty DW, Ebers GC, eds. *Multiple Sclerosis*. Philadelphia: FA Davis, 1998.

135 Smith DR, Balashov KE, Hafler DA et al. Immune deviation following pulse cyclophosphamide/methylprednisolone treatment of multiple sclerosis: increased interleukin-4 production and associated eosinophilia. *Ann Neurol* 1997; 42:313–318.

136 McCune W, Globus J, Zeldes W et al. Clinical and immunologic effects of monthly administration of intravenous cyclophosphamide in severe systemic lupus erythematosus. *N Engl J Med* 1988; 318:1423–1431.

137 Gourley M, Austin HR, Scott D et al. Methylprednisolone and cyclophosphamide, alone or in combination, in patients with lupus nephritis. A randomized controlled trial. *Ann Intern Med* 1996; 125:549–557.

138 Rott O, Cash E, Fleischer B. Phosphodiesterase inhibitor pentoxifylline, a selective suppressor of T helper type 1-but not type 2-associated lymphocyte production, prevents induction of experimental autoimmune encephalomyelitis in Lewis rats. *Eur J Immunol* 1993; 23:1745–1751.

139 Rieckmann P, Weber F, Gunther A et al. Pentoxifylline, a phosphodiesterase inhibitor, induces immune deviation in patients with multiple sclerosis. *J Neuroimmunol* 1996; 64:193–200.

140 Chao CC, Hu S, Gekker G et al. Effects of cytokine on multiplication of *Toxoplasma gondii* in microglial cells. *J Immunol* 1993; 151:328–334.

141 Reickmann P, Weber F, Gunther A, Poser S. The phosphodiesterase inhibitor pentoxifylline reduces early side effects of interferon-β1b treatment in patients with multiple sclerosis. *Neurology* 1996; 47:604.

142 Achiron A, Rotstein Z, Noy S et al. Intravenous immunoglobulin treatment in the prevention of childbirth-associated acute exacerbations in multiple sclerosis. *J Neurol* 1996; 243:25–28.

143 Confavreux C, Hutchinson M, Hours MM et al. Rate of pregnancy-related relapse in multiple sclerosis. *N Engl J Med* 1998; 339:285–291.

32

Treatment for patients with secondary progressive multiple sclerosis

Steven R Schwid

CHARACTERISTICS OF SECONDARY PROGRESSIVE MULTIPLE SCLEROSIS

Despite the endless combinations of relapses, remissions, plateaux, and progressions that can occur in the course of multiple sclerosis (MS), common patterns emerge. At least 70% of patients initially present with acute relapses separated by periods of clinical stability. Most of these patients eventually pass into a progressive phase, which is characterized by a gradually worsening baseline that may or may not be interposed with occasional relapses, minor remissions, and plateaux.[1] A recent survey of the international MS clinical research community suggested that this type of course should be designated secondary progressive MS (SPMS) to distinguish it from a relapsing–remitting course, which has a stable baseline between exacerbations, and from primary progressive MS, which has a progressive course from the onset.[2] This updated definition of SPMS therefore includes courses that would previously have been called 'chronic progressive' or 'relapsing–progressive.'

Natural history studies indicate that secondary progression may occur at any time after disease onset, with an increasing proportion of patients passing from relapsing forms of MS to SPMS with longer periods of follow-up. Studies based at MS centers suggest that approximately 30% of patients enter a secondary progressive phase within 5 years of symptom onset and that 50% enter a secondary progressive phase within 11 years.[3] Similarly, population-based studies show that over 50% of patients who initially have a relapsing course have entered a progressive phase within 10 years of disease onset, and 90% of such patients have entered a progressive phase within 25 years.[1]

Risk factors for passing from relapsing–remitting MS (RRMS) to SPMS include:[4,5]

(a) an older age at symptom onset;

(b) male sex;

(c) motor symptoms;

(d) polyregional onset;

(e) incomplete recovery from the first exacerbation;

(f) a shorter interval between the first two attacks; and

(g) frequent attacks during the first two years.

The maximum risk of transition occurs within 10–20 years for patients with onset before the age of 30 years and within 5 years for patients with disease onset after the age of 40 years.[5] Risk factors for developing more advanced disability (e.g. an inability to walk without assistance) are similar.[4–7] The strongest predictors of the development of advanced disability are higher levels of disability 5 years after disease onset and the insidious onset of a motor deficit. Both of these predictors probably indicate that a progressive phase has begun. The use of these risk factors in sophisticated multivariate prediction models indicates that the majority of patients with the greatest risk develop a progressive course within 5 years of symptom onset whereas very few of the patients with the least risk did. Nevertheless, predictions about the long-term prognosis for individual patients are still quite uncertain.[5,7]

Patients with SPMS tend to have more impairment than patients with RRMS. Approximately half of the patients enrolled in clinical trials for SPMS have expanded disability status scale[8] (EDSS) scores of 6.0 or higher, indicating that they require assistance to walk.[9] The majority of patients enrolled in trials for RRMS, on the other hand, have scores below 4.0, indicating moderate impairment but relatively intact ambulation.[10–12] Patients with SPMS are also more likely to require acute hospitalization, rehabilitation services, and long-term nursing care, resulting in greater health-care expenditures.[13] Furthermore, employment status and quality of life are reduced in patients with SPMS.[14,15] Many of these differences may simply reflect the longer mean disease duration for patients with SPMS.

Magnetic resonance imaging (MRI) studies confirm that patients with SPMS have similar but more advanced disease than patients with RRMS. Serial MRIs show that enhancing lesions, indicating localized disruption of the blood–brain barrier, occur in both RRMS and SPMS (although they are somewhat less frequent in the latter).[16,17] The distribution of lesions is similar in RRMS and SPMS, but patients with SPMS tend to have more confluent periventricular lesions and greater total lesion volumes than patients with RRMS.[16] Tissue destruction within lesions appears to be more profound in SPMS lesions, as indicated by more T1-weighted hypointensities[18] and greater decreases in N-acetyl aspartate (NAA), a neuronal marker on magnetic resonance spectroscopy.[19] Normal-appearing white matter also has lower NAA levels in SPMS patients, suggesting that these patients have more microscopic damage as well.[20,21] As a result, patients with SPMS have more atrophy of the brain and spinal cord than patients with RRMS,[22] and central motor conduction times are longer.[23,24]

Furthermore, patients with SPMS are likely to continue progressing. In one prospective study of 102 patients with progressive symptoms, only 15 remained stable during at least 2 years of follow-up, and none improved.[25] However, this study included patients with both primary progressive MS and SPMS. A recent multicenter study of interferon-β 1b in patients with secondary progressive MS found that half had sustained worsening of their EDSS scores within an average of 2.5 years of follow-up.[9] Even greater proportions of patients may be deteriorating in ways that the EDSS does not detect, since continuous scales often detect worsening in functional abilities when the EDSS score is not changing.[26]

It is still uncertain whether the transition to SPMS is a direct result of advancing neurologic damage or whether immunologic changes are also involved. Tumor necrosis factor-α levels are more often elevated[27] and interleukin-12-dependent T-helper 1-type activation is more common in patients with SPMS.[28] T cells from patients with SPMS can also develop the ability to present myelin antigens, to activate without exposure to co-stimulatory molecules, and to resist the induction of anergy.[29,30] Epitope spreading, which is known to occur in chronic forms of experimental allergic encephalomyelitis, may also be involved.[31,32]

In addition, there remains some controversy as to whether there are real biological differences between primary and progressive MS and SPMS. Some studies suggest that the mean age of transition from RRMS to SPMS (which is 36 years) is very similar to the mean age of symptom onset for patients with a primary progressive course (which is 37 years).[33] This raises the possibility that the difference between primary progressive MS and SPMS may simply be an artefact of an overlooked, forgotten, or clinically silent history of relapses in patients who appear to have symptoms that are progressive from the onset.

Other studies suggest that there are true biological differences between primary progressive (MS) and SPMS. Patients with primary progressive MS have an equal sex distribution, whereas patients with RRMS and SPMS are twice as often female. Patients with primary progressive MS are more likely to have predominantly paraparesis, whereas patients with SPMS often have prominent visual, cerebellar, and cognitive symptoms as well.[34] It is still possible that these differences could be related to under-reporting of subtle symptoms in males, but MRI studies indicate that patients with primary progressive MS have fewer brain lesions, lower total lesion volumes, and less brain atrophy than patients with SPMS.[35,36] Furthermore, patients with primary progressive MS have fewer enhancing lesions on serial MRI[37] scans and less inflammation in pathologic studies.[38] Until the pathophysiologic mechanisms of progression are understood, differences between primary progressive MS and SPMS will remain somewhat uncertain.

THE INITIATION OF TREATMENT

Given the significant disability that most patients with SPMS already have, and the likelihood that disability will worsen in the future, the rationale for treating SPMS with disease-modifying therapy is clear. In practice, however, scenarios may arise in which the need to initiate treatment is less straightforward. For example, patients passing from a relapsing to a secondary progressive phase certainly warrant disease-modifying therapy, but determining when this transition has occurred may be difficult. Patients who complain of gradually worsening symptoms or who have insidious changes on examination should be followed more closely to determine whether progression is ongoing. No formal guidelines have yet been established, but most clinical trials for SPMS have required progressive deficits over 6–12 months before initiating treatment.[9] Whether this may include deficits arising as part of an acute exacerbation that did not fully resolve has not been addressed. Many studies have also required a certain amount of progressive change, such as a deterioration of a full point on the EDSS scale, before initiating treatment.

In practice, however, determining that progressive change is ongoing is more important than quantifying the amount of change. Many patients who are passing from a relapsing course are already receiving disease-modifying therapy. As described above, it is uncertain whether significant new pathophysiologic mechanisms are beginning at this point or whether the accumulation of damage has simply led to the appearance of a change in the disease course. Whether the treatment for these patients should be changed is discussed below.

In another common scenario, patients begin to develop progressive symptoms after a period of stable disease activity. Presumably, these patients are undergoing the same type of transition as those who had a more obviously relapsing course, but their relapses probably involved fewer clinically eloquent regions. The change from a stable course to a progressive one may be more obvious than the change from a relapsing course to a progressive one, but it may also be more unexpected for both the patient and caregivers. Since the underlying disease processes are probably the same as in patients passing from an actively relapsing course to a progressive one, treatment issues are similar, except that these patients are less likely to be receiving disease-modifying therapy at the time progression becomes apparent.

MONITORING DISEASE ACTIVITY

The goal of monitoring patients with SPMS is to detect any evidence of ongoing disease activity that might require disease-modifying therapy to be initiated or changed. *Table 32.1* summarizes the advantages and disadvantages of several established monitoring methods. As in other facets of clinical neurology, obtaining a detailed history and neurological examination are the first steps towards achieving this goal. However, because the neurological examination evolved as a diagnostic tool rather than a rating scale, it can be difficult to quantify impairment in ways that foster serial comparisons. The Functional Systems of the EDSS[8] can serve this purpose and provide a semi-quantitative measure of deficits detected by examination of the visual, brainstem, pyramidal, cerebellar, sensory, and mental systems, and by a history of the bowel and bladder systems. The overall EDSS score is derived from the Functional Systems, the distance a patient can walk, and the assistance required to ambulate. A change in the EDSS score, therefore, denotes a change in the patient's impairment from MS as detected by history and neurological examination.

Simple inspection of the scale suggests that it is valid, since the degree of impairment advances steadily as the EDSS score increases. Levels reflect the usual course of impairment, initially consisting of a variety of deficits, then dominated by

Table 32.1 Methods for monitoring patients with SPMS

Method	Parameter assessed	Main advantage	Main disadvantage
EDSS	Impairment	Clear clinical relevance	Limited responsiveness
Continuous functional measures	Impairment	More responsive than EDSS	Small changes have uncertain clinical significance
MRI, evoked potentials	Pathology	Detects clinically silent lesions	Predictive value uncertain
Immunologic markers	Pathophysiology	Directly assesses disease activity	No established methods

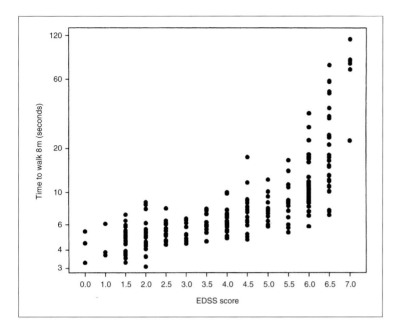

Fig. 32.1 *Time to walk 8 m in 237 ambulatory MS patients, stratified by EDSS score. There is considerable variability in the ambulatory speed within each EDSS level.[40]*

ambulatory dysfunction, and finally by paraplegia with advancing upper extremity dysfunction. Therefore, the EDSS score provides useful staging information about a patient's impairment, with higher scores indicating the development of more advanced disease. For many purposes, such as epidemiological studies, this type of staging tool is perfectly suitable.

When monitoring patients for progression, however, the EDSS is frequently insensitive to change. For example, in the milder stages, in which ambulation is not yet significantly impaired, the EDSS score is determined by the Functional System ratings. Since each of these is essentially recorded as mildly, moderately, or severely impaired, modest worsening within these ranges may be overlooked. A ceiling effect is also present, since impairment in the Functional Systems cannot raise the EDSS above 4.0 unless

ambulatory impairment is also present. Once patients are unable to walk at least 500 m, the Functional Systems do not impact on the EDSS score at all, so changes that do not affect ambulation (e.g. worsening tremor) will not be recorded. Patients requiring a walking cane (EDSS 6.0) will not register worsening on the EDSS until they begin using a walker. Patients requiring a walker (EDSS 6.5) will not register worsening until they cannot walk more than 5 m. As a result, patients tend to maintain EDSS scores of 4.0, 6.0, and 6.5 much longer than other scores,[39] and distributions of EDSS scores often have bimodal peaks at these scores.[40] Since these are very common scores for patients with SPMS, the EDSS is not responsive enough to serve as the main indicator of progressive disease.

One alternative is to focus more on continuous measures of neurological function, such as the time to walk 8 m (T8)[40] and to complete the 9-Hole Peg Test.[41] In a clinic-based sample of 237 MS patients, T8 scores ranged from 4.84 to 10.00 seconds for patients with an EDSS score of 4.0, and from 5.82 to 34.78 seconds in patients with an EDSS score of 6.0. The broad ranges of T8 scores within each EDSS level suggests that T8 might worsen considerably without the EDSS score changing (*Fig. 32.1*).[40]

As part of a pivotal trial of roquinimex in patients with SPMS, a subset of 133 patients participating at five sites of the New York State MS Consortium were evaluated for worsening on these measures regardless of treatment group assignment. During an average of 6 months' follow-up, 67% of patients had measurable worsening on a composite formed by these two functional tests, while only 25% worsened on the EDSS. Without specifically referring to these scores, the investigators reported their impression that 33% of the patients had worsened clinically. Thus, the continuous functional scales were more sensitive to worsening than the investigators' assessment, but the EDSS was less sensitive.[25]

Because continuous functional measures appear to be more sensitive to modest changes in ambulatory and upper extremity function, they could be used to monitor patients with SPMS for worsening that is related to ongoing disease activity. Continuous functional measures take only a few minutes to perform and require minimal equipment, so they could easily be incorporated into routine clinic visits. A National MS Society task force recently recommended that these tests also be used to create a Functional Composite score that could be used as the primary measure of efficacy in clinical trials.[42] Since the clinical manifestations of MS are pleomorphic, the composite would ideally include continuous measures of cognition, vision, endurance, and other measures, but optimal tests for each of these components remain to be established.

Unfortunately, the clinical significance of small changes in continuous measures is uncertain. One method of ensuring that such changes reflect progression rather than random or temporary variations is to require that changes be sustained on repeated testing.[43] The predictive value of initial changes, and those sustained for longer periods, has not yet been established empirically, but recent studies have focused on worsening impairment sustained for at least 3–6 months.[44]

Another method of ensuring clinical significance is to require a minimum threshold for changes. For example, many studies using the EDSS as the primary outcome measure have required patients to worsen by 1.0 point for baseline EDSS scores of less than 6.0 and by 0.5 points for baseline EDSS scores of 6.0 and above.[9] This convention was based on the test–retest reliability of the EDSS, which is poor for changes of 0.5 points below EDSS 6.0, and on the responsiveness of the scale, which is poor at levels 6.0 and 6.5.[45,46] Similar conventions have not yet been established for continuous scales, since the test–retest reliability of these scales has not been thoroughly examined. In an effort to characterize T8 variability, 27 patients (EDSS 2.5–6.5) had T8 measured on 5 consecutive days during a period of clinical stability. Variability in T8 was highly related to baseline walking speed, with greater variability observed in patients who walked more slowly (Spearman r = 0.83). Linear regression modeling of the data predicted that repeated T8 scores should vary by no more than 0.5 seconds (9.4%) in patients who walk 8 m in 5 seconds, 0.9 seconds (9.2%) in patients who take 10 seconds, and 1.8 seconds (12.0%) in patients who take 15 seconds.[47]

When changes beyond this predicted variation are observed in practice they represent changes beyond those observed in clinically stable patients and are therefore likely to reflect true change. In contrast, other investigators have asserted that changes in T8 should be 3 seconds or more to be considered meaningful.[48] Such a conservative threshold would reduce the sensitivity of T8 but might be appropriate when more certainty is required. Ideally, the choice of a threshold should be based on the clinical situation as well as on empirical data regarding the reliability and responsiveness of the measure.

Another alternative for monitoring patients would be to rely more on paraclinical signs of ongoing disease activity, such as changes on MRI. MRI of the brain can detect evidence of ongoing disease activity as gadolinium-enhancing lesions, an increasing number of T2-weighted lesions, or an increase in the total lesion volume.[49] As with clinical measures, issues of test–retest reliability must be addressed, especially when it is necessary to compare images obtained from different scanners or when repositioning is imprecise. In practice, comparisons are usually qualitative, since the sophisticated computer-assisted analyses that are commonly performed in clinical trials are generally not available for routine monitoring. Furthermore, changes in lesion burden must be interpreted conservatively, because some T2-weighted lesions may be reversible. Even so, the side-by-side comparison of serial MRI scans may still detect clinically unsuspected disease activity, making it particularly valuable in patients who otherwise appear stable. The predictive value of MRI changes is still controversial, because cross-sectional and longitudinal studies show weak correlations between T2-weighted lesion burden and clinical measures of disability.[16,50]

The ideal interval between serial MRI scans has not been established. However, since placebo-treated patients with SPMS have less than a 10% increase in T2-weighted lesion burden per year, more frequent scanning is unlikely to detect substantial changes.[9] Gadolinium should be administered routinely with these examinations, since even one enhancing lesion clearly indicates active disease. Magnetic resonance spectroscopy,[18] magnetization transfer,[51] T1 hypointensity,[52] and quantitative measures of brain[53] and spinal cord atrophy[54] may also provide sensitive measures of ongoing disease activity. These measures are generally better correlated with disability than the T2-weighted lesion burden, perhaps because they are more specific for axonal loss and other pathological processes that lead to progressive disability.[55] These imaging modalities are still too demanding for routine clinical practice, however, and their relative utilities have not been established.

Evoked potentials can also provide paraclinical evidence of MS lesions. The use of evoked potentials, especially in the visual system, to detect subclinical lesions for diagnostic purposes has been clearly demonstrated. Their utility for detecting subclinical disease activity in patients with SPMS, however, has not been fully established. Worsening abnormalities on visual, auditory, somatosensory, and motor evoked potentials are associated with increasing demyelination and axonal loss, but concomitant clinical changes are often apparent, obviating the need for ancillary tests.[56]

Overall, clinical measures provide the most accessible monitoring in clinical practice. The traditional neurologic examination and semi-quantitative rating scales derived from it are insensitive to change over time. Continuous measures of neurologic function are potentially more reliable and responsive, but additional data are required to establish the operating characteristics of these measures. As measures of function, they have clear clinical relevance. Ancillary tests such as MRI, evoked potentials, and immunologic measures of disease activity may prove to be more sensitive and reliable than clinical outcomes. This has been well established in clinical trials focusing on changes in large groups of patients, but their value for predicting clinically meaningful change in an individual patient is less certain.

THERAPEUTIC OPTIONS

Once it becomes clear that a patient has SPMS and ongoing disease activity, disease-modifying therapy must be considered. The goal of treatment is to prevent, or at least minimize, any further damage from MS, thus preventing worsening impairment, disability, and handicap. Treatment will probably not improve function, however, and it is important for the patient and caregivers to remember this. Such inappropriate expectations often lead to disappointment and non-compliance.[57] These expectations often prove difficult to dispel, even with explicit educational efforts.

There are several treatment options that should be considered for patients with SPMS and ongoing disease activity, many of which are discussed in earlier chapters of this text. The main categories include the use of corticosteroids, general immunosuppressants, interferon-β, glatiramer acetate, and other immunomodulatory therapies. *Table 32.2* lists treatments supported by multicenter randomized controlled clinical trials.

Table 32.2 Disease-modifying therapies for SPMS supported by multicenter randomized controlled clinical trials

Methylprednisolone[58]
Azathioprine[59]
Cyclophosphamide[60,61]
Methotrexate[62,63]
Cladribine[64,65]
Mitoxantrone[66,67]
Glatiramer[68]

Years ago, chronic low-dose corticosteroid or corticotropin treatment was dismissed as a potential treatment for progressive MS based on at least three controlled trials showing no significant therapeutic effect and numerous adverse events.[69–71] The methods and outcome measures used in these studies differed substantially from recently successful trials of interferon, however. Brief pulses of high-dose methylprednisolone have gained acceptance as treatments for acute MS exacerbations,[72] but their effect on disease progression has not been thoroughly studied (see Chapter 26). Interest in the long-term effects of corticosteroid pulses was raised again by the Optic Neuritis Treatment Trial, which suggested that a corticosteroid pulse could delay a second exacerbation of MS in patients who were treated for their first demyelinating event.[73] Since then, Goodkin and colleagues have performed a preliminary study showing that fewer patients with SPMS receiving methylprednisolone 500 mg bimonthly experienced sustained worsening compared to patients receiving 10 mg bimonthly during 2 years of treatment.[58] Based on these results, further studies of repeated corticosteroid pulses and more frequent dosing regimens (e.g. every other day) are warranted.

Several general immunosuppressants have also been studied, either as ongoing therapy or for a predetermined treatment period. Earlier studies were often performed in patients with relapsing and progressive forms of MS, and most of these studies did not distinguish between primary progressive MS and SPMS, making interpretation of the results difficult. Furthermore, the outcome measures used in these studies were often poorly defined. Azathioprine is perhaps the most thoroughly studied agent in this class, with at least seven randomized controlled trials published. Although no individual study can be considered definitive, meta-analysis demonstrated a small but statistically significant benefit.[59] The magnitude of this benefit must be weighed against the potential risk of malignancy, which may develop after years of use.[74] Cyclophosphamide has also been studied many times, but the two largest studies in progressive MS had conflicting results, leaving conclusions about efficacy uncertain.[60,61]

More recently, immunosuppressants such as methotrexate,[62,63] cladribine,[64,65] and mitoxantrone[66,67] have been studied in patients with SPMS; the results are discussed in earlier chapters. Treatments that have already proven effective for RRMS are currently being studied in SPMS; ongoing studies include several trials of interferon-β. A relatively small study of glatiramer acetate in SPMS showed mixed results,[68] dampening enthusiasm for further trials. However, a large study of glatiramer for primary progressive MS is underway, and this may rekindle interest in its use in SPMS if it is successful.

Although these treatments are all currently available, they have not yet been approved by regulatory agencies for use in SPMS and have not yet received widespread acceptance. Interferon-β is likely to be the first exception. It was recently approved for the treatment of SPMS in Europe on the basis of a successful multicenter study,[9] and it is currently under regulatory review in the USA even before confirmatory North American studies have been completed. Many other immunomodulatory agents could also be tried for SPMS, but only those with strong pharmaceutical industry support are likely to complete the pivotal multicenter trials that produce definitive data and regulatory approval. Without this, such treatments will probably not be widely used and may not be reimbursed by third-party payers.

Ideally, clinical trial results establishing the relative efficacy and safety of different therapeutic options would form the basis for appropriate treatment decisions, which could then be individualized for each patient's specific medical issues and lifestyle. Unfortunately, clinical trials are often difficult to extrapolate to specific clinical situations, and most questions have not been fully answered by trial data. For example, both methotrexate[62] and interferon-β 1a[9] have been shown to reduce the incidence of worsening neurological function patients with progressive forms of MS, but their relative efficacy and safety have not been addressed in a comparative study. Determining which of these options is superior in general or for a specific patient is not easy. First, they were studied in different numbers of patients, so confidence in the results is not equivalent. Secondly, they were studied in different patient populations, using different outcome measures. Thirdly, they have different side effect profiles and methods of administration. Fourthly, they have different costs. Each of these factors should be openly discussed with the patient, significant others, and other members of the healthcare team, and when trial data are inadequate to guide decisions, the patient's individual preferences should be given the greatest weight.

MONITORING THERAPY

After initiating disease-modifying therapy for SPMS, active follow-up is critical to promote long-term compliance, to minimize side effects, and to ensure that the desired therapeutic effect is being achieved. Compliance may be particularly difficult to maintain for treatments that require self-administered injections. For this reason, the suppliers of interferon-β 1a, interferon-β 1b, and glatiramer acetate have each developed networks to ensure that support is readily available to all patients who are prescribed these agents in the USA. Actively monitoring for side effects is another way of promoting compliance. It reinforces with patients that continuing the prescribed treatment is important and that the clinician cares about their overall well-being. Furthermore, many side effects can be minimized once they are identified, promoting compliance even more. For example, new or increased depressive symptoms occurred in 41% of MS patients in the first 6 months of treatment with interferon-β 1b. Among patients experiencing this side effect, 86% of those receiving psychotherapy continued treatment, compared to 38% of those who did not receive psychotherapy.[75]

Monitoring for the desired therapeutic effect can also help promote compliance and will allow for regular reassessment of the treatment options if the response is suboptimal. Since the goal of disease-modifying therapy is to prevent, or to at least minimize, any further damage from MS, sufficient monitoring is needed to determine whether this goal is being achieved. Earlier in this chapter, several clinical and paraclinical measures were discussed that could be used to rate the patient's current level of impairment or disease burden. Serial comparisons of these measures can provide a sensitive indicator of disease progression.

The appropriate amount of vigilance for performing serial comparisons depends on the clinical situation. For example, since any ongoing disease activity would prompt consideration of disease-modifying therapy in SPMS patients who have not yet been treated, they should be monitored very closely. On the other hand, patients who are already receiving disease-modifying therapy may still be benefiting from therapy even if they have some ongoing disease activity. Furthermore, the most appropriate therapeutic options for suboptimal responders have not been established. Monitoring of these patients may, therefore, be somewhat less aggressive.

Likewise, the definition of a suboptimal response also depends on the clinical situation. Since superior therapeutic options have not yet been established for suboptimal responders, that label should be applied conservatively, with consideration of altering disease-modifying therapy only for patients who are clearly not responding. Once options have been established, however, altering therapy will be considered more often. It is hoped that there will eventually be enough options for evidence of ongoing disease activity never to need to be tolerated.

For the time being, a conservative definition of a suboptimal response would include patients who are experiencing intolerable side effects from their present therapy or those who have sustained progression of disability. Not all disease activity or worsening impairment leads to sustained changes in disability, but these are the changes that must be taken most seriously. Thus, a change in the EDSS score from 3.5 to 4.0 may not be apparent to the patient, but a change from 4.0 to 4.5 indicates that ambulatory endurance is now significantly affected and disability has worsened. A change in T8 from 5 seconds to 6 seconds may or may not be associated with worsened disability, but such an observation should certainly prompt careful questioning to determine whether ambulatory dysfunction has worsened in a meaningful way. In practice, patients are usually aware of changes in their walking when T8 worsens by more than 10–20%.

Although increasing lesion burden or enhancing lesions detected on MRI are clear signs of ongoing disease activity, they are not always associated with worsening disability.[76] Using a conservative definition of a suboptimal response, these changes are only important to the extent that they support evidence of worsening disability. Performing serial MRIs to monitor patients receiving disease-modifying therapy would therefore not be advised. If future studies indicate that changes on MRI (or on sensitive measures of impairment) that are not associated with changes in disability are reliable predictors of worsening disability, however, more intensive monitoring may be warranted.

TREATING SUBOPTIMAL RESPONDERS

Patients with ongoing disease progression who are experiencing intolerable side effects from their current therapy should switch to another agent. Dealing with patients who are experiencing an inadequate therapeutic response, including those who are passing from RRMS to SPMS, is not as straightforward. The theoretical options would be:

(a) to increase the dosage of the current agent;
(b) to switch to another agent; or
(c) to combine the current agent with a complementary treatment.

At present, none of these options has been adequately studied to identify the most preferable strategy. Furthermore, owing to reimbursement restrictions, increasing dosages and combining expensive therapies are not usually feasible options. These restrictions make the need for studies in suboptimal responders even more important.

FUTURE ISSUES

Improved understanding of the pathophysiology that causes the transition from RRMS to SPMS and promotes further progression would probably lead to more direct methods of monitoring disease activity in these patients. This would be helpful in identifying those patients who are most in need of treatment, detecting the effects of treatment in clinical trials, and determining whether individual patients are responding as desired. Further efforts will be needed to establish the predictive value of pathophysiologic, paraclinical, and functional measures of disease activity and impairment to determine how best to monitor patients with SPMS.

Improved understanding of pathophysiologic mechanisms will also foster new ideas for disease-modifying therapies. Initial studies will be needed to establish the safety and independent effects of these therapies compared to placebo, but further studies must focus on the place for new therapies in the overall therapeutic armamentarium. Combinations of potentially synergistic therapies should also be tested, both in new SPMS patients and in patients who are experiencing a suboptimal response to their current treatment regimen. Analogous oncologic studies suggest that these may eventually lead to our greatest successes.

453

REFERENCES

1 Weinshenker BG, Bass B, Rice GPA et al. The natural history of multiple sclerosis: a geographically based study. 1. Clinical course and disability. *Brain* 1989; **112**:133–146.

2 Lublin FD, Reingold SC. Defining the clinical course of multiple sclerosis: results of an international survey. *Neurology* 1996; **46**:907–911.

3 Confavreux C, Aimard G, Devic M. Course and prognosis of multiple sclerosis assessed by the computerized data processing of 349 patients. *Brain* 1980; **103**:281–300.

4 Runmarker B, Andersen O. Prognostic factors in a multiple sclerosis incidence cohort with twenty-five years of follow-up. *Brain* 1993; **116**:117–134.

5 Runmarker B, Andersson C, Oden A, Andersen O. Prediction of outcome in multiple sclerosis based on multivariate models. *J Neurol* 1994; **241**:597–604.

6 Weinshenker BG, Bass B, Rice GPA et al. The natural history of multiple sclerosis: a geographically based study. 2. Predictive value of the early clinical course. *Brain* 1989; **112**:1419–1428.

7 Weinshenker BG, Rice GPA, Noseworthy JH, Carriere W, Baskerville J, Ebers JC. The natural history of multiple sclerosis: a geographically based study. 3. Multivariate analysis of predictive factors and models of outcome. *Brain* 1991; **114**:1045–1056.

8 Kurtzke JF. Rating neurologic impairment in multiple sclerosis: an expanded disability status scale (EDSS). *Neurology* 1983; **33**:1444–1452.

9 European Study Group on Interferon beta-1b in Secondary Progressive MS. Placebo-controlled multicentre randomised trial of interferon beta-1b in treatment of secondary progressive multiple sclerosis. *Lancet* 1998; **352**:1491–1497.

10 The IFNB Multiple Sclerosis Study Group. Interferon beta-1b is effective in relapsing–remitting multiple sclerosis: 1. Clinical results of a multicenter, randomized, double-blind, placebo-controlled trial. *Neurology* 1993; **43**:655–661.

11 Johnson KP, Brooks BR, Cohen JA et al. Copolymer 1 reduces relapse rate and improves disability in relapsing–remitting multiple sclerosis: results of a phase III multicenter, double-blind, placebo-controlled trial. *Neurology* 1995; **45**:1268–1276.

12 PRISMS (Prevention of relapses and disability by interferon beta-1a subcutaneously in multiple sclerosis) Study Group. Randomised double-blind placebo-controlled study of interferon beta-1a in relapsing/remitting multiple sclerosis. *Lancet* 1998; **352**:1498–1504.

13 Stolp-Smith KA, Atkinson EJ, Campion ME et al. Health care utilization in multiple sclerosis. A population-based study in Olmsted County, MN. *Neurology* 1998; **50**:1594–1600.

14 The Canadian Burden of Illness Study Group. Burden of illness of multiple sclerosis: Part II. Quality of life. *Can J Neurol Sci* 1998; **25**:31–38.

15 Aronson KJ. Quality of life among persons with multiple sclerosis and their caregivers. *Neurology* 1997; **48**:74–80.

16 Filippi M, Campi A, Mammi S et al. Brain magnetic imaging and multimodal evoked potentials in benign and secondary progressive multiple sclerosis. *J Neurol Neurosurg Psychiatr* 1995; **58**:31–37.

17 Tubridy N, Coles AJ, Molyneux P et al. Secondary progressive multiple sclerosis: the relationship between short-term MRI activity and clinical features. *Brain* 1998; **121**:225–231.

18 Giugni E, Pozzilli C, Bastianello S et al. MRI measures and their relations with clinical disability in relapsing–remitting and secondary progressive multiple sclerosis. *Multiple Sclerosis* 1997; **3**:221–225.

19 Matthews PM, Pioro E, Narayanan S et al. Assessment of lesion pathology in multiple sclerosis using quantitative MRI morphometry and magnetic resonance spectroscopy. *Brain* 1996; **119**:715–722.

20 Falini A, Calabrese G, Filippi M et al. Benign versus secondary progressive multiple sclerosis: the potential role of proton MR spectroscopy in defining the nature of disability. *Am J Neuroradiol* 1998; **19**:223–229.

21 Fu L, Matthews PM, De Stefano N et al. Imaging axonal damage of normal-appearing white matter in multiple sclerosis. *Brain* 1998; **121**:103–113.

22 Filippi M, Campi A, Colombo B et al. A spinal cord MRI study of benign and secondary progressive multiple sclerosis. *J Neurol* 1996; **243**:502–505.

23 Facchetti D, Mai R, Micheli A et al. Motor evoked potentials and disability in secondary progressive multiple sclerosis. *Can J Neurol Sci* 1997; **24**:332–337.

24 Kidd D, Thompson PD, Day BL et al. Central motor conduction time in progressive multiple sclerosis: correlations with MRI and disease activity. *Brain* 1998; **121**:1109–1116.

25 Patzold U, Pocklington PR. Course of multiple sclerosis: first results of a prospective study carried out on 102 MS patients from 1976–80. *Acta Neurol Scand* 1982; **65**:248–266.

26 **Schwid SR, Goodman AD, Apatoff BR et al.** Quantitative measures are more sensitive to worsening neurological function in a prospective multiple sclerosis study. *Ann Neurol* 1998; **44**:483.

27 **Sharief MK, Hentges R.** Association between tumor necrosis factor-alpha and disease progressing in patients with multiple sclerosis. *N Engl J Med* 1991; **325**:467–472.

28 **Balashov KE, Smith DR, Khoury SJ et al.** Increased interleukin 12 production in progressive multiple sclerosis: induction by activated $CD4^+$ T cells via CD40 ligand. *Proc Nat Acad Sci U S A* 1997; **94**:599–603.

29 **Correale J, Gilmore W, Lopez J et al.** Defective post-thymic tolerance mechanisms during the chronic progressive stage of multiple sclerosis. *Nature Med* 1996; **2**:1354–1360.

30 **Correale J, McMillan M, Li S et al.** Antigen presentation by autoreactive proteolipid protein peptide-specific T cell clones from chronic progressive multiple sclerosis patients: roles of co-stimulatory B7 molecules and IL-12. *J Neuroimmunol* 1997; **72**:27–43.

31 **Voskuhl RR, Farris RW, Nagasato K, McFarland HF, Dalcq MD.** Epitope spreading occurs in active but not passive EAE induced by myelin basic protein. *J Neuroimmunol* 1996; **70**:103–111.

32 **Yu M, Johnson JM, Tuohy VK.** A predictable sequential determinant spreading cascade invariably accompanies progression of experimental autoimmune encephalomyelitis: a basis for peptide-specific therapy after onset of clinical disease. *J Exp Med* 1996; **183**:1777–1788.

33 **Minderhoud JM, van der Hoeven JH, Prange AJ.** Course and prognosis of chronic progressive multiple sclerosis. *Acta Neurologica Scand* 1988; **78**:10–15.

34 **Thompson AJ, Polman CH, Miller DH et al.** Primary progressive multiple sclerosis. *Brain* 1997; **120**:1085–1096.

35 **Thompson AJ, Kermode AG, MacManus DG et al.** Patterns of disease activity in multiple sclerosis: clinical and magnetic resonance imaging study. *Br Med J* 1990; **300**:631–634.

36 **Nijeholt GJ, van Walderveen MA, Castelijns JA et al.** Brain and spinal cord abnormalities in multiple sclerosis: correlation between MRI parameters, clinical subtypes, and symptoms. *Brain* 1998; **121**:687–697.

37 **Thompson AJ, Kermode AG, Wicks D et al.** Major differences in the dynamics of primary and secondary progressive multiple sclerosis. *Ann Neurol* 1991; **29**:53–62.

38 **Revesz T, Kidd D, Thompson AJ et al.** A comparison of the pathology of primary and secondary progressive multiple sclerosis. *Brain* 1994; **117**:759–765.

39 **Weinshenker BG, Rice GPA, Noseworthy JH et al.** The natural history of multiple sclerosis: a geographically based study. 4. Applications to planning and interpretation of clinical therapeutic trials. *Brain* 1991; **114**:1057–1067.

40 **Schwid SR, Goodman AD, Mattson DH et al.** The measurement of ambulatory impairment in multiple sclerosis. *Neurology* 1997; **49**:1419–1424.

41 **Goodkin DE, Hertsgaard D, Seminary J.** Upper extremity function in multiple sclerosis: improving assessment sensitivity with box-and-block and nine-hole-peg tests. *Arch Phys Med Rehabil* 1988; **69**:850–854.

42 **Rudick R, Antel J, Confavreux C et al.** Recommendations from the National Multiple Sclerosis Society clinical outcomes assessment task force. *Ann Neurol* 1997; **42**:379–382.

43 **Weinshenker BG, Issa M, Baskerville J.** Meta-analysis of the placebo-treated groups in clinical trials of progressive MS. *Neurology* 1996; **46**:1613–1619.

44 **Rudick RA, Goodkin DE, Jacobs LD et al.** Impact of interferon beta-1a on neurologic disability in relapsing multiple sclerosis. *Neurology* 1997; **49**:358–363.

45 **Noseworthy JH, Vandervoort MK, Wong CJ et al.** Interrater variability with the Expanded Disability Status Scale (EDSS) and Functional Systems (FS) in a multiple sclerosis clinical trial. *Neurology* 1990; **40**:971–975.

46 **Francis DA, Bain P, Swan AV, Hughes RAC.** An assessment of disability rating scales used in multiple sclerosis. *Arch Neurol* 1991; **48**:299–301.

47 **Schwid SR, Bever CF, Cook SD et al.** What is a clinically significant change in a quantitative functional measure? *Neurology* 1999; **52**:A549.

48 **Goodkin DE, Priore RL, Wende KE et al.** Comparing the ability of various composite outcomes to discriminate treatment effects in MS clinical trials. *Multiple Sclerosis* 1998; **4**:480–486.

49 **Miller DH, Grossman RI, Reingold SC, McFarland HF.** The role of magnetic resonance techniques in understanding and managing multiple sclerosis. *Brain* 1998; **121**:3–24.

50 **Koziol JA, Wagner S, Adams HP.** Assessing information in T2-weighted MRI scans from secondary progressive MS patients. *Neurology* 1998; **51**:228–233.

51 **Gass A, Barker GJ, Kidd D et al.** Correlation of magnetization transfer ratio with disability in multiple sclerosis. *Ann Neurol* 1994; **36**:62–67.

52 Truyen L, van Waesberghe JHTM, van Walderveen MAA et al. Accumulation of hypointense lesions ('black holes') on T1 spin-echo MRI correlates with disease progression in multiple sclerosis. *Neurology* 1996; **47**:1469–1476.

53 Losseff NA, Wang L, Lai HM et al. Progressive cerebral atrophy in multiple sclerosis: a serial study. Brain 1996; 119: 2009–2019.

54 Losseff NA, Webb SL, O'Riordan JI et al. Spinal cord atrophy and disability in multiple sclerosis: a new reproducible and sensitive MRI method with potential to monitor disease progression. *Brain* 1996; **119**:701–708.

55 Filippi M, Iannucci G, Tortorella C et al. Comparison of MS clinical phenotypes using conventional and magnetization transfer MRI. *Neurology* 1999; **52**:588–594.

56 Nuwer MR. Evoked potentials. In: Cook SD, ed. *Handbook of Multiple Sclerosis* 2nd edn. New York: Marcel Dekker, 1996, 317–346.

57 Mohr DC, Goodkin DE, Likosky W et al. Therapeutic expectations of patients with multiple sclerosis upon initiating interferon beta-1b: relationship to adherence to treatment. *Multiple Sclerosis* 1996; **2**:222–226.

58 Goodkin DE, Kinkel RP, Weinstock-Gutmann B et al. A phase II study of IV methyprednisolone in secondary-progressive multiple sclerosis. *Neurology* 1998; **51**:239–245.

59 Yudkin PL, Ellison GW, Ghezzi A et al. Overview of azathioprine treatment in multiple sclerosis. *Lancet* 1991; **338**:1051–1055.

60 The Canadian Cooperative Multiple Sclerosis Study Group. The Canadian cooperative trial of cyclophosphamide and plasma exchange in progressive multiple sclerosis. *Lancet* 1991; **337**:441–446.

61 Weiner HL, Mackin GA, Orav EJ et al. Intermittent cyclophosphamide pulse therapy in progressive multiple sclerosis: final report of the Northeast Cooperative Multiple Sclerosis Treatment Group. *Neurology* 1993; **43**:910–918.

62 Goodkin DE, Rudick RA, Medendorp SV et al. Low-dose (7.5 mg) oral methotrexate is effective in reducing the rate of progression of neurological impairment in patients with chronic progressive multiple sclerosis. *Ann Neurol* 1995; **37**:30–40.

63 Goodkin DE, Rudick RA, Medendorp SV et al. Low-dose oral methotrexate in chronic progressive multiple

sclerosis: analyses of serial MRIs. *Neurology* 1996; **47**:1153–1157.

64 Sipe JC, Romine JS, Koziol JA et al. Cladribine in treatment of chronic progressive multiple sclerosis. *Lancet* 1994; **344**:9–13.

65 Beutler E, Sipe JC, Romine JS et al. The treatment of chronic progressive multiple sclerosis with cladribine. *Proc Nat Acad Sci U S A* 1996; **93**:1716–1720.

66 Mauch E, Kornhuber HH, Krapf H et al. Treatment of multiple sclerosis with mitoxantrone. *Eur Arch Psychiatr Clin Neurosci* 1992; **242**:96–102.

67 Edan G, Miller D, Clanet M et al. Therapeutic effect of mitoxantrone combined with methylprednisolone in multiple sclerosis: a randomised multicentre study of active disease using MRI and clinical criteria. *J Neurol Neurosurg Psychiatr* 1997; **62**:112–118.

68 Bornstein MB, Miller A, Slagle S et al. A placebo-controlled, double-blind, randomized, two-center, pilot trial of Cop 1 in chronic progressive multiple sclerosis. *Neurology* 1991; **41**:533–539.

69 Miller H, Newell DJ, Ridley A. Multiple sclerosis: trials of maintenance treatment with prednisolone and soluble aspirin. *Lancet* 1961; **1**:127–129.

70 Tourtellotte WW, Haerer AF. Use of oral corticosteroids in the treatment of multiple sclerosis: a double-blind study. *Arch Neurol* 1965; **12**:536–545.

71 Millar JHD, Vas CJ, Noronha MJ et al. Long-term treatment of multiple sclerosis with corticotropin. *Lancet* 1967; **2**:429–431.

72 Troiano R, Cook SD, Dowling PC. Steroid therapy in multiple sclerosis: point of view. *Arch Neurol* 1987; **44**:803–807.

73 Beck RW, Cleary PA, Trobe JD et al. The effect of corticosteroids for acute optic neuritis on the subsequent development of multiple sclerosis. *N Engl J Med* 1993; **329**:1764–1769.

74 Confavreux C, Saddier P, Grimaud J et al. Risk of cancer from azathioprine therapy in multiple sclerosis: a case-control study. *Neurology* 1996; **46**:1607–1612.

75 Mohr DC, Goodkin DE, Likosky W et al. Treatment of depression improves adherence to interferon beta-1b therapy for multiple sclerosis. *Arch Neurol* 1997; **54**:531–533.

76 Filippi M, Paty DW, Kappos L et al. Correlations between changes in disability and T2-weighted brain MRI activity in multiple sclerosis: a follow-up study. *Neurology* 1995; **45**:255–260.

33

Treatment for patients with primary progressive and progressive–relapsing multiple sclerosis

Siobhan M Leary and Alan J Thompson

INTRODUCTION

Patients with primary progressive multiple sclerosis (PPMS) are a unique group with atypical clinical and magnetic resonance imaging (MRI) characteristics, and this has resulted in their exclusion from the majority of therapeutic trials. This chapter discusses these characteristics and their implications for treatment and clinical trials, particularly in regard to patient selection and therapeutic monitoring. Additionally, therapeutic trials to date for PPMS are reviewed.

BACKGROUND

Approximately 10% of MS patients have PPMS, which is characterized by continuous accumulation of neurological deficits from symptom onset, without relapse or remission.[1] Occasional plateaux and temporary minor improvements are observed. There is also a small group of patients with predominantly progressive disease defined in two ways: progressive–relapsing multiple sclerosis (PRMS), which is characterized by progressive disease from onset with superimposed relapses,[2] and transitional progressive multiple

sclerosis (TPMS), which is characterized by a single relapse before or after the onset of disease progression.[3] The PPMS, PRMS,[4] and TPMS[5,6] subgroups appear to be similar to each other and should at present be considered separately from the relapsing–remitting MS (RRMS) and secondary progressive MS (SPMS) subgroups with regard to therapeutics. This chapter concentrates on PPMS, since it is presently the best characterized of these subgroups.

Differences between PPMS and RRMS have been well described. The mean age of presentation of PPMS is later than that for RRMS[7] and relatively more men are affected, resulting in an equal male:female ratio.[1] Prognosis has been considered poorer because time from disease onset to reach advanced disability is shorter than in RRMS.[8,9] However, compared with the progressive phase in SPMS, both the rate of progression[8] and the age of onset of progression are similar.[10]

MRI findings are atypical in PPMS, with a more marked discrepancy between MRI activity and disability than other groups. Patients with PPMS have a paucity of lesions, less gadolinium enhancement and fewer new lesions developing over time.[11,12] The limited enhancement on MRI suggests less inflammation, and this is supported by pathological finding of significantly less inflammation in PPMS than in SPMS.[13] Differences in immunological and genetic profiles have also been suggested but they have not been proven.

These clinical and MRI features suggest that PPMS is at least a distinct subgroup of MS. However, until recently the term 'chronic progressive' MS has often been used to describe patients in any progressive phase of the disease without distinguishing between a primary progressive or a secondary progressive course. Although there have been trials in chronic progressive MS, few have addressed PPMS specifically. This raises the question as to whether or not specific trials for PPMS are required. The answer to this is probably 'yes' if two issues are considered. First, the mechanisms that underlie impairment and disability in PPMS may be different from those in RRMS and SPMS, and this may have implications for the choice of therapeutic agent. Secondly, the atypical clinical and MRI features pose particular problems in selecting patients for treatment and in designing therapeutic trials.

The neurological deficits in RRMS result from incomplete remission from relapses, whereas deficits in PPMS arise from disease progression. These differences may relate to the occurrence of axonal loss, the probable correlate of fixed neurological deficits.[14] In RRMS, axonal loss may be related to acute inflammatory demyelination,[15] whereas in PPMS, it may result from a more diffuse low-grade inflammatory process. This is supported by the MRI finding that diffuse abnormalities of brain and spinal cord are more common in PPMS than in RRMS or SPMS.[16] Although inflammation is less in PPMS, it clearly occurs[13] and it may be that there is a different relationship between inflammation and axonal loss, perhaps with axons being more susceptible to damage. Therefore, therapeutic agents directed at both inflammation and axonal protection may be useful in this group.

Patient selection

In order to initiate treatment in any patient group a secure diagnosis should be made, and this is particularly difficult in patients with PPMS. The first step is to exclude other progressive diseases. Most patients with PPMS present with a single progressive symptom, usually implicating the spinal cord,[3,7] so other causes (e.g. compressive spinal cord lesions) must be excluded. MRI plays a particularly important role in this step.

Secondly, the certainty of the diagnosis has to be established. Conventionally the Poser criteria[17] are used, but patients with PPMS do not readily conform to these criteria. A recent retrospective study of patients with PPMS did not allow classification of any patient as having clinically definite MS, and only one third were classified as laboratory-supported definite MS.[18] Patients with only a single clinical lesion cannot be classified as having clinically definite MS and so more emphasis has to be put on the presence of oligoclonal bands and paraclinical evidence of dissemination in time and space. Without oligoclonal bands it is difficult to make a definite diagnosis according to Poser criteria. To address the problem of certainty of diagnosis in PPMS, specific diagnostic criteria have been developed.[19]

Finally, the correct classification of PPMS has to be made. This may not be possible early in the disease, as disease duration of 2 years has been suggested before making a definite diagnosis.[1] Establishing a history of gradually progressive disease may be difficult, since details of the initial presentation may fade with the passage of time and it may be difficult to distinguish retrospectively between fluctuations in function and true neurological relapses. In an ongoing study of interferon (IFN)-β 1a,[20] only 50 of 138 patients referred with a diagnosis of PPMS were enrolled. Of the 88 patients not included, 50% either clearly did not have a primary progressive course on detailed history, or else they did not fulfil the diagnostic criteria for definite MS.

The timing of the initiation of therapy also presents problems in this group. Although not universally accepted, the US National MS Society has recommended that therapy be initiated as soon as possible after the diagnosis of MS is made. However, early treatment is not possible in PPMS, since the diagnosis cannot be made for 2 years. In established disease it is not clear whether severity of disease should influence initiation of therapy. Whereas in RRMS, frequent or severe relapses or significant residual deficits often prompts treatment, the majority of patients with PPMS have a gradual course. Rate of disease progression may be a guide to treatment, since change in the expanded disability status scale (EDSS) score in the short term has been reported to predict faster disease progression in the longer term.[21]

Another problem with PPMS is the increased incidence of general medical problems caused by the higher mean age of presentation. In the study of IFN-β 1a, 12.5% of patients not entered in the study were excluded on medical grounds (e.g. because of ischemic heart disease or spinal cord compression).[20] Cervical spondylosis is also common in this age group, and spinal cord compression may be present at entry into a clinical trial or it may develop during the trial and confound clinical assessment. Patients with general medical problems may also be more sensitive to any toxic effects of therapeutic agents.

Therapeutic monitoring

In any definitive therapeutic trial in MS, the primary outcome measure has to be clinical[22] (conventionally, frequency and severity of relapses, and disease progression). In PPMS, assessment of relapses is not applicable and so the clinical outcome is limited to disease progression. Currently, the most widely used measure of disease progression is the EDSS.[23] However, there are problems with its validity and reliability,[24,25] and its responsiveness is relatively poor.[26] Responsiveness of a clinical scale is particularly important in PPMS because disease progression is gradual and small changes may be clinically significant. Despite its limitations, the EDSS remains the first choice for clinical trials until more sensitive and reliable clinical scales are validated. The recently developed Multiple Sclerosis Functional Composite Measure[27] may provide improved precision and sensitivity, but this is yet to be evaluated (see Chapter 2).

MRI outcome measures are now widely used as surrogate markers of disease activity in MS, either as a primary outcome in preliminary short-term trials in RRMS and SPMS or as a secondary outcome in definitive long-term trials in RRMS, SPMS and PPMS.[28] However, there are currently no valid MRI markers that can be used as a primary outcome in preliminary trials in PPMS.[21] Owing to the rarity of PPMS the validity and reliability of MRI markers is particularly important because multicentre trials will be necessary and markers must be robust across centres.

Therapeutic trials in RRMS and SPMS usually assess conventional MRI markers of gadolinium enhancement and changes in T2-weighted lesion volume. However, in PPMS the rate of development of new lesions is low and there are few gadolinium-enhancing lesions.[12] T2-weighted cerebral lesion load on MRI may be a responsive measure, since significant change has been demonstrated over 1 year,[29] but no correlation has been shown to date between T2 lesion load and disability in cross-sectional[3] or longitudinal studies[30] in this group. Triple-dose gadolinium (see Chapter 5) may increase the yield of enhancing lesions,[31] although this has not been confirmed[32] and fast Fluid Attenuated Inversion Recovery (FLAIR) imaging may increase detection of subcortical lesions in this group.[33] However, even with such optimization, it is likely that conventional MRI markers will prove to have limited clinical relevance in therapeutic monitoring in PPMS. Conventional imaging of the spinal cord may have been expected to be more relevant since clinical spinal cord involvement is common in PPMS, but no correlation has been demonstrated between cord lesion load and disability in cross-sectional[3,34] or longitudinal studies,[35] although results of a large serial study are awaited.[3] Further information on the responsiveness and validity of conventional MRI markers will be provided in the near future from the MAGNIMS 2-year natural history study of PPMS,[3] and 1-year data are referred to below.

It appears likely that more pathologically specific markers of tissue destruction may be more clinically relevant in PPMS (see Chapters 6, 8 and 9). Such markers include T1-weighted hypointense MRI lesions, spinal cord and cerebral atrophy, magnetization transfer ratio, proton spectroscopy and diffusion imaging. Disappointingly, T1-weighted hypointense lesion load in PPMS has not been shown to correlate with EDSS in cross-sectional[3] or longitudinal studies.[29]

Measures of atrophy appear to be a more promising marker of disease progression. Spinal cord cross-sectional area correlates strongly with disability,[36] and significant spinal cord atrophy has been demonstrated in PPMS in only 1 year.[37] A correlation of partial brain volume with disability[3] and significant cerebral atrophy over 1 year[29] have also been demonstrated in PPMS.

Owing to the paucity of lesions in PPMS, it appears likely that intrinsic changes in normal appearing white matter (NAWM) may make a major contribution to disability in this group. Magnetization transfer ratio and proton spectroscopy are potentially powerful tools to study changes in NAWM as well as lesions. A significant reduction in magnetization transfer ratio in lesions[38] and small but widespread reductions in NAWM[39] have been demonstrated in PPMS. Further work, including longitudinal studies, is required to evaluate the role of magnetization transfer ratio in monitoring disease progression. On proton spectroscopy there is a reduction in N-acetyl aspartate in lesions[40] and in NAWM[40,41] in PPMS, but longitudinal studies are required to evaluate the relationship between these changes and disability.

Finally, a preliminary study of diffusion imaging in PPMS has demonstrated increased apparent diffusion coefficient in lesions,[42] but further work is required to evaluate this as a disease marker.

THERAPEUTIC TRIALS

Currently, there is no definitively proven disease-modifying treatment available for PPMS. Several trials have been completed in chronic progressive multiple sclerosis but without clear distinction between PPMS and SPMS. Some of these trials have made reference to PPMS but there has been insufficient evidence available to recommend their use in this group of patients.

Azathioprine

Several randomized controlled trials of azathioprine in MS have been carried out. A meta-analysis of these trials confirmed a slight clinical benefit.[43] In one trial[44] a subgroup of 51 patients with progressive disease from onset were included. Although analysis of the whole group showed a small beneficial effect, no significant effects were seen in the 51 patients with progressive disease from onset.

Methorexate

A randomized, double-blind, placebo-controlled trial of low-dose oral methotrexate (7.5 mg weekly) was completed in 60 patients with chronic progressive MS.[45] Eighteen patients had PPMS defined as a progressive course since disease onset. There was significantly less progression, as judged by a newly developed composite measure, in the methotrexate group compared to the placebo group, but the result was not significant when the primary progressive group alone was considered.

Cladribine

A randomized, double-blind, placebo-controlled, cross-over study of cladribine (2-chlorodeoxyadenosine) (0.7 mg/kg via central venous line) was carried out in 51 patients with chronic progressive MS.[46] Clinical, MRI and cerebrospinal fluid parameters remained stable in patients on cladribine but deteriorated in patients on placebo. A phase 3 multicentre trial of subcutaneous cladribine was recently completed in patients with SPMS and PPMS. Preliminary reports state that no clinical efficacy was apparent, although significant effects were demonstrated on MRI parameters[47] (see Chapter 22).

Trials specifically designed for PPMS

Recently, a number of trials have been specifically designed for PPMS. These trials are currently underway but no results are available as yet.

IFN-β 1a

A small randomized, double-blind, placebo-controlled study of two doses of intramuscular IFN-β 1a (30 μg or 60 μg weekly) in 50 patients with PPMS is now in its second year.[19] The primary outcome measure is EDSS score. Secondary MRI outcomes include the conventional measures of cerebral lesion loads and new lesions in brain and spinal cord, as well as the more pathologically specific measures of cerebral and spinal cord atrophy, magnetization transfer ratio and proton spectroscopy.

IFN-β 1b

IFN-β 1b has been shown to delay disease progression in patients with SPMS, both those with and those without superimposed relapses.[48] A double-blind, placebo-controlled trial of subcutaneous IFN-β 1b (8×10^6 IU every other day) in 70 patients with PPMS and Transitional Progressive MS (TPMS) is now under way.[49] Clinical outcome measures include the EDSS score, and MRI outcome measures include lesion loads, cervical cord area, magnetization transfer ratio and magnetic resonance spectroscopy parameters.

Glatiramer acetate

A large North American study of glatiramer acetate in PPMS is about to begin. It will involve 900 patients and will have three treatment arms (two active and one placebo). Strict clinical criteria will be used and the primary outcome measure will be EDSS score, although a range of MRI outcomes will also be included.

Riluzole

A small pilot cross-over study of the neuroprotective agent riluzole has recently been completed.[50] Sixteen patients had 6-monthly clinical and MRI evaluations for 1 year untreated and 1 year on treatment. Results are currently being analysed.

CONCLUSION

Until recently, the area of therapeutic trials in PPMS has been neglected. Now, with the advent of disease-modifying drugs, this group should no longer be excluded from therapeutic trials. Further work is required to validate reliable clinical and MRI markers of disease progression to facilitate future therapeutic trials and to monitor efficacy. Further elucidation of pathophysiology is also required to guide the development of therapeutic agents. The aim of future therapeutic agents should be to target the underlying pathological process, which in PPMS may well be axonal loss.

REFERENCES

1 Thompson AJ, Polman CH, Miller DH et al. Primary progressive multiple sclerosis, *Brain* 1997; 120:1085–1096.

2 Lublin FD, Reingold SC. Defining the clinical course of multiple sclerosis: results of an international survey. *Neurology* 1996; 46:907–911.

3 Stevenson VL, Miller DH, Rovaris M et al. Primary and transitional progressive MS; a clinical and MRI cross sectional study. *Neurology* 1999; 52:839–845.

4 Kremenchutzky M, Baskerville J, Rice GPA, Ebers GC. Progressive relapsing (PR) and relapsing progressive (RP) multiple sclerosis: a re-evaluation. *Multiple Sclerosis* 1998; 4:372.

5 Filippi M, Campi A, Martinelli V et al. A brain MRI study of different types of chronic-progressive multiple sclerosis. *Acta Neurol Scand* 1995; 91:231–233.

6 Gayou A, Brochet B, Dousset V. Transitional progressive multiple sclerosis: a clinical and imaging study. *J Neurol Neurosurg Psychiatry* 1997; 63:396–398.

7 McDonnell GV, Hawkins SA. Primary progressive multiple sclerosis: a distinct syndrome? *Multiple Sclerosis* 1996; 2:137–141.

8 Runmarker B, Andersen O. Prognostic factors in a multiple sclerosis incidence cohort with twenty-five years of follow-up, *Brain* 1993; 116:117–134.

9 Weinshenker BG, Bass B, Rice GPA et al. The natural history of multiple sclerosis: a geographically based study. 1. Clinical course and disability. *Brain* 1989; 112:133–146.

12 Minderhoud JM, van der Hoeven JH, Prange AJ. Course and prognosis of chronic progressive multiple sclerosis. Results of an epidemiological study. *Acta Neurol Scand* 1988; 78:10–15.

11 Thompson AJ, Kermode AG, MacManus DG et al. Patterns of disease activity in multiple sclerosis: clinical and magnetic resonance imaging study. *Br Med J* 1990; 300:631–634.

12 Thompson AJ, Kermode AG, Wicks D et al. Major differences in the dynamics of primary and secondary progressive multiple sclerosis. *Ann Neurol* 1991; 29:53–62.

13 Revesz T, Kidd D, Thompson AJ et al. A comparison of the pathology of primary and SP-MS. *Brain* 1994; 117:759–765.

14 Trapp BD, Peterson J, Ransohoff RM et al. Axonal transection in the lesions of multiple sclerosis. *New Engl J Med* 1998; 338:278–285.

15 Ferguson B, Matysak MK, Esiri MM, Perry VH. Axonal damage in acute multiple sclerosis lesions. *Brain* 1997; 120:393–399.

16 Lycklama a Nijeholt GJ, van Walderveen AA, Castelijns JA et al. Brain and spinal cord abnormalities

in multiple sclerosis. Correlation between MRI parameters, clinical subtypes and symptoms. *Brain* 1998; **121**:687–697.

17 Poser CM, Paty DW, Scheinberg L et al. New diagnostic criteria for multiple sclerosis: guidelines for research protocols. *Ann Neurol* 1983; **13**:227–231.

18 McDonnell GV, Hawkins SA. Clinical study of PP-MS in Northern Ireland, UK. *J Neurol Neurosurg Psychiatry* 1998; **64**:451–454.

19 Thompson AJ, Montalban X, Barkhof F et al. New diagnostic criteria for primary progressive multiple sclerosis (abstract). *Ann Neurol* 1999; in press.

20 Leary SM, Stevenson VL, Miller DH, Thompson AJ. Problems in designing and recruiting to therapeutic trials in PP-MS. *J Neurol* 1999; in press.

21 Losseff NA, Kingsley DPE, McDonald WI et al. Clinical and magnetic resonance imaging predictors of disability in primary and SP-MS. *Multiple Sclerosis* 1996; **1**:218–222.

22 Whitaker JN, McFarland HF, Rudge P, Reingold SC. Outcomes assessment in multiple sclerosis clinical trials: a critical analysis. *Multiple Sclerosis* 1995; **1**:37–47.

23 Kurtzke JF. Rating neurologic impairment in multiple sclerosis: an Expanded Disability Status Scale (EDSS). *Neurology* 1983; **33**:1444–1452.

24 Willoughby EW, Paty DW. Scales for rating impairment in multiple sclerosis: a critique. *Neurology* 1988; **38**:1793–1798.

25 Noseworthy JH, Vandervoort MK, Wong CJ et al. Interrater variability with the expanded disability status scale (EDSS) and functional systems (FS) in a multiple sclerosis clinical trial. *Neurology* 1990; **40**:971–975.

26 Hobart JC, Lamping DL, Freeman JA, Thompson AJ. Reliability, validity, and responsiveness of the Kurtzke expanded disability status scale in multiple sclerosis (abstract). *J Neurol Neurosurg Psychiatry* 1997; **62**:212.

27 Cutter G, Baier M, Rudick R et al. Development of a multiple sclerosis functional composite as a clinical trial outcome measure. *Brain* 1999; **122**:871–882

28 Miller DH, Albert PS, Barkhof F et al. Guidelines for the use of magnetic resonance techniques in monitoring the treatment of multiple sclerosis. *Ann Neurol* 1996; **39**:6–16.

29 Stevenson VL, Miller DH, Leary SM et al. A one-year serial clinical and MRI study of PP-MS (abstract). *Multiple Sclerosis* 1999; in press.

30 Filippi M, Paty DW, Kappos L et al. Correlations

between changes in disability and T2-weighted brain MRI activity in multiple sclerosis: a follow-up study. *Neurology* 1995; **45**:255–260.

31 Filippi M, Campi A, Martinelli V et al. Comparison of triple dose versus standard dose gadolinium–DTPA for detection of MRI enhancing lesions in patients with PP-MS. *J Neurol Neurosurg Psychiatry* 1995; **59**:540–544.

32 Silver NC, Good CD, Barker GJ et al. Sensitivity of contrast enhanced MRI in multiple sclerosis: effects of gadolinium dose, magnetisation transfer contrast and delayed imaging. *Brain* 1997; **120**:1149–1161.

33 Gawne-Cain ML, O'Riordan JI, Thompson AJ et al. Multiple sclerosis lesion detection in the brain: a comparison of fast FLAIR and conventional T2 weighted dual spin echo. *Neurology* 1997; **49**:364–370.

34 Kidd D, Thorpe JW, Thompson AJ et al. Spinal cord MRI using multiarray coils and fast spin echo. II: findings in multiple sclerosis. *Neurology* 1993; **43**:2632–2637.

35 Kidd D, Thorpe JW, Kendall BE et al. MRI dynamics of brain and spinal cord in progressive multiple sclerosis. *J Neurol Neurosurg Psychiatry* 1996; **60**:15–19.

36 Losseff NA, Webb SL, O'Riordan JI et al. Spinal cord atrophy and disability in multiple sclerosis. A new reproducible and sensitive method with potential to monitor disease progression. *Brain* 1996; **119**:701–708.

37 Stevenson VL, Leary SM, Losseff NA et al. Spinal cord atrophy and disability in multiple sclerosis: a longitudinal study. *Neurology* 1998; **51**:234–238.

38 Gass A, Barker GJ, Kidd D et al. Correlation of magnetization transfer ratio with clinical disability in multiple sclerosis. *Ann Neurol* 1994; **36**:62–67.

39 Leary SM, Silver NC, Stevenson VL et al. Magnetisation transfer ratio of normal appearing white matter in PP-MS (abstract). *Multiple Sclerosis* 1998; **4**:297.

40 Davie CA, Barker GJ, Thompson AJ et al. ^{1}H magnetic resonance spectroscopy of chronic cerebral white matter lesions and normal appearing white matter in multiple sclerosis. *J Neurol Neurosurg Psychiatry* 1997; **63**:736–742.

41 Leary SM, Davie CA, Parker GJM et al. ^{1}H magnetic resonance spectroscopy of normal appearing white matter in PP-MS (abstract). *Ann Neurol* 1998; **44**:464.

42 Droogan AG, Clark CA, Werring DJ et al. Navigated

spin echo diffusion-weighted imaging in clinical phenotypes of multiple sclerosis (abstract). *Proc Int Soc Magn Reson Med* 1998; **1**:117.

43 Yudkin PL, Ellison GW, Ghezzi A et al. Overview of azathioprine treatment in multiple sclerosis. *Lancet* 1991; **338**:1051–1055.

44 British and Dutch Multiple Sclerosis Azathioprine Trial Group. Double-masked trial of azathioprine in multiple sclerosis. *Lancet* 1988; **ii**:179–183.

45 Goodkin DE, Rudick RA, VanderBrug Medendorp S et al. Low dose (7.5mg) oral methotrexate reduces the rate of progression in chronic progressive multiple sclerosis. *Ann Neurol* 1995; **37**:30–40.

46 Sipe JC, Romine JS, Koziol JA et al. Cladribine in treatment of chronic progressive multiple sclerosis. *Lancet* 1994; **344**:9–13.

47 Rice G, the Cladribine Study Group. Effect of cladribine on magnetic resonance imaging findings in progressive multiple sclerosis: final results of a placebo-controlled trial (abstract). *Ann Neurol* 1998; **44**:504.

48 European Study Group on Interferon Beta-1b in Secondary Progressive MS. Placebo-controlled multicentre randomized trial of interferon beta-1b in treatment of SP-MS. *Lancet* 1998; **352**:1491–1497.

49 Montalban X, Tintore M, Rio J et al. Primary progressive multiple sclerosis: description of 121 patients and study design of a controlled trial (abstract). *Multiple Sclerosis* 1998; **4**:344.

50 Kalkers NF, Bergers E, van Schijndel R et al. A pilot study of riluzole in primary progressive multiple sclerosis: effect on spinal cord atrophy on MRI. *J Neurol* 1999; **246**(suppl 1): 89.

PART V

Symptomatic drug therapy in clinical practice

34
Treatment of fatigue in multiple sclerosis

Lauren B Krupp

INTRODUCTION

Fatigue is a core feature of multiple sclerosis (MS). Over 75% of patients with MS report fatigue, and for many it is their most disabling symptom.[1–3] Unfortunately, despite its prevalence, fatigue remains a poorly understood issue. This chapter reviews what is known about fatigue in MS and the current recommendations for its management.

DEFINITION AND MEASUREMENT OF FATIGUE

There are a variety of approaches to the measurement of fatigue. These can be generally categorized according to measures of a person's performance or measures of a person's subjective experience.

Performance-based measurements

Physiologically, fatigue is defined by a reduction in power output over time. A common measurement is the time–force curve during maximal effort (e.g. sustained muscle contraction). With this approach to measurement, MS patients have been shown to have significantly greater motor fatigue than healthy controls and patients with chronic fatigue syndrome.[4] Declines in central motor drive,[5] decreased muscle torque during sustained contractions, and reduced motor evoked potentials[6–8] have all been proposed as explanations of the physiological findings.

Although more difficult to measure, cognitive functioning may also be susceptible to fatigue. In a pilot study, Caruso and colleagues[9] measured neuropsychological performances in a group of MS subjects before and after a period of physical exercise, but concluded that there was no significant decline. However, Elkins and colleagues[10] used a similar procedure but with a period of cognitive rather than physical exertion and also included a control group. In this study, the MS subjects had a striking decline on measures of memory and conceptual thinking across the testing session, whereas the controls continued to improve with practice. These preliminary findings suggest that the cognitive effects of fatigue in MS may also be identified, and future studies promise some exciting advances in this area.

Self-report measures

While physiological measurements offer the most objective findings, they do not appear to corre-

Table 34.1 Fatigue scales

Name of scale	Dimensions (number measured)	Number of items
Fatigue Impact Scale (FIS)[3]	Cognitive, psychosocial, physical (3)	21
Multidimensional Asessment of Fatigue (MAF)[12,13]	Severity, timing, distress, interference (4)	16
Checklist of Individual Strength (CIS)[14,15]	Subjective, motivation, activity, concentration (4)	24
Piper Fatigue Scale (PFS)[16]	Temporal, affective, intensity, sensory (4)	41
Multidimensional Fatigue Inventory (MFI)[17]	General, activity, mental, physical, motivation (5)	24
Fatigue Assessment Instrument (FAI) [18]	Severity, situation-specific, psychological, sleep (4)	29
Fatigue Scale (FS)[19]	Physical, mental (2)	14
Fatigue Descriptive Scale (FDS)[20]	Initiative, severity, modality, frequency, Uhthoff (5)	12
Fatigue Severity Scale (FSS)[21]	Severity on daily living (1)	9
Profile of Mood States (POMS)[22]	Tiredness–vigor (1)	
Functional Assessment of Multiple Sclerosis (FAMS)[23]	Tiredness–thinking subscale (1)	9
Rand Index of Vitality (RIV)[24]	Vitality (1)	4

spond to a person's subjective sense of fatigue.[11] Self-report measures provide an important key towards our understanding of fatigue. When patients report subjective fatigue, they usually describe an overwhelming sense of tiredness, lack of energy, or feeling of exhaustion. Patients report that fatigue is distinct from both depressed mood and from limb weakness, and compare it to a feeling of exhaustion that often accompanies a flu-like illness.

A variety of self-report instruments have been developed to assess fatigue in MS and other disorders. *Table 34.1* lists several fatigue scales that are commonly used. Multidimensional measures are designed to assess several distinct characteristics of fatigue. The Multidimensional Assessment of Fatigue (MAF)[12] is a measure of general fatigue that was developed for patients with rheumatoid arthritis[12] and has more recently been used in patients with MS.[13] The dimensions include fatigue severity and frequency, degree of interference in activities of daily living, and associated distress. The Fatigue Impact Scale (FIS) is a 40-item questionnaire that includes cognitive, psychosocial, and physical dimensions.[3] Its shorter version, the 21-item Modified Fatigue Impact Scale (MFIS), has been incorporated in the MS-specific disability measure, the MS Quality of Life (MSQOL) inventory. The FIS has been found to be a strong predictor of mental and general health in a population of 85 MS patients.[3] The Fatigue Assessment Instrument (FAI)[15] is a 28-item questionnaire that identifies a severity factor and a situation-specific factor. The situation-specific factor addresses features of fatigue that are more specific to MS, such as the exacerbating effects of heat.

Several unidimensional scales that measure fatigue intensity or severity have also been widely used in MS. The Fatigue Severity Scale (FSS)[21] is a shortened version of the FAI; it measures the effect of fatigue on activities of daily living. It has been used in a variety MS studies[21,25–27] including several treatment trials of fatigue.[11,26,28] Recently, it has been translated into several languages for international use. Other unidimensional fatigue measures are subscales from larger questionnaires. An example is the tiredness–thinking measure contained in the Functional Assessment of Multiple Sclerosis (FAMS),[23] a comprehensive disability assessment. The Rand Vitality Index is a four-item subscale of the Medical Outcome Survey (MOS and Short-Form 36).[24] The Profile of Mood States (POMS)[22] includes a tiredness–vigor subscale that has also been used in studies of MS patients.

Although all these measures have been useful for describing MS fatigue, their sensitivity to treatment effects and change over time has yet to be determined. In addition, these scales measure fatigue only at one point in time and many require that the subjects rate an individual to their fatigue severity retrospectively. Ecological momentary assessment methods, which involve frequent and random monitoring of affect and fatigue over time, may prove to be more accurate.[29]

Pathogenesis

The pathogenesis of fatigue in MS remains uncertain. Fatigue is only weakly associated with overall neurologic impairment, but it is more common in patients whose disease course is progressive.[13,21,25,27] Relapses are often associated with transient increases in fatigue. Although involvement of premotor, limbic, or brainstem areas have been suggested as a cause of decreased motivation or motor readiness, there are no established anatomic markers of fatigue. Neuroimaging studies that have attempted to identify correlates of perceived fatigue have shown conflicting findings.[26,30,31]

Immune factors may contribute to fatigue. Medications such as interferon (IFN)-α and IFN-β[26,27] produce prominent fatigue as an initial side effect. The mechanism for this effect is not known. However, the effect of interferon effects on neuroendocrine pathways or induction of other cytokines such as interleukin (IL)-6 may contribute to the production of fatigue.[34,35] In both human and animal studies, other cytokines including IL-1 and tumor necrosis factor have also been associated with either sleep induction or fatigue.[36–38]

It is possible that fatigue in MS results from disruption of the neuroendocrine or from altered cerebral metabolism. Decreases in the supply of glucose to the brain[39] could cause fatigue. A positron emission tomography study of patients with MS identified a significant correlation between perceived fatigue (as measured by the FSS) and glucose availability.[31] Disruption in neurotransmitter systems, including serotoninergic pathways, interferes with attention and could also cause cognitive fatigue.[40]

Although fatigue in MS is largely independent of depressed mood,[2,3,28] psychological factors do influence a patient's experience of fatigue. For instance, fatigue can be lessened by feelings of control and exacerbated by focusing on bodily sensations.[14] In contrast, patients who feel that they can create environments appropriate to their psychological and physical needs experience less fatigue and fatigue-related stress.[13]

TREATMENT

Treatment requires a multidisciplinary approach that considers the various factors that may contribute to fatigue. These include determining the contributions to a patient's fatigue of mood, level of physical activity, pain, side effects from medication, and sleep patterns. Once these contributing factors have been addressed and other causes have been ruled out, there are several strategies for treatment of fatigue.

Non-pharmacologic approaches

Among the non-pharmacologic treatments, education and support are very important. Patients are directly helped by validating fatigue as a genuine feature of MS. Exercise is a powerful method to combat deconditioning and enhance self-esteem. The advantages of exercise on fatigue were demonstrated in a study of 54 patients randomly assigned to either 15 weeks of aerobic training or a non-exercise group.[41] Patients in the exercise group experienced a significant reduction in fatigue as measured by the POMS[22] at week 10 and had improvement in quality of life. However, improvement was not sustained at week 15. Self-reported physical state, social interaction, emotional behavior and home management also improved. While a graded exercise program is useful, overexertion can be detrimental. Carefully timed rest periods during the work day and avoidance of environmental factors that worsen fatigue (such as heat) can lessen fatigue and enhance productivity.

A 1-year multidisciplinary rehabilitation program was found to reduce fatigue and MS symptoms in a group of 20 patients with progressive MS compared to a waiting list control group.[42] Behavioral therapy is another means of managing fatigue. When behavioral techniques have been applied to patients with chronic fatigue syndrome, there has been a significant reduction in depression and fatigue components caused by mood disorder.[43–45] Behavioral therapies on an individual or group basis can also be easily applied in MS.

Pharmacologic approaches

Non-pharmacologic measures must often be supplemented with medication. Treatments shown to be effective in randomized, double-blind, placebo-controlled trials are amantadine, an antiviral agent that also has an anti-parkinsonian effect,[28,46,47] and pemoline, a central nervous system (CNS) stimulant.[48]

In a Canadian multicenter MS fatigue treatment trial, amantadine significantly improved fatigue relative to placebo.[47] In another study comparing pemoline and placebo, no significant differences emerged but there was a trend in favor of pemoline.[48] In a placebo-controlled, randomized study comparing pemoline, amantadine, and placebo, amantadine was the most effective agent.[28] Side effects with either medication in this study were infrequent.

On the basis of relative benefit with amantadine and its low side effect profile, this is the first-line medication to use for MS fatigue. Most patients respond to amantadine 100 mg bd. A drug holiday for 2 days a week can often prolong the therapeutic effect.

If no benefit is seen, then pemoline is a second option. The optimal dose for pemoline needs to be determined on an individual basis. Many patients respond to 18.75 mg or 37.5 mg per day. Occasionally, patients require doses two to three times this range.

For patients who have not responded to amantadine and pemoline, fluoxetine may be helpful, even if the patient denies depression. Other medications for fatigue that have been found to be helpful on an anecdotal basis include CNS stimulants such as methylphenidate and dextroamphetamine. Newer treatments approved for narcolepsy are also being tested for their efficacy in MS fatigue. CNS stimulants should be used with caution but in selected cases they have value. They are contraindicated in patients with abuse potential. A potential future therapy is 4-aminopyridine. In a study that examined its long term efficacy and safety, fatigue was reported to improve with therapy.[49] A pilot study in MS with 3,4-diaminopyridine has reported subjective fatigue improvement in six of eight treated subjects but no change in physiological fatigue measures.[11] Future studies of 4-aminopyridine in the treatment of MS fatigue are under consideration.

For patients with fatigue and concurrent depression, the initial treatment of choice is an anti-depressant medication (see Chapter 37). Fatigue is likely to be resistant to all therapy if the depression is not treated first. Even patients who deny depressive symptoms may have definite responses to anti-depressant medication. Agents with the least sedating properties are preferable; these include fluoxetine, sertraline, nefazodone hydrochoride, and desipramine.

In patients in whom fatigue is associated with sleep disorder, improved sleep hygiene is important. For some patients, exercise 6 hours before sleep can help. Medications for insomnia may also lower fatigue. When fatigue is associated with anxiety, pharmacologic treatments that alleviate anxiety or panic attacks can benefit fatigue.

Other treatments for MS fatigue are under investigation. A preliminary report on the response of fatigue (measured by the FSS) to IFN-β 1a (Avonex®) in the phase 3 trial for relapsing–multiple sclerosis did not show any significant differences between the active treatment group and the placebo group.[26] The North American multicenter clinical trial using IFN-β 1b for secondary progressive MS also includes as an outcome measure fatigue as assessed by the MFIS. The results of this study should also help determine whether treatment with IFN-β lessens fatigue.

Implications for clincial practice

The clinical management of fatigue should include an assessment of the various factors that can cause fatigue as well as a step-wise treatment approach that encompasses non-pharmacologic and pharmacologic interventions. Several initial questions need to be addressed in evaluating the

MS patient with increased fatigue. Are there signs of an impending relapse? Is there an infection present or has there been increased heat exposure? Have medications been changed or added that could increase fatigue? Medications to review include anti-spasticity agents, β-blockers, tricyclic antidepressants, benzodiazepines, and anti-convulsants.

Other symptoms may also contribute to fatigue. The evaluation should include questions regarding pain, sleep, and depression. Assessment of mood is critical to the evaluation of fatigue. Most patients with MS have elevated depressive symptoms although they may not meet criteria for major depression. A simple office approach to the presence of mood disorders is to include self-report questionnaires such as the Beck Depression Inventory[50] or the Center for Epidemiologic Studies Depression Scale[51] in the initial clinical history, obtain a history for family psychiatric illness and examine the family unit and support systems.

At some point in their disease course, patients should be evaluated with a laboratory screen to exclude other fatigue-producing conditions. Testing should include thyroid function tests, full blood cell count, electrolyte and glucose measurements, tests of liver function, erythrocyte sedimentation rate, and urinalysis and urine culture.

For patients in whom overwhelming fatigue is associated with severe depression, or for patients who are refractory to all forms of fatigue therapy including exercise, medications, and behavioral interventions, psychiatric referral may be of value.

Implications for future clinical trials

Fatigue is a frequent and often disabling symptom of MS. Clinical treatment trials for fatigue are currently limited by the lack of a concise definition. As our understanding of fatigue continues to grow, improved therapies are likely to follow. Future studies may begin to examine the motor, cognitive, and subjective components separately and lead to specifically targeted interventions.

REFERENCES

1 Freal JE, Kraft GH, Coryell JK. Symptomatic fatigue in multiple sclerosis. *Arch Phys Med Rehabil* 1984; 65:135–138.

2 Krupp LB, Alvarez La, LaRocca NG, Scheinberg L. Clinical characteristics of fatigue in multiple sclerosis. *Arch Neurol* 1988; 45:435–437.

3 Fisk JD, Pontefract A, Ritvo PG et al. The impact of fatigue on patients with multiple sclerosis. *Can J Neurol Sci* 1994; 21:9–14.

4 Djaldetti R, Ziv I, Achiron A, Melamed E. Fatigue in multiple sclerosis compared with chronic fatigue syndrome: a quantitative assessment. *Neurology* 1996; 46:632–635.

5 Sheean GL, Murray MF, Rothwell SG. An electrophysiologic study of the mechanism of fatigue in MS. *Brain* 1997; 120:299–316.

6 Latash M, Kalugina E, Orpett NJ et al. Myogenic and central neurogneic factors in fatigue in multiple sclerosis. *Multiple Sclerosis* 1996; 1:236–241.

7 Kent-Braun JA, Sharma KR, Miller RG, Weiner MW. Postexercise phosphocreatine resynthesis is slowed in multiple sclerosis. *Muscle Nerve* 1994; 17:835–841.

8 Schubert M, Wohlfarth KAI, Rollnick J, Dengler R. Walking and fatigue in multiple sclerosis: the role of the corticospinal system. *Muscle Nerve* 1998; 21:1068–1070.

9 Caruso LS, LaRocca NG, Foley FW et al. Exertional fatigue fails to affect cognitive function in multiple sclerosis. *J Clin Exp Neuropsychol* 1991; 13:74.

10 Elkins LE, Pollina DA, Scheffer SR, Krupp LB. Effects of fatigue on cognitive functioning in multiple sclerosis. *Neurology* 1998; 50(suppl):A126.

11 Sheean G, Murray N, Rothwell J et al. An open labelled clinical and electrophsiological study of 3,4 diaminopyridine in the treatment of fatigue in multiple sclerosis. *Brain* 1998; 121:967–975.

12 Elza BL, Henke CJ, Yelin EH et al. Correlates of fatigue in older women with rheumatoid arthritis. *Nurs Res* 1993; **42**:93–99.

13 Schwartz CE, Coulthard-Morris L, Zeng Q. Psychosocial correlates of fatigue in multiple sclerosis. *Arch Phys Med Rehabil* 1996; **77**:165–170.

14 Vercoulen J, Hommes OR, Swanink C et al. The measurement of fatigue in patients with multiple sclerosis: a multidimensional comparison with patients with chronic fatigue syndrome and healthy subjects. *Arch Neurol* 1996, **53**:642–649.

15 Vercoulen JHMM, Swanink CMA, Fennis JFM et al. Dimensional assessment of chronic fatigue syndrome. *J Psychosom Res* 1994; **38**:383–392.

16 Piper BF, Lindsey AM, Dodd MJ et al. The development of an instrument to measure the subjective dimension of fatigue. In: Funk SG, Tornquist EM, Campagene MT et al, eds. *Key Aspects of Comfort, Management of Pain, Fatigue and Nausea*. New York: Springer, 1989.

17 Smets EMA, Garssen B, Bonke B, De Haes JCJM. The multidimensional fatigue inventory (MFI) psychometric qualities of an instrument to assess fatigue. *J Psychosom Res* 1995; **39**:315–325.

18 Schwartz J, Jandorf L, Krupp LB. The measurement of fatigue: a new scale. *J Psychosom Res* 1993; **37**:753–762.

19 Chalder T, Berelowitz G, Pawlikowska T et al. Development of a fatigue scale. *J Psychosom Res* 1993; **37**:147–153.

20 Iriarte J, Katsamakis G, De Castro P. The fatigue descriptive scale (FDS): a useful tool to evaluate fatigue in multiple sclerosis. *Multiple Sclerosis* 1999; **5**:10–16.

21 Krupp LB, LaRocca NC, Muir-Nash J, Steinberg AD. The fatigue severity scale applied to patients with multiple sclerosis and systemic lupus erythematosus. *Arch Neurol* 1989; **46**:1121–1123.

22 McNair DM, Lorr M, Droppleman LF. *Profile of Mood States (POMS)*. San Diego, California: Educational and Industrial Testing Service, 1992.

23 Cella DF, Dineen K, Arnason B et al. Validation of the functional assessment of multiple sclerosis (FAMS); quality of life instrument. *Neurology* 1996; **47**:129–139.

24 Ware JE, Kosinski M, Keller SD. *SF-36 Physical and Mental Health Summary Scales: a User's Manual*. Boston, Massachusetts: The Health Institute, New England Medical Center, 1994.

25 Bergamaschi R, Romani V, Versino M et al. Clinical aspects of fatigue in multiple sclerosis. *Funct Neurol* 1997; **12**:247–251.

26 Cookfair DL, Fischer J, Rudick R et al. Fatigue severity in low disability MS patients participating in a phase III trial of Avonex for relapsing multiple sclerosis. *Neurology* 1997; **48**:A173.

27 Grossman M, Armstrong C, Onishi K et al. Patterns of cognitive impairment in relapsing–remitting and chronic progressive multiple sclerosis. *Neuropsychiatry Neuropsychol Behav Neurol* 1994; **7**:194–210.

28 Krupp LB, Coyle PK, Doscher C et al. Fatigue therapy in multiple sclerosis: results of a double-blind randomized parallel trial of amantadine, pemoline, and placebo. *Neurology* 1995; **45**:1956–1961.

29 Stone AA, Broderick JE, Porter LS et al. Fatigue and mood in chronic fatigue syndrome patients: results of a momentary assessment protocol examining fatigue and mood levels and diurnal patterns. *Ann Behav Med* 1994; **16**:228–234.

30 Moller A, Wiedmann G, Rohde U et al. Correlates of cognitive impairment and depressive mood disorder in multiple sclerosis. *Acta Psychiatr* 1994; **89**:117–121.

31 Roelcke U, Kappos L, Lechner-Scott J et al. Reduced glucose metabolism in the frontal cortex and basal ganglia of multiple sclerosis patients with fatigue: a 18F-fluorodeoxyglucosepositron emission tomographic study. *Neurology* 1997; **48**:1566–1571.

32 Quesada JR, Guttman. Clinical toxicity of interferons in cancer patients: a review. *J Clin Oncol* 1986; **4**:234–243.

33 Neilly LK, Goodin DS, Goodkin DE, Hause SL. Side effect profile of interferon beta-1b in MS: results of an open label trial. *Neurology* 1996; **46**:552–554.

34 Jones TH, Wadler S, Hupart KH. Endocrine-mediated mechanisms of fatigue during treatment with interferon-α. *Semin Oncol* 1998; **25**:54–63.

35 Martinez EM, Rio J, Barrau M et al. Amelioration of flulike symptoms at the onset of interferon β-1b therapy in multiple sclerosis by low-dose oral steroids is related to a decrease in interleukin-6 induction. *Ann Neurol* 1998; **44**:682–685.

36 Moldofsky H, Lue FA, Eisen J et al. The relationship of interleukin-1 and immune functions to sleep in humans. *Psychosom Med* 1986; **48**:309–318.

37 Bertolone K, Coyle PK, Krupp LB et al. Cytokine correlates of fatigue in MS. *Neurology* 1993; **43**:769S.

38 Chao CC, DeLa Hunt M, Hu S et al. Immunologically mediated fatigue: a murine model. *Clin Immunopath* 1992; **64**:161–165.

39 Wei T, Lightman SL. The neuroendocrine axis in patients with multiple sclerosis. *Brain* 1997; 120:1067–1076.

40 Heilman KM, Watson RT. Fatigue. *Neurology Net Comm* 1997; 1:283–287.

41 Petajan JH, Gappmaier E, White AT et al. Impact of aerobic training on fitness and quality of life in multiple sclerosis. *Ann Neurol* 1996; 39:432–441.

42 Di Fabio RP, Soderberg, Choi T et al. Extended outpatient rehabilitation: its influence on symptom frequency, fatigue, and functional status for persons with progressive multiple sclerosis. *Arch Phys Med Rehabil* 1998; 79:141–146.

43 Deale AM, Chalder T, Marks I, Wessely S. Cognitive behavior therapy for chronic fatigue syndrome: a randomized controlled trial. *Am J Psychiatry* 1997; 54:408–414.

44 Friedberg F, Krupp LB. A comparison of cognitive behavioral treatment of chronic fatigue syndrome and primary depression. *Clin Infect Dis* 1994; 18:105–110.

45 Butler S, Chalder T, Ron M, Wessely S. Cognitive behaviour therapy in CFS. *J Neurol Neurosurg Psychiatry* 1991; 54:153–158.

46 Murray TJ. Amantadine therapy for fatigue in multiple sclerosis. *Can J Neural Sci* 1985; 12:251–254.

47 Canadian MS Research Group. A randomized controlled trial of amantadine in fatigue associated with multiple sclerosis. *Can J Neurol Sci* 1987; 14:273–278.

48 Weinshenker BG, Penman M, Bass B. A double-blind, randomized, crossover trial of pemoline in fatigue associated with multiple sclerosis. *Neurology* 1992; 42:1468–1471.

49 Polman CH, Bertelsmann FW, van Loenen AC, Koetsier JC. 4-Aminopyridine in the treatment of patients with multiple sclerosis. *Arch Neurol* 1994; 51:292–296.

50 Beck AT, Ward CH, Mendelson M. An inventory for measuring depression. *Arch Gen Psychol* 1961; 4:561–571.

51 Radloff LS. CES-D scale: a self-report depression scale for research in the general population. *Appl Psychol Meas* 1977; 1:385–401.

35
Treatment of spasticity

Mariko Kita

Spasticity is a common and disabling symptom for many patients with multiple sclerosis (MS). A classic feature of upper motor neuron dysfunction, spasticity presumably results from interruption of inhibitory descending spinal motor pathways. It has been defined as a velocity-dependent increase in tonic stretch reflexes,[1] in which faster passive movements meet with increasing resistance. A clasp-knife phenomenon may be seen with dissipation of resistance during stretch. Additional signs associated with spasticity include weakness, increased muscle tone, contractures, hyperreflexia, impaired dexterity, extensor plantar responses, and spontaneous muscle spasms.[2] Spasticity tends to affect the lower extremities more than the upper extremities[3] and it worsens in the setting of noxious stimuli such as tight or misfitting clothing or orthotics, infection, or pressure sores. These symptoms are not only uncomfortable to some patients, but they can also greatly interfere with the level of function and so compromise independence in activities of daily living (ADL).

STRUCTURES INVOLVED IN SPASTICITY

The pathophysiology of spasticity is poorly understood but the final common pathway underlying the mechanism is overactivity of the α-motor neuron. Descending spinal pathways (the corticospinal, reticulospinal and vestibulospinal pathways) exert control over α-motor neurons via mono- and polysynaptic pathways.

The muscle spindle is the complex sensory structure of the muscle that conveys information about muscle length. Spindles lie in parallel with extrafusal fibers (large muscle fibers that effect gross movement), so when the muscle is lengthened, the spindle is stretched, thereby causing Ia afferent fibers to send impulses to the spinal cord. Shortening of the extrafusal muscle results in shortening of the spindle and silencing of the Ia afferents. The intrafusal muscle fibers of the spindle complex are innervated by γ-motor neurons in the anterior horns of the spinal cord, which act to increase the tension of the intrafusal fiber when it is shortened. This resets the spindle after shortening so it is again sensitive to changes in muscle length.

When the muscle is lengthened by tendon tap or stretch, Ia afferents produce excitatory postsynaptic potentials (EPSPs) on agonist motorneurons. Although this monosynaptic connection plays a role in the stretch reflex, most excitatory activity in the reflex is mediated by oligosynaptic and polysynaptic pathways.[2] Interneurons play a major role in the reflex arc. Antagonist muscle spindles also send Ia afferents to produce EPSPs on agonist interneurons, which subsequently produce inhibitory post-synaptic potentials (IPSPs) on motor neurons. The firing of the motor neuron depends on the summation of EPSPs and IPSPs. Additional inhibitory interneurons act on Ia afferents to produce a pre-synaptic inhibition of the afferent signal. γ-Aminobutyric acid (GABA) is the neurotransmitter involved in this selective presynaptic inhibition.

The stretch reflex arc requires the participation of muscle spindles, fusimotor innervation (γ-motor neurons), Ia primary afferents, and α-motor neurons, as well as Renshaw recurrent inhibition, disynaptic reciprocal inhibition, non-reciprocal autogenic Ib inhibition, pre-synaptic inhibition, and remote inhibition–excitation of α-motor neurons.[2] Spasticity results from a prolonged disinhibition of components of this system, but the exact mechanism remains unclear.

ASSESSING SPASTICITY

Several measures have been developed to aid in quantifying spasticity and to assess efficacy of anti-spasticity agents in controlled trials as well as in clinical practice. However, there is no consensus on which of these measures or combination of tests provides the most accurate assessment of spasticity, and many of these measures have not been adequately validated. The ones most commonly used in clinical trials are presented here.

Spasticity can be assessed on an ordinal scale similar to that used to grade motor strength. The Ashworth Scale, first described in 1964,[4,5] grades muscle tone according to increasing resistance to mobilization:

1: no increase in tone;

2: slight increase in tone, giving a catch during flexion–extension;

3: more marked increase in tone, easily mobilized;

4: considerable increase in tone, passive movement difficult;

5: rigidity without any possible passive mobilization.

Although this scale may be limited by rater subjectivity, it has been reported to have low inter-rater variability and good reliability amongst experienced examiners.[6]

Penn developed an ordinal scale from 0 to 4 to reflect spasm frequency as a function of spasticity:[7]

0: no spasms;

1: mild spasms induced by stimulation;

2: infrequent full spasms occurring less than once per hour;

3: spasms occurring more than once per hour;

4: spasms occurring more than 10 times per hour.

The Wartenburg Pendulum Test quantifies the number of swings and the degree of excursion at the knee in a supine and seated patient after the leg that is hanging over the end of a table is dropped from extension.[8–10] An electrogiono-meter measures changes in knee angle and swings of the leg, and the information is transferred and analysed by computer. This test can be supplemented with the use of video and electromyographic recording of the quadriceps muscle to measure the force of muscle resistance, such as with the Cybex II isokinetic dynamometer.[11]

The Vibratory Inhibition Index (VII) is based on the finding that vibration applied to the Achilles tendon for 20 seconds in a normal subject will inhibit the H reflex.[12,13] A high VII has been associated with spasticity.[14] In this test, electrode stimulus intensity is optimized to produce a maximal amplitude of the H reflex as measured by electromyography. A 60 Hz vibrator is applied to the Achilles tendon for 20 seconds and the same intensity of stimulus is applied to evoke an H reflex during continuous vibration. The VII is calculated as:

$$VII = \frac{H \text{ reflex amplitude (vibrated)}}{H \text{ reflex amplitude (rest)}} \times 100\%$$

Finally, timed ambulation and tests of strength and co-ordination can also provide indirect assessments of spasticity.

TREATMENT OF SPASTICITY

Rationale for treatment

The goal of therapy for spasticity is to increase the patient's functional capacity and to relieve discomfort that may be associated with the symptoms. Before initiating treatment one must first evaluate the functional consequences of alleviating spasticity. For some patients with proximal leg weakness, increased extensor tone in the legs offers necessary stability and support during transferring and walking. For other patients, hyperreflexia and clonus interfere with normal ambulation. Patients with spasticity may exhibit further increase in tone or spontaneous spasm in the setting of an underlying infection such as a urinary tract infection or decubitus. Such causes should be ruled out before altering a therapeutic regimen for spasticity. The approach to treating spasticity should be multimodal and involve physiotherapy as well as pharmacotherapy. In certain cases, surgical intervention (as with posterior rhizotomy or tendon-release procedures) may be beneficial. As with any treatment

regimen, a systematic approach starting with the most conservative therapies is recommended, and in this chapter this approach is used in the presentation of physiotherapies and pharmacotherapies in the treatment of spasticity.

Physiotherapy

Physiotherapy is an essential component of antispasticity regimens. Muscle shortening increases spindle sensitivity and spasticity.[15,16] Stretching, massage, and passive range-of-motion (ROM) exercises are therefore extremely important in preventing muscle shortening and the formation of contractures. Guidance on proper positioning and posture and on how to avoid specific positions that may elicit clonus or spasms is important.

Patients and caregivers should be instructed by a physiotherapist on how to perform passive ROM and stretching exercises on a regular basis.[17] In general, joints should be supported during ROM exercises to avoid excessive motion. Limbs should be moved in a straight line from starting to ending position and all movements should be slow and consistent, avoiding rapid or abrupt motions. One should also avoid putting pressure on the ball of the foot or palm since this may elicit hyper-reflexia. If the initial movement produces clonus, it may be helpful to bend the next most proximal joint before trying again. Several ROM exercises are outlined in *Figs 35.1* and *35.2*. These exercises should be performed under the guidance of a physiotherapist.

Splinting and treatment with cold packs or transcutaneous electrical nerve stimulation may provide added benefit. Patients should also be evaluated for the need for equipment such as ambulatory aids, reachers, and other devices, and

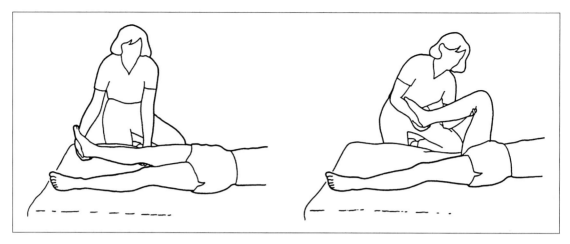

Fig. 35.1a *Hip flexion–extension*
With the patient supine, place one hand under the patient's knee and the other under the patient's heel. Move the whole leg up toward the patient's chest, bending it at the hip and knee. Return the patient's leg to the straight position. Repeat five times.

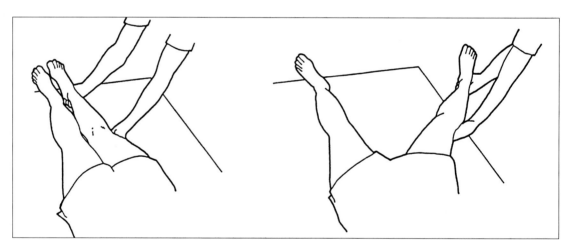

Fig. 35.1b *Hip abduction–adduction*
With the patient supine, place one hand under the patient's knee and the other under the patient's heel. Keeping the patient's leg straight, pull it away from the midline of the body until you feel resistance. Move the patient's leg back to midline. Repeat five times.

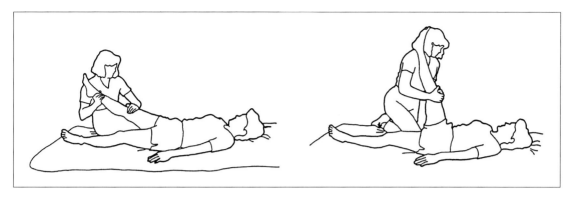

Fig. 35.1c Hamstring stretch
Start with the patient supine with his or her legs straight. Kneel beside the patient's leg and place one hand under the ankle. Place your other hand on top of the patient's knee. Lift the patient's leg straight into the air, and reposition yourself to place the ankle on your shoulder. Place both hands on top of the patient's knee. Lean forward to lift the patient's leg higher into a stretch. Stretch the patient's leg until you meet with resistance or the patient expresses discomfort. Hold for 10 seconds, then lower the patient's leg and relax. Repeat for the other leg. Do five cycles.

Fig. 35.1 *Passive range-of-motion exercises at the hip. From Bezner J. Adult Exercise Instruction Sheets. Home Exercises for Rehabilitation. 1989. Copyright © 1988 by Therapy Skill Builders, a division of The Psychological Corporation. Reproduced by permission. All rights reserved.*

they should be instructed on the appropriate use of these tools. Direct effects of muscle relaxation from physiotherapy are often short-lived and, for many patients, these conservative measures alone are insufficient to treat their symptoms. In most patients, adjunctive pharmacologic therapy is necessary.

Pharmacotherapy

Oral medications that are typically used in the treatment of spasticity include baclofen, benzo-diazepines, and tizanidine. Other medications include clonidine, dantrolene, gabapentin, and botulinum toxin. Of these, only baclofen, diazepam, tizanidine, and dantrolene are approved for the treatment of spasticity in the USA. A general rule with any of these medications is to initiate treatment at low doses and increase gradually, using the lowest dose that proves to be effective for an individual patient.

Baclofen
Baclofen is a structural analog of GABA. It binds the GABA-b receptor, which is coupled to calcium and potassium channels and occurs both pre- and post-synaptically.[18] Binding at the pre-synaptic site increases potassium conductance (and so hyperpolarizes the membrane)

479

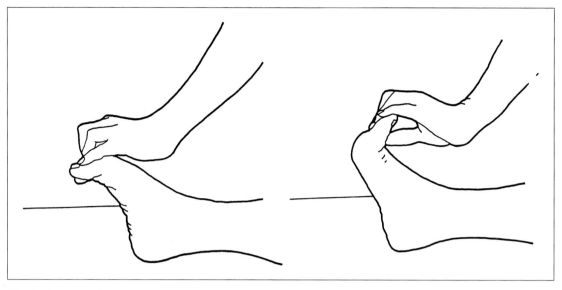

Toe flexion–extension

In the supine patient, support the patient's foot near the ankle with one hand. Place the palm of your other hand on the patient's toes and push them up toward the knee. Repeat five times.

Fig. 35.2 *Passive range-of-motion exercise for the foot. From Bezner J. Adult Exercise Instruction Sheets. Home Exercises for Rehabilitation. 1989.*

and restricts calcium influx into pre-synaptic terminals. The end result is a decrease in neurotransmitter release in excitatory spinal pathways and a decrease in α-motor neuron activity.[19] Activation of GABA-b receptors may also result in inhibition of γ-motor neuron activity and decreased muscle spindle sensitivity.[20]

Several trials have been conducted to test the efficacy of baclofen in treating spasticity in MS, but comparison of these studies and interpretation of results is difficult because of heterogeneous study populations and variable assessment methods.[21–24] Pinto and colleagues[25] summarized international clinical trial experience up to 1972 in a total of 343 MS patients. They reported that baclofen improved spasticity in approximately 70% of these patients, reduced spasticity in approximately 58%, and reduced flexor spasms in approximately 70%.[25]

In 1978, Feldman and colleagues[26] published results of a 10-week double-blind, cross-over study in 23 MS patients and a subsequent 3-year open-label extension study in nine of these patients. Therapeutic response was measured by counting the frequency of spasms, passive resistance to movement, presence and degree of clonus, and ability to ambulate and transfer.

Baclofen recipients in the cross-over study showed a significant reduction in the frequency and severity of spasms and in the severity of clonus. During the open-label phase of the study, the only benefit maintained for the 3-year period was reduction in total number of daily spasms, but it was a benefit appreciated by every participant.

More recently, Brar and colleagues[27] conducted a 10-week masked cross-over study in 30 patients with MS. Patients were randomized to baclofen alone, a stretching regimen with placebo, placebo alone, or stretching with baclofen. The maximum dose of baclofen given was 20 mg/day. Measures to assess efficacy included the Ashworth scale, quadriceps tone as measured by the Cybex II isokinetic unit, timed ambulation and the patient's assessment of function. Cybex flexion scores were significantly improved both after baclofen and after combination baclofen and stretching compared to placebo. A trend for positive effect was noted in combination therapy when compared to baclofen alone. Stretching exercises alone (1.5 minutes/day per muscle group) did not significantly alter spasticity, although patients reported a subjective improvement in symptoms with stretching.[27]

Baclofen is rapidly absorbed after oral administration but penetration into the central nervous system is relatively limited. The mean half-life is fairly short, averaging approximately 3.5 hours. Since it is partially metabolized by the liver (15%) and is excreted by the kidney, the dose should be decreased in patients with known hepatic or renal impairment. There have been reports of elevated liver enzymes in patients taking baclofen. As such, screening of liver function tests should be performed when initiating treatment and then every 6 months. Doses are

often initiated at 5 mg/day, increasing to three times daily as tolerated. Thereafter, doses can be increased slowly at increments of 5 mg/day as needed. It may be helpful to initiate doses and increases at night to minimize experience of side effects. The highest recommended dosage is 80 mg daily in divided doses, but for some patients, this dose may not be sufficient to relieve symptoms. Higher doses should be attempted with caution since side effects are likely to be more prominent. Typical side effects are related to central depression and include drowsiness, fatigue, weakness, nausea, and dizziness. Abrupt cessation of sustained treatment should be avoided because sudden withdrawal of baclofen has been associated with seizures.

Diazepam

The action of the benzodiazepines is mediated by the coupling of the benzodiazepine–GABA-a receptor–chloride ionophore complex.[28] Binding of benzodiazepine to the GABA-a receptor increases chloride conductance, which results in pre-synaptic inhibition in the spinal cord.[29,30] Diazepam is the most commonly used benzodiazepine in the treatment of spasticity.

Early trials have demonstrated efficacy in treating spasticity in patients with spinal cord injury, hemiplegia, and MS.[31–34] From and colleagues[35] studied 17 patients with MS in a double-blind, cross-over trial with baclofen and diazepam. Each patient received 4 weeks of therapy with each drug. No differences were seen in efficacy of reducing spasticity, clonus, or flexor spasms or in improvement in gait or bladder function. The side effect profile of the two drugs differed slightly, with more patients reporting sedation while on diazepam, but the severity of side effects was similar in both groups. When patients, still masked to treatment assignment, were asked which agent they preferred, baclofen was significantly favored.

Other studies[36,37] have confirmed the similar anti-spasticity effects of baclofen and diazepam in reducing muscle tone and the frequency of spasms. However, in these trials, baclofen was not necessarily favored by patients over diazepam. In clinical practice, diazepam is frequently used as an adjunct to baclofen in treating spasticity in MS patients[38] and less commonly used as a single agent.

Diazepam is well absorbed orally and reaches a peak level in approximately 1 hour. It is 98% protein bound and is metabolized by the liver to the active compounds nordazepam and oxazepam. The total half-life ranges between 20 and 80 hours. Doses are initiated at 2 mg daily increasing as needed to a desired effect. Side effects include sedation and cognitive impairment, and there is a potential for dependence. A withdrawal syndrome is associated with the benzodiazepines, and abrupt cessation of diazepam has been associated with seizures.

Tizanidine

Tizanidine is an imidazole derivative. It is a centrally acting α_2-adrenergic agonist that inhibits the release of excitatory amino acids in spinal interneurons and may facilitate the action of glycine. Tizanidine has demonstrated potent muscle-relaxing properties in animal models of spasticity.[39] In the spinal-transected cat, tizanidine was found to suppress the polysynaptic reflex.[40,41] Furthermore, tizanidine has been shown to enhance vibratory inhibition of the H reflex in humans and to reduce abnormal co-contraction, which may partly contribute to its anti-spasticity effects.[42] Early studies of tizanidine in MS have shown efficacy, and when tizanidine has been compared to baclofen in several

trials, similar efficacy and tolerability have been demonstrated.[44–48] In 1994, results of two double-blind placebo controlled trials were published.[49,50]

The United States Tizanidine Study Group conducted a 15-week, multicenter trial[49] of tizanidine in 159 patients (76 taking placebo, 83 taking tizanidine). Primary outcome measures for this study were Ashworth scores and type and frequency of muscle spasms based on historical account using patient diaries. While tizanidine significantly reduced spasms and clonus reported by patients, no significant differences were seen in the Ashworth scores of tizanidine versus the Ashworth scores of the placebo recipients. Sub-analysis of this study showed that stratifying for the timing of the examination (examinations were performed between 1 and 6 hours after drug administration) uncovered a trend for improvement in the group examined within 3 hours of drug administration. This is relevant when it is remembered that peak levels of the drug occur 1 hour after administration and the half-life of tizanidine is 2.5 hours.

The United Kingdom Tizanidine Study Group performed a 9-week, double-blind, placebo-controlled trial[50] in 187 MS patients (94 taking tizanidine, 93 taking placebo) with expanded disability status scale (EDSS) scores ranging from 1.5 to 9.5. The primary outcome measure in this study was score on the Ashworth scale. Using intention-to-treat analysis, the tizanidine recipients experienced a 21% reduction in mean Ashworth scale scores and placebo recipients experienced a 9% decrease. This difference was statistically significant. In addition, no significant difference in muscle strength was noted between the two groups. Despite improvement in spasticity without compromising muscle strength, there was no significant difference between tizanidine and placebo in functional measures, such as timed ambulation, upper extremity function, or activities necessary in ADL.

Tizanidine undergoes first-pass hepatic metabolism and is subsequently eliminated by the kidney. Its half-life is approximately 2.5 hours and its peak effect is seen 1–2 hours after dosage. Liver function tests should be checked at baseline, in months 1, 3, and 6 of treatment, and periodically after that. Doses are initiated at 2–4 mg daily, increasing every 3 days by 2–4 mg. Total dose should not exceed 36 mg/day in three divided doses. There is little experience with single doses greater than 8 mg. Side effects include dry mouth (45% of patients), drowsiness (54%) and dizziness (19%), and these were seen primarily with doses exceeding 24 mg per day. Visual hallucinations (3%) and elevated liver function tests (5%) were reversible with dose reduction.[50] Tizanidine has not been found to have consistent effects on blood pressure, but because of its central α_2-adrenergic activity and the risk of potential hypotension, concomitant use of anti-hypertensives, and especially clonidine, should be avoided. When tizanidine was compared to baclofen, night-time insomnia was reported more frequently with tizanidine; and weakness was also reported, but less frequently than with baclofen.[43] There have been no controlled trials investigating the use of tizanidine in combination with baclofen.

Clonidine

Clonidine is a centrally acting α_2-adrenergic agonist that is frequently used to treat hypertension as well as opiate withdrawal. The central α_2-adrenergic activation is thought to decrease sympathetic outflow. Clonidine has been shown to decrease the vibratory inhibition index in spinal cord patients[51] and to reduce muscle tone

in brain-injured patients (e.g. those with stroke, trauma, hematoma, or cerebral palsy),[52] and has shown modest benefit as an add-on agent to baclofen.[53] Clonidine is rarely used as a single agent in the treatment of spasticity. It is available in tablets of 0.1 mg, but the patch formulation (0.1 mg and 0.2 mg) is designed to deliver the specified daily dose and must be changed every 7 days. Side effects include bradycardia, hypotension, dry mouth, drowsiness, constipation, dizziness, and depression.

Dantrolene sodium

Dantrolene sodium is a hydantoin derivative. It acts directly on muscle contractile elements to decrease the release of calcium from skeletal muscle sarcoplasmic reticulum. This interferes with the excitation–contraction coupling that is necessary to produce muscle contraction.[54–56] The effect is most pronounced on extrafusal fibers, but there is a minor effect on intrafusal fibers as well. Whether this effect alters spindle sensitivity is unclear.[57] Dantrolene sodium has a greater effect on fast-twitch fibers (those that produce rapid contraction and high tension but that fatigue relatively easily) than on slow-twitch fibers (those that contract tonically and produce less tension but are more resistant to fatigue).[58] Studies of dantrolene sodium in MS have been limited but show modest efficacy as an anti-spasticity agent.[59,60] When dantrolene sodium was compared to diazepam in a double-blind, cross-over trial in 42 MS patients, both drugs were found to decrease spasticity, clonus and hyperreflexia, as well as diminish muscle stiffness and cramping.[61]

The half-life of oral dantrolene sodium is approximately 15 hours, with peak concentrations occurring 3–6 hours after ingestion. It is metabolized largely by the liver. Treatment with dantrolene sodium is initiated at 25 mg/day and the dose should be increased slowly in increments of 25 mg/day every 5–7 days, with a recommended maximum of 400 mg/day in divided doses. Because its site of action is peripheral, the most common side effect of dantrolene sodium is weakness (the mechanism by which it achieves its anti-spasticity effects). For this reason, dantrolene sodium may be most appropriate for those patients who are non-ambulatory and who have severe spasticity. Other side effects include drowsiness, diarrhea, and malaise. Hepatotoxicity, which can be irreversible, is the major concern with dantrolene sodium, and those patients who are being considered for therapy should have liver function tests checked before therapy is started and then regularly every 3 months.

Gabapentin

Gabapentin was first introduced in 1994 as a new treatment option for patients with partial seizures.[62] It is structurally similar to GABA and exerts GABA-ergic activity by binding receptors in the neocortex and hippocampus. However, it does not bind conventional GABA-a, GABA-b, glycine, glutamate, benzodiazepine, or *N*-methyl aspartate receptors.[63,64] It is easily absorbed and reaches peak plasma concentrations in 2–3 hours. It is not protein-bound, does not undergo metabolism, and is excreted unchanged in the urine. It is well tolerated in doses up to 3600 mg per day.[65] Recent studies and reports have suggested that it might be effective as another tool in treating spasticity.[65,66] Further studies are necessary to confirm efficacy in MS patients.

Botulinum toxin

Botulinum toxin is a product of *Clostridium botulinum*. Botulism results when *C. botulinum* or its spores are ingested. Botulinum toxin blocks pre-synaptic release of acetylcholine from nerve terminals. Seven immunologically distinct toxins (types A–G) have been purified. Local intramuscular injection of botulinum toxin A has been approved in the USA for the treatment of strabismus and blepharospasm associated with dystonia. When injected, the agent spreads through muscle and fascia approximately 30 mm from the site of the injection, binding pre-synaptic cholinergic nerve terminals, resulting in a chemical denervation.

Botulinum toxin injection has been studied as a treatment for severe spasticity resulting from stroke, traumatic brain injury, and other causes.[67–70] It has been found to be effective in reducing muscle tone and spasms. Snow and colleagues[71] studied botulinum toxin A in nine patients with advanced MS (wheelchair-bound or bed-bound) in a randomized, cross-over, double-blind study. Muscle tone, frequency of spasms, and hygiene and self-care scores were used to assess efficacy. Botulinum toxin injection produced a significant reduction in spasticity and improvement in ease of nursing care, with no adverse effects. More recently Kerty and Stein[72] reported their experience in five patients with advanced MS who received botulinum toxin injections for adductor spasticity. Three patients showed no response, but two experienced a marked and sustained improvement.

Although botulinum toxin injection is 'off-label' for treatment of spasticity in MS, it may be an appropriate option for selected patients with severe spasms, and physicians should be trained in its use, with attention given to relevant topical anatomy and kinesiology. Onset of focal muscle fiber paralysis begins in 24–72 hours, with a maximal effect at 5–14 days. The paralysis is transient but lasts 12–16 weeks. Localizing specific muscles with electromyographic guidance may be necessary to produce optimal effects. Injection site reactions can occur and antibodies may develop to specific immunologic strains, which can limit efficacy. Because the delivery of toxin is not entirely contained, the paralysis of muscles may not be exact. Excessive weakness, though ultimately reversible, may result.

Intrathecal baclofen

When treatment with oral medication fails in a patient with persistent severe spasticity, intrathecal administration of baclofen should be considered. A pump with a reservoir is surgically implanted in the subcutaneous tissue of the abdominal wall. A catheter is threaded into the subarachnoid space, allowing delivery of baclofen directly into the cerebrospinal fluid. This allows as much as four times the level of drug to be delivered at only 1% of the oral dose without concomitant elevation of serum levels, thereby reducing unwanted side effects.[73] Penn and colleagues[73] conducted a double-blind, placebo-controlled, 3-day cross-over study in 20 patients (10 with MS and 10 with spinal cord injury). All patients had decreased muscle tone and frequency of spasms when they were treated with baclofen. All patients were subsequently enrolled in a long-term open trial of continuous infusion, with a mean follow-up period of 19 months. Using the Ashworth scale all patients exhibited normal tone, and spasm frequency was diminished to the point that there was no interference with ADL. Seven out of eight patients also experienced improvement in bladder function. Other studies have found equally dramatic results.[74–76] Safe and effective long-term follow-up has been reported in patients up to 84 months.[77]

Pump implantation is considered only after a patient undergoes a trial of intrathecal baclofen to establish responsiveness. Starting doses are 25 μg/day up to an average of 400–500 μg/day, although doses as high as 1500 μg/day have been reported.[78] The half-life of intrathecal baclofen is approximately 5 hours. Many patients require increased dosing in the first 6 months and tolerance has been reported.[74,79] Most side effects tend to occur during the titration phase; they include drowsiness, headache, nausea, weakness, and hypotension. Reversible coma has been reported in baclofen overdosing.[80] Other complications may be due to mechanical problems (dislodgement, disconnection, kinking, or blockage), pump failure, or infection.

SUMMARY

Although spasticity remains a very troubling symptom for many patients with MS, most patients experience symptomatic improvement with physiotherapy in combination with one or more anti-spasticity agents. Patients who are refractory to these treatment options may respond to intrathecal baclofen. An understanding of the mechanisms of these therapies should aid in developing individualized regimens.

REFERENCES

1 **Lance JW.** Symposium synopsis. In: Feldman RG, Young RR, Koella WP, eds. *Spasticity: Disordered Motor Control.* Chicago: Year Book, 1980, 485–494.
2 **Young RR.** Spasticity: a review. *Neurology* 1994; **44(suppl 9)**: S12–S20.
3 **Thompson AJ.** Multiple sclerosis: symptomatic treatment. *J Neurol* 1996; 243:559–565.
4 **Ashworth B.** Preliminary trial of carisprodol in multiple sclerosis. *Practitioner* 1964; **192**:540–542.
5 **Lee KC, Carson L, Kinnin E, Patterson.** The Ashworth

Scale: a reliable and reproducible method of measuring spasticity. *J Neurol Rehabil* 1989; **3**: 205–209.

6 Bohannon RX, Smith MB. Interrater reliability of a modified Ashworth scale of muscle spasticity. *Phys Ther* 1987; **67**:206–207.

7 Penn RD. Intrathecal infusion of baclofen for spasticity: the RUSH and the US multicenter studies. In: Sindou M, Abbot R, Keravel Y, eds. *Neurosurgery for Spasticity*. Vienna: Springer, 1991, 103–109.

8 Wartenburg R. Pendulousness of the legs as a diagnostic test. *Neurology* 1951; **1**:18–24.

9 Bajd T, Vodovnik L. Pendulum testing of spasticity. *J Biomed Eng* 1984; **6**:9–16.

10 Boczko M, Mumenthaler M. Modified pendulousness test to assess tonus of thigh muscles in spasticity. *Neurol* 1954; **8**:846–851.

11 Knutsson E, Martensson A. Dynamic motor capacity in spastic paresis and its relation to prime move dysfunction, spastic reflexes and antagonistic co-activation. *Scand J Rehabil Med* 1980; **12**:83–106.

12 Delwaide PJ. Human monosynaptic reflexes and presynaptic inhibition: an interpretation of spastic hyperreflexia. In: Desmedt JE, ed. *New Developments in Electromyography and Clinical Neurophysiology.* Basel, Switzerland: Karger, 1973, 486–507.

13 Lance JW, Burke D, Andrews CJ. The reflex effects of muscle vibration. In: Desmedt JE, ed. *New Developments in Electromyography and Clinical Neurophysiology.* Basel, Switzerland: Karger, 1973, 444–462.

14 Delwaide PJ. Human monosynaptic reflexes and presynaptic inhibition: an interpretation of spastic hyperreflexia. In: Desmedt JE, ed. *New Developments in Electromyography and Clinical Neurophysiology.* Basel, Switzerland: Karger: 1973, 508–522.

15 Williams RG. Sensitivity changes shown by spindle receptors in chronically immobilized skeletal muscle. *J Physiol* 1980; **306**:26P–27P.

16 Gious M, Petit J. Effects of immobilizing the cat peroneus longus muscle on the activity of its own spindles. *J Appl Physiol* 1993; **75**:2629–2635.

17 Bezner J. *Adult Exercise Instruction Sheets, Home Exercises for Rehabilitation*. Tuscon, Arizona: Therapy Skill Builders, 1989.

18 Bormann J. Electrophysiology of Gaba-a and Gaba-b receptor subtypes. *Trends Neurol Sci* 1988; **11**:112–116.

19 Davidoff RA. Antispasticity drugs: mechanism of action. *Ann Neurol* 1985; **17**:107–117.

20 Van Hemet JCJ. A double-blind comparison of baclofen and placebo in patients with spasticity of cerebral origin. In: Feldman RG, Young RR, Koella, eds. *Spasticity: Disordered Motor Control*. Chicago: Year Book, 1980.

21 Jerusalem F. A double-blind study on the antispastic action of beta-(4-chlorophenyl)-gamma-amino butyric acid in multiple sclerosis. *Nervenarzt* 1968; **39**:515.

22 Basmajan JV. Lioresal (baclofen) treatment of spasticity in multiple sclerosis. *Am J Phys Med* 1975; **54**:175–177.

23 Sawa GM, Paty DW. The use of baclofen in treatment of spasticity in multiple sclerosis. *Can J Neurol Sci* 1979; **6**:351–354.

24 Smith CR, LaRocca NG, Giesser BS, Scheinberg L. High dose oral baclofen: experience in patients with multiple sclerosis. *Neurology* 1991; **41**:1829–1831.

25 Pinto ODS, Polikar M, Debono G. Results of international clinical trials with Lioresal. *Postgrad Med J* 1972; **48** (suppl 5): 18–23.

26 Feldman RG, Kelly-Hayes M, Conomy JP, Foley JM. Baclofen for spasticity in multiple sclerosis: double blind crossover and three year study. *Neurology* 1978; **28**:1094–1098.

27 Brar SP, Smith MB, Nelson LM et al. Evaluation of treatment protocols on minimal to moderate spasticity in multiple sclerosis. *Arch Phys Med Rehabil* 1991; **72**:186–189.

28 Costa E, Guidotti A. Molecular mechanisms in the receptor action of the benzodiazepines. *Annu Rev Toxicol* 1979; **19**:531–545.

29 Schwarz M, Turski L, Janiszewski W, Sontag KH. Is the muscle relaxant effect of diazepam in spastic mutant rats mediated through GABA-independent benzodiazepine receptors? *Neurosci Lett* 1983; **36**:175–180.

30 Pedersen E. Clinical assessment and pharmacologic therapy of spasticity. *Arch Phys Med Rehabil* 1974; **55**:344–354.

31 Kendall PH. The use of diazepam in hemiplegia. *Ann Phys Med* 1964; **7**:225–228.

32 Neill RW. Diazepam in the relief of muscle spasm resulting from spinal-cord lesions. *Ann Phys Med* 1964; **7**(suppl):33–38.

33 Nathan PW. The action of diazepam in neurological disorders with excessive motor activity. *J Neurol Sci* 1970; **10**:33–50.

34 Corbett M, Frankel HL, Michaelis L. A double blind cross-over trial of Valium in the treatment of spasticity. *Paraplegia* 1972; **10**:19–22.

35 From A, Heltberg A. A double-blind trial with

baclofen and diazepam in spasticity due to multiple sclerosis. *Acta Neurol Scand* 1975; **51**:158–166.

36 **Roussan M, Terrence C, Fromm G.** Baclofen versus diazepam for the treatment of spasticity and long term follow-up of baclofen therapy. *Pharmatherapeutica* 1987; **4**:278–284.

37 **Cartlidge NEF, Hudgson P, Weightman D.** A comparison of baclofen and diazepam in the treatment of spasticity. *J Neurol Sci* 1974; **23**:17–24.

38 **Mitchell G.** Update on multiple sclerosis therapy. *Med Clin North Am* 1993; **77**:231–249.

39 **Coward DM.** Selective muscle relaxant properties of tizanidine and an examination of its mode of action. *Triangle* 1981; **20**:151–158.

40 **Davies J.** Selective depression of synaptic transmission of spinal neurones in the cat by a new centrally acting muscle relaxant, 5-chloro-4-(2-imidazolin-2-yl-amino)-2,1,3-benzothiadazole (DS 103 282). *Br J Pharmacol* 1982; **76**:473–481.

41 **Newman PM, Nogues M, Newman PK et al.** Tizanidine in the treatment of spasticity. *Eur J Clin Pharmacol* 1982; **23**:31–35.

42 **Delwaide PJ.** Electrophysiological testing of spastic patients: its potential usefulness and limitations. In: Delwaide PJ, Young RR, eds. *Clinical Neurophysiology in Spasticity.* Amsterdam: Elsevier, 1985, 185–203.

43 **Bass B, Weinshenker B, Rice GPA et al.** Tizanidine versus baclofen in the treatment of spasticity in patients with multiple sclerosis. *Can J Sci* 1988; **15**:15–19.

44 **Stein R, Nordal HJ, Oftendal SI, Slebetto M.** The treatment of spasticity in multiple sclerosis: a double-blind clinical trial of a new anti-spasticity drug tizanidine compared with baclofen. *Acta Neurol Scand* 1987; **75**:190–194.

45 **Smolenski C, Muff S, Smolenski-Kauts S.** A double-blind comparative trial of a new muscle-relaxant, tizanidine (DS102-282) and baclofen in the treatment of chronic spasticity in multiple sclerosis. *Curr Med Res Opin* 1981; **7**:374–383.

46 **Hoorgstraten MC, van der Ploeg RJO, Van der Burg W et al.** Tizanidine versus baclofen in the treatment of multiple sclerosis patients. *Acta Neurol Scand* 1988; **77**:224–230.

47 **Eyssette M, Rohmer F, Serratrice G et al.** Multi-centre, double-blind trial of a novel antispastic agent, tizanidine, in spasticity associated with multiple sclerosis. *Curr Med Res Opin* 1988; **10**:699–708.

48 **Lapierre Y, Bouchard S, Tansey C et al.** Treatment of spasticity with tizanidine in multiple sclerosis. *Can J Neurol Sci* 1987; **14**:513–517.

49 **Smith C, Birnbaum G, Carter JL et al.** Tizanidine treatment of spasticity caused by multiple sclerosis: results of a double-blind, placebo controlled trial. US Tizanidine Study Group. *Neurology* 1994; **44 (suppl 9)**:34–44.

50 **The United Kingdom Tizanidine Study Group.** A double-blind placebo-controlled trial of tizanidine in the treatment of spasticity caused by multiple sclerosis. *Neurology* 1994; **44 (suppl 9)**: 70–79.

51 **Nance PW, Shears AH, Nance DM.** Reflex changes induced by clonidine in spinal cord injured patients. *Paraplegia*, 1989; **4**:296–301.

52 **Dall JT, Harmon RL, Quinn CM.** Use of clonidine for treatment of spasticity arising from various forms of brain injury: a case series. *Brain Inj* 1996; **10**:453–458.

53 **Donovan WH, Carter RE, Rossi CD, Wilkerson MA.** Clonidine effect on spasticity: a clinical trial. *Arch Phys Med Rehabil* 1988; **69**:193–194.

54 **Herman R, Mayer N, Mecomber SA.** Clinical pharmaco-physiology of dantrolene sodium. *Am J Phys Med* 1972; **51**(suppl 6):296–311.

55 **Ellis KO, Carpenter JF.** Mechanisms of control of skeletal muscle contraction by dantrolene sodium. *Arch Phys Med Rehabil* 1974; **55**:362–369.

56 **Pinder RM, Brodgen RN, Speight TM, Avery GS.** Dantrolene sodium: a review of its pharmacological properties and therapeutic efficacy in spasticity. *Drugs* 1977; **13**:3–23.

57 **Whyte J, Robinson KM.** Pharmacologic management. In: Glenn M, Whyte J, eds. *The Practical Management of Spasticity in Children and Adults.* Philadelphia: Lea and Febinger, 1990.

58 **Monster AW, Tamai Y, McHenry J.** Dantrolene sodium in spasticity. *Acta Neurol Scand* 1979; **59**:309–316.

59 **Gelenberg AJ, Poskanzer DC.** The effect of dantrolene sodium on spasticity in multiple sclerosis. *Neurology* 1973; **23**:1313–1315.

60 **Tolosa ES, Soll RW, Loewenson R.** Treatment of spasticity in multiple sclerosis with dantrolene. *JAMA* 1975; **233**: 1046.

61 **Schmidt RT, Lee RH, Spehlman R.** Comparison of dantrolene sodium and diazepam in the treatment of spasticity. *J Neurol Neurosurg Psychiatry* 1976; **39**:350–356.

62 **The long-term safety and efficacy of gabapentin (Neurontin) as add-on therapy in drug-resistant partial epilepsy. The US Gabapentin Study Group.** *Epilepsy Res* 1994; **18**:67–73.

63 **Fromm GH.** Gabapentin. *Epilepsia* 1995; **36 (suppl 5)**:S77–S80.

64 **McLean MJ.** Gabapentin. *Epilepsia* 1995; **36 (suppl 2)**:S73–S86.

65 **Priebe MM, Sherwood AM, Graves DE et al.** Effectiveness of gabapentin in controlling spasticity: a quantitative study. *Spinal Cord* 1997; **35**:171–175.

66 **Dunevsky A, Perel A.** Gabapentin for relief of spasticity associated with multiple sclerosis. *Am J Phys Med Rehabil* 1998; **77**:451–454.

67 **Yablon SA, Agana BT, Ivanhoe CB, Boake C.** Botulinum toxin in severe upper extremity spasticity among patients with traumatic brain injury: an open label trial. *Neurology* 1996; **47**:939–944.

68 **Simpson DM, Alexander DN, O'Brien CF et al.** Botulinum toxin type A in the treatment of upper extremity spasticity: a randomized, double-blind, placebo-controlled trial. *Neurology* 1996; **46**:1306–1310.

69 **Burbaud P, Wiart L, Dubos JL et al.** A randomized, double blind placebo controlled trial of botulinum toxin in the treatment of spastic foot in hemiparetic patients. *J Neurol Neurosurg Psychiatry* 1996; **61**:265–269.

70 **Das TK, Park DM.** Effect of treatment with botulinum toxin on spasticity. *Postgrad Med J* 1989; **65**:208–210.

71 **Snow BJ, Tsui JKC, Bhatt MH et al.** Treatment of spasticity with botulinum toxin: a double-blind study. *Ann Neurol* 1990; **28**:512–515.

72 **Kerty E, Stein R.** Treatment of spasticity with botulinum toxin. *Tidsskr Nor Laegeforen* 1997; **117**:2022–2024.

73 **Penn RD, Savoy SM, Corcos D et al.** Intrathecal baclofen for severe spinal spasticity. *N Engl J Med* 1989; **320**:1517–1521.

74 **Ochs G, Struppler A, Meyerson BA et al.** Intrathecal baclofen for long-term treatment of spasticity: a multi-centre study. *J Neurol Neurosurg Psychiatry* 1989; **52**:933–939.

75 **Albright AL, Barron WB, Fasick MP et al.** Continuous intrathecal baclofen infusion for spasticity of cerebral origin. *JAMA* 1993; **270**:2475–2477.

76 **Dralle D, Muller H, Zierski J, Klug N.** Intrathecal baclofen for spasticity. *Lancet* 1985; **2**:1003.

77 **Penn RD.** Intrathecal baclofen for spasticity of spinal origin: seven years experience. *J Neurosurg* 1992; **77**:236–240.

78 **Nance PW, Schryvers OI, Schmidt BJ et al.** Intrathecal baclofen therapy for adults with spinal spasticity: therapeutic efficacy and effect on hospital admission. *Can J Neurol Sci* 1995; **22**:122–129.

79 **Nanninga JB, Frost F, Penn R.** Effect of intrathecal baclofen on bladder and sphincter function. *J Urol* 1989; **142**:101–105.

80 **Siegfried J, Rea GL.** Intrathecal application of drugs for muscle hypertonus. *Scand J Rehabil Med* 1988; **17 (suppl)**:145–148.

36
Treatment of bladder and sexual dysfunction

Scott E Litwiller

Over 80% of patients with multiple sclerosis (MS) have symptoms of lower genitourinary tract dysfunction. Over 96% of patients who have had the disease for more than 10 years have had urologic problems at some time.[1–4] The effect of MS on the genitourinary tract ranges from bladder and urethral dysfunction to impotence. Consequently, genitourinary symptoms are often a major source of frustration and distress for patients. Urologic involvement most commonly presents as lower urinary tract (bladder and urethral) dysfunction (LUTD) or sexual dysfunction. Knowledge of pathophysiology, evaluation, and treatment of these conditions is essential for the MS specialist because LUTD and sexual dysfunction can have a significant impact on the patient's quality of life and because the MS specialist is often called upon to manage these severe, debilitating symptoms.

NEUROLOGIC EFFECTS OF MS ON THE URINARY TRACT

Although MS plaques can be seen anywhere in the central nervous system (CNS), there is a documented prevalence of the disease in the cervical spinal cord, predominantly the lateral corticospinal (pyramidal) and reticulospinal tracts.[5–9] Because innervation of the detrusor and external urethral sphincter is mediated by these tracts, most MS patients experience LUTD.[10–20]

Suprasacral spinal cord effects

Autopsy studies by Oppenheimer[6] showed that lesions of the suprasacral spinal cord are extremely common in MS patients. Cervical cord plaques are the commonest, occurring in up to 80% of patients.[20,21] Accordingly, patients with MS may lack supraspinal suppression of autonomous bladder contractions, resulting in detrusor hyperactivity (detrusor hyper-reflexia) and urgency incontinence in the majority (> 60%). Spinal lesions may also disrupt reticulospinal pathways from the pons that are involved in the synergic integration of urethral sphincteric and detrusor activity.[10,11,22,23] This disruption may result in a continuum of three main abnormalities: detrusor sphincter dyssynergia (DSD), incomplete sphincteric relaxation (ISR), or sphincteric paralysis.[11,12,14,20,21]

Sacral cord effects

Lower motor neuron symptoms associated with presumed demyelination of the sacral cord and conus medullaris have been reported in up to 63% of patients.[1–3] In contrast, autopsy studies by Philip and colleagues[16] showed only an 18% incidence of sacral plaques. Mayo and Chetner[14] found 63% of patients with detrusor hypocontractility, but only 5% displayed bona fide areflexia.[14] This has led some authors to question the contribution of sacral plaques to overall symptoms of LUTD.[13–15] In animal studies, Kruse and colleagues[18,19] have demonstrated that intact spinal afferents and efferents are crucial to the facilitation of sustained detrusor contractions.[18,19] Plaques in these afferent or efferent pathways may inhibit facilitated contractions, thereby causing impaired emptying and urinary retention. As a result, some patients may suffer from paradoxical detrusor hyperactivity in the absence of a co-ordinated detrusor contraction that fails to empty the bladder. Although abnormal sacral nerve function (as demonstrated by prolonged reflex latencies) has been documented by several authors and may help secure the diagnosis of MS, the sole contribution of these reflex pathways to bladder dysfunction remains uncertain.[1,3,18–21]

Intracranial plaques

Intracranial plaques are common in MS and have been reported in between 60 and 90% of patients.[21–24] Although the most commonly involved area is the periventricular white matter, plaques have been reported in nearly all areas of the intracranial white matter. Accordingly, the presence of disease in the supraspinal CNS may account for urologic dysfunction (detrusor hyperreflexia). In 90 MS patients studied by Kim and colleagues,[25] there was no correlation between MRI findings (atrophy, number of lesions, nature or size of a lesion) and any specific urodynamic parameters. Pozzilli and colleagues,[26,27] however, demonstrated a statistically significant correlation ($p < 0.001$) between urinary symptoms and midbrain lesions seen on T2-weighted imaging. Although lesions in the midbrain are highly correlated with urologic disease, the urologic significance of clinically isolated pontine lesions in the absence pyramidal findings remains in question.[28,29]

CLINICAL PRESENTATIONS

Lower urinary tract dysfunction

Lower urinary tract symptoms are varied and range from frequency and urgency (in 31–85% of patients) and incontinence (in 37–72% of patients) to obstructive symptoms with urinary retention (in 2–52% of patients).[1–9] Although the incidence of lower urinary tract symptoms ranges from 52 to 97%, the presence or absence of symptoms is an unreliable indicator of the extent of vesical dysfunction.[4,12,30,31] Betts and colleagues[13] found that only 47% of patients with elevated post-void residual volumes had the sensation of incomplete emptying. Conversely, they found that 83% of patients who complained of incomplete emptying had post-void residual volumes greater than 100 ml. Koldewijn and colleagues[4] noted urodynamic evidence of urinary tract dysfunction in 100% of patients with urologic symptoms and 52% of patients without symptoms.

Although several investigators' studies have

shown that duration of disease, increased age at diagnosis, and the degree of motor or sensory dysfunction correlate well with the degree of urologic impairment, LUTD is best correlated with pyramidal tract involvement and overall disability as measured by the Expanded Disability Status Scale (EDSS).[4,28,31–36] In contrast, Awad and colleagues[15] found that pyramidal tract dysfunction, independent of the level of disability (as measured by the EDSS), was most closely related to lower urinary tract dysfunction. As such, a history of ataxia, gait disturbances, unexplained lower extremity weakness, numbness, or paresthesias may suggest occult urologic dysfunction. Thus, the degree of lower extremity motor dysfunction may be the best predictor of urologic and bladder dysfunction. This correlation is so significant that LUTD is rarely seen in the absence of pyramidal dysfunction.[4,35] In assessing different types of MS, secondary progressive MS is the only course of disease associated with an increased risk of progressively deteriorating bladder function (p < 0.05).[4]

Urinary symptoms may be age-related and follow a bimodal distribution. Patients under the age of 40 years are most bothered by bladder storage and voiding symptoms, although these findings may be related to the inherently higher expectations of younger patients compared to their older counterparts. Patients over the age of 50 years are also greatly bothered with bladder symptoms, which may be related to their longer duration of disease or the cumulative effect of other causes of bladder dysfunction, such as benign prostatic hyperplasia in males or genuine stress incontinence in females.[31] Although increasing duration of disease is linked to increased frequency of overall symptoms, no single symptom is more prevalent in patients with longstanding disease. No significant relationship has been found between the incidence of overall symptoms and sex. However, men with MS report a higher incidence of obstructive symptoms than women do, which may be related to age-related changes in the prostate or the severity of DSD in males.[4] As a result of urinary tract dysfunction and stasis of urine, patients may develop bladder calculi or renal calculi or suffer from frequent urinary tract infections, often involving atypical organisms.[37]

Evaluation of voiding dysfunction

History

Clearly, a history of lower extremity sensory or motor loss (pyramidal tract dysfunction) can be a sign of unrecognized urological pathology.[15] A history of visual disturbance (e.g. diplopia or oscillopsia) or dizziness may point to pontine pathology (e.g. internuclear ophthalmoplegia). Since the central co-ordinating center for bladder and sphincter integration lies in the pontine tegmentum, a history suggestive of pontine pathology may be pertinent to the diagnosis of occult bladder and sphincteric dysfunction. Patients should be asked about the frequency of daytime urination, nocturia, degree of bladder emptying, and the ease with which micturition is achieved. Patients should also be questioned about urgency and urge or stress incontinence. The disparity in symptoms and underlying pathology gives support for the objective measurement of post-voiding residual volumes (see Ancillary Testing p. 493). Patients who strain or push in order to urinate may also suffer from lower urinary tract dysfunction and incomplete emptying, thereby placing themselves at risk of other urologic complications such as bladder calculi, infection, bladder diverticuli, and lower urinary tract

491

decompensation. The need for protective devices should be determined and an incontinence-specific quality-of-life instrument may be of benefit to assess the overall daily impact of the urinary symptoms.[38,39] Assessment of the fluid intake is also important since many patients attempt to remedy their bladder symptoms by decreasing their fluid intake, which may cause hyperconcentration of urine and thereby cause more irritative symptoms. To help in this assessment, a fluid intake and voiding diary are beneficial.

A current and past medication profile should be obtained, since many medications that are used to treat MS have neuroleptic or anticholinergic side effects (e.g. anti-depressant and anti-psychotic agents). These medications may cause inappropriate bladder relaxation and exacerbate urinary retention. α-Adrenergic agonists used as decongestants in many preparations for colds may impair bladder emptying by stimulating α-receptors in the bladder neck or prostate. In women, α-blockers used as anti-hypertensives may exacerbate stress incontinence. Because bladder cancer has been linked to the use of cyclophosphamide, a patient's medication history should be thorough and include dates and courses of treatments and whether Mesna was given concomitantly. The wide use of corticosteroids and immunosupressive agents in the MS population may also contribute to urinary tract infections caused by especially virulent organisms.[37]

Past medical and surgical history is especially important in the MS patient, since competing pathologies may have an impact on lower urinary tract dysfunction. A history of previous urethral instrumentation (including catheterization) or urethral injury may suggest the presence of urethral stricture as a cause of voiding dysfunction.

A history of previous prostate or urethral surgery may alert to the possibility of post-operative urethral stricture. In males who are aged over 40 years, benign prostatic hyperplasia may act as a confounding variable and mimic neurologic bladder dysfunction. In both sexes, diabetic cystopathy may adversely affect bladder emptying and predispose the patient to urinary tract infections and complicate the diagnosis or treatment.

Women with MS should similarly be questioned about their surgical and medical history. A history of previous incontinence surgery or for vaginal prolapse may raise a suspicion of concomitant anatomic factors affecting continence (e.g. urethral hypermobility, urethral stricture, or obstruction). Those with a history of incontinence surgery, hysterectomy, abdominal–perineal resection, or urethropelvic surgery are at increased risk of having a combined anatomic and neurologic deficit. Obstetric history is important, including any history of birth-related trauma or complications. Women may note a cyclical nature to their MS symptoms with worsening symptoms during the week before the week of their menstrual period. Many women with MS note the regulating effect of oral contraceptive preparations on their MS symptoms. Gastrointestinal disturbances may be reported and may have a significant effect on voiding dysfunction. A history of chronic constipation may contribute significantly to incontinence not only from mechanical compression but also from sacral nerve feedback.

The general physical examination is of significant help in the management of urologic dysfunction. The abdominal examination may reveal surgical scars, denoting previous urologic or gynecologic surgery. Fecal impaction may be detected on abdominal examination as well as on digital rectal examination. Rectal tone should be assessed, as should the bulbocavernosus reflex as a measure of sacral reflex integrity. In men, rectal examination also aids in assessing prostate size and its possible contribution to voiding dysfunction. A testicular examination is also important to aid in cancer screening. In women, the vaginal examination aids in excluding co-existing vaginal pathology (e.g. pelvic prolapse, urethral hypermobility, cystocele, rectocele, urethral diverticulum, or atrophic vaginitis). Co-existing vaginal pathology may significantly contribute to both incontinence and voiding dysfunction. Examination of the genitalia is crucial, since patients who are managed with an indwelling catheter may develop traumatic hypospadias (in males) or urethral erosion (in females).

Physical examination

A directed neurological examination to assess the first lumbar to the fourth sacral levels may help to reveal the extent of urologic dysfunction. In addition to the high correlation between lower extremity dysfunction and bladder dysfunction, cerebellar signs (such as ataxia and dysdiadochokinesis) are correlated with detrusor areflexia.[15] Extensor plantar responses (the Babinski reflex) may be seen in 70–95% of patients with bladder dysfunction and in 70% of those with detrusor sphincter dys-synergia; however, poor specificity limits the use of this sign as a diagnostic tool. Similarly, many patients display hyperactive deep tendon reflexes, but this finding is also a poor specific indicator of detrusor hyper-reflexia or bladder dysfunction (sensitivity 76%, specificity 58%).[1]

Sensory abnormalities may also be seen in association with bladder dysfunction, especially abnormalities of lower extremity vibratory sensation.[36] An assessment of upper extremity

strength and dexterity is important, since this may play an integral role in determining the options for bladder management in the impaired patient.

The association between cranial nerve findings and urinary tract abnormalities is not well established. Betts and colleagues[13] evaluated 16 patients and found that the presence of internuclear ophthalmoplegia correlated with bladder dysfunction. However, most of these patients demonstrated concomitant pyramidal tract dysfunction, raising a question as to the significance of isolated Internuclear ophthalmoplegia. In similar work at the author's institution, the incidence of vesicourethral dysfunction (DSD) in patients with internuclear ophthalmoplegia approaches 97%.

Ancillary testing

URINALYSIS

Urinalysis is an integral and important part of the urologic evaluation. In most instances, a multicomponent dip-stick suffices for screening. The method of urine collection is of prime importance since many patients are treated inappropriately because of a falsely contaminated specimen. Urine should be collected as a mid-stream, clean-catch specimen; however, because of spasticity or obesity, most patients are unable to provide a truly clean and uncontaminated specimen. In these instances, or in patients with repeated infections, sterile catheterization provides the most reliable way of ensuring proper specimen collection.

Leukocyte esterase and nitrite are often good screening measures for urinary tract infection. The specificity of these tests is fairly high and presence of infection in their absence is rare. Urine specific gravity is a useful test for determining the state of hydration, since many patients with MS restrict their fluids in an attempt to control incontinence and frequency. The presence of blood in the urine, although often seen with infection, is a worrying sign and may raise the suspicion of a bladder stone or tumor, especially in patients who have had multiple courses of cyclophosphamide.

UPPER URINARY TRACT IMAGING

Baseline radiographic assessment of the MS patient remains an integral part of the initial urologic evaluation. In a review of 14 series comprising 2076 patients,[4] Koldewijn and colleagues found the incidence of hydronephrosis or renal complication to be 0.34%; all seven affected patients had DSD. Although there are isolated reports of severe morbidity and mortality from upper tract disease in MS,[40,41] progression to upper tract deterioration is the exception rather than the rule.[4,17,31] Studies advocating initial surgical intervention for mild hydronephrosis are largely historical and often antedate the widespread acceptance of clean intermittent catheterization as a treatment alternative.[40,42] Upper tract deterioration may be linked to at least two risk factors: DSD in the male, and the presence of an indwelling catheter (1.7%).[3,12,22] In these high-risk patients, a baseline renal ultrasound is advisable since it may diagnose clinically silent calculi, identify parenchymal scarring, and provide comparison for longitudinal monitoring.

LOWER URINARY TRACT IMAGING

In the incontinent or otherwise symptomatic female, an initial lateral voiding cystourethrogram or videourodynamics (urodynamic evaluation performed with concomitant fluoroscopic bladder imaging) may aid in the assessment of the bladder neck support, urethral hypermobility and bladder diverticuli. Because patients with MS are frequently at an age where they may have competing symptomatologies, such as genuine stress incontinence and urge incontinence, this type of imaging may be beneficial in determining the relative contribution of anatomic factors (such as urethral hypermobility or cystocele) relative to voiding dysfunction or incontinence. Videourodynamics may also be of benefit in the more accurate determination of DSD (*Fig. 36.1*). In the patient with no stress incontinence or with good pelvic floor support on physical examination, lower tract radiologic imaging may not be necessary.

URODYNAMIC EVALUATION

The urodynamic evaluation of the patient with MS not only allows for proper identification of any underlying bladder and sphincteric abnormalities but also aids in the individualization of bladder management. During this study, the bladder is filled via a small (6–7 French) multilumen catheter. Measurements of bladder pressure are continuously made during both filling and voiding. Concomitant rectal manometry is performed to record and correct for the effect of intra-abdominal contents on bladder pressure. Electromyelographic monitoring of the external sphincter is also performed during the study to assess bladder and sphincteric co-ordination (*Fig. 36.2*).

Blaivas and colleagues[10] found that 73% of MS patients who had not had urodynamic evaluation were treated inappropriately. Indeed, 73% of patients with symptoms suggestive of obstruction were found to have detrusor areflexia. In equivocal cases, urodynamic evaluation may lend support to a suspected diagnosis of MS in 10–14% of patients.[1,13,31] Within the MS patient population, the incidence of abnormal urodynamic findings may be as high as 100% in some series.[3] In a meta-analysis of 22 series and

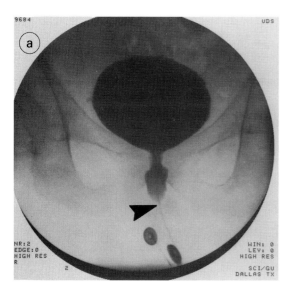

Fig. 36.1 *Detrusor Sphincter Dyssynergia (DSD) This cystourethrogram reveals DSD in a 40 year old male with relapsing remitting MS who presented with poor bladder emptying. Note the columnation of the radiographic contrast down to the external sphincter. (Bold arrow) The two round densities at the bottom of the screen are EMG leads. In the accompanying urodynamic tracing, sphincter activity increases dramatically and is accompanied by attempted voiding at a detrusor pressure of over 45 cm H_2O. Note the virtual absence of flow and near complete retention.*

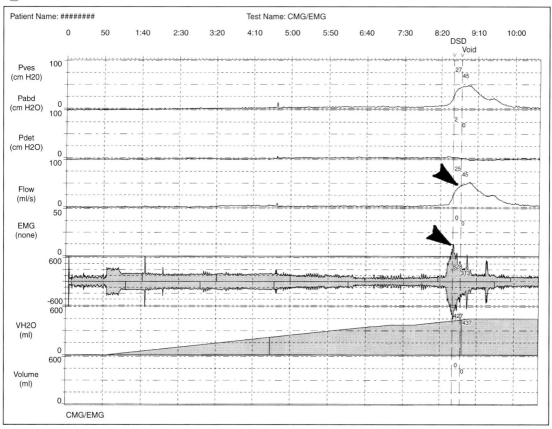

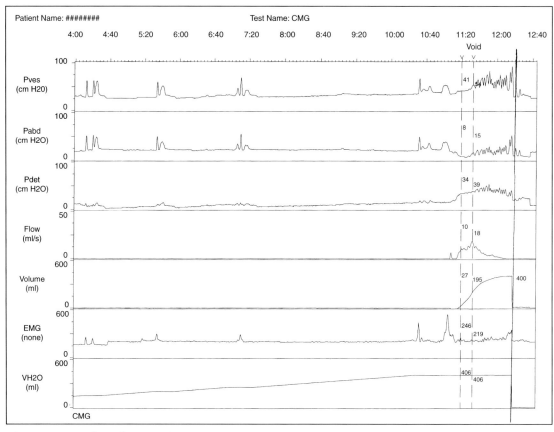

Fig. 36.2 *Normal Urodynamic Tracing*

Note how the bladder accommodates a large volume at a very low pressure.

P ves *represents total bladder pressure (vesical pressure, cm/H_2O) and is a measured value from the dual lumen urethral catheter.*

P abd *represents abdominal pressure and is measured value derived from a rectal catheter (cm/H_2O).*

Pdet *is a calculated pressure derived by subtracting (Pves − Pabd) and represents the true detrusor pressure in the absence of abdominal effects (cm/H_2O).*

Flow *represents the rate of urinary flow (cc/second).*

VH$_2$O *is the volume infused (ml).*

Volume *represents volume voided (ml).*

EMG *represents activity of the pelvic floor and external sphincter.*

1882 patients,[43] the incidence of normal urodynamic findings was 9% (*Table 36.1*). However, because most published series deal with symptomatic patients referred specifically for urologic evaluation, there has been a significant reporting bias towards patients with advanced disease and

Table 36.1 Published series of urodynamic findings in MS

Series	N=	Hyper-reflexia		DESD		Hyporeflexia		Normal	
		Number of Patients	%	Number of patients	%	Number of patients	%	Number of patients	%
Andersen, Bradley 1976[2]	52	33	63	16	31	21	40	2	4
Awad et al 1984[15]	57	38	66	30	52	12	21	7	12
Beck et al 1981[33]	46	40	87	–	–	6	13	–	–
Betts et al 1993[13]	70	63	91	–	–	0	0	7	10
Blaivas et al 1979[10]	41	23	56	12	30	16	40	2	4
Bradley et al 1973[44]	99	58	60	20	20.2	40	40	1	1
Bradley 1978[3]	302	127	62	–	–	103	34	10	24
Eardley et al 1991[45]	24	15	63	6	27	3	13	6	25
Goldstein et al 1982[1]	86	65	76	57	66	16	19	5	5.8
Gonor et al 1985[46]	64	40	78	8	12	13	20	1	2
Hinson, Boone 1996[17]	70	44	63	15	21	20	28	6	9
Koldewijn et al 1995[4]	212	72	34	27	12.7	32	8	76	36
Mayo, Chetner 1992[14]	89	69	78	5	6	5	6	11	12
McGuire, Savastano 1984[12]	46	33	72	21	46	13	28	0	0
Peterson, Pederson 1984[47]	88	73	83	36	41	14	16	1	1
Philip et al 1981[16]	52	51	99	16	37	0	0	1	1.9
Piazza, Diokno 1979[48]	31	23	74	9	47	2	6	3	9
Schoenberg et al 1979[49]	39	27	69	20	5	2	6	6	15
Sirls et al 1993[50]	113	79	70	15	27.8	17	15	7	6
Summers 1978[51]	50	26	52	6	12	6	12	9	18
Van Poppel, Baert 1987[37]	160	105	66	38	24	38	24	16	10
Weinstein et al 1988[52]	91	64	70	16	18	15	16	11	12
Total	1882	1194	62.10%	373/1464	25.40%	394	20.1%	188	10%

pyramidal dysfunction. To date there have been few prospective studies dealing with asymptomatic bladder dysfunction. In one prospective study,[22] 52% of patients (21 of 40) demonstrated silent urodynamic abnormalities. The incidence of positive urodynamic findings in patients with lower urinary tract complaints, however, was 98%.[22] Once a urodynamic diagnosis is made, therapy may be tailored to each patient's storage and emptying function, thereby eliminating a trial-and-error method of management.

Detrusor hyper-reflexia

Detrusor hyper-reflexia (DH), defined as bladder overactivity resulting from disturbance of nervous control mechanisms, is the most commonly encountered urodynamic abnormality seen in MS (*Fig. 36.3*; see *Table 36.1*). The incidence of DH varies directly with the level of the neurologic lesion:[23] patients with a higher predominance of cervical plaques have a higher incidence of DH. In 22 published series evaluating primarily symptomatic MS patients, 62% of patients (1194 of 1882) were found to have detrusor hyper-reflexia (DH) as their primary urodynamic diagnosis (see *Table 36.1*). This is not, however, surprising given the high incidence of cervical and intracranial plaque formation in MS.[10,19,20,31] DH is commonly manifest as urgency, frequency, and generalized irritative symptoms. Among patients with DH, 67% display synergic voiding and 43% display

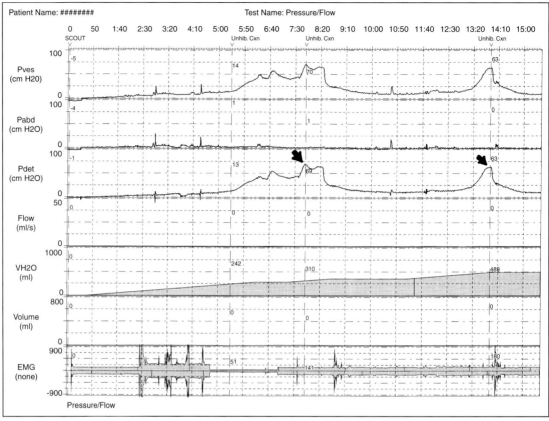

Fig. 36.3 *Detrusor Hyperreflexia*

Detrusor hyperreflexia in a 50 year old woman with MS and severe urinary urgency. Note the rise in bladder pressure and detrusor pressure in the absence of abdominal pressure. The sphincter is quiet during these contractions, denoting the absence of DSD. This patient was effectively treated with oral anticholinergic medications.

detrusor sphincter dyssynergia.[53] Patients in the latter group may paradoxically suffer from both storage and emptying failure, further complicating their management.

Detrusor hypocontractility

Although detrusor hypocontractility may be seen in up to 63% of patients with or without associ- ated hyper-reflexia, true areflexia is only seen in 20% of patients and may be associated with hesitancy and elevated residuals (see *Table 36.1*). Hypocontractility may be related to cerebellar plaque involvement, lack of cortical facilitary input, or sacral cord involvement.[3,13,16] Some evidence suggests that areflexia is a temporary condition that may progress to hyper-reflexia in 57–100% of patients.[1,54]

Urethral dysfunction and dyssynergia

Urethral dysfunction (DSD or ISR or flacidity) represents a continuum that may be seen in 12–84% (mean 25.4%) of patients (see *Table 36.1* and *Fig. 36.1*)[10,13,46] Consequently, a variety of clinical effects may be seen, ranging from retention to complete incontinence. DSD has been highly correlated with cervical plaque formation as well as with increased levels of CSF myelin basic protein (p < 0.05).[1,4,23] Most commonly, DSD presents with incomplete emptying and stranguria (symptoms also seen with hypocontractility). DSD is the most extreme defect in this continuum and is seen when a detrusor voiding contraction is accompanied by concomitant contraction of the internal sphincter, the external sphincter, or both.[10] In sharp contrast to the dys-synergia seen in patients with spinal cord injury, DSD in the MS population is rarely associated with upper tract dysfunction but rather with local symptoms of incomplete emptying, elevated post-void residual volumes, bladder calculi and infection.[4,10,33,41,46,55] The reason for this difference is unclear, but it may be related to the protective effect of the poorly sustained detrusor contractions that are seen in up to 50% of MS patients with detrusor hyper-reflexia. Alternatively, the hyper-reflexia and degree of external sphincter spasm seen in MS may be less severe than that seen in spinal cord injury.[46,50,55]

Although the diagnosis of DSD is most commonly made by electromyography, the proper method for the diagnosis of DSD is unclear.[56] The use of urethral versus anal electromyelography, wire or patch electrodes, urethral pressure gradients and videourodynamic urethral assessment is also debated.[10,11,57–61] The necessity for sphincteric assessment and diagnosis of DSD has been questioned.[10,12,22,33] Sirls and col-

leagues[31] found sphincteric evaluation by electromyelography unhelpful in the management of 15 patients with DSD and they felt that its only utility was in securing the diagnosis of MS.

ISR is similar to DSD but is of lesser magnitude and is less commonly associated with lower urinary tract complications. Rather, ISR may be manifested by weak force of stream or stranguria. Sphincteric paralysis (flacidity) is seen in less than 15% of patients and may manifest as sphincteric incontinence.[2]

Stability of urodynamic findings

Since MS is a dynamic disease characterized by exacerbations and remissions, changes in lower urinary tract function over time and in response to therapy can occur. In studies of selected patients, 15–55% of patients demonstrate changes on repeat urodynamic testing.[54] It is of note that once DSD is found on urodynamic evaluation it rarely remits.[10,54] However, there have been few studies evaluating the natural progression of urologic findings in patients who are mildly symptomatic or asymptomatic. Furthermore, longitudinal studies following MS patients over time and in response to systemic treatment are currently lacking.

MANAGEMENT

Urologic treatment and therapeutic guidelines

Currently, most authors cite a low incidence of renal complications and upper tract deterioration in low-risk patients (those without indwelling catheters or DSD).[4,15,31,36] These findings may support a rather conservative approach to upper tract management, discouraging the routine use of yearly upper urinary tract monitoring except in high-risk patients, patients with a changing clinical course, and patients with progression of disease.[13,17,31,32] Aggressive surgical management for mild hydronephrosis, as practiced in the past, has largely been replaced by clean intermittant catheterization.[40,42] Although pyelonephritis is rare, its treatment may be complicated by atypical organisms. In 34% of cases *Pseudomonas* spp. is a causative factor for pyelenophritis; in 31% of cases it is *Proteus* spp. and in 25% of cases it is *Providencia* spp.[37]

Treatment decisions should take into account the patient's level of disability and his or her ability to function independently, manual dexterity, competing medical problems, and social support networks. A team approach involving the patient's treating neurologist, urologist and rehabilitation specialist is essential to optimize patient care. An empiric trial-and-error method is discouraged since it may be time consuming and costly and leave many patients improperly treated and at risk of potential complications.[10,22] Rather, a clear understanding of each patient's underlying pathology should be established on the basis of objective parameters such as flow rate, residual urine volumes, and urodynamic evaluation. For treatment purposes, patients may be separated into those with storage problems, those with emptying problems, and those with both. In most patients, conservative measures are an effective means of primary management.

Medical management

Bladder storage disorders

Symptoms arising from storage disorders (fre-quency, urgency, nocturia, and incontinence) are the commonest reasons for urologic consultation. Since nearly two thirds of patients suffer from detrusor hyper-reflexia, treatment involves pharmacologic therapy to suppress uninhibited bladder contractions. Traditionally, the use of atropine-like drugs that competitively bind the acetylcholine receptor, thereby blocking muscarinic effects, have represented the cornerstone of treatment. A variety of drugs can be used (*Table 36.2*)[26,62–66] Dosages of these drugs may be titrated to therapeutic response or until anticholinergic side effects become intolerable.[67] The use of imipramine in MS may be tempered by its α-agonistic properties, which impair bladder emptying in patients with DSD.[68] Concomitant use of other anti-depressants in MS also limits the effective use of imipramine. When monotherapy fails to improve detrusor storage, medications with pure anti-cholinergic properties (e.g. hyoscyamine, propantheline) may be combined with those that have additional direct smooth muscle relaxant properties (e.g. oxybutynin, flavoxate).[63,64,69–71]

Oxybutynin chloride is one of the most widely prescribed of these medications and has shown fair-to-good results in 67–80% of MS patients. Anti-cholinergic side effects (decreased salivation, blurred vision, and constipation), which occur in 57–94% of patients, have had a significant effect on long-term patient compliance. Attrition rates of up to 50% have been reported in long-term studies.[72–74] These side effects are especially troublesome in MS patients because blurry vision may be mistaken for deterioration caused by optic neuritis and because constipation is a significant problem for most MS patients.[75]

New selective muscarinic receptor blockers such as tolterodine may show promise in reliev-

Table 36.2 Pharmacotherapy for bladder dysfunction

	Class of drug	How supplied	Use	Dose	Side effects
Hyoscyamine	Anticholinergic	Sublingual	Detrusor hyper-reflexia	0.125 mg q4 hrs	dry mouth, blurred vision,
		Extended release		0.375 mg q12 hrs	constipation, dizziness,
Probanthine	Anticholinergic	Oral	Detrusor hyper-reflexia	7.5–15 mg q8 hrs	nausea, urinary retention,
Flavoxate	Musculotropic		Detrusor hyper-reflexia	100–200 mg q8–12 hrs	
Oxbutynin	Anticholinergic/	Oral	Detrusor hyper-reflexia	2.5–5 mg q8 hrs	
	Muscolotropic	Extended release		5–30 mg qday	
		Intravesical		5–10 mg q8–12 hrs	
Tolterodine	Antimuscarinic	Oral	Detrusor hyper-reflexia	2 mg q12 hrs	
Imipramine	Tricyclic	Oral	Detrusor hyper-reflexia	25 mg q8 hrs or	anticholinergic side effects
	Antidepressan			50 mg qhs	orthostasis, esthenia
					drowsiness, weakness
DDAVP	Vasopressin	Intranasal	Nocturia or frequency	1–2 puffs qhs	edema, hyponatremia,
	Analog	Oral		0.05–0.5 mg q12 hrs	headache, weight gain
Doxazosin	Alpha Blocker	Oral	Sphincter Dyssynergia	4–12 mg qhs	orthostatic hypotension,
Terazosin				5–10 mg qhs	esthenia, incontinence
Tizanidine (Experimental)	Alpha 2 Agonist (Spasmolytic)	Oral	Sphincter Dyssynergia	8 mg q8 hrs	esthnia, drowsiness, weakness

ing urgency and frequency with a lower incidence of anti-cholinergic side effects.[76,77] In some patients, clean intermittent catheterization may be combined with anti-cholinergic therapy; this may be especially beneficial in patients with both storage and emptying failure. In these patients, urinary retention is promoted by anti-cholinergic agents, thus alleviating storage problems, while emptying is provided solely by intermittent catheterization.

In an attempt to avoid anti-cholinergic side effects from oral medications, a variety of intravesical medications (e.g. verapamil, lidocaine, oxybutynin) have been tested for treatment of detrusor hyper-reflexia.[78–84] These agents are crushed, suspended, and instilled into the bladder via sterile catheterization. The most commonly used intravesical agent is oxybutynin. The therapeutic response to intravesical oxybutynin in MS patients has exceeded 86% in selected studies; however, the inconvenience of this route of administration has contributed to a high attrition rate and has tempered enthusiasm for this treatment method.[84] Nevertheless, in selected patients who are already using intermittent catheterization, intravesical oxybutynin may lead to a significant improvement in continence but with fewer side effects than oral oxybutynin.

Newer intravesical medications—resiniferatoxin and capsaicin—also show promise for the intravesical treatment of detrusor hyperactivity. These compounds exert a selective action on C sensory fiber axons, which are thought to play an important role in bladder reflex pathways after insult to the spinal cord. When instilled intravesically, capsaicin exerts a neurotoxic effect on afferent C fiber axons, causing depletion of substance P and calcitonin gene-related peptide (CGRP).[85–91] In a study of 18 patients,[89] 61% of the patients treated with capsaicin demonstrated excellent results and 17% demonstrated clinical improvement. The duration of patient response in this study ranged from 3–6 months. Optimism for capsaicin has been tempered by its pungent effects and because of pain on instillation.

Because resiniferatoxin lacks these side effects and is 1000 times more potent than capsaicin, it may represent a more attractive form of intravesical therapy. In studies evaluating the effect of resiniferatoxin, the mean bladder volume at initial urge was not affected, although total bladder capacity was increased by an average of 105 ml (p < 0.001).[91] These preliminary results suggest a difference in the urodynamic effect between resiniferatoxin and capsaicin that merits further evaluation. As capsaicin and resiniferatoxin are industrial reagents rather than drugs approved by the Food and Drug Administration, their use in the USA at the present time is limited to investigational protocols.

Detrusor hyper-reflexia (especially nocturia) may also be treated effectively by decreasing the production of urine. In multiple placebo-controlled trials evaluating MS patients, 1 desamino-8-D-vasopressin (DDAVP) nasal spray has shown significant efficacy in reducing the incidence of nocturia and nocturnal enuresis and in increasing the duration of sleep.[92–95] The use of DDAVP may be especially helpful in the management of patients with detrusor hyper-reflexia who cannot tolerate anti-cholinergic medication or who suffer from concomitant emptying failure due to DSD or hypocontractility. In a phase 1 trial,[94] doses of 10–20 µg were found to provide a signifi-

cant decrease in nocturnal urinary volumes without hyponatremia. Increased doses to 60 µg were no more efficacious and were accompanied by a trend towards lower serum sodium levels. Recently, DDAVP has become available in a tablet preparation, which may be more convenient for some patients (see *Table 36.2*).

Emptying failure (hypocontractility and sphincter dys-synergia)

Despite problems encountered with storage failure (detrusor hyper-reflexia), 42% of MS patients may also suffer from emptying difficulties caused by DSD, unsustained voiding contractions, or detrusor hypocontractility (see *Table 36.1*). In a small, selected group of MS patients, timed voiding or double voiding may be sufficient for adequate emptying. However, in most patients, intervention is required to prevent infections, calculi, or overflow incontinence. Attempts to manage these patients conservatively with α-1 blocking agents (e.g. prazosin, terazosin, doxazosin) and muscle relaxants (e.g. diazepam, lioresal, dantrolene sodium) have had mixed results (see *Table 36.2*).[96,97] Anecdotal success has been reported with the use of tizanidine, a new spasmolytic with centrally acting α-2 adrenergic properties. The use of α-blockers and muscle relaxants in patients with emptying failure should, however, be limited to patients with urodynamically proven DSD and not detrusor hypocontractility.

Clean intermittent catheterization has been the primary means of management for patients with emptying difficulties and it may aid in bladder rehabilitation.[98] Urodynamic evaluation may facilitate the decision for clean intermittent catheterization by defining bladder storage capabilities and selecting the optimum catheterization interval.

Surgical management

Bladder dysfunction

When conservative management fails in the management of LUTD, more aggressive surgical options may be entertained. A variety of factors should be considered, including the degree of manual dexterity, social support systems, disability status, life expectancy of another 20–50 years, and urodynamic parameters. Thus, short-term solutions may need to be dismissed in favor of a more comprehensive long-term approach. Surgical options include suprapubic cystostomy, sphincterotomy, sphincteric stents, augmentation cystoplasty (surgical enlargement using an intestinal patch) with or without a catheterizable limb, incontinent vesicostomy, or supravesical diversion (*Figs 36.4* and *36.5*).[40,99–101]

Suprapubic cystostomy (SP tube) may be an attractive initial plan for patients who fail conservative management since it has several distinct advantages over a conventional indwelling catheter. Urethral erosion (in female patients) and traumatic hypospadias (in male patients), which are often seen with chronic Foley catheterization (prompted by the use of successively larger catheters) are avoided. Personal hygiene and catheter care is simplified because catheter position is readily accessible and remote from vaginal and perineal soilage. Commonly, the tube can be placed percutaneously under local anesthesia. This decision is reversible because the tube may be removed without difficulty and the site will heal in 1–2 days. The SP tube may not be a good long-term option for younger patients because of the risk of bladder calculi, infection and the development of squamous cell carcinoma.[102–104]

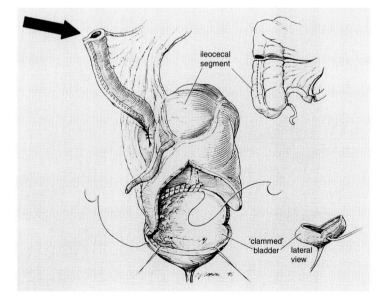

Fig. 36.4 Catheterizable Augmentation Cystoplasty
An ileocecal segment is used to not only augment existing bladder capacity, but the plicated ileum acts as a catheterizable abdominal stoma, allowing the patient to empty their bladder while standing or sitting in a wheelchair. This tapered ileal segment (bold arrow) may be exteriorized in the right lower quadrant or to the umbilicus, allowing for maximal cosmesis.
(From: Sutton MA, Hinson JL, Nickell KG, Boone TB, Continent ileocecal augmentation cystoplasty, *Spinal Cord 36:246–251, 1998)*

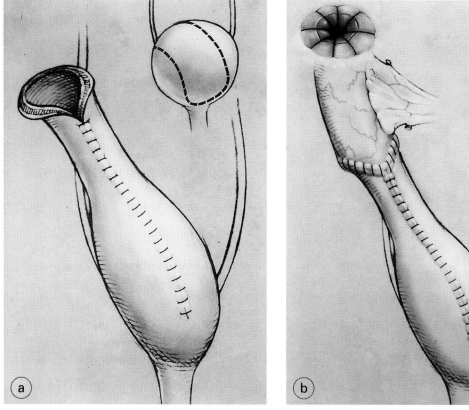

Fig. 36.5 *Ileovesicostomy*

The ileovesicostomy allows the bladder to be tubularized and brought toward the abdominal wall. As the bladder will rarely reach the skin on its own, an interposed segment of ileum is used to bridge this gap. The bladder is allowed to drain freely and a relatively maintenance free appliance is placed on the skin.

In the male patient with detrusor hyperactivity and DSD who cannot be managed by conservative measures, an outlet reducing procedure such as a sphincterotomy (endoscopically cutting the external sphincter) or a urethral stent may be of benefit to facilitate bladder emptying. In both treatment options, a condom catheter may be necessary to manage the resulting incontinence. These procedures are best reserved for the patient with limited hand function for whom CIC is not an option. Documentation of adequate detrusor contractility is imperative as patients with hypocontractile bladders may carry an unacceptably high residual volume even after the procedure.[100,101]

Surgical augmentation for detrusor dysfunction is usually reserved for the patient in whom all other conservative options have been exhausted. As the course of MS is by nature dynamic and progressive, permanent procedures using intestinal segments should be undertaken only after careful consideration of the current course of disease (relapsing or progressive) and overall prognosis. Patients undergoing augmentation cystoplasty should be assessed for manual dexterity because most will continue to require some degree of intermittent catheterization.[67] In most cases, surgical augmentation is combined with a catheterizable abdominal stoma, which allows easy catheterization, especially in the chair-bound patient, the patient with lower extremity spasticity, and the patient with poor dexterity who cannot perform urethral catheterization (see *Fig. 36.4*).

When neither the patient nor a family member or caretaker can perform intermittent catheterization and conservative management has failed, a cutaneous ileovesicostomy has been used successfully for both storage and emptying abnormalities in the MS patient (see *Fig. 36.5*) In this procedure, a segment of ileum is used to construct a chimney emanating from the bladder to allow cutaneous drainage to an external collection device[99] (PE Zwemmer; personal communication). The advantages of this procedure over supravesical diversion are preservation of the bladder and ureterovesical junctions (if competent), lack of a defunctionalized bladder, and decreased blood loss. Although some patients are reluctant to proceed with major surgical intervention, most are pleasantly surprised post-operatively with the improvement that this procedure provides in quality of life and daily management of their incontinence.

Urethral incompetence

The treatment for urethral incompetence has been previously described[58,105,106] and includes the use of injectable bulking agents (e.g. collagen, polytetrafluoroethylene, fat), urethral inserts, conventional bladder suspension procedures, and compressive slings. In female patients with urethral incompetence or destruction resulting from

indwelling catheterization, transvaginal bladder neck closure and suprapubic drainage may serve as a minimally invasive way of dealing with intractable incontinence. Surgical intervention for urethral insufficiency should consider a variety of factors: voiding efficiency, ability to perform intermittant catheterization, stability of disease, and general overall health. Patients should be informed of the risk of post-surgical urinary retention, since this may adversely affect the amount of nursing care required and the quality of life.

The artificial urinary sphincter has had a limited role in the management of incontinence in MS. This is primarily due to the significant incidence of detrusor hyper-reflexia in MS and its association with upper tract deterioration in patients undergoing artificial urinary sphincter placement.[109] Before any outlet-enhancing procedure is performed, bladder storage and voiding function should be assessed since patients with poorly sustained voiding contractions may be at increased risk of post-operative urinary retention.

SEXUAL DYSFUNCTION

Because MS affects patients in mid-life, issues concerning sexual dysfunction become an increasingly important factor in enhancing patient quality of life as patients in this age group still desire to be sexually active. Studies have shown that MS adversely effects sexual functioning in up to 91% of males and 72% of females. In 64% of males and 39% of females with MS, sexual activity ceases or is unsatisfactory.[108–111] In addition to physiological disturbances, psychosocial stressors can influence sexual functioning. Mattson and colleagues[114] found associated marital relationship problems in 71% of MS patients with complaints of primary sexual dysfunction.

Male sexual dysfunction

Men with MS report a variety of adverse symptoms, including erectile dysfunction, decreased sensation, fatigue, and decreased libido resulting in orgasmic dysfunction.[113] The onset of erectile dysfunction has been reported from 3.7–9.0 years after diagnosis.[109,110] Yet, despite impotence rates as high as 80%, more than 75% of patients report a continued interest in sexual activity.[108] Sexual dysfunction has been shown by some to parallel the level of overall disability.[108,113,114] However, other studies demonstrated that erectile dysfunction is independent of disability and more closely related to bladder and pyramidal dysfunction alone.[110,111,115] In a study by Betts and colleagues,[110] 100% of 48 patients with erectile dysfunction were found to have concomitant bladder dysfunction. However, the absence of bladder or pyramidal dysfunction does not ensure adequate sexual function, since up to 50% of patients without pyramidal symptoms suffer from sexual impairment.[113]

Several authors have studied the physiologic basis of erectile dysfunction using pudendal reflex latencies and tibial, pudendal and cortical evoked potentials. These studies have shown consistent deficits in cortical and pudendal evoked potentials without consistent changes in the evaluation of bulbocavernosus reflex latency.[110,111,115] Thus, it is thought that impotence in MS is related to suprasacral mechanisms. Abnormal pudendal evoked potentials are also shown to be predictive of ejaculatory dysfunction.[110] In addition to neurophysiologic abnormalities, nocturnal penile tumescence studies have demonstrated a significant psychogenic component in over 50% of patients.[111] In these patients, marital and sexual counseling may be beneficial.

Evaluation of male sexual dysfunction

The evaluation of male sexual dysfunction should begin with a thorough sexual and urologic history. Patients should be questioned about a variety of topics. A number of patients complain of decreased libido; however, close questioning may discriminate patients who have a physiologically decreased desire for sex from those in whom MS has made sexual activity an anxiety-laden burden. If morning erectile activity is present, this may confirm erectile integrity. Erections that occur and then spontaneously undergo detumescence may lend suspicion to the possibility of a venous leak or a steal phenomenon. Spasticity and fatigue are often severely limiting factors for sexual activity and may play a role both in patient positioning and in the desire for sex. The importance of an understanding stable partner cannot be overestimated, making it preferable to have the partner present for this portion of the office visit. Physiological evaluation of erectile dysfunction has centered around the use of penile doppler flow evaluation and nocturnal penile tumescence monitoring. Although these are helpful in selected patients, many physicians have gone to a more practical approach for a number of reasons: these tests may be expensive and have a variable degree of false-positive and false-negative results; they may not accurately reproduce what happens in a patient's sexual encounter at home; and the options for management are often not altered by the results of the testing. The one clear benefit to these tests is their ability to discern psychogenic impotence from physiologic dysfunction.

Treatment of male sexual dysfunction

Treatment of male sexual dysfunction (*Table 36.3, Fig. 36.6*) should take into account a variety of factors, including the degree of manual

Table 36.3 Treatment of sexual dysfunction

	Sex	*Cost*	*Covered by insurance*	*Pros*	*Cons*
Sexual counseling	M/F	$50–100/hr	no	promotes a healthy relationship, helps partner, fosters intimacy	none
Vibratory stimulation	M/F	$25–350	no	inexpensive	none
Yohimbine	M	$100/month	sometimes	natural and spontaneous	poor efficacy in organic erectile dysfunction, cost
Sildenafil *(Viagra™)*	M/??F	$9–11/dose	sometimes	spontaneous and easily taken	cost, contraindicated in pts with nitrates or cardiac disease, may need vibratory assistance
Vacuum erection devices	M	$250–350/unit	usually	one time cost, few complications	penis feels cool, may look blue, less spontaneous, may need partner assistance
Injection Pharmacotherapy	M	$10–20/dose	usually	provides a reliable firm erection	penile fibrosis, acute priapism, pain, may need partner assistance, high attrition rate (50–80%)
Penile prosthesis	M	$8–10,000	usually	high patient and partner satisfaction, most reliable erection	risk of infection or mechanical failure, may require partner assistance, may not revert to other therapies

dexterity, the stability of the patient's current relationship, the degree of disability, and the course of disease. The approach to treatment should involve the neurologist, the rehabilitation physician, and the urologist. An initial course of sexual counseling may aid in treating any psychologic factors and also help to develop a better understanding between partners, thereby promoting intimacy. There are few studies involving impotence treatment specifically in the MS patient, and much of what is known is extrapolated from general studies involving neurogenic impotence.[116,117] Although the possibility for recovery of erectile activity is low (2%), non-surgical options such as oral agents (e.g. sildenafil), vacuum erection devices, and intracorporal

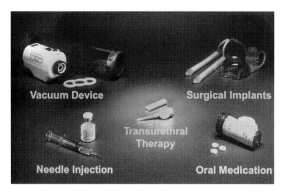

Fig. 36.6 *Examples of Treatments for Erectile Dysfunction.*

injection therapy (prostaglandin E1 or papaverine), play a more prominent role than prosthetic implantation since most patients are reluctant to undergo surgery for impotence.

Oral therapy for impotence, although receiving recent interest, is not a new concept. Probably the oldest oral treatment available is yohimbine, which first saw clinical use in the 1950s. Since that time, a variety of clinical studies have presented data with varied results. In a meta-analysis, yohimbine was found to be slightly superior to placebo (odds ratio 3.85; 95% CI 2.2–6.7).[118,119] However, the American Urological Association's guidelines panel on erectile dysfunction has recommended that yohimbine should not be used as treatment for organic erectile dysfunction.[120] The use of yohimbine in MS patients has never been tested and with the advent of newer oral agents it has become a seldom-used option. Side effects include anxiety (in 18% of patients), headache (in 13% of patients), urinary frequency (in 32% of patients), and vertigo (in 14% of patients).[119]

With the recent advent of newer oral therapy for erectile dysfunction (e.g. sildenafil), most patients will elect to pursue this option first. Current studies are under way to evaluate the use of oral sildenafil in men with MS; however, studies in the spinal cord injury population have shown a nearly 70% success rate when used in combination with vibratory stimulation.[121] Sildenafil (50–100 mg) is taken 1 hour before sexual intercourse and is ineffective in the absence of psychologic or tactile stimulation. Caution should be exercised with the use of oral sildenafil since there are a number of drug interactions (e.g. with macrolide antibiotics, cimetidine, and oral anti-fungal agents) that should be borne in mind, and its use in patients with known cardiac disease is severely cautioned against. The use of sildenafil in patients who are taking topical or oral nitrate therapy is absolutely contraindicated. Side effects are usually limited to nasal congestion, headache, flushing, and dyspepsia and are seen in 6–18% of patients.[122]

Although there are no studies in men with MS, vibratory stimulation may be used as an adjunct to virtually any type of erectile therapy and has been well studied in patients with spinal cord injuries.[123] Vibratory stimulation may enhance erections and may be used to decrease the orgasmic threshold for both men and women.

Vacuum erection devices have been used successfully in a variety of patients with erectile dysfunction including MS.[124] When this form of therapy is used, a plastic tube is placed over the penis and a pump is used to create a vacuum, drawing blood into the penis. A silicone or latex ring is then slipped over the base of the penis to maintain the erection (*Fig. 36.7*). Although results in some studies are promising, the attrition rate may be high in improperly selected patients. Many patients find that with the use of vacuum erection devices, their penis is cold and

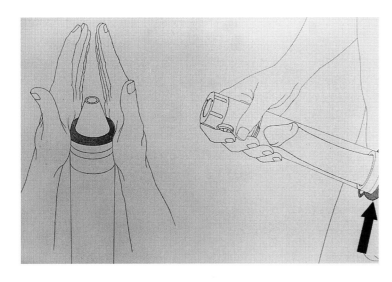

Fig. 36.7 *The Vacuum Erection Device*
When using a vacuum erection device, a constriction ring is first placed on the base of the vacuum tube. The tube is then placed over the penis and the manual or battery operated vacuum pump is activated, drawing blood into the penis. The elastic ring (arrow) is then slipped off the tube to constrict the base of the penis and prevent egress of blood. After intercourse, the constriction ring is removed allowing detumescence.

painful, and many patients feel that this option is less natural than other options. Patients may require partner assistance in operating the device because some degree of dexterity is required. Vacuum erection devices are, however, relatively inexpensive and have few associated risks.

The injection of vasoactive substances into the penis has been in use for nearly 20 years and may take one of two forms: intraurethral suppositories (prostaglandin E1) and injected suspensions (prostaglandin E1 or papavarine). These medications, although fairly reliable, carry with them a risk of priapism (0.8–1.5%) (a painful prolonged erection accompanied by corporal hypoxia), pain at the injection site, and chronic penile fibrosis (0.5%).[125] Interestingly, despite a better than 95% initial success rate with injection therapy, the attrition rate at 2 years in MS patients is 39–80%.[110,125,126]

The use of penile prostheses in MS patients has also been reported for over 20 years[127] and may take one of two forms: inflatable and semi-rigid prostheses or malleable prostheses. Although the inflatable prosthesis provides a more natural-looking and more esthetic erection, it does require manual dexterity by either the patient or the partner to activate its use. Infection rates range from 1.2 to 1.8% and the need for revision ranges from 4.5 to 7.7%.[128,129] In a study by Sexton and colleagues,[130] a 5-year comparison was made of patients undergoing penile prosthesis with those undergoing injection therapy. Interestingly, patients undergoing prosthesis insertion had sex twice as often as patients who used injection therapy. They also reported significantly higher patient satisfaction (77% versus 70%) and partner satisfaction rates (88% versus 67%) over patients on injection therapy.

Female sexual dysfunction

Although the majority of females with MS wish to remain sexually active, sexual dysfunction is a significant problem for 56–72% of patients.[113,130] The most common reasons for sexual dysfunction in females are: fatigue (in 68% of patients), decreased sensation (in 48% of patients), decreased or absent orgasm (in 72% of patients), difficulty with arousal (in 35% of patients) and frequent urinary tract infections (in 21% of patients).[113] Vaginal dryness is also a frequently reported complaint and it may be related to anti-cholinergic medications.

The evaluation of the female with sexual dysfunction should begin with a thorough sexual history. Patients should be questioned about their sexual activity and sexual satisfaction before MS as well as about their present symptoms and their current methods of coping. Since the sexual response in female is less dependent on the mechanics of erection or sexual performance and more dependent on the dynamics of a loving relationship, sufficient time should be spent discussing the way the patient and her partner relate both sexually and non-sexually. A helpful way of assessing the female sexual response is often with the use of a validated questionnaire.[132] These may allow the practitioner to distinguish physiologic from psychosocial factors involved in the sexual response. A complete medication history is also of prime importance because a number of drugs (especially serotonin-reuptake inhibitors) used in the MS population may have adverse effects on sexual functioning especially on libido and orgasm.[133]

The physical examination of the female MS patient with sexual dysfunction remains an integral part of the overall evaluation for sexual dysfunction. Since sexual dysfunction may be closely associated with bladder dysfunction,[113,114] a careful vaginal and pelvic examination is important to rule out the co-existence of urogenital pathology, such as a cystocele, enterocele, rectocele, or urethral diverticulum. Perineal and perianal sensation should also be assessed because decreased sensation is reported by up to half of patients.[113,114]

The laboratory evaluation of these patients is limited. Though normal values for testosterone have been established in healthy females, the use of testosterone as an adjunct to diagnosis and treatment of sexual dysfunction is not established and unsupported.

Treatment of female sexual dysfunction

Treatment of female sexual dysfunction may take many forms. First and foremost the importance of a loving and supportive partner cannot be overestimated. In nearly all relationships, sexual dysfunction can be a major stressor. For that reason, sexual counseling by a registered therapist can prove invaluable.

Symptomatic treatment is also of great benefit. Vaginal dryness can be effectively treated with water-soluble vaginal moisturizers or lubricants. For patients with orgasmic dysfunction, vibratory stimuli may aid in decreasing the orgasmic threshold. The use of oral sildenafil in females with sexual dysfunction, although not formally tested, may hold promise for patients with symptomatic sexual dysfunction including anorgasmia, hypoesthesia and vaginal dryness. The basis for its use lies in the homologous nature of the male and female genitalia and the presence of type 5 phosphodiesterase activity in the genital tissues of both men and women. In patients with decreased mobility, sexual positioning may be altered to aid in patient comfort. Involvement of the patient's neurologist and careful attention to overall systemic treatment can alleviate many somatic symptoms related to sexual dysfunction (e.g. fatigue, spasticity).

Historically, oral or parenteral testosterone has been used in an effort to improve libido and sexual response. However, since the female sex drive is not dependent on testosterone, few patients will actually benefit from this type of therapy. Testosterone suppplementation is also not without risk or side effects. Patients may note mood swings and growth of facial or body hair. Systemic complications of testosterone therapy include hepatic or renal damage, an increased risk of stroke, and suppression of the hypothalamic–pituitary axis. In the majority of cases, loss of libido is more closely related to frustration and feelings of hopelessness over relationship issues and lack of sexual responsiveness than physiologically decreased sexual desire.

SUMMARY

MS is a devastating disease that affects 0.1% of the population in the prime years of their life. During the course of the disease, nearly all patients manifest lower urinary tract symptoms, sexual dysfunction, or both. Although these symptoms are rarely life threatening, they nonetheless have a significant impact on a patient's quality of life. Consequently, the neurologist may be called on to assist in the care of these patients. In order to treat these problems effectively and intelligently, the neurologist must have a fundamental working knowledge of the disease process itself and of its effects on the genitourinary system. Using this knowledge, a logical and individualized treatment plan can be formulated.

REFERENCES

1 Goldstein I, Siroky MB, Sax S, Krane RJ. Neurourologic abnormalities in multiple Sclerosis. *J Urol* 1982; **128**:541–545.

2 Andersen JT, Bradley WE. Abnormalities of detrusor and sphincter function in multiple sclerosis. *Br J Urol* 1976; **48**:193–198.

3 Bradley WF. Urinary bladder dysfunction in multiple sclerosis. *Neurology* 1978; **29**:52–58.

4 Koldewijn EL, Homme OR, Lemmens WA et al. Relationship between lower urinary tract abnormalities and disease related parameters in multiple sclerosis. *J Urol* 1995; **154**:169.

5 Fog T. Topographic distribution of plaques in the spinal cord in multiple sclerosis. *Arch Neurol Psychol* 1950; **63**:382–414.

6 Oppenheimer DR. The cervical cord in multiple sclerosis. *Neuropathol Appl Neurobiol* 1978; **4**:151–162.

7 Nathan PW, Smith MC. The centrifugal pathway for micturition within the spinal cord. *J Neurol* 1958; **21**:177–189.

8 Blaivas JG, Barbalias GA. Detrusor external sphincter dyssynergia in men with multiple sclerosis: an ominous urologic condition. *J Urol* 1984; **131**:91–94.

9 Blaivas JG. The neurophysiology of micturition: a clinical study of 550 patients. *J Urol* 1982; **127**:958–963.

10 Blaivas JG, Bhimani G, Labib KB. Vesicourethral dysfunction in multiple sclerosis. *J Urol* 1979; **122**:342–347.

11 Siroky MB, Krane RJ. Neurologic aspects of detrusor–sphincter dyssynergia, with reference to the guarding reflex. *J Urol* 1982; **127**:953–957.

12 McGuire EJ, Savastano JA. Urodynamic findings and long term outcome management of patients with multiple sclerosis-induced lower urinary tract dysfunction. *J Urol* 1984; **132**:713–715.

13 Betts CD, D'Mellow MT, Fowler CJ. Urinary symptoms and neurological features of bladder dysfunction in multiple sclerosis. *J Neurol* 1993; **56**:245–250.

14 Mayo ME, Chetner MP. Lower urinary tract dysfunction in multiple sclerosis. *Urol* 1992; **39**:67–70.

15 Awad SA, Gajewski JB, Sogbein SK et al. Relationship between neurological and urological status in patients with multiple sclerosis. *J Urol* 1984; **139**:499.

16 Philip T, Read DJ, Higson RH. The urodynamic characteristic of multiple sclerosis. *Br J Urol* 1981; 53:672–675.

17 Hinson JL, Boone TB. Urodynamics and multiple sclerosis. *Urol Clin North Am* 1996; 23:475–481.

18 Kruse MN, Mallory NH, Roppolo JR, DeGroat WC. Modulation of the spinobulbospinal micturition reflex pathway in cats. *Am J Physiol* 1992; 262:478–484.

19 Kruse MN, Mallory BS, Noto H. Properties of the descending limb of the spinal–bulbospinal reflex pathway in the cat. *Brain Res* 1991; 556:6–12.

20 Andersen JT, Bradley WF. Bladder and urethral innervation in multiple sclerosis. *Br J Urol* 1976; 48:239–243.

21 Eardley I, Nagendran, Lecky B et al. Neurophysiology of the striated sphincter in multiple sclerosis. *Br J Urol* 1991; 68:81–88.

22 Bemmelmans BLH, Hommes OR, Van Kerrebroek PEV et al. Evidence for early lower urinary tract dysfunction in clinically silent multiple sclerosis. *J Urol* 1991; 145:1219–1224.

23 Francis GS, Evans AC, Arnold DL. Neuroimaging in multiple sclerosis. *Neurol Clin* 1995; 13:147–171.

24 Filippi M, Miller DH. Magnetic resonance imaging in the differential diagnosis and monitoring of the treatment of multiple sclerosis. *Curr Opin Neurol* 1996; 9:178–186.

25 Kim YH, Goodman C, Omessi E et al. The correlation of urodynamic findings with cranial magnetic resonance imaging findings in multiple sclerosis. *J Urol* 1998; 159:972–976.

26 Pozilli C, Grasso MG, Bastianello S, Anzini A. Structural correlates of neurourologic abnormalities in multiple sclerosis. *Eur Neurol* 1992; 32:228–230.

27 Stevens JC, Kinkel WR, Polachini I. Clinical correlation in 64 patients with multiple sclerosis. *J Neurol* 1986; 43:1145–1148.

28 Huber SJ, Paulson GW, Chakeres D et al. Magnetic resonance imaging and clinical correlations in multiple sclerosis. *J Neurol Sci* 1988; 86:1–12.

29 Baumhefner RW, Tourtellotte WW. Quantitative multiple sclerosis plaque assessment with magnetic resonance imaging. *Arch Neurol* 1990; 47:19–26.

30 Rao SM, Leo GJ, Haughton VM et al. Correlation of magnetic resonance imaging with neuropsychological testing in multiple sclerosis. *Neurol* 1989; 39:161–166.

31 Sirls LT, Zimmern PE, Leach GE. Role of limited evaluation and aggressive medical management in

multiple sclerosis: a review of 113 patients. *J Urol* 1994; 151:946.

32 Bakke A, Myhr KM, Gronning M, Nyland H. Bladder, bowel and sexual dysfunction in patients with multiple sclerosis: a cohort study. *Scand J Urol Nephrol Suppl* 1996; 179:61–66.

33 Beck RP, Warren KG, Whitman P. Urodynamic studies in female patients with multiple sclerosis. *Am J Obstet Gynecol* 1981; 139:273.

34 Blaivas JG, Holland NJ, Geisser B et al. Multiple sclerosis bladder: studies and care. *Ann N Y Acad Sci* 1984; 436:328–346.

35 Kurtzke JF. Rating disability in multiple sclerosis: an expanded disability status scale (EDSS). *Neurology* 1983; 33:1444.

36 Fowler CJ. Bladder dysfunction in multiple sclerosis: causes and treatment. *Int M S J* 1996; 1:431–440.

37 Van Poppel H, Baert L. Treatment of multi-resistant urinary infections in patients with multiple sclerosis. *Pharm Weekbl* 1987; 9 (suppl):76–77.

38 Shumaker SA, Wyman JF, Uebersax JS et al. Health related quality of life measures for women with urinary incontinence: the incontinence impact questionnaire and the urogenital distress inventory. *Qual Life Res* 1994; 3:291–306.

39 Raz S, Erickson DR. SEAPI QMM incontinence classification system. *Neurourol Urodynamics* 1992; 11:187–199.

40 Samellas W, Rubin B. Management of upper urinary tract complications of multiple sclerosis by means of urinary diversion to an ileal conduit. *J Urol* 1965; 93:169.

41 Franz DA, Towler MA, Edlich RF, Steers WD. Functional urinary outlet obstruction causing urosepsis in a male multiple sclerosis patient. *J Emerg Med* 1992; 10:284.

42 Webb RJ, Lawson AL, Neal DE. Clean intermittent self-catheterisation in 172 adults. *Br J Urol* 1990; 65:20–23.

43 Litiwiller SE, Frohman EM, Zimmern PE. Multiple Sclerosis and the Urologist. *J Urol* 1999; 161:743–757.

44 Bradley WE, Logothetis JL, Timm GW. Cystometric and sphincter abnormalities in multiple sclerosis. *Neurol* 1973; 23:1131–1139.

45 Eardley I, Nagendran, Lecky B et al. Neurophysiology of the striated sphincter in multiple sclerosis. *Br J Urol* 1991; 68:81–88.

46 Gonor SE, Carroll DJ, Metcalfe JB. Vesical dysfunction in multiple sclerosis. *Urology* 1985;

128:541–545.

47 **Peterson T, Pederson E.** Neurourodynamic evaluation of voiding dysfunction in multiple sclerosis. *Acta Neurol Scand* 1984; **69**:402–411.

48 **Piazza DH, Diokno AC.** Review of neurogenic bladder in multiple sclerosis. *Urology* 1979; **14**:33–35.

49 **Schoenberg HW, Gutrich J, Banno J.** Urodynamic patterns in multiple sclerosis. *J Urol* 1979; **122**:648–650.

50 **Sirls L, Weese D, Zimmern PE et al.** Intravesical oxybutynin for refractory detrusor over activity. Annual meeting of the Urodynamics Society, San Antonio, Texas, May, 1993.

51 **Summers JL.** Neurogenic bladder in the women with multiple sclerosis. *J Urol* 1978; **120**:555–556.

52 **Weinstein MS, Cardenas DD, O'Shaughnessy EJ, Catanzaro ML.** Carbon dioxide cystometry and postural changes in patients with multiple sclerosis. *Arch Phys Med Rehabil* 1988; **69**(11):923–927.

53 **Chancellor MB, Blaivas JG.** Multiple sclerosis and diabetic neurogenic bladder. In: Blaivas JG, Chancellor MB, eds. *Atlas of Urodynamics* 1st edn, vol 1, 1995, 187–189.

54 **Wheeler JS, Siroky MB, Pavlakis AJ et al.** The changing neurourologic pattern of multiple sclerosis. *J Urol* 1983; **130**:1123–1126.

55 **Blaivas JG, Sinha HP, Zayed AA, Labib KB.** Detrusor external sphincter dyssynergia. *J Urol* 1981; **125**:542–544.

56 **Dibenedetto M, Yalla SV.** Electrodiagnosis of striated urethral sphincter dysfunction. *J Urol* 1978; **122**:361–365.

57 **McGuire EJ, Fitzpatrick CC, Wan J et al.** Clinical assessment of urethral sphincteric function. *J Urol* 1993; **150**:1452–1454.

58 **McGuire EJ, Gormley AE.** Clinical assessment of urethral sphincter and conduit function by measurement of abdominal and detrusor pressures required to induce leakage. In: Raz S, ed. *Female Urology* 2nd edn. Philadelphia: WB Saunders, 1996, 106–114.

59 **Swift SE, Ostergard DR.** Evaluation of current urodynamic testing methods in the diagnosis of genuine stress incontinence. *Obstet Gynecol* 1995; **86**:85–91.

60 **Horbach N, Ostergard DR.** Predicting intrinsic sphincteric dysfunction in women with stress urinary incontinence. *Obstet Gynecol* 1994; **84**:188–192.

61 **Miklos JR, Sze EH, Karram MM.** A critical appraisal of the methods of measuring leak point pressures in women with stress incontinence. *Obstet Gynecol* 1995; **86**:349–352.

62 **Miller H, Simpson CA, Yeates WK.** Bladder dysfunction in multiple sclerosis. *Br Med J* 1965; **1**:1265–1269.

63 **Hebjorn S.** Treatment of detrusor hyperreflexia in multiple sclerosis: a double blind crossover clinical trial comparing methantheline bromide (Banthine), flavoxate chloride (Urispas) and meladrazine tartarate (Lisidonil). *Urol Int* 1977; **32**:209.

64 **Rabey JM, Moriel EZ, Farkas A et al.** Detrusor hyperreflexia in multiple sclerosis, alleviation by combination of imipramine and propantheline, a clinico-laboratory study. *Eur Neurol* 1979; **18**:33–37.

65 **Schoenberg HW, Gutrich JM.** Management of vesical dysfunction in multiple sclerosis: the role of drug therapy. *Urology* 1980; **16**:444.

66 **Awad SA, Wilson JW, Fenmore J, Kiruluta HG.** Dysfunction of the detrusor and urethra in multiple sclerosis: the role of drug therapy. *Can J Surg* 1982; **25**:259.

67 **Blaivas JG, Kaplan SA.** Urologic dysfunction in patients with multiple sclerosis. *Semin Neurol* 1988; **8**:159–165.

68 **Wein AJ.** Pharmacologic approaches to the management of bladder dysfunction. *J Continuing UC Ed Urol* 1979; **18**:17.

69 **Diokno AC, Lapides J.** Oxybutynin: a new drug with analgesic and anticholinergic properties. *J Urol* 1972; **108**:307–309.

70 **Thompson IM, Lauvetz R.** Oxybutynin in bladder spasms, neurogenic bladder and eneuresis. *Urol* 1976; **8**:452–454.

71 **Brooks ME, Braf ZF.** Oxybutynin chloride (ditropan) clinical uses and applications. *Paraplegia* 1980; **18**:64–68.

72 **Moisey CU, Stephenson TP, Brendler CB.** The urodynamic and subjective results of treatment of detrusor instability with oxybutynin chloride. *Br J Urol* 1980; **52**:472–475.

73 **Thuroff JW, Bunke B, Ebner A et al.** Randomized, double blind multi center trial on the treatment of frequency, urgency, and incontinence related to detrusor hyperactivity: oxybutynin versus propantheline versus placebo. *J Urol* 1991; **145**:813–817.

74 **Tapp AJ, Cardozo LD, Versi D, Cooper D.** The treatment of detrusor instability in post menopausal women with oxybutynin hydrochloride, a double

blind placebo controlled study. *Br J Obstet Gynecol* 1990; **97**:521.

75 Fowler CJ, Van Kerrebroek EV, Nordenbo A, Van Poppel H. Treatment of lower urinary tract dysfunction in patients with multiple sclerosis. *J Neurol* 1992; **55**:986–989.

76 Nilvebrant L, Hallen B, Larsson G. Tolterodine—a new bladder selective muscarinic receptor antagonist: preclinical pharmacological and clinical data. *Life Sci* 1997; **60**:1129–1136.

77 Jonas U, Hofner K, Madersbacher H, Holmdhal TH. Efficacy and safety of two doses of tolterodine versus placebo in patients with detrusor over activity and symptoms of frequency, urge incontinence and urgency: urodynamic evaluation. *World J Urol* 1997; **15**:144–151.

78 Madersbacher H, Jilg G. Control of detrusor hyperreflexia by the intravesical instillation of oxybutyin hydrochloride. *Paraplegia* 1991; **28**:84–90.

79 Greenfield SP, Fera M. Intravesical oxybutynin in children with neurogenic bladder. *J Urol* 1991; **146**:532–534.

80 Mohler JL. Relaxation of intestinal bladders by intravesical oxybutynin chloride. *Neurourol Urodynamics* 1990; **9**:179–182.

81 Brendler CB, Radebaugh LC, Mohler JL. Topical oxybutynin chloride for relaxation of dysfunctional bladders. *J Urol* 1989; **141**:350–352

82 Higson RH, Smith JC, Hills W. Intravesical lidocaine and detrusor instability. *Br J Urol* 1979; **51**:500–503.

83 Mattiasson A, Ekstrom B, Anderson KE. Effects of intravesical instillation of verapamil into patients with detrusor hyperactivity. *Neurourol Urodynamics* 1987; **6**:253–256.

84 Weese DL, Rosenkamp DA, Zimmern PE. Intravesical oxybutynin: experience with 42 patients, *Urology* 1993; **41**:527–530.

85 Sharkey KA, Williams RG, Schultzberg WM, Dockray GJ. Sensory substance P-innervation of the urinary bladder: possible site of action of capsaicin in causing urinary retention in rats. *Neuroscience* 1983; **10**:861–868.

86 Szallasi A, Blumberg P. Resiniferatoxin and its analogs provide novel insights into the pharmacology of the vanilloid (capsaicin) receptor. *Life Sci* 1990; **47**:1399–408.

87 Maggi CA, Barbanti G, Santiciolici P et al. Cystometric evidence that capsaicin sensitive nerves modulate the afferent branch of the micturition reflex in humans. *J Urol* 1989; **142**:150–154.

88 De Ridder D, Chandiramani V, Dasgupta P et al. Intravesical capsaicin as a treatment for refractory detrusor hyperreflexia: a dual center study with long term follow up. *J Urol* 1997; **158**:2087–2092.

89 Fowler CJ, Beck RO, Gerrerd S et al. Intravesical capsaicin for the treatment of detrusor hyperreflexia. *J Neurol Neurosurg Psychiatry* 1994; **57**:169–173.

90 Fowler CJ, Jewkes D, McDonald WI et al. Intravesical capsaicin for neurogenic bladder dysfunction. *Lancet* 1992; **339**:1239.

91 Lazzeri M, Beneforti P, Turini D. Urodynamic effects of intravesical resiniferatoxin in humans: preliminary results in stable and unstable detrusor. *J Urol* 1997; **158**:2093–2096.

92 Hilton P, Hertogs K, Stanton SL. The use of desmopressin for nocturia in women with multiple sclerosis. *J Neurol Neurosurg Psychiatry* 1983; **46**:854–855.

93 Kinn AC, Larsson PO. Desmopressin: a new principle for symptomatic treatment of urgency and incontinence in patients with multiple sclerosis. *Scand J Urol Nephrol* 1990; **24**:109–112.

94 Eckford SD, Carter PG, Jackson SR et al. An open in-patient incremental safety study of desmopressin in women with multiple sclerosis and nocturia study. *Br J Urol* 1995; **76**:459–463.

95 Valiquette G, Herbert J, D'Alisera PM. Desmopressin in the management of nocturia in patients with multiple sclerosis. *Arch Neurol* 1996; **53**:1270–1275.

96 Nordling J. Alpha blockers and urethral pressure in neurological patients. *Urol Int* 1978; **33**:304–309.

97 O'Roirdan JI, Doherty C, Javed M et al. Do alpha blockers have a role in lower urinary tract dysfunction in multiple sclerosis? *J Urol* 1995; **153**:1114–1116.

98 Kornhuber HH, Schutz A. Efficient treatment of neurogenic bladder disorders in multiple sclerosis with intermittent catheterization and ultrasound controlled training. *Eur Neurol* 1990; **30**:260–267.

99 Schwartz SL, Kennelly MJ, McGuire EJ, Faerber GJ. Incontinent ileo-vesicostomy urinary diversion in the treatment of lower urinary tract dysfunction. *J Urol* 1994; **152**:99–102.

100 Juma S, Niku SD, Brodak PP, Joseph AC. Urolume urethral wallstent in the treatment of detrusor sphincter dyssynergia. *Paraplegia* 1994; **32**:616–621.

101 Sauerwein D, Gross AJ, Kutzenberger J, Ringert RH. Wallstents in patients with detrusor sphincter

dyssynergia. *J Urol* 1995; **154**:495–497.

102 Maruf NJ, Godec CJ, Strom RL et al. Unusual therapeutic response of massive squamous cell carcinoma of the bladder to aggressive radiation and surgery. *J Urol* 1982; **128**:1313–1315.

103 Broecher BH, Klein FA, Hackler RH. Cancer of the bladder in spinal cord injury patients. *J Urol* 1981; **125**:196–197.

104 Bejany EC, Lockhart JL, Rhamy RK. Malignant vesical tumors following spinal cord injury. *J Urol* 1987; **138**:1390–1392.

105 Haab F, Zimmern PE, Leach GE. Female stress incontinence due to intrinsic sphincteric deficiency: recognition and management. *J Urol* 1996; **156**:3–17.

106 Winters JC, Appell R. Periurethral injection of collagen in the treatment of intrinsic sphincteric deficiency in the female patient. In: Kluke C, Raz S, eds. *Evaluation and Treatment of the Incontinent Female Patient. The Urologic Clinics of North America* vol 22. Philadelphia: WB Saunders, 1995, 673–678.

107 Light JK, Pietro T. Alteration in detrusor behavior and the effect on renal function following insertion of the artificial urinary sphincter. *J Urol* 1986; **136**:632–635.

108 Lilius HG, Valtonen EJ, Wikstrom J. Sexual problems in patients suffering from multiple sclerosis. *J Chron Dis* 1976; **29**:643–647.

109 Vas CJ. Sexual impotence and some autonomic disturbances in men with multiple sclerosis. *Acta Neurol Scand* 1969; **45**:166–182.

110 Betts CD, Jones SJ, Fowler CG, Fowler CJ. Erectile dysfunction in multiple sclerosis: associated neurological deficits and treatment of the condition. *Brain* 1994; **117**:1303–1310.

111 Ghezzi A, Malvestii GM, Baldini S et al. Erectile impotence in multiple sclerosis: a neurophysiological study. *J Neurol* 1994; **242**:123–126.

112 Mattson D, Petrie M, Strivastava DK, McDermott M. Multiple sclerosis and its response to medications. *Arch Neurol* 1995; **52**:862–868.

113 Valleroy ML, Kraft GH. Sexual dysfunction in multiple sclerosis. *Arch Phys Med Rehabil* 1984; **65**:125–128.

114 Lundberg PO. Sexual dysfunction in patients with multiple sclerosis. *Sex Disabl* 1978; **1**:218–222.

115 Kirkeby HJ, Poulsen EU, Derup J. Erectile dysfunction in multiple sclerosis. *Neurology* 1988; **38**:1366–1374.

116 Heller L, Keren O, Aloni R, Davidoff G. An open

trial of vacuum penile tumescence constriction therapy for neurological impotence. *Paraplegia* 1992; **30**:550–553.

117 Hirsch JH, Smith RL, Chancellor MB et al. Use of intracavernous injection of prostaglandin E1 for neuropathic erectile dysfunction. *Paraplegia* 1994; **32**:661–664.

118 Ernst R, Pittler MH. Yohimbine for erectile dysfunction: a systematic review and meta-analysis of randomized clinical trials. *J Urol* 1998; **159**:433–436.

119 Teloken C, Rhoden EL, Sogari P et al. Therapeutic effects of high dose yohimbime hydrochloride on organic erectile dysfunction. *J Urol* 1998; **159**:122–124.

120 Montague DK, Barada JH, Belker A et al. Clinical guidelines on erectile dysfunction: summary report on the treatment of organic erectile dysfunction. *J Urol* 1996; **154**:1–5.

121 Derry F, Gardner BP, Glass C et al. Sildenafil (Viagra™): a double blind, placebo controlled single dose two way cross-over study in men with erectile dysfunction caused by traumatic spinal cord injury (abstract). *J Urol* 1997; **154**:181.

122 Goldstein I, Lue TF, Padma-Nathan H et al. Oral sildenafil in the treatment of erectile dysfunction. Sildenafil Study Group. *N Engl J Med* 1998; **338**:1397–1404.

123 Sonksen J, Biering-Sorensen F, Kristensen JK. Ejaculation induced by penile vibratory stimulation in men with spinal cord injuries. The importance of the vibratory amplitude. *Paraplegia* 1994; **32**:651–660.

124 Heller L, Keren O, Aloni R, Davidoff G. An open trial of vacuum penile tumescence: constriction therapy for neurological impotence. *Paraplegia* 1992; **30**:550–553.

125 Flynn RJ, Williams G. Longterm followup of patients with erectile dysfunction commenced on self injection with intracavernosal papaverine with or without phentolamine. *Br J Urol* 1996; **78**:628–631.

126 Weiss JN, Ravelli R, Brettschneider N, Badlani GH. Reasons for high dropout rate with self injection therapy for impotence. *J Urol* 1992; **147**:309A.

127 Massey EW, Pleet AB. Penile prosthesis for impotence in multiple sclerosis. *Ann Neurol* 1978; **5**:451–454.

128 Goldstein I, Newman L, Baum N et al. Safety and effecacy of Mentor alpha-1 inflatable penile

prosthesis implantation for impotence treatment. *J Urol* 1997; **157**:833–839.

129 **Randrup E, Wilson S, Mobley D et al.** Clinical experience with the Mentor alpha 1 inflatable penile prosthesis. *Urology* 1993; **42**:305–308.

130 **Sexton WJ, Benedict JF, Jarow JP.** Comparison of long term outcomes of penile prosthesis and intracavernosal injection therapy. *J Urol* 1998; **159**:811–815.

131 **Minderhound JM, Leemhuis JG, Kremer J et al.** Sexual disturbances arising from multiple sclerosis. *Acta Neurol Scand* 1984; **70**:299–306.

132 **Hudson WW, Harrison DF, Crosscup PC.** A short form scale to measure sexual dyscord in dyadic relationships. *J Sex Res* 1981; **17**:157–174.

133 **Langworthy OR.** Disturbances in micturition associated with disseminated sclerosis. *J Nerv Ment Dis* 1938; **88**:760–770.

37
Treatment of mood and affective disorders

Sarah L Minden

INTRODUCTION

Emotional disturbances are common in multiple sclerosis (MS).[1–4] They consist of disturbances of mood (which refers to a sustained and pervasive emotion that influences perception of self, others, and the world), such as depression, elation (mania), and anxiety, and disturbances of affect, which refers to more fluctuating changes in the outward expression of inner feeling states, and in which emotional expression may be blunted, flat, inappropriate, or labile.[5] The terms mood and affect are often used interchangeably, but differences between them are important and have etiologic, diagnostic, and treatment implications. The relationship between mood disorders (major depressive disorder, dysthymic disorder, bipolar disorder, panic disorder, and generalized anxiety disorder) and MS is multifactorial and complex, and the extent to which mood disorders are direct consequences of the disease process or psychological reactions to it remains unclear. Whatever their cause, mood disorders in MS are phenomenologically no different from mood disorders more generally, and they respond similarly to standard treatments. By contrast, disorders of affect (euphoria, pathological laughing and weeping, and other frontal lobe syndromes) result from the pathologic process in

MS, are among the characteristic symptoms of MS, and have implications for treatment that are similar to those for other aspects of the disease.

Although mood disorders can be diagnosed and treated effectively using customary psychiatric procedures, non-mental health-care providers too often fail to identify, diagnose, and treat them appropriately.[6–9] Patients and family members may have trouble acknowledging emotional difficulties, discussing them with health-care providers, and following recommendations for psychiatric consultation and treatment.[10] Although disorders of affect may be more obvious than disorders of mood, it can be difficult to distinguish them diagnostically. Effective treatments have been established only for pathological laughing and weeping; for people with euphoria and other frontal lobe syndromes, treatment consists mainly of providing education, coping strategies, and support.

Over the past 25 years there has been a major advance in the classification of mental disorders, primarily due to the establishment of explicit definitions of terms and diagnostic criteria. The current nomenclature, as outlined in the fourth edition of the American Psychiatric Association's *Diagnostic and Statistical Manual of Mental Disorders* (DSM-IV),[5] is neutral in regard to etiology and is based on empirical evidence collected with reliable and valid diagnostic tools (i.e. semi-structured interviews and symptom rating scales). A systematic approach and the use of accepted criteria should help practitioners reach an accurate diagnosis of mood disorders; treatment then follows logically from the diagnosis.[11]

The mental health field makes an important distinction between symptoms and disorders. Symptoms can be elicited through an unstructured clinical interview, through a semi-structured research interview such as the Schedule for Affective Disorders and Schizophrenia (SADS), the Structured Clinical Interview for DSM (SCID), the Diagnostic Interview Schedule (DIS), the Hamilton Rating Scale for Depression (HRSD), or through a symptom rating scale such as the Beck Depression Inventory (BDI), the General Health Questionnaire (GHQ), the Center for Epidemiologic Studies Depression Scale (CES-D), the Zung Self-Rating Depression Scale, and the Symptom Checklist (SCL-90). These scales can also indicate the intensity of the symptom(s). However, a mental disorder can be diagnosed only if specified criteria are met in regard to the number, duration, and intensity of symptoms and to their impact on functioning; symptoms must not be due to the direct physiological effects of a substance or a general medical condition, and they must not be better accounted for by a recent life event. Hence, in the words of DSM-IV (page xxi),[5] a mental disorder is 'a clinically significant behavioral or psychological syndrome or pattern that occurs in an individual and ... is associated with present distress (e.g. a painful symptom) or disability (i.e. impairment in one or more important areas of functioning) or with a significantly increased risk of suffering death, pain, disability, or an important loss of freedom ... [which is not] merely an expectable and culturally sanctioned response to a particular event, for example, the death of a loved one.'

Following this model, evaluation of a patient with an emotional disturbance begins with:

(a) identifying symptoms;

(b) determining their duration, intensity, and impact on functioning; and

(c) excluding alternative explanations such as physiological disturbances or life events.

For people with MS, it is necessary to distinguish between symptoms caused by a mood disorder and symptoms caused by MS, such as fatigue and diminished ability to think or concentrate. With this systematically acquired information, it becomes possible to decide whether criteria have been met for a particular mental disorder or whether the person is suffering various symptoms that do not currently meet those standards or from an MS-related disorder of affect. This diagnostic decision is critical since it determines treatment: once made, evidence-based and consensus-based practice guidelines are available to indicate the most effective pharmacologic and psychosocial interventions for virtually all mental disorders.[11] Therefore, this chapter describes the symptoms and diagnostic criteria for mood disorders and affective disturbances; the focus is on diagnostic decision making since treatments for mood disorders are virtually the same for people with and without MS, except for a few caveats in regard to minimizing potential adverse effects. It is expected that readers are familiar with accepted practices for treatment of mental disorders and that they routinely consult standard texts and the literature. Data from relevant epidemiologic and pathophysiological studies of mood and affective disorders in MS are also presented, treatment options are outlined, and implications for clinical practice and future research are discussed. DSM-IV diagnostic criteria for all disorders mentioned in this chapter are summarized in the glossary below.

MOOD DISORDERS

The mood disorders that are seen most commonly in MS are depressive disorders (major depressive disorder, dysthymic disorder, bipolar disorder) and generalized anxiety disorder. The literature contains reports of psychotic disorders, and people with MS may develop any of the other mental conditions in the nomenclature.

Major depressive disorder and dysthymic disorder

There are no population-based estimates of the prevalence of depressive disorders in MS, but investigators have estimated their prevalence from clinical samples. As a result of differences in definitions, instruments, and samples used, there is enormous variation. The prevalence rates for depression range from 6–57%, with rates of 10–54% for depression developing after the onset of MS.[1] Investigators who used more reliable, valid measurement techniques (i.e. semi-structured interviews) to determine whether patients met formal diagnostic criteria, estimated prevalence rates of major depressive disorder at 14%,[12] 22%,[13] 24%,[14] 34%,[15] 40%,[16] and 37%[17] and lifetime prevalence rates at 42%,[12] 50%,[18] and 54%.[15] The rate of major depression in one group of MS patients before the onset of their disease did not differ from the rate reported for a community sample with the same age distribution, but the rate after the onset of the MS was significantly higher than the age-adjusted lifetime rate for the community sample.[15,19] Lifetime rates of major depression or occurrence of depressive episodes have been shown to be higher in MS patients than in patients with general medical conditions,[15] other

chronic neurologic conditions[20] and in some (but not all[21]) groups of patients with chronic fatigue syndrome.[22] The rate of depression among a group of MS patients discharged from hospital was significantly higher than for non-MS hospital users.[23] Studies of the frequency of attempted and completed suicide suggest that rates are substantially higher for the MS population than for the general population.[23,24]

Depression rating scales have been used by many investigators to indicate the severity of depressive symptoms. Beck Depression Inventory mean scores were reported by different investigators to be 11.1 ($\pm$8.5),[12] 12.7 ($\pm$8.4),[15] and 22.03 ($\pm$11.4).[25] These were significantly higher than scores found in samples of patients with general medical conditions,[15,26] cancer,[15] and in normal controls.[27,28] Scores were not higher that those of patients with chronic fatigue syndrome,[27,29,30] spinal cord injury,[31] or motor neuron disease.[32]

Investigators have hypothesized that if depression is more prevalent or severe in people with MS than in people with other medical conditions, particularly non-central nervous system disabling disorders,[33,34] then it is less likely to be a psychological reaction to illness and more likely to be related to the disease process. To test this hypothesis, the relationship between depression and various disease parameters has been examined, but results are inconsistent and not conclusive. There were no observed correlations between depression and MS disease duration,[14,15,20,35] severity and type of disability,[14,15,35,36] cognitive impairment,[14,37–39] various magnetic resonance imaging (MRI) measures,[14,37–41] fatigue,[14] disease activity,[42] or course of illness.[14,15] Other investigators reported a significant correlation between depression and MS disease duration,[25] degree of neurological impairment,[20,25,31,32,43] progressive MS,[31,44] cognitive impairment,[31,36,44] enlargement of the ventricles,[31] lesions in the frontal and temporal lobes and paraventricular areas,[45] left hemisphere,[46] and left arcuate fasciculus region,[47] and regional cerebral blood flow asymmetries in the limbic cortex.[39] Associations have also been reported between depression and sleep disturbance,[48,49] fatigue,[50] relapses,[34,35,51] sexual dysfunction,[40] low melatonin secretion and circadian phase lability,[52] lower $CD8^+$ T-cell numbers and higher CD4:CD8 ratio, and higher $CD4^+$ T-cell numbers,[53] high plasma cortisol levels but normal responses to provocative tests of hypothalamic–pituitary–adrenal axis function,[54] and failure to suppress cortisol release after dexamethasone challenge.[55] There appears to be no higher risk of depression among first-degree relatives of depressed MS patients, making a genetic susceptibility to depression unlikely.[12,15,18] Suicide in male MS patients has been associated with age (40–49 years), previous suicidal behavior and mental disorder, recent worsening of MS, and moderate disability; risk factors were less clear for women, but for all patients a more severe disease course was associated with higher risk.[56]

Bipolar disorder

The literature contains case reports of mania in patients with MS,[57–63] and three studies found the rate of bipolar disorder to be significantly higher in MS patients than in the general population.[12,23,64] Some investigators have suggested a genetic relationship between these disorders on the basis of findings of familial clustering of MS and bipolar disorder and certain major histocompatibility class II markers.[65,66] Hypomania and

mania may be precipitated by corticotropin and prednisone, primarily with higher doses and particularly in patients with a previous history of depression and a family history of depression or alcoholism.[67,68]

Anxiety disorders

There are fewer studies of anxiety than depression in MS. Noy and colleagues[35] found that the rate of anxiety was higher than the rate of depression (90% versus 50%) among 20 patients with relapsing–remitting MS; anxiety was associated with disease activity but not with disease duration or severity. Stenager and colleagues[69] reported elevated scores on measures of both state anxiety (i.e. anxiety at the time of assessment) and trait anxiety (i.e. anxiety as an enduring characteristic) in a sample of MS patients; anxiety correlated significantly with neurologic disability but not with disease course or cognitive impairment. Indeed, this group of researchers and others observed that it is the moderately disabled patients who are the most anxious and most depressed, who are at highest risk of suicide, and who are most likely to have difficulty carrying out usual social roles[70] and maintaining leisure activities.[69–72] Panic attacks have also been reported in MS.[73,74]

Adjustment disorders

People with MS develop adjustment disorders with depressed or anxious mood, or both. There are no systematic studies of these disorders, but clinical experience suggests that they tend to occur at characteristic times, namely in association with diagnosis, exacerbations, and significant changes in clinical status that require use of an ambulatory aid. They also occur in response to MS-related life events, namely withdrawal from the labor force, dissolution of a marriage, and entry into a long-term care facility. Several studies have explored how people with MS adjust to and cope with their illness, and these studies have identified factors associated with successful or unsuccessful coping.[25,43,75–79] Patients who are hospitalized for an exacerbation reported that the most disturbing aspects were fatigue, inability to walk, and uncertainty about the future. They coped primarily by using self-reliance and humor, and by trying to learn more about their disease. Optimistic coping was associated with less depression.[80] People with MS use coping strategies that are similar in type and effectiveness to those used by normal controls, and they modify their coping strategies to deal with different types of stressors.[81] Depression has been associated with illness representations,[82] perceived uncertainty, and perceived unsupportiveness of social network interactions.[83] Past performance was the best predictor of ability to control mood and maintain social activity; self-efficacy and disability level also contributed.[84]

AFFECTIVE DISORDERS

Pathological laughing and weeping

Estimates of the prevalence of pathological laughing and weeping in MS are highly variable—7%,[85] 10%,[86] 51%,[87] 79%,[88] 95%[89] —as a result of different definitions, incommensurate samples, and variable evaluation methods. In a recent study, Feinstein and colleagues[9] discussed the diagnostic problems that arise from the absence of a systematic definition: imprecise

terminology (e.g. 'pseudobulbar affect,' 'emotional dyscontrol,' 'emotional incontinence,' 'excessive emotionality,' and 'emotionalism') and lumping together of patients with different problems (e.g. those with difficulty controlling facial musculature who have displays of crying without subjective feelings of sadness and those who are depressed and have bouts of crying that appear excessive). Using explicit criteria (sudden loss of emotional control (crying or laughing or both) on multiple occasions over 1 month that occurs in response to nonspecific stimuli and lacks an associative, matching mood state)[91] and a validated rating scale (the Pathological Laughing and Crying Scale[92]), they estimated a prevalence rate of 10%. The disorder was related to chronic progressive MS, greater intellectual impairment and physical disability, and longer duration compared to controls, but not to relapse, depression or anxiety scale scores, or pre-morbid or family history of mental illness.[90] Pathological laughing and weeping has been associated with diffuse, bilateral cerebral disease,[93–95] which is presumed to interrupt corticobulbar tracts involved in control of emotional expression,[92] right hemisphere damage,[96] and lesions in the pons or connectons between the middle right cerebral hemispheres and the pons.[97,98]

Euphoria

Euphoria is different from both pathological laughing and mania. Whereas pathological laughing refers to outbursts of laughter without an underlying joyous mood state and mania describes an elated mood with hyperactivity, pressured speech, and racing thoughts, euphoria is a sustained 'mental state of cheerfulness, happiness, [and] ease' in which patients appear 'serene and cheerful,' report feeling physically fit and healthy, and display 'an optimism as to the future and the prospects of ultimate recovery which is out of place and incongruous.'[89] Euphoria is not an episodic emotional expression like pathological laughing or a reversible mood like mania. It is a persistent frame of mind or outlook, perhaps best characterized as a permanent change in personality. Patients with euphoria are different from the way they had been; and there is an apparent disconnection between their intellectual understanding of their condition and the emotional response that one would expect to accompany it. Note, however, that investigators who explored underlying feeling states more closely found significant unhappiness and depression in patients with euphoria.[86,88]

Prevalence rates for euphoria are highly variable—0,[99] 5%,[100] 7%,[87] 10%,[101] 13%,[85] 26%,[86] 48%,[31] 54%,[88] 63%[89]—again resulting from differences in assessment methods and in severity and duration of illness across samples.

Euphoria is a neurologically-based emotional state, the result of the pathologic process in the brain. Euphoric MS patients are more likely to have brain involvement, progressive MS, enlarged ventricles, and more cognitive impairment than non-euphoric MS patients.[31] In one study relapsing–progressive patients with euphoria had significantly larger lesions in the parietal region and relatively smaller lesions in the temporal region than relapsing–remitting patients. Among patients with combined euphoria and depression, relapsing–progressive patients had larger lesions in the parietal and occipital areas and relapsing–remitting patients had larger lesions in the temporal area.[102]

Psychotic and organic mental disorders

Psychiatric nomenclature clearly distinguishes mood from psychotic disorders (schizophrenia, schizoaffective disorder, delusional disorder, brief psychotic disorder, and psychotic disorders resulting from a general medical condition, medication, drug of abuse, or toxin exposure). A distinction is also made between mood disorders and what formerly were called 'organic mental disorders', now classified under the rubric 'delirium, dementia, and amnestic and other cognitive disorders.'[5] People with MS are at no higher risk of schizophrenia and schizoaffective disorder than the general population, but case reports describe delusions and other psychotic symptoms. It is sometimes difficult to determine from these reports whether patients were psychotic or had one of the affective disorders, dementia, or delirium.[58,103–107] Clinically, these disorders should be distinguished with a careful mental status examination since treatment approaches are different.

TREATMENT OPTIONS

The three stages of successful management are:
1 Make the correct diagnosis
2 Select the appropriate treatment
3 Consult with and refer to specialists

Making the correct diagnosis

Effective treatment depends above all else on an accurate diagnosis. For people with MS, diagnostic decision making should proceed as indicated in *Fig. 37.1*.

Conflicting results from studies of depressive

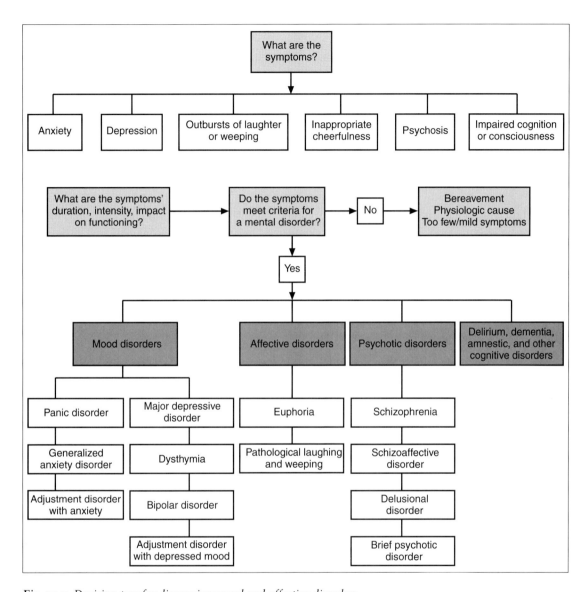

Fig. 37.1 *Decision-tree for diagnosing mood and affective disorders*

disorders should not be discouraging. Rather, they support our current understanding of mood disorders as being heterogeneous in regard to symptoms, course, outcomes, and etiolo-gies.[108,109] With the wide array of efficacious treatment options now available, the clinical focus should be on identifying symptoms, making the correct diagnosis, providing appropriate treatment, and closely monitoring the response to therapy.

When clinicians talk empathically and listen carefully to their patients, it is not difficult to elicit symptoms of emotional distress. Further inquiry will determine precipitants, associated symptoms, and whether the duration, intensity, and impact of the symptoms meet criteria for a mental disorder. A review of systems, physical examination, and laboratory assessment will rule out medical conditions that mimic or are associated with abnormal mood states (e.g. thyroid or other endocrine disorders, malignancy, and autoimmune disease) and the use of medications or substances (i.e. alcohol and drug intoxication or withdrawal) that could produce these symptoms.

Distinction must be made between mood disorders and normal or expected responses to life experiences. Grief over the loss of a loved person, the ability to carry out desired activities or a sense of oneself as whole and intact involves sadness and affects appetite, sleep, and concentration. Major depression and dysthymia can be distinguished from grief by the intensity of the symptoms and their failure to diminish over time. While grief always has a precipitant, major depression and dysthymia may or may not be related to life events. Loss of interest in formerly pleasurable activities and diminished capacity for enjoyment occur in both grief and depression but are far more characteristic of depressive states. Grief does not involve loss of self-esteem, pessimism, self-reproach or suicidal thoughts, unlike depression.

In all patients, but particularly the elderly and those with neurological conditions such as MS, care must be taken to assess the true import of 'diminished ability to think or concentrate' or of 'indecisiveness.' Pseudodementia of depression

(i.e. reversible cognitive deficits secondary to depressive illness) has been well-described[110] but must be distinguished from the irreversible cognitive deficits commonly found in people with MS. Ultimately, the only reliable 'test' is that depression-related deficits will resolve with treatment and MS-related deficits will not.

The presence of various risk factors makes the diagnosis of a mood disorder more likely than not. These factors include family history of the disorder, including alcoholism for major depressive disorder, and previous episodes of mood disorder. Affective disorders are associated with longer duration of illness, progressive course, and high lesion load, particularly in frontal areas.

Screening instruments such as the Beck Depression Inventory (BDI) or the Symptom Checklist (SCL-90) are useful, but the overlap between MS and certain depressive symptoms may falsely inflate the scores.[111] For example, Mohr and colleagues[28] found that items that measure work difficulty, fatigue, and concerns about health contributed significantly more to total BDI scores in patients with MS than in patients with major depression and normal controls, and they recommended eliminating these three confounding items from the scale. Minden and colleagues[15] reported psychological and somatic scores as well as total scores to separate items that could be confounded by physical symptoms from purely psychological ones. These authors also recommended eliminating confounding items such as fatigue and slowed thinking from formal diagnostic criteria. Rating scales, in general, 'have unduly low positive predictive power for purposes of generating a diagnosis. However, high-scoring patients should be given a more thorough clinical assessment to ascertain whether they are true or false positives for depression.'[8]

Selecting the appropriate treatment

Major depressive disorder and dysthymia

In general, combined psychotherapy and pharmacotherapy is more effective than either modality alone for treatment of depressive disorders (or, indeed, any mental disorder).[112] Anti-depressants, including heterocyclics and tricyclics (TCAs), monoamine oxidase inhibitors (MAOIs), and selective serotonin reuptake inhibitors (SSRIs), provide effective treatment for both major depressive disorder and dysthymia.[108,109] Depression occurs in many neurologic disorders in which pharmacologic treatments have been shown to be safe and efficacious.[113] Individual and group psychotherapy are particularly useful in helping patients to adjust to MS and in minimizing the sequelae of depressive disorders. They are also effective treatments for problems in living and personality issues that are unrelated to MS.[114]

There are few systematic studies of pharmacologic treatment of depression in MS. Schiffer and Wineman[115] conducted a double-blind, placebo-controlled trial of desipramine in 28 patients with MS and major depressive disorder and found significantly greater improvement as assessed by clinical judgment and scores from the Hamilton Rating Scale for Depression. Unfortunately, almost 40% of patients experienced side effects with doses of 125 mg per day or higher. Scott and colleagues[42] conducted a retrospective review of affective disturbances in 238 MS patients seen over a 6-month period. they found that 22% received pharmacologic treatment for depressive symptoms during the 6 months or within 4 years and that 7% received treatment for rapid mood swings. Therapeutic response to medication was high, and side effects were tolerable; the relapse rate for depressive symptomatology after discontinuing medication was 59%.

The same group conducted an open-label trial[116] of sertraline 100 mg per day in 11 patients with MS. One patient discontinued treatment because of perceived lack of efficacy; the remainder continued for at least 3 months, showed significant improvement in depressive symptoms on the Carroll Scale, and had no side effects.

Clinical experience suggests that any of the currently available anti-depressants are effective in treating depressive disorders in people with MS. Side effects are the same for people with MS as for other patients, although they may occur at lower doses and anti-cholinergic side effects of urinary retention, blurred vision, and dry mouth may be more problematic. The clinician should assume, even without systematic study, that people with MS will be more vulnerable to such symptoms, and that consequences may be more profound (e.g. urinary tract infection and tremors). SSRIs, unlike TCAs, tend not to have these problems and, clinically, they appear to be safe and effective for people with MS at standard doses. The dietary restrictions, potential drug interactions, and wide range of serious and discomforting adverse effects of MAOIs make them poor candidates for use in MS. Readers should refer to standard psychopharmacology texts and the literature for discussions of available medications, dosages, and adverse effects.[117] *Table 37.1* lists the more commonly used anti-depressants, their potential for sedation and anti-cholinergic effects, and the dosages recommended by one group of experts.

A general approach to pharmacologic treatment of depression in a person with MS is outlined in *Table 37.2*. The basic elements of this approach—careful evaluation and diagnosis, thoughtful patient-specific selection of medication, careful monitoring, and a strong

Table 37.1 Commonly used anti-depressants[118]

Generic name	Sedative effect	Anti-cholinergic effect	Initial daily dose	Usual therapeutic dose
Amitriptyline	High	High	25–75 mg	150–300 mg
Imipramine	Moderate	High	25–75 mg	150–300 mg
Doxepin	High	High	25–75 mg	150–300 mg
Nortiptyline	Moderate	Moderate	20–40 mg	75–150 mg
Desipramine	Low	Low	25–75 mg	75–200 mg
Protriptyline	Low	Low	10–20 mg	20–60 mg
Trimipramine	High	High	25–75 mg	75–300 mg
Amoxapine	Moderate	Moderate	50–150 mg	150–600 mg
Maprotiline	Moderate	Moderate	25–75 mg	75–225 mg
Trazadone	High	Very low	50–100 mg	150–600 mg
Fluoxetine	Low	Very low	20 mg	20 mg
Bupropion	Low	Very low	75 mg tid or 100 mg bid	450 mg
Sertraline	Moderate	Very low	25–50 mg	50–250 mg
Paroxetine	Low	Very low	20 mg	50 mg
Fluvoxamine	Low	Very low	50 mg	100–300 mg
Nefazadone	Low	Very low	100 mg bid	200–600 mg
Venlafaxine	Low	Very low	75 mg	75–225 mg

patient–doctor relationship—apply as well to treatment of anxiety and other mood disorders and are not be repeated in those sections.

Psychotherapy is an important component of treatment. Schiffer described four interpersonal management strategies that non-psychiatric physicians can use in treating depressed MS patients.[119] Crawford and McIvor[120] found that patients in insight-oriented group psy-chotherapy were significantly less depressed than patients in a current events group and patients who had no treatment. Participation in the struc-tured current events group itself alone resulted in an improvement in emotional state compared to no treatment. Other kinds of group thera-pies[121,122] and individual and group cognitive behavioral therapy are also helpful.[123,124]

Whether the physician who treats the MS

Table 37.2 Approach to the pharmacologic treatment of depression[120]

1   Take a thorough medical history and perform a thorough examination (including cardiac history and examination), review organ systems and current medication, and take a psychiatric history regarding past episodes, treatments, and responses (including adverse reactions).

2   Choose a drug based on the following considerations: least problematic adverse effects and interactions (i.e. cardiovascular, anti-cholinergic, sedation) given the patient's age, medical history, clinical status, and other medications; desirable effects such as sedation for an agitated patient; a drug that was previously effective for the patient or a family member. The SSRIs (fluoxetine, sertraline, paroxetine) are typically tried first for mild to moderately severe depression, then venlafaxine and nefazodone, with buproprion reserved for later trials because of an increased risk of seizures. TCAs (especially the secondary amines nortriptyline and desipramine) are also used as first-line agents for people with previous positive responses and for severe depressions, but because even they may not be well tolerated and can be lethal in overdose, clinicians tend to prefer to start with an SSRI.

3   Talk with the patient and family members about the recommended treatment and the rationale, risks and benefits, alternatives, and possible adverse effects; establish rapport and engage patient and family in a collaborative treatment process.

4   Develop a plan to monitor effects closely and to provide support and reassurance (e.g. access to physician by telephone to answer questions about effects; regular weekly contact by phone or in person for the first several weeks, then monthly in-person contact for several months until stabilized, followed by second-monthly visits; steady state blood levels for TCAs after dosage changes).

5   Begin with the lowest possible dose and increase very slowly to minimize adverse effects. Advise patients that it takes several weeks to achieve therapeutic levels of almost all antidepressants and several weeks thereafter to achieve full anti-depressant effect. Tailor the dosage to each patient: there is considerable variation among patients in their sensitivity and responsiveness to anti-depressants with some requiring doses much lower and others requiring doses much higher than standard regimens.

6   Monitor for adverse effects caused by drug interactions: additive adverse effects such as sedation, stimulation, and sexual dysfunction; potentially fatal interactions with MAOIs; changes in concentrations of either the anti-depressant or the other medication(s) resulting from inhibition or induction of hepatic enzyme systems or effects on absorption, distribution, and biotransformation.

7   Assess the patient regularly for suicidal ideas and take precautions regarding availability of medications, particularly those that are life threatening when taken in an overdose.

8   Monitor the patient for response to treatment. Talk with the patient and family about treatment with any anti-depressant being a 'trial': if one does not work, another should, but all of them usually take several weeks to be effective. While some patients may notice a partial response after 1 week, most do not experience the full effect for 6–8 weeks.

9   The goal should be complete remission of an acute depression: if the dose has been gradually increased to the maximum (perhaps higher in consultation with a psychopharmacologist) and there has been no response after 4–5 weeks, incomplete response after 6–8 weeks, or intolerable side effects, then another drug should be tried. Sometimes combinations of drugs or adjunctive treatment with lithium or tri-iodothyronine are used, but this should probably be tried only after consultation with a specialist.

10 Once effective, treatment should be continued for about 6 months and then re-evaluated. Some patients may do well on lower doses, others may continue free of depression if the drug is gradually tapered off and discontinued, while still others may need ongoing treatment at the same dose. With SSRIs, some patients reach a plateau and need an increase in dose. Between 70 and 85% of patients with depression have a recurrent course and may need treatment reinstated; if recurrences are frequent, ongoing treatment may be indicated.

should also provide psychotherapy depends on several factors, primarily the physician's interest and skill, the severity and complexity of the patient's problems, and the patient's preference.[114] Regardless of who provides psychotherapy or who manages anti-depressant medication, a strong and consistent relationship between the patient and family and the MS physician is key to successful management of mood and affective disorders. Patients and family members should feel comfortable and secure enough with their MS physician to talk openly about the stresses associated with the MS and to seek help for painful and disruptive emotional symptoms. Physicians should know their patients well enough to detect subtle changes in mood and to offer counsel and assistance. They should talk frankly with their patients about referrals to mental health professionals for consultation and treatment, being sensitive to concerns that people have that they are being 'got rid of' or considered 'crazy'. Physicians can help patients to recognize that referral to a mental health provider is intended to provide them with the best possible care by being clear about the reasons for the referral, by addressing patients' concerns directly, and by telling patients what they may expect at the initial visit and over the long term. When mental health professionals become involved in the patient's care, close communication between them and the primary physician is essential.[114,125]

Bipolar disorder

There have been no systematic studies of treatment of bipolar disorder in MS. In two reported cases, lithium carbonate was as effective for mania in MS patients as it was in non-MS patients, but in a third, it was not.[57,59,63] Lithium has also been used successfully to prevent psychiatric reactions to corticotropin.[126] There is no reason to believe that other treatments, including carbamezapine, valproic acid, and lamotragine, would not be effective in people with MS. MS physicians are advised to consult with a psychiatrist for assessment, diagnosis, and assistance with the long-term management of patients with bipolar disorder.

Anxiety disorders

There are even fewer studies of treatment of anxiety disorders in MS. In one case report, an MS patient with panic attacks during a depressive episode was treated effectively with clonazepam and chlormipramene.[73] There are, however, reports of making MS symptoms worse with psychotropic medications.[73,127,128] As with depression, MS patients with generalized anxiety disorder or panic disorder have been treated effectively with a combination of psychotherapy and medication. For generalized anxiety disorder, the many available benzodiazepines, buspirone, and the SSRIs are effective (*Table 37.3*).[129] Barbiturates (e.g. phenobarbital) and propanediols (e.g. meprobamate) are no longer indicated for the treatment of anxiety, and anti-histamines (e.g. hydroxyzine) should be used only for persons at risk of addiction to benzodiazepines (i.e. those with a history of dependence on alcohol, sedative–hypnotics, opiates or cocaine). When used in therapeutic doses for short-term treatment (less than a few weeks), the benzodiazepines provide significant relief from painful symptoms and are not associated with dependence. They are of particular value in helping people cope with a life crisis such as the diagnosis of MS. Long-term treatment (more than a few months) produces tolerance and withdrawal symptoms upon discontinuation but may be necessary for patients with generalized anxiety

Table 37.3 Medications used to treat generalized anxiety disorder[130,131]

Generic name	Usual dose	Half-life
Alprazolam	0.25–0.5 mg tid	Short
Chlordiazepoxide	5–10 mg tid or qid	Long (30–200 hours)
Clonazepam	0.5 mg bid or tid	Long (18–50 hours)
Clorazepate	15–30 mg/day	Long (30–200 hours)
Diazepam	2–10 mg bid, tid or qid	Long (30–200 hours)
Halazepam	20–40 mg tid or qid	Long (30–200 hours)
Lorazepam	1 mg bid or tid	Short (10–20 hours)
Oxazepam	10–15 mg tid or qid	Short
Prazepam	30–60 mg/day	Long (30–200 hours)
Buspirone	5–20 mg tid	Not applicable
Hydroxyzine	50–100 mg qid	Not applicable

disorder, social phobia, or panic disorder. Withdrawal generally occurs with high doses for long periods of time, but can occur after a relatively brief period of use with the short-acting agents.

Buspirone is not sedating, does not affect arousal, attention, or reaction time, and does not lead to abuse, tolerance, or withdrawal. However, it takes 2–4 weeks to work and many patients discontinue use before it becomes effective. Studies have shown trazadone and imipramine to be efficacious in treating generalized anxiety, and clinicians are increasingly using the SSRIs as well.

Panic disorder in people with MS responds to standard treatments including the benzodiazepines, certain anti-depressants (imipramine, clomipramine, fluoxetine, sertraline, and paroxetine) and the MAOIs. Other anti-depressants may cause a paradoxical activation and increase anxiety, panic, and sleeplessness. The major advantage of the anti-depressants is that they can treat co-existing depression, are taken once per day, have no addictive or abuse potential, and do not produce withdrawal symptoms. The anti-depressants are prescribed at the same starting doses and increased to the same maintenance doses as for depression (see *Table 37.1*). Alprazolam (starting at 0.25 mg qid and increasing to 0.5–2.0 mg qid), clonazepam (starting at 0.25–0.5 mg bid and increasing to 1–4 mg bid), and lorazepam (starting at 0.5 mg qid and increasing to 1–4 mg qid) have also been used for panic disorder.[129]

As with all mood disorders, physiological causes of anxiety should be ruled out; such causes include endocrine, metabolic, cardiovascular, and respiratory disorders, and intoxication with or withdrawal from medications and other substances.

Pathological laughing and weeping

Schiffer and colleagues[130] conducted a double-blind, cross-over study that compared amitriptyline and placebo in 12 patients with pathological laughing and weeping. Eight patients improved dramatically on an average dose of 57.8 mg/day (maximum dose 75 mg/day). Improvement was unrelated to change in concurrent measurements of mood. There are reports of levodopa being effective[132,133] as well as desipramine[91] and fluoxetine[134] in other patient groups. Fluvoxamine 100 mg at bed time was used successfully to treat emotional lability/incontinence in 10 patients with amyotrophic lateral sclerosis, MS, and stroke; within 2–6 days the number of emotional outbursts dropped from more than 30 per day to between none and five per day.[135] In addition to medication, it is important to explain the nature of this syndrome to patients and families to help them cope with it.

Euphoria

There is no known treatment for euphoria. However, explaining the condition to family members and caregivers can enhance their understanding and their capacity for empathy and support for the person with MS.

Other treatments

Sandyk[52] reported that extracerebral applications of pulsed electromagnetic fields in the pico tesla range improved depression and suicidal behavior in three patients, an effect that was presumably mediated by augmentation of serotonin neurotransmission and resynchronization of circadian melatonin secretion.[136–138] Lithium or bright light therapy may also be effective through mechanisms related to melatonin secretion and circadian phase lability.[52]

Garland and Zis[139] reported two cases to illustrate the difficulties in distinguishing organic and functional illness and suggested that anti-inflammatory agents may be required to manage acute psychiatric symptoms, in spite of the risk of precipitating psychosis.

Consultation with and referral to specialists

Consultation with a psychiatrist is advisable for patients whose diagnoses are not clear-cut, whose symptoms are severe, disruptive, or life-threatening, and who do not respond to standard treatments and usual doses. The psychiatrist may evaluate the patient and make recommendations for treatment that is then carried out by the primary care physician or neurologist. Alternatively, the psychiatrist may assume responsibility for treating the mental disorder, either alone, or in combination with a non-physician mental-health practitioner (e.g. a psychologist, social worker, or psychiatric nurse). As discussed above, patients and family members should be active participants in the treatment process. They should be made aware of the reasons for the consultation, informed about what will happen, and advised of the results. They should participate fully in decision making about what the treatment will entail and who will provide care. The better the communication among the referring physician, the psychiatrist and other mental health caregivers, and the patient and family, the better the results in treating mood and affective disorders in MS.

IMPLICATIONS FOR PRACTICE

The literature suggests that people with MS are not adequately treated for their mood disorders.

Minden and colleagues[15] found that although 40 out of a sample of 50 patients met diagnostic criteria for major depression in the preceding year, only 24 received some sort of psychiatric treatment. Moreover, many of the treatments were not appropriate for the disorder.

Research has shown that depression has a significant adverse effect on patients' work, family functioning, and leisure activities. Even with successful treatment, these areas of life may continue to be impaired for up to 1 year after the depressive symptoms resolve. Many studies have shown that treatment of mental disorders improves functional status and 'how patients feel about themselves, their lives, and the efficacy of their health care.'[140] Mohr and colleagues found that treatment of depression improved adherence to interferon-β 1b therapy.[141] It is clear, then, that early detection and effective treatment of mood disorders relieves pain and suffering and enhances patients' levels of functioning and quality of life. Given the high rate of mood disorders in MS and the morbidity associated with them, the quality of care of people with MS depends on physicians being able to diagnose and treat these conditions. Many decision-making aids are now available to non-psychiatric physicians; these include clinical practice guidelines for primary care physicians[142,143] and screening instruments for detecting mental disorders in primary care settings.[144] Psychiatric and psychopharmacologic specialists are widely available for consultation.[145] The SSRIs are so clearly safe, efficacious, and well tolerated that clinicians should have a low threshold for initiating pharmacologic treatment of depression in their MS patients. Similarly, mood disturbances associated with high-dose corticosteroids are so clearly preventable with lithium carbonate that clinicians should not hesitate to use this drug prophylactically in patients at risk.

While this chapter has emphasized underdiagnosis and undertreatment of mood disorders in MS, the opposite problem can also occur. Only the mental disorder may be diagnosed, and MS may go unrecognized and untreated.[146–148] In some cases, this is simply an error, while in other cases, physical signs and symptoms of MS are apparently absent[149] or the cognitive and affective impairments overshadow mild and intermittent evidence of neurologic disease.[150]

IMPLICATIONS FOR FUTURE RESEARCH

Our understanding of mood and affective disorders in MS has advanced considerably over the past 15 years. Areas for future research include instrument development, population-based prevalence studies, randomized clinical trials of the relative efficacy of different treatments, and clinical–pathological correlations.

Reliable and valid instruments for the diagnosis of euphoria and pathological laughing and weeping are prerequisites for prevalence studies and clinical trials. The Pathological Laughing and Crying Scale[91] is now available, but a standardized definition and tool to measure euphoria is needed. The semi-structured interviews and rating scales used in psychiatric research are adequate for detecting symptoms and diagnosing mood disorders in people with MS, although they must be modified to account for overlap in symptoms.

Studies with small clinical samples have been used to enable the researchers to infer the prevalence of mood and affective disorders in MS. Larger clinical samples are available through MS databases such as COSTAR, EDMUS, and the New York State Registry, but their data collection procedures do not include systematic evaluation of mood and affective disorders. Medical claims files and other administrative databases (e.g. the Veterans Administration in the USA) can be searched for MS cases, but they do not contain reliable data on mood disorders. Large, population-based samples are needed to determine the true prevalence of these disorders among people with MS. While people with MS can be identified among the randomly selected respondents to population surveys such as the National Health Interview Survey,[151] mental health data are not routinely collected and the numbers of people with MS are too small to examine such characteristics. A representative sample, such as that being developed by the National Multiple Sclerosis Society, and careful baseline and longitudinal assessment of emotional and affective functioning, should provide answers to some of the questions raised in this chapter.

It appears that standard pharmacologic treatments are as efficacious for mood disorders in people with MS as they are for others. With the SSRIs, adverse effects are uncommon and less likely to interfere with effective treatment. With the ongoing development of pharmacologic agents and with increasing understanding of the neurotransmitters associated with mood disorders and of the pathophysiology of MS, more specific and targeted treatments may be possible. Much more work is needed to clarify the mechanisms underlying the affective disorders and to explore different treatment options.

Health services researchers should study the economic and social consequences of mood disorders, particularly their impact on employment, income, and quality of life. Given the prevalence of mood and other mental disorders in MS, people with MS in the USA are doubly vulnerable to issues such as denial of health insurance because of pre-existing illness, lack of parity for medical and mental illnesses, and limited mental health benefits under managed care. People with MS encounter the same obstacles to high-quality health and mental health care as do people with other chronic medical conditions and people with serious and persistent mental illness. Policy analyses are needed to examine these obstacles and identify solutions. Advocates for all these groups have much in common and can learn from each other; working together, they can enhance access to high-quality care for persons with a wide variety of chronic and disabling conditions.

GLOSSARY

The terms in this glossary are based on DSM-IV.[5]

Adjustment disorder Development of emotional or behavioral symptoms (i.e. anxiety and depression) in response to and within 3 months of an identifiable stressor that are clinically significant as evidenced by marked distress and/or impairment in social or occupational functioning; criteria for another mood disorder are not met; the symptoms resolve within 6 months after the stress ends; and the symptoms do not represent bereavement.

Affect Fluctuating changes in the outward expression of inner feeling states. Affect may be blunted (significant reduction in the intensity of emotional expression), flat (absence of emotional expression), inappropriate (mismatch between what is felt, said, and/or thought), labile (rapid and sudden shifts in emotional expression).

Bipolar disorder One or more manic

episodes usually accompanied by major depressive episodes.

Delirium   Developing over a short period of time (hours to days) with a tendency to fluctuate over the course of the day, the following symptoms: a disturbance of consciousness (i.e. reduced clarity of awareness of the environment), reduced ability to focus, sustain or shift attention; a change in cognition (i.e. memory deficit, disorientation, language disturbance) or development of a perceptual disturbance; and evidence of a direct physiological cause.

Dementia   Gradual onset and continuing worsening of the following symptoms: memory impairment (impaired ability to learn new information or recall previously learned information) and one or more of aphasia (language disturbance), apraxia (impaired ability to carry out motor activities despite intact motor function), agnosia (failure to recognize or identify objects despite intact sensory function), or disturbance in executive functioning (planning, organization, sequencing, abstracting); and evidence of a direct physiological cause.

Dysthymic disorder   At least 2 years of depressed mood for more days than not, accompanied by at least two of the following symptoms: poor appetite or overeating, insomnia or hypersomnia, low energy or fatigue, low self-esteem, poor concentration or difficulty making decisions, feelings of hopelessness. The symptoms cause clinically significant distress or impairment in social, occupational, or other important areas of functioning and are not due to the direct physiological effects of a substance or a medical condition.

Generalized anxiety disorder   Anxiety and worry are associated with at least three of the following symptoms for at least 6 months and cause clinically significant distress or impairment in social, occupational, or other important areas of functioning: restlessness or feeling keyed up or on edge; easy fatigability; difficulty concentrating or mind going blank; irritability; muscle tension; trouble falling or staying asleep or restless unsatisfying sleep. The symptoms are not due to the direct physiological effects of a substance or medical condition.

Major depressive disorder   One or more major depressive episodes involving at least 2 weeks of depressed mood or loss of interest accompanied by at least four additional symptoms nearly every day including significant weight loss or weight gain or decrease or increase in appetite; insomnia or hypersomnia; psychomotor agitation or retardation; fatigue or loss of energy; feelings of worthlessness or excessive or inappropriate guilt; diminished ability to think or concentrate or indecisiveness; recurrent thoughts of death, recurrent suicidal ideation without a specific plan, or a suicide attempt with a specific plan. Symptoms cause clinically significant distress or impairment in social, occupational, or other important areas of functioning and are not due to the direct physiological effects of a substance, a medical condition, or to bereavement.

Manic episode   A distinct period of abnormally and persistently elevated, expansive or irritable mood for at least 1 week in association with three or more symptoms including inflated self-esteem or grandiosity; decreased need for sleep; more talkative than usual or pressure to keep talking; flight of ideas or racing thoughts; distractibility; increase in goal-directed activity or psychomotor agitation; excessive involvement in pleasurable activities that have a high potential for painful consequences. Symptoms cause marked impairment in social or occupational functioning, necessitate hospitalization, or have psychotic features; and are not due to the direct physiological effects of a substance or a medical condition.

Mood disorder   A sustained and pervasive emotion that influences perception of self, others, and the world.

Panic attack   A discrete period of intense fear or discomfort with abrupt and rapid development (i.e. within 10 minutes) of at least four of the following symptoms: palpitations, pounding heart, accelerated heart rate; sweating; trembling or shaking; sensations of shortness of breath or smothering; feeling of choking; chest pain or discomfort; nausea or abdominal distress; feeling dizzy, unsteady, lighteaded, or faint; feelings of unreality or being detached from oneself; fear of losing control or going crazy; fear of dying; numbness or tingling sensations; chills or hot flashes.

Panic disorder   Recurrent and unexpected panic attacks, and at least one attack that has been followed by 1 or more months of persistent concern about having additional attacks, and/or worry that the attack signifies losing control, having a heart attack, or 'going crazy,' and/or significant change in behavior. Attacks are not due to the direct physiological effects of a substance or medical condition. Agoraphobia (i.e. anxiety about being in places or situations from which escape might be difficult or embarrassing, as in a crowd or tunnel or on a bridge, and which are avoided or endured only with marked distress or a companion) may or may not be present.

REFERENCES

1   Minden SL, Schiffer RB. Affective disorders in multiple sclerosis. Review and recommendations for clinical research. *Arch Neurol* 1990; 47:98–104.

2   Petersen RC, Kokmen E. Cognitive and psychiatric abnormalities in multiple sclerosis. *Mayo Clin Proc* 1989; 64:657–663.

3   Minden SL. Neuropsychiatric aspects of multiple sclerosis. *Curr Opin Psychiatry* 1996; 9:93–97.

4   Ron MA. Multiple sclerosis: psychiatric and psychometric abnormalities. *Psychosom Res* 1986; 30:3–11.

5   American Psychiatric Association. *Diagnostic and Statistical Manual of Mental Disorders*, 4th edn. (Washington, DC: American Psychiatric Association, 1994).

6   Gerber P, Barrett J, Barrett J et al. Recognition of depression by internists in primary care: A comparison of internist and 'gold standard' psychiatric assessments. *J Gen Intern Med* 1989; 4:7–13.

7   Perez-Stable E, Miranda J, Munoz R, Ying YW. Depression in medical outpatients: underrecognition and misdiagnosis. *Arch Intern Med* 1990; 150:1083–1088.

8   Schulberg H, Saul M, McClelland M et al. Assessing depression in primary medical and psychiatric practice. *Arch Gen Psychiatry* 1985; 42:1164–1170.

9   Badger L, deGruy F, Plant M et al. Patient presentation, interview content, and the detection of depression in primary care physicians. *Psychosom Med* 1994; 56(2):128–135.

10   Matas M, Staley D, Griffin W. A profile of the noncompliant patient: a thirty-month review of outpatient psychiatry referrals. *Gen Hosp Psychiatry* 1992; 14:124–130.

11   Schulberg HC, Rush JA. Clinical practice guidelines in managing major depression in primary care practice. *Am Psychol* 1994; 49:34–41.

12   Joffe RT, Lipppert GP, Gray TA et al. Mood disorder and multiple sclerosis. *Arch Neurol* 1987; 44:376–378.

13   Areas Bal MA, Vazquez-Barquero JL, Pena C, Berciano JA. Psychiatric aspects of multiple sclerosis. *Acta Psychiatr Scand* 1991; 83:292–296.

14   Moller A, Wiedman G, Rohde U et al. Correlates of cognitive impairment and depressive mood disorder in multiple sclerosis. *Acta Psychiatr Scand* 1994; 89:117–121.

15   Minden SL, Orav J, Reich P. Depression in multiple sclerosis. *Gen Hosp Psychiatry* 1987; 9:426–434.

16   Sullivan MJ, Weinshenker B, Mikail S, Bishop SR. Screening for major depression in the early stages of multiple sclerosis. *Can J Neurol Sci* 1995; 22:228–231.

17   Schiffer RB, Caine ED, Bamford KA, Levy S.

Depressive episodes in patients with multiple sclerosis. *Am J Psychiatry* 1983; **140**:1498–1500.

18 Sadovnick AD, Remick RA, Allen J et al. Depression and multiple sclerosis. *Neurology* 1996; **46**:628–632.

19 Weissman MM, Myers JK. Affective disorders in a U.S. urban community. The use of research diagnostic criteria in an epidemiological survey. *Arch Gen Psychiatry* 1978; **35**:1304–1311.

20 Whitlock FA, Siskind MM. Depression as a major symptom of multiple sclerosis. *J Neurol Neurosurg Psychiatry* 1980; **43**:861–865.

21 Pepper CM, Krupp LB, Friedberg F et al. A comparison of neuropsychiatric characteristics in chronic fatigue syndrome, multiple sclerosis, and major depression. *J Neuropsychiatry Clin Neurosci* 1993; **5**:200–205.

22 Krupp LB, Sliwinski M, Masur DM et al. Cognitive functioning and depression in patients with chronic fatigue syndrome and multiple sclerosis. *Arch Neurol* 1994; **51**:705–710.

23 Fisk JD, Morehouse SA, Brown MG et al. Hospital-based psychiatric service utilization and morbidity in multiple sclerosis. *Can J Neurol Sci* 1998; **25**:230–235.

24 Kahana E, Liebowtiz U, Alter M. Cerebral multiple sclerosis. *Neurology* 1971; **21**:1179–1185.

25 McIvor GP, Riklan M, Reznikoff M. Depression in multiple sclerosis as a function of length and severity of illness, age, remissions, and perceived social support. *J Clin Psychol* 1984; **40**:1028–1033.

26 Schubert DS, Foliart RH. Increased depression in multiple sclerosis. A meta-analysis. *Psychosomatics* 1993; **34**:124–130.

27 DeLuca J, Johnson SK, Natelson BH. Information processing efficiency in chronic fatigue syndrome and multiple sclerosis. *Arch Neurol* 1993; **50**:301–304.

28 Mohr DC, Goodkin DE, Likosky W et al. Identification of Beck Depression Inventory items related to multiple sclerosis. *J Behav Med* 1997; **20**:407–414.

29 Natelson BH, Johnson SK, DeLuca J et al. Reducing heterogeneity in chronic fatigue syndrome: a comparison with depression and multiple sclerosis. *Clin Infect Dis* 1995; **21**:1204–1210.

30 Johnson SK, DeLuca J, Natelson BH. Depression in fatiguing illness: comparing ptients with chronic fatigue syndrome, multiple sclerosis and depression. *J Affective Disord* 1996; **39**:21–30.

31 Rabins PV, Brooks BR, O'Donnell P et al. Structural

brain correlates of emotional disorder in multiple sclerosis. *Brain* 1986; **109**:585–597.

32 Tedman BM, Young CA, Williams IR. Assessment of depression in patients with motor neuron disease and other neurologically disabling illness. *J Neurol Sci* 1997; **152** (suppl 1):S75–S79.

33 Schiffer RB, Babigian HM. Behavioral disorders in multiple sclerosis, temporal lobe epilepsy, and amyotrophic lateral sclerosis: an epidemiologic study. *Arch Neurol* 1984; **41**:1067–1069.

34 Dalos NP, Rabins PV, Brooks BR, O'Donnell P. Disease activity and emotional state in multiple sclerosis. *Ann Neurol* 1983; **13**:573–583.

35 Noy S, Achiron A, Gabbay U et al. A new approach to affective symptoms in relapsing–remitting multiple sclerosis. *Compr Psychiatry* 1995; **36**:390–395.

36 Gilchrist AC, Creed FH. Depression, cognitive impairment and social stress in multiple sclerosis. *J Pscyhosom Res* 1994; **38**:193–201.

37 Clark CM, James G, Li D et al. Ventricular size, cognitive function and depression in patients with multiple sclerosis. *Can J Neurol Sci* 1992; **19**:352–356.

38 Schiffer RB, Caine ED. The interaction between depressive affective disorder and neuropsychological test performance in multiple sclerosis patients. *J Neuropsychiatry Clin Neurosci* 1991; **3**:28–32.

39 Sabitini U, Pozzilli C, Pantano P et al. Involvement of the limbic system in multiple sclerosis patients with depressive disorders. *Biol Psychiatry* 1996; **39**:970–975.

40 Barak Y, Achiron A, Elizur A et al. Sexual dysfunction in relapsing–remitting multiple sclerosis: magnetic resonance imaging, clinical, and psychological correlates. *J Psychiatry Neurosci* 1996; **21**:255–258.

41 Tsolaki M, Drevelegas A, Karachristianous et al. Correlation of dementia, neuropsychological and MRI findings in multiple sclerosis. *Dementia* 1994; **5**:48–52.

42 Scott TF, Allen D, Price TR et al. Characterization of major depression symptoms in multiple sclerosis patients. *J Neuropsychiatry Clin Neurosci* 1996; **8**:318–323.

43 Mohr DC, Goodkin DE, Gatto N, Van der Wende J. Depression, coping and level of neurological impairment in multiple sclerosis. *Multiple Sclerosis* 1997; **3**:254–258.

44 Filippi M, Alveroni M, Martinelli V et al. Influence of

clinical variables on neuropsychological performance in multiple sclerosis. *Eur Neurol* 1994; **34**:324–328.

45 Honer WG, Hurwitz Y, Li DKB. Temporal lobe involvement in multiple sclerosis patients with psychiatric disorders. *Arch Neurol* 1987; **447**:187–190.

46 George MS, Kellner CH, Berstein H, Goust JM. A magnetic resonance imagining investigation into mood disorders in multiple sclerosis: a pilot study. *J Nerv Ment Dis* 1994; **182**:410–412.

47 Pujol J, Bello J, Deus J et al. Lesions in the left arcuate fasciculus region and depressive symptoms in multiple sclerosis. *Neurology* 1997; **49**:1105–1110.

48 Clark CM, Fleming JA, Li D et al. Sleep disturbance, depression, and lesion site in patients with multiple sclerosis. *Arch Neurol* 1992; **49**:641–643.

49 Devins GM, Edworthy SM, Paul LC et al. Restless sleep, illness intrusiveness, and depressive symptoms in three chronic illness conditions: rheumatoid arthritis, end-stage renal disease, and multiple sclerosis. *J Psychosom Res* 1993; **37**:163–170.

50 Schwartz CE, Coulthard-Morris L, Zeng Q. Psychosocial correlates of fatigue in multiple sclerosis. *Arch Phys Med Rehabil* 1996; **77**:165–170.

51 Cleeland CS, Matthews CG, Hopper CL. MMPI profiles in exacerbation and remission of multiple sclerosis. *Psychol Rep* 1970; **41**:373–374.

52 Sandyk R, Awerbuch GI. Nocturnal melatonin secretion in multiple sclerosis patients with affective disorders. *Int J Neurosci* 1993; **68**:227–240.

53 Foley FW, Traugott U, LaRocca NG et al. A prospective study of depression and immune dysregulation in multiple sclerosis. *Arch Neurol* 1992; **49**:238–244.

54 Sternberg EM, Gold PW. Multiple sclerosis is associated with alternations in hypothalamic–pituitary–adrenal axis function. *J Clin Endocrinol Metab* 1994; **79**:848–853.

55 Fassbender K, Schmidt R, Mossner R et al. Mood disorders and dysfunction of the hypothalamic–pituitary–adrenal axis in multiple sclerosis: association with cerebral inflammation. *Arch Neurol* 1998; **55**:66–72.

56 Stenager EN, Koch-Henriksen N. Stenager E. Risk factors for suicide in multiple sclersosis. *Psychother Psychosom* 1996; **65**:86–90.

57 Kellner CH, Davenport Y, Post RM, Ross RJ. Rapidly cycling bipolar disorder and multiple sclerosis. *Am J Psychiatry* 1982; **141**:112–113.

58 Matthews B. Multiple sclerosis presenting with acute remitting psychiatric symptoms. *Neurol Neurosurg Psychiatry* 1979; **42**:859–863.

59 Peselow ED, Fieve RR, Deutsch SI, Kaufman M. Coexistent manic symptoms and multiple sclerosis. *Psychosomatics* 1981; **22**:824–825.

60 Garfield DAS. Multiple sclerosis and affective disorders: 2 cases of mania with psychosis. *Psychother Psychosom* 1985; **44**:22–33.

61 Mapelli G, Ramelli E. Manic syndrome associated with multiple sclerosis:secondary mania? *Acta Pscyhiatr Scand* 1981; **81**:337–349.

62 Solomon JG. Multiple sclerosis masquerading as lithium toxicity. *J Nerv Ment Dis* 1978; **166**:663–665.

63 Kemp K, Lion JR, Magram G. Lithium in the treatment of a manic patient with multiple sclerosis: a case report. *Dis Nerv Syst* 1977; **38**:210–211.

64 Schiffer RB, Wineman NM, Weirkamp LR. Association between bipolar affective disorder and multiple sclerosis. *Am J Psychiatry* 1986; **143**:94–95.

65 Schiffer RB, Weitkamp LR, Wineman, NM, Guttormsen S. Multiple sclerosis and affective disorder, family history, sex, and HLA-DR antigens. *Arch Neurol* 1988; **45**:1345–1348.

66 Cazzullo CL, Smeraldi E, Gasperini M, Caputo D. Preliminary correlation between primary affective disorders and multiple sclerosis. In: Cazzullo CL, Caputo D, Ghezzi A, eds. *New Trends in Multiple Sclerosis Research*, New York: Masson, 1983: 57–62.

67 Minden SL, Orav J, Schildkraut JJ. Hypomanic reastions to ACTH and prednisone treatment for multiple sclerosis. *Neurology* 1988; **38**:1631–1634.

68 Cass LJ, Alexander L, Enders M. Complications of corticotropin therapy in multiple sclerosis. *JAMA* 1966; **197**:105–111.

69 Stenager E, Knudsen L, Jensen K. Multiple sclerosis: correlation of anxiety, physical impairment and cognitive dysfunction. *Ital J Neurol Sci* 1994; **15**:97–101.

70 Rao SM, Leo GJ, Ellington I et al. Cognitive dysfunction in multiple sclerosis. *Neurology* 1991; **41**:692–696.

71 Stenager E, Knudsen L, Jensen K. Correlation of Beck Depression Inventory score, Kurtzke Disability Status Scale and cognitive functioning in multiple sclerosis. In: Jensen K, Knudsen I, Stenager E, Grant I, eds. *Mental Disorders and Cognitive Deficits in Multiple Sclerosis*. London: John Libbey, 1989: 147–151.

72 Stenager E, Knudsen L, Jensen K. Multiple sclerosis: the impact of physical impairment and cognitive

dysfunction on social and sparetime activities. *Psychother Psychosom* 1991; **56**:123–138.

73 **Andreatini R, Sartori VA, Leslie JR, Oliveira ASB.** Panic attacks in a multiple sclerosis patient. *Biol Psychiatry* 1994; **35**:133–134.

74 **Ontiveros A, Fontaine R.** Panic attacks and multiple sclerosis. *Biol Psychiatry* 1990; **27**:672–673.

75 **Brooks NA, Matson RR.** Social-psychological adjustment to multiple sclerosis:a longitudinal study. *Soc Sci Med* 1982; **16**:2129–2135.

76 **Counte MA, Bieliauskas LA, Pavlou M.** Stress and personal attitude in chronic illness. *Arch Phys Med Rehabil* 1983; **64**:272–275.

77 **Maybury C, Brewin C.** Social relationships, knowledge and adjustment to multiple sclerosis. *J Neurol Neurosurg Psychiatry* 1984; **47**:372–376.

78 **Zeldow PB, Pavlou M.** Physical disability, life stress, and psychological adjustment in multiple sclerosis. *J Nerv Ment Dis* 1984; **172**:80–84.

79 **Lindgren CL, Burke ML, Hainsworth MA, Eakes GG.** Chronic sorrow:a lifespan concept. *Sch Inq Nurs Pract* 1992; **6**:27–40.

80 **Buelow JM.** A correlational study of disabilities, stressors and coping methods in victims of multiple sclerosis. *J Neurosci Nurs* 1991; **23**:247–252.

81 **Jean VM, Beatty WW, Paul RH, Mullins L.** Coping with general and disease-related stressors by patients with multiple sclerosis: relationship to psychological distress. *Multiple Sclerosis* 1997; **3**:191–196.

82 **Schiaffino KM, Shawaryn MA, Blum D.** Examining the impact of illness representations on psychological adjustment to chronic illness. *Health Psychol* 1998; **17**:262–268.

83 **Wineman NM.** Adaptation to multiple sclerosis: the role of social support, functional disability, and perceived uncertainty. *Nurs Res* 1990; **39**:294–299.

84 **Barnwell AM, Kavanagh DJ.** Prediction of psychological adjustment to multiple sclerosis. *Soc Sci Med* 1997; **45**:411–418.

85 **Langworthy OR, Kolb LC, Androp S.** Disturbances of behavior in patients with disseminated sclerosis. *Am J Psychiatry* 1941; **98**:243–249.

86 **Surridge D.** An investigation into some psychiatric aspects of multiple sclerosis. *Br J Psychiatry* 1969; **115**:749–764.

87 **Pratt RTC.** An investigation of the psychiatric aspects of disseminated sclerosis. *J Neurol Neurosurg Psychiatry* 1951; **14**:326–335.

88 **Sugar C, Nadell R.** Mental symptoms in multiple sclerosis. *J Nerv Ment Dis* 1943; **98**:267–280.

89 **Cottrell SS, Wilson SAK.** The affective symptomatology of disseminated sclerosis. *J Neurol Psychopathol* 1926; **7**:1–30.

90 **Feinstein A, Feinstein K, Gray T, O'Connor P.** Prevalence and neurobehavioral correlates of pathological laughing and crying in multiple sclerosis. *Arch Neurol* 1997; **54**:1116–1121.

91 **Poeck K.** Pathophysiology of emotional disorders associated with brain damage. In: Vinken PJ, Bruyn GW, eds. *Handbook of Clinical Neurology.* Amsterdam: North Holland Publishing, 1969, 227–231.

92 **Robinson RG, Parikh RM, Lipsey JR et al.** Pathological laughing and crying following stroke: validation of a measurement scale and double-blind treatment study. *Am J Psychiatry* 1993; **150**:286–293.

93 **Black DW.** Pathologic laughter: a review of the literature. *J Nerv Ment Dis* 1982; **170**:67–71.

94 **Ironside R.** Disorders of laughter due to brain lesions. *Brain* 1956; **79**:589–609.

95 **Langworthy OR, Hesser FH.** Syndrome of pseudobulbar palsy: an anatomic and physiologic analysis. *Arch Intern Med* 1940; **65**:106–121.

96 **Sackheim HA, Greenberg MS, Weinman AL et al.** Hemisphere asymmetry in the expression of positive and negative emotions. *Arch Neurol* 1982; **39**:210–218.

97 **Tatemichi TK, Nichols FT, Mohr JP.** Pathological crying: a pontine pseudobulbar syndrome (abstract). *Ann Neurol* 1987; **22**:133.

98 **Yarnell PR.** Pathological crying localization (abstract). *Ann Neurol* 1987; **22**:133.

99 **Baldwin MV.** A clinico-experimental investigation into the psychologic aspects of multiple sclerosis. *J Nerv Ment Dis* 1952; **115**:299–342.

100 **Kahana E, Leibowitz U, Alter M.** Cerebral multiple sclerosis. *Neurology* 1971; **21**:1179–1185.

101 **Braceland FJ, Giffin ME.** The mental changes associated with multiple sclerosis (an interim report). *Res Publ Assoc Res Nerv Ment Dis* 1950; **28**:450–455.

102 **Gonzalez CF, Swirsky-Sacchetti T, Mitchell D et al.** Distributional patterns of multiple sclerosis brain lesions. Magnetic resonance imaging—clinical correlation. *J Neuroimaging* 1994; **4**:188–195.

103 **Young AC, Saunders J, Ponsford JR.** Mental change as an early feature of multiple sclerosis. *J Neurol Neurosurg Psychiatry* 1976; **39**:1008–1013.

104 **Awad A.** Schizophrenia and multiple sclerosis. Single case study. *J Nerv Ment Dis* 1983; **171**:323–324.

105 Geocaris K. Psychotic episodes heralding the diagnosis of multiple sclerosis. *Bull Menninger Clin* 1957; **21**:107–116.

106 Mur J, Kumpel G, Dostal S. An anergic phase of disseminated sclerosis with psychotic course. *Confin Neurol* 1966; **28**:37–49.

107 O'Malley PP. Severe mental symptoms in disseminated sclerosis: a neuro-pathological study. *J Ir Med Assoc* 1966; **58**:115–127.

108 Keller MB (ed). Mood disorders. *Psychiatr Clin North Am* 1996; **19**(1):1–178.

109 Amsterdam JD, Hornig-Rohan M. Treatment algorithms in treatment-resistant depression. *Psychiatr Clin North Am* 1996; **19**(2):371–386.

110 Caine ED. Pseudodementia. *Arch Gen Psychiatry* 1981; **38**:1359–1364.

111 Nyenhuis DL, Rao SM, Zajecka JM et al. Mood disturbance versus other symptoms of depression in multiple sclerosis. *J Int Neuropsychol Sco* 1995; **1**:291–296.

112 Weissman MM. The psychological treatment of depression. Evidence for the efficacy of psychotherapy alone, in comparison with, and in combination with pharmacotherapy. *Arch Gen Psychiatry* 1979; **36**:1261–1269.

113 Silver JM, Hales RE, Yudofsky SC. Psychopharmacology of depression in neurologic disorders. *J Clin Psychiatry* 1990; **51** (Suppl):33–39.

114 Minden SL. Psychotherapy for people with multiple sclerosis. *J Neuropsychiatry Clin Neurosci* 1992; **4**:1–16.

115 Schiffer RB, Wineman NM. Antidepressant pharmacotherapy of depression associated with multiple sclerosis. *Am J Psychiatry* 1990; **147**:1493–1497.

116 Scott TF, Nussbaum P, McConnell H, Brill P. Measurement of treatment response to sertraline in depressed multiple sclerosis using the Carroll scale. *Neurol Res* 1995; **17**:421–422.

117 Gelenberg AJ, Bassuk EL. *The Practitioner's Guide to Psychoactive Drugs* 4th edn. New York: Plenum Medical Book Company, 1997.

118 Gelenberg AJ, Delgado PL. Depression. In: Gelenberg AJ, Bassuk EL, eds. *The Practitioner's Guide to Psychoactive Drugs* 4th edn. New York: Plenum Medical Book Company, 1997, 19–97.

119 Schiffer RB. The spectrum of depression in multiple sclerosis. An approach for clinical management. *Arch Neurol* 1987; **44**:596–599.

120 Crawford JD, McIvor GP. Group psychotherapy: benefits in multiple sclerosis. *Arch Phys Med Rehabil* 1985; **66**:810–813.

121 Hartings MF, Pavlou MM, Davis FA. Group counseling of MS patients. *J Chron Dis* 1976; **29**:65–73.

122 Pavlou M, Hartings M, Davis FA. Discussion groups for medical patients. *Psychother Psychsom* 1978; **30**:105–115.

123 Bates A, Burns DD, Moorey S. Medical illness and the acceptance of suffering. *Int J Psychiatry Med* 1989; **19**:269–280.

124 Laracombe NA, Wilson PH. An evaluation of cognitive–behavior therapy for depression in patients with multiple sclerosis. *Br J Psychiatry* 1984; **145**:366–371.

125 Minden SL, Moes E. A psychiatric perspective. In: Rao SM, ed. *Neurobehavioral Aspects of Multiple Sclerosis*. New York: Oxford University Press, 1990: 230–250.

126 Falk WE, Mahnke MW, Poskanzer DC. Lithium prophylaxis of corticotropin-induced psychosis. *JAMA* 1979; **241**:1011–1012.

127 Browning WN. Exacerbation of symptoms of multiple sclerosis in a patient taking fluoxetine (letter). *Am J Psychiatry* 1990; **147**:1089.

128 Flax JW, Gray J, Herbert J. Effect of fluoxetine on patients with multiple sclerosis (letter). *Am J Psychiatry* 1991; **148**:1603.

129 Reiman EM. Anxiety, In: Gelenberg AJ, Bassuk EL, eds. *The Practitioner's Guide to Psychoactive Drugs* 4th edn. New York: Plenum Medical Book Company, 1997: 213–264.

130 Schiffer RB, Herndon RM, Rudick RA. Treatment of pathologic laughing and weeping with amitriptyline. *N Engl J Med* 1985; **312**:1480–1482.

131 Minden SL, Fife A. Anxiety disorders. In: Branch WT. *Office Practice of Medicine*, 3rd edn. Philadelphia: WB Saunders, 1994, 999–1011.

132 Wolf JK, Santana HB, Thorpy M. Treatment of 'emotional incontinence' with levodopa. *Neurology* 1979; **29**:1435–1436.

133 Udaka F, Yamao S, Nagata H et al. Pathologic laughing and crying treated with levodopa. *Arch Neurol* 1984; **41**:1095–1096.

134 Seliger GM, Hornstein A, Flax J et al. Fluoxetine improves emotional incontinence. *Brain Inj* 1992; **6**:267–270.

135 Iannaccone S, Ferini-Strambi L. Pharmacologic treatment of emotional lability. *Clin Neuropharmacol* 1996; **19**:532–535.

136 **Sandyk R.** Suicidal behavior is attenuated in patients with multiple sclerosis by treatment with electromagnetic fields. *Int J Neurosci* 1996; **87**:5–15.

137 **Sandyk R.** Further observations on the effects of external picoTesla range magnetic fields on visual memory and visuospatial functions in multiple sclerosis. *Int J Neurosci* 1994; **77**:203–227.

138 **Sandyk R.** Rapid normalization of visual evoked protentials by picoTesla range magnetic fields in chronic progressive multiple sclerosis. *Int J Neurosci* 1994; **77**:243–259.

139 **Garland EJ, Zis AP.** Multiple sclerosis and affective disorders. *Can J Psychiatry* 1991; **36**:112–117.

140 **Spitzer RL, Kroenke K, Linzer M et al.** Health-related quality of life in primary care patients with mental disorders. Results from the PRIME-MD 1000 study. *JAMA* 1995; **274**:1511–1517.

141 **Mohr DC, Goodkin DE, Likosky W et al.** Treatment of depression improves adherence to interferon beta-1b therapy for multiple sclerosis. *Arch Neurol* 1997; **54**:531–533.

142 **Depression Guideline Panel.** *Depression in Primary Care, Vol 2. Detection and Diagnosis.* Clinical Practice Guideline, No 5, AHCPR Pub No 93–0550. Rockville, Maryland: US Department of Health and Human Services, Public Health Service, Agency for Health Care Policy and Research, 1993.

143 **Depression Guideline Panel.** *Depression in Primary Care, Vol 2. Treatment of Major Depression.* Clinical Practice Guideline, No 5, AHCPR Pub No 93-0551.

Rockville, Maryland: US Department of Health and Human Services, Public Health Service, Agency for Health Care Policy and Research, 1993.

144 **Mulrow CD, Williams JW, Gerety MB et al.** Case-finding instruments for depression in primary care settings. *Ann Intern Med* 1995; **122**:913–921.

145 **Cohen-Cole S, Friedman C.** Attitudes of nonpsychiatric physicians toward psychiatric consultation. *Hosp Community Psychiatry* 1982; **33**:1002–1006.

146 **Skegg K, Corwin PA, Skegg DCG.** How often is multiple sclerosis mistaken for a psychiatric disorder? *Psychol Med* 1988; **18**:733–736.

147 **Tomsyck RR, Jenkins PL.** Psychiatric aspects of multiple sclerosis (clinical conference). *Gen Hosp Psychiatry* 1987; **9**:294–301.

148 **Salloway S, Price LH, Charney DS, Shapiro M.** Multiple sclerosis presenting as major depression: a diagnosis suggested by MRI scan but not by CT scan. *J Clin Psychiatry* 1988; **49**:364–366.

149 **Mendez MF.** The neuropsychiatry of multiple sclerosis. *Int J Psychiatry Med* 1995; **25**:123–130.

150 **Hotoff MH, Pollock S, Lishman WA.** An unusual presentation of multiple sclerosis. *Psychol Med* 1994; **24**:525–528.

151 **Minden SL, Marder W.** *Multiple Sclerosis:A Statistical Portrait. A Compendium of Data on Demographics, Disability, and Health Services Utilization in the United States.* Report to the National Multiple Sclerosis Society, August 1993.

38
Treatment of chronic pain

Ronald Kanner

INTRODUCTION

Pain is a common occurrence in multiple sclerosis (MS), with a reported prevalence of 29–86%,[1,2] depending on the study design. The low figures are derived from retrospective chart reviews, while the high figures are from interviews of patients with active disease. The most widely accepted figure is about 55%. The prevalence does not seem to vary with disease type or duration.[3] Pain is the initial complaint in 11% of MS patients.[4]

Despite the large number of patients suffering from pain and its concomitant social and physical disability, there is a dearth of published literature specifically addressing pain management in MS. A Medline search from 1966 up to February 1999 revealed 420 articles that mentioned pain and MS—239 had pain and MS as major subject headings, 43 actually focused on pain issues specific to MS, and 13 cited specific treatment modalities. There were only two prospective, controlled medication studies, both of which dealt with paroxysmal pains.

Given the paucity of hard data on the management of pain in MS, an evidence-based medicine approach is impossible. The most fruitful approach is to identify specific pain syndromes in MS and use information gathered from similar pain states in other diseases to guide treatment.

PAIN SYNDROMES IN MS

On the basis of their inferred pathophysiology, pain syndromes in MS can be classified as (*Table 38.1*):

(a) neuropathic;
(b) somatic nociceptive;
(c) visceral nociceptive; or
(d) psychogenic.

Table 38.1 Pain syndromes in MS

Neuropathic syndromes
Spinal cord
Dysesthetic limbs
Somatic nociceptive syndromes
Back pain
Degenerative disease
Osteoporosis
Fractures
Painful spasms*
Visceral nociceptive syndromes
Bladder spasms
Pelvic pain
Psychogenic syndromes
Depression
Anxiety

* Painful spasms are due to nervous system injury and may respond to anti-convulsants and anti-depressants, but the pain itself originates in the muscles and is considered somatic.

Neuropathic pain can be caused by injury any-where in the nervous system. The clinical hall-marks are burning, dysesthetic pains, spontaneous paroxysms of pain (lancinating pains) and painful responses to non-noxious stimuli (allodynia). Somatic, nociceptive pain is due to ongoing noxious stimulation that origi-nates in muscles, bones, and connective tissue. It is generally described as being aching and well localized. Visceral nociceptive pain is due to acti-vation of nociceptors in a hollow viscus (bowel or bladder). Visceral pain is often referred to cutaneous sites, is cramping in nature, and waxes and wanes with time. A psychogenic origin is inferred when no causative lesion can be found or when the reaction to the pain is out of propor-tion to the underlying problem. This is the least satisfying of the diagnoses and should be sup-ported by a clear psychological diagnosis and a thorough attempt to identify other explanations. Although this classification has received broad acceptance in the cancer pain literature,[5] only a few of the MS case series make these distinctions clearly.[6]

Neuropathic pain syndromes

Neuropathic pain syndromes constitute the most common pathophysiologic group in multiple sclerosis.[7,8] Within neuropathic pain, syndromes may be defined further by either their temporal course or their physical distribution.

Acute neuropathic syndromes generally present in the distribution of a nerve or a nerve root. Trigeminal neuralgia (TN) is the most widely recognized of these syndromes. TN in MS differs from the idiopathic form in that the patients are usually younger (if they have TN as a first manifestation) and bilateral disease is more commonly seen in MS. MS should be considered in anyone under 40 years of age presenting with TN. As a late symptom, it affects about 2–4% of MS patients.[9,10] The causative lesion is believed to be a demyelinating plaque in the pons,[11] but vascular and tumor-related compressive lesions have also been demonstrated.[12] As with idio-pathic TN, carbamazepine has been shown to be effective in reducing the severity and frequency of attacks in TN associated with MS.[13] Gabapentin[14] and lamotrigine[15] have also been reported to be effective, but only in open-label trials.

Acute radicular syndromes are less common, but have been reported as both an early and late symptom of MS.[16] Approximately half of the patients in this series had no history of trauma at the onset of the radiculopathy, and imaging pro-cedures ruled out compressive causes in all cases. The differentiating factors in these patients was that they had a higher than expected number of associated neurological signs and plaques detected on magnetic resonance imaging, although not always at the site of pain.

Pain from optic neuritis is subacute in course. It is localized to the affected eye and increases with eye movement. Minor analgesics are helpful and corticosteroids usually eliminate the pain in short order. The discomfort resolves with resolu-tion of the neuritis.

Chronic neuropathic pains are almost invari-ably associated with spinal cord lesions.[10] Chronic intractable pain may rarely be the pre-senting symptom of MS,[17] but it more com-monly appears later in the disease, after spinal cord lesions have been established.[2,10] Chronic, painful dysesthesias in the limbs are the most prevalent and disabling pains.[18] They are usually associated with some degree of sensory loss in the area. Extrapolating from neuropathic pains in other conditions, these syndromes are commonly treated with tricyclic anti-depressants, but the results are less than satisfactory.[8,19] Gabapentin[20] and mexiletine[21] have been reported anecdotally as relieving painful dysesthesias in open-label trials.

Assessment and treatment of neuropathic pain

Neuropathic pain is different in character and time course from other pains. Assessment depends on defining the severity and duration of specific symptoms (spontaneous burning, lancinating jabs, evoked pains) as a guide to appropriate therapy.[22] Tricyclic anti-depressants are the most widely used medications for chronic, burning neuropathic pain. However, a systematic review of their use revealed that, when compared with placebo, only about 30% of patients could be expected to achieve greater than 50% pain relief and that 30% of patients would have side effects.[19] By extrapolation from the success of carbamazepine in the treatment of idiopathic trigeminal neuralgia, it has been used for many other lancinating pains. By extrapolation from that use, other anticonvulsants (most recently gabapentin[23]) have been used in the same way. These levels of abstraction do not provide scientific reliability and it is unclear whether anti-depressants, or anti-convulsants should be first-line drugs for neuropathic pain.

Recent studies have proposed that central neuropathic pain is the result of a relative imbalance between glutamate transmission and GABAergic function,[24] lending support to the use of GABAergic agents or N-methyl D-aspartate (NMDA) blockers.[25] However, firm guidelines cannot be provided without appropriately controlled testing in clinical settings, and this testing is lacking.[26]

At present, it is probably prudent to follow the World Health Organization guidelines for the treatment of neuropathic pain in cancer (*Table 38.2*)[27] and apply those principles to the management of neuropathic pain in multiple sclerosis.

Somatic nociceptive pain

Back pain and painful tonic spasms are the most common types of somatic nociceptive pain seen in MS.[18] Back pain affects about 20% of patients with MS.[10] It is generally aching and localized, although radicular radiation may occur. It tends to be a late manifestation of the disease, appearing after neurological disability has taken its toll on the spine. Treatment is designed in a rehabilitative model, correcting

Table 38.2 World Health Organization Cancer Pain Treatment Guidelines

Step I: Mild to moderate pain

    Non-opioid analgesics

    ± 'adjuvant' drugs*

Step II: Moderate pain

    Non-opioid analgesic

    + 'Weak' opioid[†]

    ± Adjuvant drugs

Step III: Severe pain

    Non-opioid analgesic

    + 'Potent' opioid[‡]

    ± Adjuvant drugs

* Adjuvant drugs are medications such as the anti-depressants, anti-convulsants, corticosteroids, and systemically administered anesthetics, which are not primarily analgesics but may relieve pain in certain clinical circumstances. They may often be used as first line drugs for neuropathic pain.
† Weak analgesics are those that, after a certain dose, have increasing side effects without added efficacy (ceiling dose). Examples are codeine and the oxycodone combinations.
‡ The potent opioids, such as morphine and methadone, have no ceiling effect and may be increased as pain or tolerance increase.

abnormal postures and stretching and strengthening paraspinal muscles. Non-steroidal anti-inflammatory drugs are the first line of pharmacological therapy. Orthotic devices should be used only sparingly.

Osteoporosis is a frequent complication of MS, mainly because of inactivity and the relatively high proportion of women affected. Corticosteroid use may contribute to its development but it does not appear to be a primary factor in most cases.[28] Osteoporotic back pain is even more localized than pain due to degenerative disease of the spine and it is exquisitely sensitive to changes in position. The combination of osteoporosis and the risk of falls makes MS patients particularly vulnerable to vertebral and hip fractures, as well as fractures of the ribs and pelvis.[29] If the hip fracture occurs on a side with significant sensory loss, it may produce a nondescript and poorly localized pain. Patients with severe disability and pain anywhere around the hip should be investigated for fractures.

A combination of non-steroidal anti-inflammatory drugs and opioids may provide enough pain relief to allow for rehabilitation exercises. Short serum half-life opioids may be administered just before a physical therapy session and a period of rest provided after the session. The goal is for increased weight bearing and movement.

Painful tonic spasms can affect any extremity. They present as slow, painful writhing movements. Pain is due to forced muscular contraction. The events are short-lived, lasting only many seconds to a few minutes. Although the pain is nociceptive, the causative lesion is in the brain or spinal cord. Treatment is directed at reducing spasticity, generally with benzodiazepines. Spinal procedures, such as intrathecal baclofen and epidural stimulation, appear to be more effective in relieving spasticity than in con-trolling pain. Gabapentin[30] and other anticonvulsants are also widely used. The episodes themselves are so brief in duration that they render analgesic treatment ineffective. Hypnosis may also be a useful adjunctive therapy.[31]

As interferon has become more widely used as a therapy for MS, treatment-related pain syndromes have emerged. The two most common are local pain at the injection site and diffuse muscle pains ('interferon flu'). The muscular pains are self-limited and rarely require more than aspirin for treatment. Application of topical lidocaine preparations can reduce injection pain, but persistent pain at the injection site should raise the suspicion of sterile abscess.

Visceral nociceptive pain

The most common visceral nociceptive pain in MS is painful bladder spasm. It presents as a crampy pelvic pain that appears intermittently and may be accompanied by incontinence. It is invariably associated with spinal cord dysfunction. In open studies, intrathecal baclofen and intravesicular denervation have been reported to be effective. Occasionally, pelvic pain may be paroxysmal in nature, in which case it may respond to carbamazepine.[32]

Psychogenic pain

Pure psychogenic pain is uncommon. Vermote and colleagues[6] reported that two of their 45 MS patients with pain had a presumed psychogenic origin; one with 'psychosis' and the other with 'hysteria'. Much more commonly, chronic disease takes its toll on the psyche in the form of depression or anxiety, or an underlying psychological condition makes the pain less tolerable. MS patients with chronic pain report greater disability and social dysfunction than similarly affected patients without pain.[3] Part of this increased disability is due to depression, which should be treated aggressively.[33]

Headache

Headache is listed separately because, while there is an increased prevalence of headache in MS, the etiology is unclear.[34] In a prospective, detailed analysis, 52% of MS patients were found to have headache, compared with 18% in matched general neurology patients.[35] Rarely, a vascular headache may be the presenting symptom of MS or herald an exacerbation.[36] While there are case reports of single lesions causing headache[37] and of apopleptic headache as a presenting symptom,[38] headaches are usually of the tension type or migrainous and do not necessarily correlate with disease activity. In a relatively large sample, Rolak[35] was unable to detect any clear 'MS headache.' There is no evidence to suggest that headaches in MS should be treated any differently from similar headache syndromes in patients without underlying disease.

CONCLUSION

Firm guidelines for the treatment of pain in multiple sclerosis cannot be drawn up until the mechanisms of pain are elucidated and appropriately controlled and blinded studies are completed.

REFERENCES

1 **Clifford DB, Trotter JL.** Pain in multiple sclerosis. *Arch Neurol* 1984; **41**:1270–1272.

2 **Stenager E, Knudsen L, Jensen K.** Acute and chronic pain syndromes in multiple sclerosis. A 5-year follow-up study. *Ital J Neurol Sci* 1995; **16**:529–532.

3 **Archibald CJ, McGrath PJ, Ritvo PG et al.** Pain prevalence, severity and impact in a clinic sample of multiple sclerosis patients. *Pain* 1994; **58**:89–93.

4 **Paty DW, Ebers GC.** Clinical features. In: Paty DW, Ebers GC, eds. *Multiple Sclerosis.* Contemporary Neurology Series. Philadelphia: FA Davis, 1998.

5 **Portenoy RK, Kanner RM.** Definition and assessment of pain. In: Portenoy RK, Kanner RM, eds. *Pain Management: Theory and Practice.* Contemporary Neurology Series. Philadelphia: FA Davis, 1996.

6 **Vermote R, Ketelaer P, Carton H.** Pain in multiple sclerosis patients: a prospective study using the McGill Pain Questionnaire. *Clin Neurol Neurosurg* 1986; **88**:87–93.

7 **Warnell P.** The pain experience of a multiple sclerosis population: a descriptive study. *Axone* 1991; **13**:26–28.

8 **Moulin DE, Foley KM, Ebers, GC.** Pain syndromes in multiple sclerosis. *Neurology* 1988; **38**:1830–1834.

9 **Hooge JP, Redekop WK.** Trigeminal neuralgia in multiple sclerosis. *Neurology* 1995; **45**:1294–1296.

10 **Moulin DE.** Pain in central and peripheral demyelinating disorders. *Neurol Clin* 1998; **16**:889–897.

11 **Gass A, Kitchen N, MacManus DG et al.** Trigeminal neuralgia in patients with multiple sclerosis: lesion localization with magnetic resonance imaging. *Neurology* 1997; **49**:1142–1144.

12 **Meaney JF, Watt JW, Eldridge PR et al.** Association between trigeminal neuralgia and multiple sclerosis: role of magnetic resonance imaging. *J Neurol Neurosurg Psychiatry* 1995; **59**:253–259.

13 **Espir ML, Millac P.** Treatment of paroxysmal disorders in multiple sclerosis with carbamazepine (Tegretol). *J Neurol Neurosurg Psychiatry* 1970; **33**:528–531.

14 **Houtchens MK, Richert JR, Sami A, Rose JW.** Open label gabapentin treatment for pain in multiple sclerosis. *Multiple Sclerosis* 1997; **3**:250–253.

15 **Lunardi G, Leandri M, Albano C et al.** Clinical effectiveness of lamotrigine and plasma levels in essential and symptomatic trigeminal neuralgia. *Neurology* 1997; **48**:1714–1717.

16 Ramirez-Lassepas M, Tulloch JW, Quinones MR, Snyder BD. Acute radicular pain as a presenting symptom in multiple sclerosis. *Arch Neurol* 1992; 49:255–258.

17 Portenoy RK, Yang K, Thornton D. Chronic intractable pain: an atypical presentation of multiple sclerosis. *J Neurol* 1998; 235:226–228.

18 Indaco A, Iachetta C, Nappi C et al. Chronic and acute pain syndromes in patients with multiple sclerosis. *Acta Neurol Napoli* 1994; 16:97–102.

19 McQuay HJ, Tramer M, Nye BA et al. A systematic review of antidepressants in neuropathic pain. *Pain* 1996; 68:217–227.

20 Samkoff LM, Daras M, Tuchman AJ, Koppel BS. Amelioration of refractory dysesthetic limb pain in multiple sclerosis by gabapentin. *Neurology* 1997; 49:304–305.

21 Okada S, Kinoshita M, Fujioka T, Yoshimura M. Two cases of multiple sclerosis with painful tonic seizures and dysesthesia ameliorated by the administration of mexiletine. *Jpn J Med* 1991; 30:373–375.

22 Galer BS, Jensen MP. Development and preliminary validation of a pain measure specific to neuropathic pain: the Neuropathic Pain Scale. *Neurology* 1997; 48:332–338.

23 Attal N, Brasseur L, Parker F et al. Effects of gabapentin on the different components of peripheral and central neuropathic pain syndromes: a pilot study. *Eur Neurol* 1998; 40:191–200.

24 Canavero S, Bonicalzi V. The neurochemistry of central pain: evidence from clinical studies, hypothesis and therapeutic implications. *Pain* 1998; 74:109–114.

25 Felsby S, Nielsen J, Arent-Nielsen L, Jensen TS. NMDA receptor blockade in chronic neuropathic pain: a comparison of ketamine and magnesium chloride. *Pain* 1996; 64:283–291.

26 Portenoy RK. Neuropathic pain. In: Portenoy RK, Kanner RM, eds. *Pain Management: Theory and Practice*. Contemporary Neurology Series Vol 48. Philadelphia: FA Davis, 1996, 83–124.

27 Grond S, Radbruch L, Meuser T et al. Assessment and treatment of neuropathic cancer pain following WHO guidelines. *Pain* 1999; 79:15–20.

28 Nieves J, Cosman F, Herbert J et al. High prevalence of vitamin D deficiency and reduced bone mass in multiple sclerosis. *Neurology* 1994; 44:1687–1692.

29 Troiano RA, Jotkowitz A, Cook SA et al. Rate and types of fractures in corticosteroid-treated multiple sclerosis patients. *Neurology* 1992; 42:1389–1391.

30 Solaro C, Lunardi GL, Capello E et al. An open label trial of gabapentin treatment of paroxysmal symptoms in multiple sclerosis patients. *Neurology* 1998; 51:609–611.

31 Dane JR. Hypnosis for pain and neuromuscular rehabilitation with multiple sclerosis: case summary, literature review, and analysis of outcomes. *Int J Clin Exp Hypn* 1996; 44:208–231.

32 Miro J, Garcia-Monco C, Leno C, Berciano J. Pelvic pain: an undescribed paroxysmal manifestation of multiple sclerosis. *Pain* 1988; 32:73–75.

33 Taylor A, Taylor RS. Neuropsychologic aspects of multiple sclerosis. *Phys Med Rehabil Clin N Am* 1998; 9:643–657.

34 Sandyk R, Awerbuch GI. The co-occurrence of multiple sclerosis and migraine headache: the serotoninergic link. *Int J Neurosci* 1994; 76:249–257.

35 Rolak LA, Brown S. Headache and multiple sclerosis: a clinical study and review of the literature. *J Neurol* 1990; 237:300–302.

36 Freedman MS, Gray TA. Vascular headache: a presenting symptom of multiple sclerosis. *Can J Neurol Sci* 1989; 16:63–66.

37 Haas DC, Kent PF, Friedman DI. Headache caused by a single lesion of multiple sclerosis in the periaqueductal gray area. *Headache* 1993; 33:452–455.

38 Galer BS, Lipton RB, Weinstein S et al. Apopleptic headache and oculomotor nerve palsy: an unusual presentation of multiple sclerosis. *Neurology* 1990; 40:1465–1466.

39
Treatment of paroxysmal symptoms

William H Stuart

INTRODUCTION

The majority of patients with multiple sclerosis (MS) have ongoing or recurrent symptoms that emanate from a variety of causes. These symptoms may be paroxysmal in nature. The pattern of symptom expression does not necessarily reflect disease activity. While many symptoms are secondary to fixed areas of pre-existing MS injury, other symptoms can be related to relapses or secondary to complicating medical conditions. Fifteen percent of MS patients develop paroxysmal symptoms, which at times can be temporarily disabling and for which the cause is more obscure.

Since many MS symptoms are clinically similar, separating them by etiology requires a thorough understanding of the mechanisms by which MS symptoms occur. This can be challenging clinical work in the case of paroxysmal symptoms, and misdiagnosis, particularly by physicians who are not widely experienced in MS care, often results. The disease mechanisms by which symptoms occur in multiple sclerosis patients are presented in *Table 39.1*.

This chapter deals with the unique characteristics of paroxysmal symptoms in MS patients and their management.

Table 39.1 Causes of symptoms in MS

Disease relapse or progression
Pre-existing demyelination or axonal injury
Infection or fever (pseudorelapse)
Physiological causes (i.e. exercise)
Co-morbidity (e.g. arthritis, diabetes mellitus)
Paroxysmal (transient) symptoms

PATTERNS OF PAROXYSMAL SYMPTOMS IN MS

While many paroxysmal events in multiple sclerosis have clinically distinct patterns, the author's experience has shown that a large number of paroxysmal events are subtle and are clinically or historically poorly defined. Even when paroxysmal events occur in the presence of the examining physician, they may be ill-defined and not create a major clinical impact in the patient.

There are, however, certain common characteristics that describe these symptoms (*Table 39.2*). Although paroxysmal events have been described as the initial clinical event in multiple sclerosis, they occur more commonly in known disease. When these clinical events occur, they are often very transient, lasting only seconds to minutes, and they are often repetitive, occurring in clusters of four or five times a day or occasionally as several hundred events in a single 24-hour period. Paroxysmal symptoms are generally self-limiting; they may last over a period of several days to weeks and are commonly triggered by anxiety, stress, sensory stimuli, movement, or hyperventilation. In many instances, no triggering event can be defined. Misdiagnosis is common, leading to excessive or improper testing and treatment or to a diagnosis of psychological impairment.

Clinical patterns

The clinical patterns of paroxysmal symptoms in MS can be broadly categorized into sensory, motor, and miscellaneous. The miscellaneous category encompasses a broad range of paroxysmal events described in MS that do not fit readily into the more common paroxysmal sensory and motor symptoms.

Sensory paroxysmal symptoms

Lhermitte's sign is perhaps the most common paroxysmal event in MS (*Table 39.3*). It is the central nervous system equivalent of Tinel's sign. It is a symptom generally associated with posterior column spinal cord involvement that results in a sense of 'electrical' stimulation down the spine out into the arms or down into the legs. It is frequently triggered by neck or thoracic spine movement. This symptom can be an early presenting sign of new disease but more commonly it reflects resolving or fixed disease in the posterior column of the spinal cord.

Pruritus is another sensory distortion that occurs paroxysmally in MS patients. It can occur at segmental levels or in a limb distribution. The pruritus can at times be intense and result in self-induced trauma to the skin.

Pain patterns are also frequent paroxysmal events in MS. The occurrence of typical trigeminal neuralgia is readily recognized, but more atypical pain syndromes and radicular pain patterns that reflect disease of nerve entry zone areas often occur. Atypical trunk, chest, and pelvic

Table 39.2 Characteristics of paroxysmal symptoms in MS

They may be initial presenting event

They are usually very transient, lasting seconds to minutes

They are repetitive, from several to several hundred events daily

They are generally self-limiting, continuing for days to weeks

Triggering events are common (movements, stress, sensory stimuli, and hyperventilation)

They are commonly misdiagnosed and considered psychological

Table 39.3 Sensory manifestations of paroxysmal symptoms in MS

Lhermitte's sign

Pruritus

Neuralgic phenomena

    Trigeminal neuralgia

    Atypical facial pain

    Radicular pain (nerve entry zone disease)

    Atypical trunk pain (chest, abdominal and pelvic pain)

Paresthetic phenomena

    Painful

    Non-painful

pain patterns will often result in evaluation and treatment for chest or abdominal diseases that are not present.

Paresthetic sensory distortions over the face, trunk and limbs, both painful and non-painful, are commonly seen paroxysmally in MS patients.

Motor paroxysmal symptoms

Table 39.4 summarizes the motor manifestations of paroxysmal MS symptoms. Most of these motor abnormalities have been described in individual case reports in the literature. Common to these motor abnormalities is the presence of a spasm or segmental contraction of muscle or the displacement of a limb in a ballistic, dystonic or choreiform posturing. The unique nature of MS as it effects each individual patient contributes to the protean character of these motor events. Although individual syndromes have been described, in the clinical setting a partial or incompletely recognized example of these syndromes more commonly occurs. Pain is often an associated symptom, although usually no significant sensory distortion occurs at the time.

Miscellaneous paroxysmal symptoms

The miscellaneous paroxysmal symptoms are listed in *Table 39.5*. Most common among these is the Uhthoff phenomenon, which was originally described in patients with significant optic nerve disease. This paroxysmal fading or obscuring of vision is generally brought on by exercise or increased temperature; Uhthoff's phenomenon can also result in dysarthria and hypophonia.

Paroxysmal abnormalities of ocular motility have occurred but they are very rare. Seizures also occur in MS with a low frequency. They are generally associated with cortical or subcortical

Table 39.4 Motor manifestations of paroxysmal symptoms in MS

Movement disorders
  Tonic spasms
  Myoclonus
    Segmental
    Palatal
  Dystonic
  Choreiform
  Ballism
Paroxysmal dysarthria and ataxia
Paroxysmal dystonia and tremor
Hiccups
Facial myokymia
Pyramidal tract claudication

Table 39.5 Miscellaneous manifestations of paroxysmal symptoms in MS

Oculomotor phenomena
  Ocular ataxia
  Convergence spasm
  Paroxysmal superior rectus and levator spasm
Uhthoff's phenomenon
  Visual
  Laryngeal
  Sensorimotor
Autonomic phenomena
  Paroxysmal urinary incontinence
  Paroxysmal bowel incontinence
  Dysregulation of respirations, pulse, and blood
    pressure
Seizures
Cataplexy
Periodic leg movements during sleep
Pathological laughing or weeping

lesions and are readily controlled with anti-convulsant medication.

The autonomic symptoms that occur in MS are only now being described. This is a large untapped area of research and few data are available. It would, however, be incongruous not to expect involvement of the autonomic nervous system in MS, comparable to the spinal cord injury seen in the disease. Early reports of paroxysmal autonomic symptoms affecting the bladder and bowel have been described and it is probable that future reports of dysreflexia and dysregulation of blood pressure and pulse will be described.

Paroxysmal cerebral symptoms, such as pathological laughing and weeping and word dysfunction, are also seen in MS.

PATHOPHYSIOLOGY

The presumed mechanisms of paroxysmal symptoms in MS are listed in *Table 39.6*. At present there is little proof for any of these presumed mechanisms. There are no clinical–pathological correlation studies in the literature and only limited magnetic resonance imaging (MRI) correlations have been described.

Table 39.6 Presumed mechanisms of paroxysmal symptoms in MS

Ephaptic (cross-talk) transmission (in old lesions)
Acute demyelination
Movement induced
Temperature increase
  Exercise
  Fever (disease induced)
  Environmental

The concept of ephatic (cross-talk) transmission as a cause for paroxysmal MS symptoms has been extrapolated from the presumed mechanism seen in trigeminal neuralgia and facial hemispasm. It is a probable cause for many of the paroxysmal symptoms but most likely not the sole cause. The dramatic response to carbamazepine and gabapentin in patients with these symptoms lends credibility to the mechanism of ephatic transmission. Temperature-related symptoms have long been observed and may well represent the most frequent trigger for paroxysmal symptoms. Beyond this, movement-induced (kinesogenic) symptoms have been described. Areas of micro-relapse almost certainly contribute to many of these paroxysmal events. Limited MRI correlations have supported this assertion, and the response of sustained paroxysmal symptoms to corticosteroids has added further confirmation.

PHARMACOLOGIC INTERVENTIONS

Once paroxysmal symptoms have been clinically identified their treatment is generally successful (*Table 39.7*). Surprisingly low doses of carbamazepine and gabapentin are usually successful in rapidly controlling paroxysmal MS symptoms. When low doses are not successful, the dosage should be gradually increased to therapeutic levels or until tolerance is reached. If this is unsuccessful in bringing a conclusion to the paroxysmal event, then a course of intravenous methylprednisolone is strongly recommended.

Secondary treatment measures, including Dilantin, phenobarbital, clonazepam, amitriptyline, baclofen, and acetazolamide, have been described, but they are generally not necessary; by the time these secondary treatments are

Table 39.7 Pharmacologic treatment of paroxysmal symptoms in MS

Primary (most successful) treatments

    Carbemazepine 50–100 mg tid

    Gabapentin 100–300 mg tid

    Methylprednisolone 1000 mg/day intravenously for 3–5
      days

Secondary (less successful) treatments

    Phenytoin

    Phenobarbital

    Clonazepam

    Amitriptyline

    Baclofen

    Acetazolamide

brought into use, the clinical event is usually beginning to subside of its own accord.

DISCUSSION AND FUTURE DIRECTIONS

Virtually all of the information available in the literature regarding paroxysmal MS symptoms is anecdotal, experiential, or reports of single cases. A few open-label trials and multi-patient observations are reported. The very transient nature of these events makes it difficult to establish pathogenic mechanisms or to perform any type of blinded placebo-controlled treatment protocols. Pathological correlations have not been made and only recently some limited correlations with MRI abnormalities have been described in individual case reports. Newer MRI techniques and measures of cytokine levels may in the future establish surrogate markers that can be used to characterize paroxysmal symptoms in MS

further. Open-label studies on treatments can and should be done now that more MS patients are concentrated in large treatment centers. It is probable, however, that most of our information regarding these events will remain based on solid clinical experience presented by observant clinicians.

CONCLUSION

Paroxysmal events in MS patients are extremely common. The common estimate that 15–20% of MS patients are affected is probably far below the true figure. Many of the paroxysmal events that MS patients experience go undescribed to the physician because of their brief nature. Others produce no significant functional change but enhance levels of anxiety in patients because of their concern about relapse. Other paroxysmal events are more severe and require treatment, which is generally very successful. The neurologist who treats MS patients must have a thorough understanding of the varied nature of paroxysmal symptoms in MS in order to avoid pitfalls in the long-term care of these patients.

REFERENCES

1 Yamamoto M, Yabuki S, Hayabara T et al. Paroxysmal itching in MS. *Neurol Neurosurg Psychiatry* 1981; **44**:19–22.

2 Keoppel MC, Bramont C, Ceccaldi M et al. Paroxysmal pruritus and multiple sclerosis. *Br J Dermatol* 1993; **129**:597–598.

3 Ramirez-Lassepas M, Tulloch JW, Quisnones MR et al. Acute radicular pain as a presenting symptom in multiple sclerosis. *Arch Neurol* 1992; **49**:255–258.

4 Moulin DE, Foley KM, Ebers GC. Pain syndromes in multiple sclerosis. *Neurology* 1988; **38**:1830–1834.

5 Brisman R. Trigeminal neuralgia and multiple sclerosis. *Arch Neurol* 1987; **44**:379–381.

6 Sanders E, Arts R. Paraesthesiae in multiple sclerosis. *J Neurol Sci* 1986; 72:297–305.

7 Berger J, Sheremata W, Melamed E. Paroxysmal dystonia as the initial manifestations of multiple sclerosis. *Arch Neurol* 1984; 41:747–750.

8 Toyokua Y, Sakuta M, Nakanishi T. Painful tonic seizures in multiple sclerosis. *Neurology* 1976; 30:17–19.

9 Jacobs L, Kaba S, Pullicino P. *Arch Neurol* 1994; 51:1115–1119.

10 Masucci E, Saini N, Kurtzko J. Bilateral ballism in multiple sclerosis. *Neurology* 1989; 39: 1641–1642.

11 Kapoor R, Brown P, Thompson D et al. Propriospinal myoclonus in multiple sclerosis. *J Neurol Neurosurg Psychiatry* 1992; 55:1086–1088.

12 Skillned P, Goldstein M. Paroxysmal limb hemiataxia with crossed facial paresthesia in multiple sclerosis. *JAMA* 1983; 250:2843–2844.

13 Cosentino C, Torres L, Flores M et al. Paroxysmal kinesigenic dystonia and spinal cord lesion. *Mov Disord* 1996; 11:453–455.

14 Tranchant C, Bhatia K, Marsden C. Movement disorders in multiple sclerosis. *Mov Disord* 1995; 10:418–423.

15 Yoshimura N, Nagahama Y, Ueda T et al. Paroxysmal urinary incontinence associated with multiple sclerosis. *Urol Int* 1997; 59:197–199.

16 Posterb T, McMonagle U, Buttner T et al. Paroxysmal convergence spasm in multiple sclerosis. *Acta Neurol Scand* 1996; 94:35–37.

17 Ezra E. Paroxysmal superior rectus and levator palpebrae spasm: a unique presentation of multiple sclerosis. *Br J Ophthalmol* 1996; 80:187–188.

18 Schroth W, Tenner S, Rappaport B et al. Multiple sclerosis as a cause of atrial fibrillation and electrocardiographic changes. *Arch Neurol* 1992; 49:422–424.

19 Ghezzi A, Montanini R, Basso PF et al. Epilepsy in multiple sclerosis. *Eur Neurol* 1990; 30:218–223.

20 McFarling DA, Susac JO. Hoquet diabolique: intractable hiccups as a manifestation of multiple sclerosis. *Neurology* 1979; 29:797–801.

21 Thompson A, Kermode A, Mosely I et al. Seizures due to multiple sclerosis: seven patients with MRI correlations. *J Neuro Neurosurg Psychiatry* 1993; 56:1317–1320.

22 Schiffer RB, Herndon RM, Rudick RA. Treatment of pathological laughing and weeping with amitriptyline. *N Engl J Med* 1985; 312:1480–1482.

40
Treatment of tremor

François Bethoux

INTRODUCTION

Tremor is the most common movement disorder in multiple sclerosis (MS).[1] Severe tremor may, by itself, preclude effective use of the extremities, although it is most often associated with other impairments. Unfortunately, medical and rehabilitative therapies for MS tremor are of limited efficacy. Thalamic surgery, originally developed for other types of tremor, has been used with some success in carefully selected patients.

DEFINITION AND PATHOPHYSIOLOGY

A tremor is a rhythmic involuntary oscillating movement.[2] The tremor of MS is usually identified as a cerebellar intention and postural tremor.[3,4] Action tremor occurs during a targeted voluntary movement (e.g. finger-to-nose or heel-to-shin testing) with a frequency of 3–5 Hz.[5,6] Postural tremor is observed when a limb is maintained in a fixed position against gravity, with proximal large oscillations or distal, more rapid, oscillations, or both.[3] Axial tremor, with titubation of the head and trunk, and other cerebellar symptoms such as dysmetria may also

be present.[6] The term 'rubral tremor' designates a combination of rest, postural, and action tremor caused by midbrain lesions in the vicinity of the red nucleus.[5]

The pathophysiology of MS tremor is not completely elucidated. It is most likely related to lesions in the cerebellar nuclei and cerebellar efferent pathways, particularly in the dentato-rubrothalamic pathways.[4,7–9] The role of the thalamus in the genesis and control of MS tremor has been more extensively explored since the development of thalamic surgery and micro-electrode neuronal recording and stimulation.[10] It is hypothesized that cerebellar tremor is the result of abnormal oscillations in sensorimotor loops.[5,6] The nucleus ventralis intermedius of the thalamus, which has been identified as the most effective target for relief of intention tremor, is considered as a proprioceptive relay for one or several of these feedback loops.[10–13] Destruction or high-frequency stimulation of the ventralis intermedius suppresses these oscillations, thus controlling the tremor.[14] The presence of rhythmic activity in kinesthetic ventralis intermedius neurons concomitant with or even preceding the onset of tremor supports this model.[10,11] However, the exact role of thalamic nuclei in the genesis of tremor remains uncertain.

ASSESSMENT TOOLS

The consequences of MS tremor can be assessed in terms of impairments, disabilities, and handicaps, following the World Health Organization's conceptual framework.[15] MS tremor limits or precludes completion of activities of daily living (e.g. writing, feeding, or dressing) and may significantly reduce social participation. Its impact on self-esteem and quality of life is extremely significant.

Impairment is the first parameter used to evaluate the effect of therapies for MS tremor.[3] Qualitative assessment of tremor is based on standardized clinical examination, sometimes using videotapes to allow comparison of tremor severity over time or by independent observers.[16] Fahn's Tremor Rating Scale is a widely used ordinal scale for the assessment of tremor severity, with good inter-rater and intrarater reliability.[17,18] Quantitative measurement of tremor can be achieved with accelerometers.[4,9,19–21]

Independent assessment of disability is at least equally important, since satisfactory control of tremor does not necessarily translate into functional improvement.[10,22,23] Extensively validated generic or disease-specific disability scales are not very helpful in detecting modest changes secondary to reduction of tremor, especially in patients who are already severely disabled as a result of other impairments.[24] Fahn's Tremor Rating Scale also includes a subjective assessment of disability by the patient.[17,18,25] Most authors design their own scale for the purpose of a particular study,[9,24] or use non-standardized descriptive terms to reflect improvement.[23]

The global impact treatment on handicap and quality of life, which integrates tremor reduction, functional gains, and side effects, is the patient's global life situation and expectations. This has

not been commonly evaluated in research into MS tremor, and it has been reported only anecdotally.[24,26] The anecdotal reports are interesting, however. For example, Speelman and van Manen[24] reported that four MS patients out of a sample of 11 had a negative opinion of thalamotomy, despite objective tremor improvement in three of the patients. Tremor improved in 10 of 12 patients treated with isoniazid, but only one patient chose to continue isoniazid at the end of the trial.[27]

TREATMENT OPTIONS

Medications

Isoniazid

Sabra and colleagues[23] reported improvement of disabling action tremor associated with functional improvement in four MS patients treated with isoniazid, 800–1200 mg/day and pyridoxine, 100 mg/day.[23] Morrow and colleagues[28] reported short-term benefit from isoniazid in four of five patients, and long-term benefit in one of five. Duquette and colleagues[27] observed partial improvement of tremor in 10 of 12 patients (83%). Other authors have failed to duplicate these results, and they concluded that isoniazid was not effective.[9,29] Two double-blind, cross-over trials of isoniazid versus placebo showed improvement of postural tremor but no significant benefit on intention tremor.[8,16]

The dose of isoniazid used in published studies was 800–1200 mg/day. Some authors modify the daily dose on the basis of the acetylator phenotype of the patient (12 mg/kg per day for slow acetylators, 20 mg/kg per day for rapid acetylators).[8]

Reported side effects are usually mild.

Reversible perturbations of liver function tests were reported in 0[8,16] to 33%[23] of patients. Other side effects included sleepiness, fever, rash, nausea, dysphagia, and increased bronchial secretions.[27–29] Upper motor neuron weakness was also noted, probably unmasked by the reduction of tremor.[28]

The mechanism of action of isoniazid on tremor is not known. Sabra and colleagues[23] postulated that isoniazid increases brain γ-aminobutyric acid (GABA) content by inhibition of GABA aminotransferase. Bozek and colleagues[8] reported elevation of GABA, ornithine, and homocarnosine in all patients who underwent cerebrospinal fluid analysis and an elevation of blood ornithine levels in eight of nine patients.[8] Inhibition of monoamine oxidase or the action of one or more therapeutic metabolites have also been mentioned as possible mechanisms.[27,30]

Other medications

Other medications, including gluthetimide,[31] oral tetrahydrocannabinol,[32] primidone,[33] carbamazepine,[6] L-tryptophan,[34] and clonazepam,[35] have been found to be at least partially effective on tremor in open studies on small samples of MS patients. Propranolol is usually not effective for intention tremor.[36] Intravenous injections of 50 ml of 10% solution of ethanol failed to produce any significant short-term improvement of MS tremor.[37]

Thalamic surgery

Thalamotomy

Stereotactic thalamotomy has been used in the treatment of hyperkinetic movement disorders since the late 1940s, primarily in Parkinson's disease and essential tremor.[14] In MS, immediate relief following thalamotomy is obtained in between 90%[4,38] and 100%[24,26] of patients. Long-term results are less satisfying or unknown because of the lack of follow-up. In 1960, Cooper[4] reported complete relief of intention tremor lasting at least 1 year in 72% of patients, and a partial improvement in 13% of cases in a series of 32 MS patients who underwent thalamotomy between 1950 and 1960. More recently, other authors have obtained similar results, with variable length of follow-up.[22,24,25,39] Wester and Hauglie-Hanssen,[26] in a series of nine patients, reported a moderate or good long-term result of the surgery in only 45% of cases, based on ratings by the patient's treating neurologist. Functional improvement, when reported, is observed in between 37[22] and 54%[24] of patients. Patients selected for thalamotomy are usually severely disabled because of multiple impairments before surgery, and this limits the potential for dramatic functional improvement.[24,26] Ambulatory patients appear to have a better functional outcome.[22] Complications occur in between 20[4] and 55%[26] of patients; these include new symptoms or worsening of existing symptoms (including hemiparesis, dysphagia, and speech disorders), worsening of cognitive deficit,[40] bladder dysfunction, and post-surgical Guillain–Barré syndrome.[41] Speelman and colleagues[24] reported a worsening of expanded disability status scale scores in four of 11 patients after thalamotomy. Complications are transient in the majority of patients, but permanent deficits have been reported in 22% of patients.[11] Death can occur in the post-operative period, although its relationship with the surgery is not always established.[4]

Deep brain stimulation

Deep brain stimulation was more recently introduced as an alternative to thalamotomy in the treatment of essential tremor and the tremor of Parkinson's Disease.[14] The development of magnetic resonance imaging and computed tomography to guide stereotactic surgery and the advent of microneuronal recordings allow very precise localization of the target before electrode implantation.[13] The site of stimulation is usually the nucleus ventralis intermedius of the thalamus,[10,12–14] although other areas have been targeted.[14] Immediate relief of tremor is obtained in almost 100% of cases, and this usually persists when the stimulator is turned off. This phenomenon is attributed to the 'microthalamotomy' effect (i.e. reversible injury to the tissue surrounding the electrode), and usually lasts 2–3 weeks.[13] Later, the tremor is controlled when the stimulator is on but recurs after a short delay when the stimulator is turned off.[14] Stimulation parameters, including voltage, pulse width, and frequency, must be adjusted to obtain the best response. Frequencies are usually between 130 and 185 Hz.[14]

Long-term results of deep brain stimulation are theoretically more promising than those of thalamotomy, since it is possible to adapt the parameters of stimulation when the benefit decreases. Montgomery and colleagues,[13] in a series of 14 patients followed up to 1 year, observed a significant reduction in postural and intention tremor and in the ability to bring a cup to the lips. The optimal response to stimulation (i.e. the best response obtained after adjustment of the stimulation parameters) did not change significantly over time (*Figs 40.1 and 40.2*). However, the benefit on action tremor and functional tasks decreased between stimulator adjustments. Geny and colleagues[12] reported improvement of tremor in 69% of patients undergoing deep brain stimulation; this improvement was more pronounced on proximal tremor than on distal tremor.[12] Functional improvement also occurred in a majority of patients, but was less dramatic. Complications are rare and usually transient.[10,12,13] Paresthesias at the onset of stimulation are reported by almost all patients, but they are well tolerated.

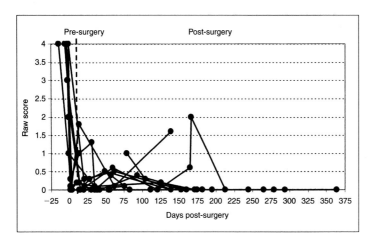

Fig. 40.1 *Postural tremor: best response (after adjustment of stimulation parameters) in a series of 14 MS patients followed for up to 1 year after implantation of a deep brain stimulator. CTRS: Clinical Tremor Rating Scale (adapted from Montgomery et al,[13] with permission). The tremor was rated clinically after adjustment of stimulation parameters (0 = no tremor, 1 = minimal or intermittent tremor, 2 = tremor amplitude < 2 cm, 3 = amplitude from 2 to 4 cm, 4 = amplitude > 4 cm or unable to perform the task).*

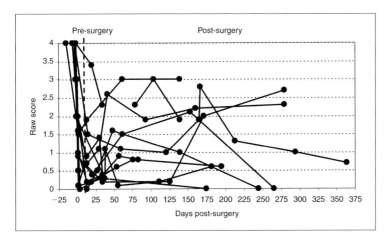

Fig. 40.2 Action tremor: best response (after adjustment of stimulation parameters) in a series of 14 MS patients followed for up to 1 year after implantation of a deep brain stimulator. CTRS: Clinical Tremor Rating Scale (adapted from Montgomery et al,[13] with permission).

Rehabilitative therapies

Comprehensive rehabilitation, focusing on compensation strategies, stabilization of the joints, and co-ordination exercises, aims at maximizing functional performances for a given level of impairment; however, it is of limited efficacy.[35] Hewer and colleagues[42] reported objective reduction of tremor in four of 10 MS patients after applying weights (480–600 g) to the wrist.[42] However, the use of weights is limited by weakness and fatiguability and it sometimes results in increased tremor.[20,42] There is no linear relationship between the amount of weight applied and the clinical benefit, and viscous loads appear to be more effective than weights.[20]

Javidan and colleagues[43] studied the efficacy of functional electrical stimulation (the use of neuromuscular electrical stimulation for functional purposes) on different types of tremors. These authors used concomitant flexor and extensor surface stimulation at the wrist or elbow, with a closed-loop control system. Attenuation of tremor in five MS patients ranged from 0 to 68%. A more consistent benefit was obtained in patients with essential tremor and Parkinsonian tremor.

IMPLICATIONS FOR CLINICAL PRACTICE

The use of evidence-based medicine in the treatment of MS tremor is limited. There are few controlled studies. Those that exist are probably underpowered to detect small changes, and follow-up data are not always available. In most cases, the assessment of functional results is not standardized or is carried out with tools that are not validated. The intrinsic variability of the disease, and the presence of multiple associated impairments, limit our ability to compare results from different studies, and to predict results of treatments.

Overall, the efficacy of medications for postural and intention tremor in MS is reported only anecdotally and is not confirmed by controlled studies. In every individual case, the side effects must be weighed against the potential therapeutic effect. Sedation and weakness are probably the most significant concerns in this regard, since many patients with severe cerebellar tremor have advanced disease. Nevertheless, empirical use of medications together with rehabilitative techniques remain the first line of treatment.

Despite recent technical improvements, thalamotomy is not yet as effective in the MS population as in patients with Parkinson's disease or essential tremor. Deep brain stimulation appears more promising, considering the reversibility and adaptability of the stimulation, the lower rate of complications, and the possibility of bilateral stimulation (whereas bilateral thalamotomy carries considerable risk).[3,10,12,13] Both procedures have benefited from the advent of microelectrode recordings and stimulation, which allow a more precise localization of the target, therefore reducing the risk of complications and increasing the success rate, compared to the use of stereotactic techniques alone.[13] The indications for deep brain stimulation could potentially be extended to less severely disabled patients, in whom the potential for functional improvement may be greater. However, careful selection of patients is still required. In particular, associated motor and proprioceptive deficits in the targeted limb must be carefully assessed. Deep brain stimulation is more costly than thalamotomy, requires highly skilled personnel, and necessitates follow-up visits for the adjustment of parameters.[14]

Rehabilitative interventions primarily target disability, with no or little effect on impairment. The efficacy of compensation strategies is limited by the presence of other deficits, and the benefit associated with the use of weights is controversial. The efficacy of functional electrical stimulation in controlling MS tremor still needs to be demonstrated. As a general rule, in MS and other progressive diseases of the central nervous system, the usefulness of rehabilitation is enhanced when it is integrated into a comprehensive care approach. In particular, rehabilitative interventions can be an effective complement to other therapies in an effort to optimize functional gain after reduction of impairment.

IMPLICATIONS FOR FUTURE RESEARCH

Further understanding of the pathophysiology of MS tremor is certainly necessary to enhance current therapeutic approaches and to develop new therapies. Montgomery and colleagues[13] observed discrepancies between the results of microelectrode recordings and stimulation during surgery for deep brain stimulation: when neuronal activity was recorded by touching one area of the body, microstimulation of the same neurons produced a sensation in a different part of the body in half of the patients. Whittle and Haddow[44] also reported unusual responses to low frequency microstimulation before thalamotomy. These observations suggest that changes in the somatotopy of thalamic nuclei occur in MS patients.

Well-designed clinical trials that involve multiple centers in order to achieve larger sample sizes are required to define the indications of anti-tremor medications. For this purpose, valid, reliable, and sensitive assessment tools are needed, particularly for disability. With the increasing use of surgical treatments, criteria for patient selection will be refined, and new anatomical targets may be identified.[14] Finally, adjunctive therapies such as rehabilitation would benefit from a more scientific evaluation, in order to optimize their use in a comprehensive care model.

REFERENCES

1 **Tranchant C, Bhatia KP, Marsden CD.** Movement disorders in multiple sclerosis. *Mov Disord* 1995; 10:418–423.

2 **Johnson DS, Montgomery EB.** Pathophysiology of cerebellar disorders. In: Watts RL, Koller WC, eds. *Movement Disorders: Neurologic Principles and Practice.* New York: McGraw-Hill, 1997: 587–610.

3 **Nguyen JP, Feve A, Keravel Y.** Is electrostimulation preferable to surgery for upper limb ataxia? *Curr Opin Neurol* 1996; 9:445–450.

4 **Cooper IS.** Relief of intention tremor of multiple sclerosis by thalamic surgery. *JAMA* 1967; 199:689–694.

5 **Elble RJ.** The pathophysiology of tremor. In: Watts RL, Koller WC, eds. *Movement Disorders: Neurologic Principles and Practice.* New York: McGraw-Hill, 1997: 405–417.

6 **Deuschl G, Krack P.** Tremors:differential diagnosis, neurophysiology, and pharmacology. In: Jankovic J, Tolosa E, eds. *Parkinson's Disease and Movement Disorders* 3rd edn. Baltimore: Williams and Wilkins, 1998: 419–452.

7 **Arsalo A, Hanninen A, Laitinen L.** Functional neurosurgery in the treatment of multiple sclerosis. *Ann Clin Res* 1973; 5:74–79.

8 **Bozek CB, Kastrukoff LF, Wright JM et al.** A controlled trial of isoniazid therapy for action tremor in multiple sclerosis. *J Neurol* 1987; 234:36–39.

9 **Koller WC.** Pharmacologic trials in the treatment of cerebellar tremor. *Arch Neurol* 1984; 41:280–281.

10 **Benabid AL, Pollak P, Dongming G et al.** Chronic electrical stimulation of the ventralis intermedius nucleus of the thalamus as a treatment of movement disorders. *J Neurosurg* 1996; 84:203–214.

11 **Kraus JK, Grossman RG.** Surgery for hyperkinetic movement disorders. In: Jankovic J, Tolosa E, eds. *Parkinson's Disease and Movement Disorders* 3rd edn. Baltimore: Williams and Wilkins, 1998: 1017–1047.

12 **Geny C, Nguyen JP, Pollin B et al.** Improvement of severe postural cerebellar tremor in multiple sclerosis by chronic thalamic stimulation. *Mov Disord* 1996; 11:489–494.

13 **Montgomery EB Jr, Baker KB, Kinkle RP, Barnett G.** Chronic thalamic stimulation for the tremor of multiple sclerosis. *Neurology*; in press.

14 **Pollak P, Benabid AL, Krack P et al.** Deep brain stimulation. In: Jankovic J, Tolosa E, eds. *Parkinson's Disease and Movement Disorders* 3rd edn. Baltimore: Williams and Wilkins, 1998: 1085–1101.

15 **World Health Organization.** *International Classification of Impairments, Disabilities, and Handicap.* Geneva: World Health Organization, 1980.

16 **Hallett M, Lindsey JW, Adelstein BD, Riley PO.** Controlled trial of isoniazid therapy for severe postural cerebellar tremor in multiple sclerosis. *Neurology* 1985; 35:1374–1377.

17 **Fahn S, Tolosa E, Marin C.** Clinical rating scale for tremor. In: Jankovic J, Tolosa E, eds. *Parkinson's Disease and Movement Disorders* 2nd edn. Edinburgh: Churchill Livingstone, 1991: 271–280.

18 **Hooper J, Taylor R, Pentland B, Whittle IR.** Rater reliability of Fahn's tremor rating scale in patients with multiple sclerosis. *Arch Phys Med Rehabil* 1998; 79:1076–1079.

19 **Morgan MH, Hewer RL, Cooper R.** A method of recording and analysing intention tremor. *Brain* 1972; 95:573–578.

20 **Sanes JN, LeWitt PA, Mauritz KH.** Visual and mechanical control of postural and kinetic tremor in cerebellar system disorders. *J Neurol Neurosurg Psychiatry* 1988; 51:934–943.

21 **Potvin AR, Tourtellotte WW, Snyder DN et al.** Validity of quantitative tests measuring tremor. *Am J Phys Med* 1975; 54:243–252.

22 **Barnett GH, Kinkel RP, Bhasin C et al.** Stereotactic thalamotomy for intractable tremor in multiple sclerosis (MS) (abstract). *Neurology* 1992; 42 (suppl 3):327.

23 **Sabra AF, Hallett M, Sudarsky L, Mullally W.** Treatment of action tremor in multiple sclerosis with isoniazid. *Neurology* 1982; 32:912–913.

24 **Speelman JD, Van Manen J.** Stereotactic thalamotomy for the relief of intention tremor of multiple sclerosis. *J Neurol Neurosurg Psychiatry* 1984; 47:596–599.

25 **Goldman MS, Jelly PJ.** Symptomatic and functional outcome of stereotactic ventralis lateralis thalamotomy for intention tremor. *J Neurosurg* 1992; 77:223–229.

26 **Wester K, Hauglie-Hanssen E.** Stereotaxic thalamotomy: experiences from the levodopa era. *J Neurol Neurosurg Psychiatry* 1990; 53:427–430.

27 **Duquette P, Pleines J, du Souich P.** Isoniazid for tremor in multiple sclerosis:a controlled trial. *Neurology* 1985; 35:1772–1775.

28 **Morrow J, McDowell H, Ritchie C, Patterson V.** Isoniazid and action tremor in multiple sclerosis (letter). *J Neurol Neurosurg Psychiatry* 1985; 48:282–283.

29 Scheinberg L, Giesser BS. INH in multiple sclerosis (letter). *Neurology* 1984; 34:134–135.

30 Francis DA, Grundy D, Heron JR. The response to isoniazid of action tremor in multiple sclerosis and its assessment using polarised light goniometry. *J Neurol Neurosurg Psychiatry* 1986; 49:87–89.

31 Aisen ML, Holzer M, Rosen M et al. Glutethimide treatment of disabling action tremor in patients with multiple sclerosis and traumatic brain injury. *Arch Neurol* 1991; 48:513–515.

32 Clifford DB. Tetrahydrocannabinol for tremor in multiple sclerosis. *Ann Neurol* 1983; 13:669–671.

33 Henkin Y, Herishanu YO. Primidone as a treatment for cerebellar tremor in multiple sclerosis: two case reports. *Isr J Med Sci* 1989; 25:720–721.

34 Trouillas P, Brudon F, Adeleine P. Improvement of cerebellar ataxia with levorotary form of 5-hydroxytryptophan. *Arch Neurol* 1988; 45:1217–1222.

35 Cobble ND, Dietz MA, Grigsby J, Kennedy PM. Rehabilitation of the patient with multiple sclerosis. In: DeLisa JA, ed. *Rehabilitation Medicine: Principles and Practice* 2nd edn. Philadelphia: JB Lippincott, 1993: 861–885.

36 Ebadi M. Management of tremor by beta adrenergic blocking agents. *Gen Pharmacol* 1980; 11:257–260.

37 Koller WC, Biary N. Effect of alcohol on tremors: comparison with propranolol. *Neurology* 1984; 34: 221–222.

38 Laitinen L, Arsalo A, Hanninen A. Combination of thalamotomy and longitudinal myelotomy in the treatment of multiple sclerosis. *Acta Neurochir (Wien)* 1974; 21(suppl):89–91.

39 Shahzadi S, Tasker RR, Lozano A. Thalamotomy for essential and cerebellar tremor. *Stereotact Funct Neurosurg* 1995; 65:11–17.

40 Modesti LM, Blumetti AE. Long term effects of stereotaxic thalamotomy on parameters of cognitive functioning. *Acta Neurochir (Wien)* 1980; 30(suppl):401–403.

41 McCabe PH, Blakeslee MA, Tenser RB. Guillain–Barré syndrome after thalamotomy for tremor in MS. *Neurology* 1998; 51:1229.

42 Hewer RL, Cooper R, Morgan MH. An investigation into the value of treating intention tremor by weighting the affected limb. *Brain* 1972; 95:579–590.

43 Javidan M, Elek J, Prochazka A. Attenuation of pathological tremors by functional electrical stimulation. II: Clinical evaluation. *Ann Biomed Eng* 1992; 20:225–236.

44 Whittle IR, Haddow LJ. CT guided thalamotomy for movement disorders in multiple sclerosis: problems and paradoxes. *Acta Neurochir (Wien)* 1995; 64(suppl):13–16.

Index